D1161463

Understanding Anesthesia Equipment

Construction, Care and Complications

SECOND EDITION

Understanding Anesthesia Equipment

Construction, Care and Complications

SECOND EDITION

Jerry A. Dorsch, M.D.

St. Vincent's Medical Center
Jacksonville, Florida

Susan E. Dorsch, M.D.

Riverside Hospital
Jacksonville, Florida

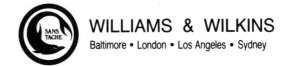

WILLIAMS & WILKINS

Baltimore • London • Los Angeles • Sydney

Editor: Toni M. Tracy
Associate Editor: Jonathan W. Pine, Jr.
Copy Editor: Leilani Ellison
Design: Bert Smith
Production: Carol L. Eckhart

Accurate indications, adverse reactions, and dosage schedules for drugs are provided in this book, but it is possible that they may change. The reader is urged to review the package information data of the manufacturers of the medications mentioned.

Made in the United States of America

First Edition, 1975

Library of Congress Cataloging in Publication Data

Dorsch, Jerry A.
    Understanding anesthesia equipment.

    Includes bibliographical references and index.
    1. Anesthesiology—Apparatus and instruments. I. Dorsch, Susan E. II. Title.
[DNLM: 1. Anesthesiology—Instrumentation. WO 240 D717u]
RD78.8.D67 1984   617'.96'028   83-23605
ISBN 0-683-02615-1

Composed and printed at the
Waverly Press, Inc.   85 86 87 88 89   10 9 8 7 6 5 4 3

*To our children
David and Alycia,
who added new dimensions
to our lives
and whose sacrifices made
this book possible.*

Foreword to the First Edition

The importance of his instruments to the anesthesiologist cannot be overestimated. The practice of anesthesia is evolving along sound modern physiological and pharmacological lines, and the demand for reliable instruments constructed to the highest engineering and physical standards is continuously increasing. Yet, if his sophisticated flowmeters, valves, vaporizers, lung ventilators, breathing equipment and "black boxes" of all sorts are to be used intelligently and safely, and if the information they supply is to be correctly interpreted and wisely applied, the anesthesiologist must have access to equally sophisticated and reliable information about the construction and functioning of these instruments. It is not enough to refer to a book on physics written for physicists, or to a manual on engineering for engineers, or a compendium on electronics, or one on hydraulics, or mechanics or physiology. The anesthesiologist needs a book which builds a bridge of relevance between these highly specialized fields and his everyday clinical work. This book by Drs. Susan and Jerry Dorsch provides exactly what he needs. They have brought together an intimate knowledge of clinical anesthesia and the physical sciences and technologies on which their functioning depends.

The information herein is not only for anesthesiologists. It must surely become an essential source of reference to all who work in the anesthesia instrument industry, for it gives them the clinical environment and its problems without which the instrument designer cannot function. The inhalational therapist, the clinical physiologist and even the experimental animal physiologist and pharmacologist—all whose work brings them up against problems involving breathing equipment, anesthetic instruments, compressed medical gases, and similar matters, will sooner or later need to use this book.

I congratulate Drs. Susan and Jerry Dorsch for having completed a work for which a wide range of medical and other specialists will be grateful. Whether for study or reference this book is commended as a substantial addition to the really useful literature on clinical anesthesiology.

William W. Mushin
Professor of Anaesthetics
Welsh National School of Medicine
University of Wales
Cardiff, Wales

Preface to the Second Edition

In the years since the first edition of this book was published numerous developments have occurred and much new information has become available concerning anesthesia equipment. Many changes, including some standardization, have been made in the equipment discussed in the first edition. At the same time rapidly developing technology has made available new devices, many of them more complex and sophisticated than those used previously. It is essential that users have sufficient knowledge of all apparatus, both old and new, to use it properly and safely.

Every piece of equipment has hazards associated with it. In this edition an entire chapter has been devoted to potential mishaps associated with anesthesia machines and breathing systems. Since most of these problems are avoidable, accident prevention has been emphasized.

Another new chapter in this edition is concerned with checking of equipment before use. Even the best equipment can fail. Proper checking will reveal most problems before harm comes to the patient. Because of increasing medicolegal problems and requirements by accreditation agencies, a section on record keeping has been added.

In the years since the first edition was published, great interest has been shown in the potential hazards of operating room pollution by anesthetic agents and methods to scavenge these gases. This was considered only very briefly in the first edition. The large amount of material published and the many developments led us to the decision that it deserved a separate chapter.

Another important change in anesthesia has been the increasing use of vigilance aids. There can be no doubt that use of these contributes greatly to patient safety. Accordingly, we have included sections on equipment for monitoring anesthetic agents, oxygen, carbon dioxide, and breathing system pressures.

It has been our goal to provide an easily understood text that will be especially helpful to individuals with little or no prior experience with anesthesia equipment. We hope it will help them gain a level of expertise that will permit them to use equipment confidently and competently, avoiding complications associated with its use. There is emerging in our profession a growing realization that anesthesia equipment deserves recognition as a subject in its own right. In the past, teaching of equipment use and care has often been delegated to anyone who, willing or unwilling, would accept the task. All too often, this individual received little or no recognition. It is time that teaching and study of equipment receive the same emphasis in anesthesia training as such topics as anatomy, pharmacology, and physiology.

We also hope this edition will become a source of continuing education for those who have completed their formal training and who face the dual task of retaining older information and supplementing it with new knowledge. Hopefully, these individuals will find in this work a few new "tricks of the trade" which will result in better patient care and less frustration and wasted time.

Finally, we hope that this edition will stimulate individuals to do research and continue to work on developing easier-to-use, more efficient, and above all, safer equipment.

Jerry A. Dorsch, M.D.
Susan E. Dorsch, M.D.
2941 Greenridge Road
Orange Park, Florida

Preface to the First Edition

As in most areas of medicine the anesthesiologist and nurse anesthetist are finding it necessary to rely more and more upon increasingly sophisticated equipment. While this increased reliability allows the practitioner more flexibility in technique and more accuracy, it also requires a thorough understanding of the equipment. The responsibility of the practitioner for the safe and efficient performance of his equipment should be a fundamental consideration in his care for patients.

Most anesthesia equipment does not come with an instruction manual, or if it does, it is soon lost in a busy department. Most general anesthesia textbooks cover some pieces of equipment, often in a fair degree of detail. However, components are often treated individually with no attempt to bring them together into a comprehensive whole. A working knowledge of one's equipment, therefore, must usually come from practice or be imparted by those with experience in its use. Unfortunately, this experience is usually incomplete and lacking in true understanding.

This book has been written to fulfill a need to inform practitioners in anesthesia about their equipment. The authors feel that an understanding of commonly used equipment is not prevalent and this lack causes incorrect selection and use. Accordingly, we have selected for discussion the equipment about which the least information is readily available in the literature. Equipment which has been covered well in other books, e.g., ventilators, monitors, etc., has not been included. While we feel that all practitioners of anesthesia will be benefited by it, it should be especially useful to the resident anesthesiologist or student nurse anesthetist who is faced with a bewildering assortment of strange gadgets.

A final word of caution should be issued to the readers. Proper use of equipment is but one facet in the safe administration of anesthesia. There is always a danger that attention to the equipment may replace attention to the patient. Even with the finest equipment, vigilance is still necessary to prevent accidents that result in patient mortality and morbidity. Horton summed it up very well: "The value of an adequate physical environment is not that it makes vigilance unnecessary, but that it makes it effective."*

---

* National Fire Protection Association: Recommended safe practice for hospital operating rooms. Bulletin No. 56, July, 1956.

Acknowledgments

The authors wish to express our sincere gratitude to the many people who have helped and supported us in the preparation of this book.

Literature searches and reprints were furnished by the Borland Medical Library of Jacksonville.

Mr. Cuyler Ewing provided editorial and proofreading assistance.

Mr. and Mrs. Carl Dorsch furnished an ideal setting to concentrate on creative writing.

It would not have been possible to write this edition without cooperation from the makers of the various anesthesia products.

We wish to give special thanks to James F. Ferguson, Joseph Rosano, C. R. Tobin, Chalmers Goodyear, Peter Schreiber, Ronald J. Luich, Michael Marker, Ernest R. Savidge, Thomas Burns, and Hartly C. Erickson, all of whom reviewed various sections of this book.

We are particularly grateful to Dr. Robert L. Rayburn, who was kind enough to review the chapter on Mapleson systems, Dr. Andranik Ovassapian for assistance with the section on fiberoptic laryngoscopy, and Jeffrey B. Cooper for his help on the section on oxygen analyzers.

Contents

Foreword to the First Edition vii
Preface to the Second Edition ix
Preface to the First Edition xi
Acknowledgments xiii
1   Compressed Gas Containers 1
2   Medical Gas Piping Systems 16
3   The Anesthesia Machine 38
4   Vaporizers 77
5   The Breathing System. I. General Considerations 136
6   The Breathing System. II. The Mapleson Systems 182
7   The Breathing System. III. Systems Employing Non-Rebreathing Valves . . . 197
8   The Breathing System. IV. The Circle System 210
9   Controlling Trace Gas Levels 247
10   Hazards of Anesthesia Machines and Breathing Systems 289
11   Face Masks and Airways 326
12   Laryngoscopes 338
13   Endotracheal Tubes 353
14   Equipment Checking and Maintenance 401
15   Cleaning and Sterilization 415
Index 443

CHAPTER 1

Compressed Gas Containers

The gases used by the anesthesiologist may come from either of two sources: gas cylinders or the hospital piping system. Even when a piping system is present, cylinders are needed for an emergency supply for the anesthesia machine and for patient transport and resuscitation. Every anesthesiologist should be familiar with gas cylinders and their use.

The National Fire Protection Association (NFPA) and the Compressed Gas Association (CGA) publish a number of pamphlets and standards on safe practices (1–19). Anyone using compressed gases should read these publications.

DEFINITIONS

A compressed gas is defined as "any material or mixture having in the container either a pressure exceeding 40 psia* (275.6 kPa) at 70°F or, regardless of the pressure at 70°F, having a pressure exceeding 104 psia (716.56 kPa), at 130°F or any liquid flammable material having a vapor pressure exceeding 40 psia (275.6 kPa) at 100°F" (1). A liquified compressed gas is a gas which, under the charging pressure, is partially liquified at a temperature of 70°F (5).

Medical gases are prepared under carefully controlled conditions to meet the purity specifications prescribed in the *Pharmacopoeia of the United States* or the *National Formulary*. They are also subject to regulations of the Food and Drug Administration.

The Department of Transportation has established requirements for the design, construction, testing, marking, labeling, filling, storage, handling, maintenance, and transportation of compressed gas cylinders.

CONSTRUCTION

Medical gas cylinders are constructed of steel with walls 5/64 to 1/4 inches thick. Alloys containing molybdenum and/or chronium may be used to minimize weight and wall thickness.

SIZES AND CAPACITIES

Cylinder sizes are designated according to the alphabet, with size A being the smallest cylinder. Table 1.1 gives the approximate dimensions and capacities for the commonly used cylinders. There is some variation in cylinder sizes and capacities among the various manufacturers. Size E is the cylinder most commonly used on anesthesia machines for gases other than cyclopropane, for which a size D or DD cylinder is commonly used.

CONTENTS AND PRESSURE

As illustrated in Figure 1.1, in a cylinder containing a nonliquified gas such as oxygen, the pressure in the cylinder declines steadily as the contents are withdrawn. Therefore the pressure can be used to measure the cylinder contents. The weight of the cylinder can also be used as a measure of the contents.

In a cylinder containing a liquified gas such as nitrous oxide, the pressure in the cylinder depends on the vapor pressure of the liquefied gas and is not an indication of the contents of the cylinder if part of the contents is in the liquid phase. This pressure remains nearly constant (if the temperature remains constant) until all the liquid has evaporated, after which the pressure declines until the cylinder is exhausted. In actual use, the temperature is not likely to remain constant. The evaporation of the liquid in the cylinder requires energy in the form of heat, which is supplied mainly by the liquid in the cylinder. This results in cooling of the liquid. As the temperature falls, the vapor pressure of

---

* "Psia" stands for pounds per square inch absolute, which is the pressure difference between the measured pressure and that at "absolute zero." "Psig" stands for pounds per square inch gauge, which is the difference between the measured pressure and surrounding atmospheric pressure. For example, under normal circumstances on the ground we are at 0 psig (since most gauges are constructed to read 0 at atmospheric pressure), but we are at 14.7 psia.

Table 1.1.
Typical Medical Gas Cylinders

Cylinder Dimensions	Capacity	Carbon dioxide	Cyclopropane	Helium	Nitrous Oxide	Oxygen	Helium-Oxygen Mixtures	CO₂-Oxygen Mixtures	Wt (lb) Empty Cylinder
A (3″ o.d. × 7″)	Lb	0.8	0.6	0.02	0.8	0.23			
	Liters	189	151	57	189	76	57	76	3
	Gal	50	40	15	50	20	15	20	
B (3½″ o.d. × 13″)	Lb	1.6	1.5	0.06	1.5	0.6			
	Liters	378	378	148	378	196	113	150	6
	Gal	100	100	39	100	52	40	40	
D (4¼″ o.d. × 17″)	Lb	3.8	3.3	0.1	3.8	1.2			
	Liters	946	871	299	946	396	299	396	10
	Gal	250	230	79	250	105	79	105	
E (4¼″ o.d. × 26″)	Lb	6.6	5.5	0.2	6.4	1.9			
	Liters	1,590	1,438	496	1,590	659	496	659	13
	Gal	420	380	131	420	174	131	174	
F (5½″ o.d. × 51″)	Lb	20		0.6	21.0	6.0			
	Liters	4,800		1,585	5,260	2,062	1,640	2,062	67
	Gal	1,270		420	1,400	545	433	545	
M (7″ o.d. × 43″)	Lb	30.6		0.9	30.6	8.8			
	Liters	7,570		2,263	7,570	3,000	2,263	3,000	70
	Gal	2,000		598	2,000	800	598	800	
G (8½″ o.d. × 51″)	Lb	50		1.5	56.0	15.5			
	Liters	12,358		4,016	13,836	5,331	4,016	5,300	110
	Gal	3,260		1,061	3,655	1,408	1,061	1,400	
H & K (9¼″ o.d. × 51″)	Lb				64.3	16–22			
	Liters				15,899	5,570–7,500			130
	Gal				4,200	1,470–2,000			
AA* (2¾″ o.d. × 11″)	Lb		0.6						
	Liters		150						3
	Gal		40						
BB* (2¾″ o.d. × 19¾″)	Lb		1.25						
	Liters		377						4
	Gal		100						
DD* (3¾″ o.d. × 23¼″)	Lb		3.3						
	Liters		850						8
	Gal		220						

* Chromium-plated cylinders.

the liquid also falls, so that a progressive fall in pressure accompanies the release of gas from the cylinder at constant flow. The rate at which the pressure declines is related to the flow rate (20). Frost may develop on the outer surface of cylinder containing liquified gas. This is not related to the state of emptiness of the cylinder, but does indicate that at the time of its development there is residual liquid left in the cylinder.

TESTING

U.S. Department of Transportation regulations set forth manufacturing and testing specifications for medical gas cylinders. CGA pamphlets C-1 (11), C-2 (12), C-5 (13), C-6 (14); and C-8 (15) also guide industry practices. A cylinder must be subjected periodically to visual examination and must be subjected to internal hydrostatic pressure testing at least every five years or, with special permit, up to every ten years. A cylinder is checked for leaks and to determine retention of structural strength by testing to a minimum of ⁵⁄₃ (1.66) times its service pressure. The service pressure is the maximum pressure to which the cylinder may be filled at 70°F. Table 1.2 gives the service pressure for the gases commonly used in anesthesia. The test date (month and year) of a cylinder must be permanently stamped on the cylinder.

CGA pamphlet C-6 (14) has been prepared as

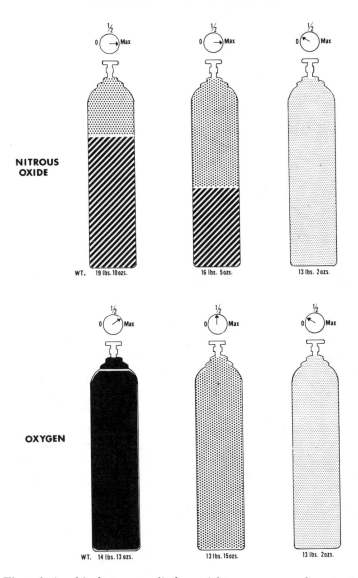

Figure 1.1. The relationship between cylinder weight, pressure, and contents. A gas stored partially in liquid form, such as nitrous oxide, will show a constant pressure (assuming constant temperature) until all the liquid has evaporated, at which time the pressure will drop in direct proportion to the rate at which gas is withdrawn. A non-liquified gas such as oxygen will show a steady decline in pressure until the cylinder is evacuated. Each cylinder, however, will show a steady decline in weight as gas is discharged.

a guide to cylinder users for their own visual inspection of cylinders. In general the features to be watched for are corrosion (especially in a narrow line or crevice configuration), pitting, cuts, gouges, dings, dents, bulges, cracks, fire damage, leaks, and general distortion. The bottom of the cylinder should always be checked since it is most susceptible to damage. Doubtful containers should be returned to the supplier.

FILLING LIMITS

Whenever a gas is confined in a closed container, a rise in the temperature will cause a rise in pressure. Thus if a cylinder containing gas under a safe pressure at normal temperatures is subjected to higher temperatures, the pressure may increase to a dangerous level. To prevent this, the Department of Transportation has es-

Table 1.2.
Medical Gases Color Code

Gas	Formula	United States	International	70° Service Pressure in psig (kPa × 100)	State in Cylinder	Filling Density
Oxygen	O_2	Green	White	1900–2200 (130–150)*	Gas†	
Carbon dioxide	CO_2	Gray	Gray	838 (57)	Liquid <88°	68%
Nitrous oxide	N_2O	Blue	Blue	745 (50)	Liquid <98°	68%
Cyclopropane	C_3H_6	Orange	Orange	75 (5)	Liquid	55%
Helium	He	Brown	Brown	1600–2000 (110–136)*	Gas	
Nitrogen	N_2	Black	Black	1800–2200 (122–150)*	Gas	
Air		Yellow‡	White & black	1800 (122)	Gas	

* Depending on type of cylinder.
† Special containers for liquid oxygen are discussed in Chapter 2.
‡ Air, including mixtures of oxygen with nitrogen containing 19.5–23.5% oxygen, is color-coded yellow. Mixtures of nitrogen and oxygen other than those containing 19.5–23.5% oxygen are color-coded black and green.

tablished regulations limiting the amount of gas a cylinder may contain.

1. The pressure in the filled cylinder at 70°F may not exceed the service pressure marked on the cylinder except for some nonliquified, nonflammable gases such as oxygen, helium, carbon dioxide-oxygen mixtures and helium-oxygen mixtures which may be allowed an additional 10% (2).

2. At 130°F, the pressure in cylinders containing gases other than nitrous oxide and carbon dioxide may not exceed 1¼ times the maximum permitted filling pressure at 70°F (2).

3. As illustrated in Figure 1.1, in a cylinder containing a liquified gas, the pressure will remain nearly constant as long as there is liquid in the cylinder. Thus, if only the pressure was limited on these cylinders, they could be filled with any amount of liquid. To prevent a cylinder containing a liquified gas from being overfilled, the maximum amount of gas that can be contained is defined by a "filling density" (filling ratio) for each gas. The filling density is defined as "the percent ratio of the weight of gas in the container to the weight of water that the container would hold at 60°F (2)." The filling densities of gases commonly used in anesthesia are shown in Table 1.2.

The filling density is not the same as the volume of the full cylinder occupied by the liquid phase. For example, in a full nitrous oxide cylinder, the liquid phase occupies about 90 to 95%

of the total cylinder volume, while the filling density is 68%.

COLOR CODING (10)

Because of the number of medical gases available, accidental confusion of cylinders is a significant problem (21). To combat this hazard, a color code was established (22).

There is no mandatory color code for medical gas cylinders in the United States. However, most manufacturers use the color code shown in Table 1.2.

The top and shoulder of each cylinder is painted the color assigned to the gas it contains, except for chromium-plated cylinders for cyclopropane. Since paint does not adhere well to polished metal surfaces, chromium-plated cylinders for cyclopropane must bear labels which prominently display the color orange. A cylinder containing a mixture of two gases is painted the two colors corresponding to the gases in the cylinder.

An International Color Code (Table 1.2) has been adopted in several countries. This system differs from the one used in the United States in that oxygen's color code is white and air is black and white rather than yellow (23). There are several countries other than the United States which follow color codes differing from the International Code. Therefore color should be regarded only as an aid to gas identification and no more. It cannot be relied upon to identify cylinder contents. The label is the primary means of identification.

MARKING AND LABELING (2, 4, 7, 11)

Department of Transportation regulations require specific markings to be stamped on the top or neck of each cylinder. Representative markings are shown in Figure 1.2. The first number is the DOT specification number, followed by the service pressure for the cylinder. Next is a serial number and identifying mark of the purchaser, user, or manufacturer of the cylinder. The mark must be registered with the Bureau of Explosives. The original test date appears last with the inspector's mark between the month and year of the test date. Certain other markings may be present. The word "spun" or "plug" refers to the method used to manufacture the cylinder. The maximum allowable expansion in cubic centimeters may appear. Materials used in manufacture may be noted. If a cylinder has

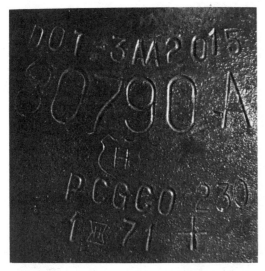

Figure 1.2. Cylinder markings. DOT-3AA is the Department of Transportation specification number. 3AA indicates the type of steel. 2015 is the service pressure in psig. 80790-A is the serial number. The mark below the serial number identifies the manufacturer. PCGCO is the purchaser's name. 230 is the maximum allowable expansion is cubic centimeters. 1-71 is the original testing date. The symbol between 1 and 71 is the testing facility symbol. The + after the test date means that the cylinder complied with the requirements of the test.

been retested, the retest date and testing facility must appear.

Each cylinder must bear in a conspicuous place a label showing the name and having the color code of the contained gas or gas mixture, CGA pamphlet C-7 (4) contains guidelines for the preparation of cylinder labels. The label serves to identify the cylinder contents and give warning of the principal hazards associated with the cylinder and/or its contents.

Figure 1.3 shows a typical cylinder label, which utilizes the CGA basic marking system. This consists of a diamond-shaped figure denoting the hazard class of the contained gas combined with a panel containing the proper shipping name of the gas to the left. In addition, a signal word (DANGER, WARNING, or CAUTION, depending on whether the release of gas would create an immediate, less than immediate, or no immediate hazard to health or property) is present. A statement of hazard follows the signal word and gives notice of the hazards present in connection with the customary or reasonably anticipated handling or use of the product. Precautionary measures may also be present. These are intended to supplement the statement of hazard by setting forth measures to be taken to avoid injury or damage.

The label should contain the name and address of the cylinder manufacturer or distributor. Other information such as cylinder weight when empty and full may also be present.

Tags normally bear the same color as the cylinder. A tag usually has three sections connected by perforations. The sections are labeled FULL, IN USE, and EMPTY. When a cylinder is first opened the FULL portion of the tag should be detached. When the cylinder is empty, the IN USE portion should be removed. The tag sometimes contains a washer to fit between the cylinder valve and the yoke or regulator.

CYLINDER VALVES

Cylinders are charged and discharged through a cylinder valve which is attached to the cylinder neck by means of a tapered thread. Each valve consists of several parts: (a) the body, which forms the basic structure; (b) the port, which is the point of exit for the gas; (c) the stem or shaft, which, when opened, allows the gas to flow to the port; (d) a handle or handwheel for turning the valve stem; (e) the safety relief device which allows discharge of cylinder contents

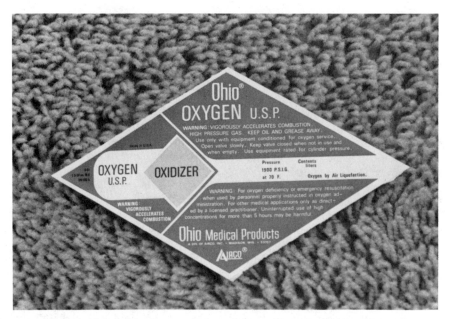

Figure 1.3. Cylinder label. The diamond-shaped figure denotes the hazard class, with the name of the gas to the left. The signal word, WARNING, is followed by the statement of hazard (VIGOROUSLY ACCELERATES COMBUSTION). Various precautionary measures are suggested on the label.

to the atmosphere under certain conditions of exposure; (*f*) the conical depression (on small cylinder valves) which receives the retaining screw of the yoke, and (*g*) the noninterchangeable safety systems which prevent attachment of the incorrect cylinder to the yoke or regulator.

The Body

There are two kinds of cylinder valves in general use. Small cylinder valves (flush valves) are used for cylinder sizes A to E (Table 1.1). Large cylinder valves are used on cylinder sizes F to H (Table 1.1). Both are made of brass and usually are chromium plated. They are fitted into the cylinder neck by a threaded connection. The valve should never be removed from the cylinder except by the supplier.

The Port

The port is the point of exit for the cylinder contents. It fits over the nipple of the yoke (on small cylinders) or the regulator (on large cylinders). It should be protected in transit by a covering. When installing a small cylinder on the machine it is important not to mistake the port for the conical depression on the opposite side of the valve. Inserting the retaining screw

into the port may damage the port and the index pins. Damage to the port may prevent a tight seal or result in a leak.

The Stem

Each valve contains a stem which closes the valve by sealing against the seat. Most cylinder valves are of the packed type. (Figs. 1.5 and 1.6). In these the stem is sealed by a resilient packing such as Teflon. This type of valve is also called a direct-acting valve because turning the stem causes the seat to turn. In the large cylinder valve, the force is transmitted by means of a driver square. (Fig. 1.6). The packed valve offers a good performance with gases under high pressure.

A second type of valve, the diaphragm valve, acts indirectly in that turning the stem either raises or lowers a metal diaphragm (Figs. 1.7 and 1.8). The downward force of the stem is opposed by a spring acting on the seat assembly. Turning the stem clockwise lowers the diaphragm; this, in turn, lowers the seat assembly and closes the valve. When the stem is turned counterclockwise, the diaphragm is raised and the force of the spring raises the seat assembly, opening the valve. This valve is more expensive than the packed type and usually is used for

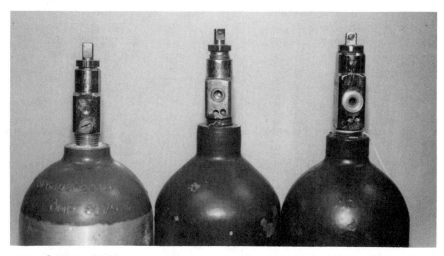

Figure 1.4. Small cylinder valves. At center, showing port and pin index holes. The valve on the right has a sealing washer in place over the port. The valve on the left shows the conical depression above the safety relief device.

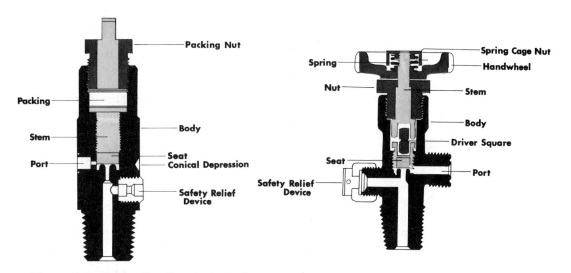

Figure 1.5 (*left*). Small packed cylinder valve. Most commonly used type of valve. The packing seals the stem and prevents leaks. (From a drawing furnished by Puritan-Bennett Corporation.)
Figure 1.6 (*right*). Large packed valve. Turning the stem counterclockwise forces the driver square downward and turns the seat in its thread, opening the valve. (From a drawing furnished by Puritan-Bennett Corporation.)

gases such as nitrous oxide and cyclopropane which liquify under pressure. Some manufacturers feel that these valves operate better under the low temperature conditions produced when these gases are liberated. They can be turned on fully in a one-half to three-fourths turn while the packed valve requires two or three full turns. Less wear and tear on the seat results. These valves are also said to be tighter at the stem and consequently are less susceptible to leaks and possible explosion (24).

The Handle

In order to open or close a cylinder valve, a handle or handwheel is used. It is turned counterclockwise to open the valve. Small cylinder valves have a detachable handle which slips onto

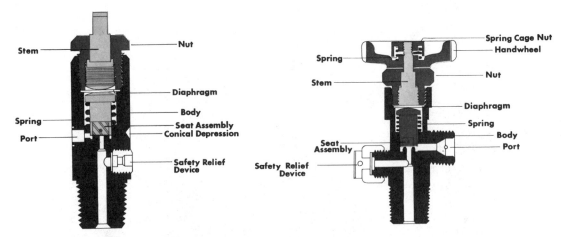

Figure 1.7 (*left*).   Small diaphragm valve. Turning the handle clockwise forces the diaphragm downward and closes the seat. Upon opening the valve the upward force of the spring opens the seat. (From a drawing furnished by Puritan-Bennett Corporation.)

Figure 1.8 (*right*).   Large diaphragm valve. See text for details. (From a drawing furnished by Puritan-Bennett Corporation.)

the top of the stem and comes in a variety of styles (Fig. 1.9). A good practice is to chain a handle to the anesthesia machine. Some handles, such as the one in the middle of Figure 1.9, have, in addition, a hexagonal opening which fits the packing nut (gland nut) of the valve (Fig. 1.5). This may be used to tighten the nut should it become loose and allow the cylinder valve to leak. A hazard using this handle has been described (25). A person unacquainted with cylinders could loosen the packing nut with the handle under the mistaken impression that he was opening the valve. This could cause the valve stem and retaining nut to be shot off the cylinder with great force. The large cylinder valve has a permanently attached handwheel which utilizes a spring and nut to hold it firmly in place (Figs. 1.6 and 1.8).

The Safety Relief Device (5)

An integral part of each cylinder valve is the safety relief device which is designed to prevent rupture of the cylinder under certain conditions of exposure. The three types of safety relief devices are the frangible disc assembly, the fusible plug, and the safety relief valve.

THE FRANGIBLE DISC ASSEMBLY (6)

The frangible disc assembly (Fig. 1.10) consists of a frangible disc and a safety cap whose ports may be filled with a fusible alloy. The disc itself is usually made of copper and closes the discharge channel, preventing release of the contained gas. The pressure opening is the orifice against which the frangible disc functions. The rated bursting pressure is the minimum pressure for which the disc is designed to burst. When this pressure is exceeded, the disc bursts and gas escapes through the discharge channel. A reinforced disc is thickened in the center and the diameter of the reinforced part corresponds to that of the pressure opening.

THE FUSIBLE PLUG (8)

The fusible plug (Fig. 1.4, *left side*) is made of a low-melting-point material, usually a metal alloy, which occludes the discharge channel and melts at a predetermined temperature. The alloy is usually composed of varying percentages of bismuth, lead, tin and cadmium. A commonly used one is called Wood's metal. The yield temperature of the fusible plug is that temperature at which the alloy will melt. A reinforced fusible plug consists of a core having a high yield temperature surrounded by a metal of low yield temperature. There are two temperature ranges of fusible plugs employed. One melts in the 157–170°F range and the other in the 208–220°F range.

A combination of frangible disc and low-melting-point fusible plug is available which pre-

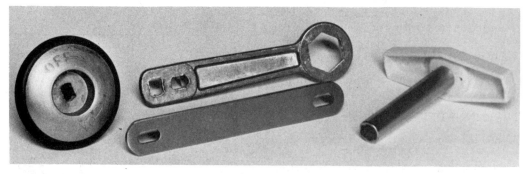

Figure 1.9. Representative small cylinder valve handles. The hexagonal opening at the end of the upper middle handle is used to tighten the packing nut on the valve.

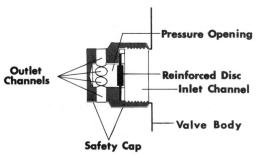

Figure 1.10. Frangible disc assembly. When the rated bursting pressure is exceeded the disc ruptures and gas flows from the inlet channel into the pressure opening and to the atmosphere through the outlet channels. (From a drawing in Compressed Gas Association pamphlet S-3, p. 4.)

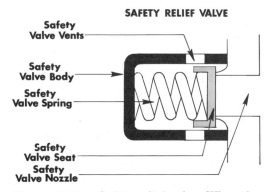

Figure 1.11. Safety relief valve. When the set pressure is exceeded, the pressure in the cylinder forces the spring to the left and gas flows around the seat of the safety valve vents. When the excess pressure is relieved the spring closes the valve. (From a drawing by Ohio Medical Products.)

vents bursting at a predetermined pressure unless the melting temperature has also been attained.

THE SAFETY RELIEF VALVE (5)

The safety relief valve (Fig. 1.11) consists of a safety valve seat held by a spring in a position occluding the discharge channel. When the pressure for which the device is set is exceeded, the valve opens and gas escapes through the safety valve vents until the pressure is reduced and the valve closes again. This may be used in combination with a fusible plug, with the safety valve vents filled with a low- or high-melting-point material.

The Conical Depression

Above the safety relief device on small cylinders is the conical depression which receives the retaining screw from the yoke (Fig. 1.4, *left*). It should be distinguished from the safety relief device. If the retaining screw is tightened into the safety relief device, the plug may be damaged and the cylinder contents escape (26–28).

The Noninterchangeable Safety Systems (9)

With the widespread use of cylinders containing different gases, a potential hazard arose in that an incorrect cylinder could be connected to equipment intended for a different gas. To help solve this problem, color coding of cylinders was developed (Table 1.2). However, this did not give complete protection against human error. Through the cooperation of the CGA and others, two systems were developed to help resolve this problem. Both of these systems are located between the cylinder valve and the regulator and should not be confused with the Diameter Index Safety System which is on the low pressure side of the regulator and will be discussed in Chapter 2.

THE PIN INDEX SAFETY SYSTEM

The Pin Index Safety System is used on small cylinder valves (size E or less) with yoke-type connections and consists of two pins projecting from the inner surface of the yoke (Figs. 1.12 and 3.2) and so positioned as to fit into two corresponding holes drilled into the cylinder valve (Fig. 1.4). Unless the pins and holes are aligned, the port will not seat against the washer of the yoke. It is possible for a yoke that is not pin indexed to receive any cylinder valve, but ordinarily it is not possible for an undrilled cylinder valve to be placed in a yoke containing pins. Combinations of pins assigned to gases or gas mixtures in anesthesia are shown in Table 1.3.

The use of the Pin Index Safety System was begun in 1952. Most anesthetic apparatus produced after 1953 incorporates the Pin Index System (9). A conversion unit can and should

Table 1.3.
Pin Index System

Gas	Index Pins	CGA Connection No.
Oxygen	2–5	870
Nitrous oxide	3–5	910
Cyclopropane	3–6	920
O_2-CO_2 ($CO_2 < 7.5\%$)	2–6	880
O_2-CO_2 ($CO_2 > 7.5\%$)	1–6	940
O_2-He (He $> 80.5\%$)	4–6	930
O_2-He (He $< 80.5\%$)	2–4	890
Air	1–5	950
Nitrogen	1–4	960
N_2O-O_2 (N_2O 47.5–52.5%)	7	965

be applied to yokes of machines produced prior to this time.

VALVE OUTLET CONNECTIONS FOR LARGE CYLINDERS

A large cylinder cannot connect directly to a yoke, so the Pin-Index System cannot be used. A different system (9) for these valves was developed, the essential components of which are shown in Figure 1.13. The cylinder valve has a threaded outlet. When the threads of this outlet mesh with those of the nut, the nut may be tightened by turning it clockwise, causing the nipple to seat against the valve outlet. In this way the gas channel of the valve is aligned with the channel of the nipple. The threaded outlets are separated into four basic dimensions—internal, external, right hand, and left hand. Further separation is made within each division by varying the diameter of the threads. Still further separation is made by varying the size and shape of seats and nipples for any given thread size. Table 1.4 gives the CGA connection numbers and the thread types for the valve outlets. The first three numbers of the thread refer to the major thread diameter in inches and the second to the number of threads per inch. NGO signifies that it is a National Gas Outlet type and the last five letters refer to whether the threads are right hand or left hand and external or internal.

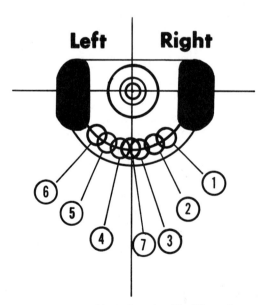

Left   Right

Figure 1.12. Pin index pins. Positions shown are as if looking directly at the yoke. (Redrawn from Compressed Gas Association pamphlet V-1, pp. 38–39.)

RULES FOR SAFE USE OF CYLINDERS (1–3, 17, 18, 21, 22, 29–35)

1. Gas cylinders should be stored in a cool, dry, clean, well-ventilated room which is, if prac-

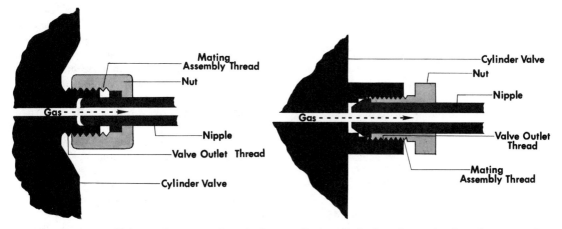

Figure 1.13. Valve outlet connections for large cylinders. *Left*, the valve outlet thread is external, that is, the threads are on the outside of the cylinder valve outlet and the nut screws over the valve outlet. (Redrawn courtesy of Compressed Gas Association.) *Right*, the value outlet thread is internal, so that the nut screws into the outlet. (Redrawn from Compressed Gas Association pamphlet V-1.)

Table 1.4.
American Standard Compressed Gas Cylinder Valve Outlet Connections for G, H, M, and K Cylinders

Gas	CGA Connection No.	Valve Outlet
Air	346 (formerly 1340)	0.825-14NGO-RH-EXT
O_2-CO_2 ($CO_2 >$ 7.5%)	500	0.885-14NGO-RH-INT
O_2-He (He > 80.5%)		(bullet nipple)
Cyclopropane	510	0.885-14NGO-LH-INT
CO_2	320	0.825-14NGO-RH-EXT
O_2	540	0.903-14NGO-RH-EXT
O_2-CO_2 ($CO_2 <$ 7.5%)	280	0.745-14NGO-RH-EXT
O_2-He (He < 80.5)		
N_2O	326	0.825-14NGO-RH-EXT (small round nipple)
Helium	580	0.965-14NGO-RH-INT
Nitrogen		
N_2O-O_2 (N_2O 47.5–52.5%)	280	0.745-14NGO-RH-EXT

tical, fireproof. Conductive flooring must be present where flammable gases are stored. The room should be vented to the outside so that if there is a leak in a cylinder gas will not accumulate in the room. Cylinders should not be stored in an operating room, corridor, heavy traffic area, or where heavy moving objects may strike or fall on them.

Easily visible signs with texts such as "GAS CYLINDERS. REMOVE TO A SAFE PLACE IN THE EVENT OF FIRE" and "OFF LIMITS TO UNAUTHORIZED PERSONNEL" should be set up outside the cylinder room. Signs reading "NO SMOKING," "NO OPEN FLAMES OR SPARKS," "NO OIL OR GREASE," and "NO COMBUSTIBLE MATERIALS" should be posted inside the room and on the door.

2. Cylinders may be stored in the open, but must be protected from the ground beneath, accumulation of snow and ice, and from the sun's direct rays, since the labels and identification colors will deteriorate under climatic conditions and could lead to mistakes in identification.

3. Cylinders should not be stored near flammable materials, especially oil or grease, as oxygen or gas mixtures containing oxygen may cause such materials to ignite.

4. Cylinders should not be exposed to extremes of heat or cold or allowed to become wet or dirty. They should be kept away from any

source of heat (such as a radiator or hot pipe), sparks or flames. No part of the cylinder should ever be subjected to a temperature above 130°F (1). Should a valve outlet become clogged with ice, it should be thawed at room temperature or with water at a temperature not exceeding 130°F.

5. Cylinders should not be exposed to continuous dampness, corrosive chemicals, or fumes, since these may cause rusting which will damage the cylinders and valves and cause the valve protection caps to stick.

6. Paper or plastic covers should be removed from cylinders before storage. The presence of these in the storage area is undesirable since they are dirty from transportation, provide a combustible medium, and conceal the cylinder labels.

7. Cylinders should not be covered with drapes. Combustible mixtures may accumulate under a drape and its removal could provide the electrostatic spark that ignites the mixture trapped beneath.

8. Cylinders should be properly secured at all times both while in storage and while in use to prevent them from falling or being knocked over. A large amount of energy is stored in a compressed gas cylinder. If the cylinder valve is struck (or strikes something else) hard enough to break the valve, the contents of the cylinder may be discharged with sufficient force to impart a dangerous reactive movement to the cylinder.

Small cylinders are best stored upright or horizontally in bins or racks constructed of a nonflammable material that will not damage the surfaces of the cylinders when they are moved. Large cylinders should be placed upright against a wall and chained in place.

9. The valve is the most easily damaged part of the cylinder. Valve protection caps, metal caps which screw over the valve on large cylinders, are available and should be in place and hand tightened when the cylinders are not connected for use.

10. Full cylinders should be stored so that they are used in the order they were received from the supplier and grouped according to their contents. Empty cylinders should be marked as such and stored separately from full cylinders to avoid confusion and delay if a full cylinder is needed immediately.

11. Cylinders containing nonflammable oxidizing gases which support combustion, such as nitrous oxide and oxygen, should be stored separately from cylinders containing flammable gases. Should the flammable gases escape from their cylinders and become ignited, the oxidizing gases would support their combustion. Conversely, cylinders containing carbon dioxide should be stored in the same areas as flammable gases, since carbon dioxide acts as a fire extinguisher.

12. Cylinders should be cleaned before being taken into the operating room area.

13. The valve protection cap or the covering over the port should be left on during transportation and removed only when the cylinder is to be used.

14. Cylinders should be handled with care and not dropped, violently struck, dragged, rolled, slid, or used as supports. They should never be allowed to come into violent contact with one another or with any hard object. Carriers are available for moving both large and small cylinders and should always be used. The retaining chain or fastener, on large cylinder carriers should be secured before transport.

15. Before a cylinder is connected for use it should be inspected. Only approved cylinders with the letters "DOT" or "ICC" should be used. In Canada equivalent cylinders are marked "BTC" or "CRC." A cylinder that does not show evidence of inspection within the required period should not be used. The cylinder valve, especially the safety relief valve and the pin index holes, should be checked for damage. A cylinder with worn pin index holes may accommodate an incorrect yoke (36). Any defective cylinder should be clearly marked "defective" and returned to the vendor as such. No repairs or modifications should ever be performed on any part of the cylinder or its valve by a user. Any cylinder whose proper function is in doubt for any reason should be returned to the supplier.

16. The gas contents must be identified by the label or cylinder markings. If a cylinder's contents are not identifiable by these means the cylinder must be returned to the supplier without use. Cylinder color must not be relied upon for identification of contents.

17. Cylinders should never be repainted or the markings repainted, removed, obscured or altered. Labels, tags or the upper half of a DOT Red or Green label should not be defaced or removed.

18. Full cylinders are usually supplied with a

plastic cover over the outlet to prevent dirt from entering the outlet. This should be removed immediately before fitting the cylinder. Also just before any fitting is applied to the cylinder, particles of dust should be cleared from the cylinder by slightly opening and closing the valve ("cracking the valve") with the port pointed away from anyone in the area (29). This clearing reduces the possibility of a flash fire or explosion when the valve is later opened with the fittings in place; also the dust will not be blown into the anesthesia machine or other equipment where it could clog filters or interfere with internal workings.

19. With the possible exception of cyclopropane and, in certain instances, carbon dioxide, a cylinder should not be used unless its pressure is reduced through a suitable pressure-reducing device and there is a means for controlling gas flow. For small cylinders attached to an anesthesia machine, both of these functions are performed by the anesthesia machine. Most portable regulators perform both functions.

20. Regulators should be kept in good condition and stored in plastic bags to avoid contamination with dirt or oil. Yokes should not be left empty. Either a full cylinder or a yoke plug (see page 41) should always be in place.

21. Oil, grease or other readily combustible materials should not be allowed to come into contact with valves, washers, gauges, regulators, or other equipment associated with the use of compressed gases. Cylinders should not be handled with rags, hands, gloves, or other clothing which contain grease, oil, acids, or corrosive substances.

22. One should never attempt to substitute regulators or other appliances designed for use with one gas with similar gas equipment intended for use with another gas.

23. The threads on the regulator or pins on the yoke must correspond to those on the cylinder valve. Connections that do not fit must never be forced. A cylinder with a valve that does not correspond to its label should not be used.

24. Wrenches or tools other than those provided by the manufacturer should not be used. Wrenches with misaligned jaws should not be used as they may damage the equipment or slip and injure personnel. The sealing washers must be in good condition.

25. A sealing washer should always be used with small cylinder valves. It fits over the port (Fig. 1.4). After the washer is in place the regulator or yoke can be attached. Connections should be made tight to prevent leakage but only a reasonable amount of effort should be used. Excessive force may damage threads and valve seats.

26. After a cylinder is attached to a regulator, but before its valve is opened, the pressure-adjusting screw of the regulator should be turned OFF by turning counterclockwise until it turns freely.

27. When a cylinder is attached to the yoke of an anesthesia machine the flow control valve on the machine should be closed before the cylinder valve is opened. Otherwise the pressure of the cylinder directed into the machine may damage the flowmeter.

28. A cylinder valve should always be opened SLOWLY (37) by turning counterclockwise. If this is not done slowly and gas passes quickly into the space between the cylinder valve and the yoke or regulator, the instantaneous recompression in this space will generate large amounts of heat. Since there is little time for dissipation of this heat, this constitutes an adiabatic process (one in which heat is neither lost nor gained from its environment). Particles of dust, grease, etc. present in this space may be ignited by the heat, causing a flash fire or explosion (38, 39). By opening the valve slowly the time of recompression is prolonged, permitting some of the heat to dissipate. Also very rapid opening of a valve may damage sensitive instruments connected to the cylinder.

29. The person opening a cylinder valve should position his face and trunk well away from the valve for 5–10 sec to allow pressure equilibration and to avoid direct impact from an explosion should one occur.

30. The handle or handwheel should not be hammered when attempting to open or close the valve. If a cylinder valve cannot be opened by hand or is otherwise inoperable, it should not be tampered with, but returned to the supplier.

31. If a hissing sound is heard when the cylinder valve is opened, a large leak exists and the connection should be tightened. If the sound does not disappear, the sealing washer should be replaced (in the case of a small cylinder valve). However, under no circumstances should more than one washer be used. If the hissing sound persists, soapy water or a commercial leak detection fluid should be applied to all the joints and parts. Bubbles will appear at the site of the

leak(s). An open flame should never be used for this purpose.

Should a leak be found in the cylinder valve itself, it may be possible to tighten the packing nut by turning it slightly in a clockwise direction (see special handle in Fig. 1.9), unless the manufacturer recommends otherwise.

If the leak cannot be remedied easily, the cylinder valve should be closed, the cylinder marked "defective" and returned to the supplier, with a note indicating the fault.

32. If no hissing sound is audible when the valve is opened, a slow leak may be present and should be suspected if there is loss of pressure when no gas is being used. These leaks should be located and remedied as indicated above.

33. Any hoses used between a cylinder and dispensing equipment should be kept in good condition and checked periodically for leaks.

34. After the cylinder valve is opened the pressure should be checked. A cylinder arriving with a pressure substantially greater than the service pressure should not be used, but marked and returned to the supplier. A cylinder arriving with a pressure substantially below the service pressure should be checked carefully for leaks.

35. The cylinder valve should always be fully open when the cylinder is in use. Marginal opening of the valve may result in failure to deliver adequate gas. Death due to anoxia from this error has been reported (40).

36. Measures should be taken to prevent a cylinder from being knocked over when connected to utilization equipment.

37. The user should notify the owner or supplier of a cylinder immediately if it is believed that any potentially harmful foreign substances may have entered a cylinder or if the contents are suspect for any reason.

38. When work is finished the cylinder valve should be closed completely and all pressure released from the system. Only sufficient force should be used to close a cylinder valve. Excessive force may result in damage.

39. An empty cylinder should not be left on an anesthesia machine. A defective check valve in the yoke could result in accidental filling of the cylinder if the cylinder valve is left open. Also the presence of an empty cylinder may create a false sense of security in the user by deluding him into thinking an emergency supply is present. An empty cylinder may be replaced with a yoke plug (see page 41) if a full cylinder is not available.

40. Before removing a cylinder from a regulator or yoke the cylinder valve should be closed and all pressure released.

41. When a cylinder is empty, the lower part of the tag should be removed. A DOT Green or Red label should be covered with an Empty label.

42. Valves should be completely closed on all empty cylinders. Valve protection caps and outlet caps or plugs, if used, should be replaced before shipment. Often cylinders are not completely empty and accidents have resulted from release of gas from a supposedly empty cylinder. Also keeping the valve closed prevents contamination of the valve and cylinder by dirt and/or moisture.

TRANSFILLING

This practice is mentioned only to be condemned. When small cylinders are transfilled from large cylinders containing gas at high pressure, rapid recompression of the gas in the small cylinder may cause the temperature to rise abruptly, resulting in an explosion (23). Since filling conditions vary for cylinders of different manufacturers, the hazard of overfilling a cylinder is always present (41). Cylinders used for one type of gas may accidentally be recharged with a gas other than that originally contained in the cylinder, resulting in a dangerous mixture of gases, for example, if a flammable and an oxidizing gas are mixed. Such an error, which occurred when a cyclopropane cylinder was filled with oxygen and cyclopropane, resulted in an explosion that caused multiple deaths and injuries (42).

References

1. *Safe Handling of Compressed Gases in Containers.* Pamphlet P-1, Compressed Gas Association, Inc., 500 Fifth Ave., New York, N.Y. 10036, 1974.
2. *Characteristics and Safe Handling of Medical Gases.* Pamphlet P-2, Compressed Gas Association, Inc., 500 Fifth Ave., New York, N.Y. 10036, 1978.
3. *Oxygen.* Pamphlet G-4, Compressed Gas Association, Inc., 500 Fifth Ave., New York, N.Y. 10036, 1972.
4. *Guide to the Preparation of Precautionary Labeling and Marking of Compressed Gas Containers.* Pamphlet C-7, Compressed Gas Association, Inc., 500 Fifth Ave., New York, N.Y. 10036, 1976.
5. *Safety Relief Device Standards.* Part 1: *Cylinders for Compressed Gases.* Pamphlet S-1.1, Compressed Gas Association Inc., 500 Fifth Ave., New York, N.Y. 10036, 1969.

6. *Frangible Disc Safety Device Assembly.* Pamphlet S-3, Compressed Gas Association Inc., 500 Fifth Ave., New York, N.Y. 10036.
7. *Method of Marking Portable Compressed Gas Containers to Identify the Material Contained.* Pamphlet C-4, Compressed Gas Association, Inc., 500 Fifth Ave., New York, N.Y. 10036, 1971.
8. *Recommended Practice for the Manufacture of Fusible Plugs.* Pamphlet S-4, Compressed Gas Association, Inc., 500 Fifth Ave., New York, N.Y. 10036, 1967.
9. *Compressed Gas Cylinder Valve Outlet and Inlet Connections.* Pamphlet V-1, Compressed Gas Association, Inc., 500 Fifth Ave., New York, N.Y. 10036, 1977.
10. *Standard Color-Marking of Compressed Gas Cylinders Intended for Medical Use in the United States.* Pamphlet C-9, Compressed Gas Association, Inc., 500 Fifth Ave., New York, N.Y. 10036, 1973.
11. *Methods for Hydrostatic Testing of Compressed Gas Cylinders.* Pamphlet C-1, Compressed Gas Association, Inc., 500 Fifth Ave., New York, N.Y. 10036, 1975.
12. *Recommendations for the Disposition of Unserviceable Compressed Gas Cylinders.* Pamphlet C-2, Compressed Gas Association, Inc., 500 Fifth Ave., New York, N.Y. 10036, 1976.
13. *Cylinder Service Life—Seamless, High-Pressure Cylinders.* Pamphlet C-5, Compressed Gas Association, Inc., 500 Fifth Ave., New York, N.Y. 10036, 1976.
14. *Standards for Visual Inspection of Compressed Gas Cylinders.* Pamphlet C-6, Compressed Gas Association, Inc., 500 Fifth Ave., New York, N.Y. 10036, 1975.
15. *Standard for Requalification of DOT-3HT Cylinders.* Pamphlet C-8, Compressed Gas Association, Inc., 500 Fifth Ave., New York, N.Y. 10036, 1978.
16. *Standard for the Installation of Nitrous Oxide Systems at Consumer Sites.* Pamphlet G-8.1, Compressed Gas Association, Inc., 500 Fifth Ave., New York, N.Y. 10036, 1964.
17. *Standard for the Use of Inhalation Anesthetics.* NFPA 56A, National Fire Protection Association, 470 Atlantic Ave., Boston, Mass. 02210, 1973.
18. *Respiratory Therapy.* NFPA 56B, National Fire Protection Association, 470 Atlantic Ave., Boston, Mass. 02210, 1976.
19. *Nonflammable Medical Gas Systems.* NFPA 56F, National Fire Protection Association, 470 Atlantic Ave., Boston, Mass. 02210, 1977.
20. Jones PL: Some observations on nitrous oxide cylinders during emptying. *Br J Anaesth* 46:534–538, 1974.
21. Anonymous: Medico-legal: identification of gas cylinders. *Br Med J* 1:381, 1945.
22. Grove DD, Covintree GE: Precautions with gases used by the anesthesiologist (exclusive of fire and explosion hazards). *Anesth Analg* 32:145–158, 1953.
23. *Medical Gas Cylinders and Anaesthetic Apparatus.* British Standard 1319. British Standards Institution, British Standards House, 2 Park St., London W. 1, 1955. (Available from the American National Standards Institute, 1430 Broadway, New York, N.Y.)
24. Tristram GV: Personal communication, Puritan-Bennett Corporation.
25. Finch JS: A report on a possible hazard of gas cylinder tanks. *Anesthesiology* 33:467, 1970.
26. Fox JWC, Fox EJ: An unusual occurrence with a cyclopropane cylinder. *Anesth Analg* 47:624–626, 1968.
27. Milliken RA: Correspondence. *Anesth Analg* 50:775 1971.
28. Milliken RA: An explosion hazard due to an imperfect design. *Arch Surg* 105:125–127, 1972.
29. Eger EI, Epstein RM: Hazards of anesthetic equipment. *Anesthesiology* 25:490–504, 1964.
30. Collins VJ: *Principles of Anesthesiology.* Philadelphia, Lea & Febiger, 1966.
31. *Inhalation Anesthetics.* NFPA 56A, National Fire Protection Association, 470 Atlantic Ave., Boston, Mass. 02210.
32. American Association for Inhalation Therapy: *Safety Code Manual,* 1970.
33. *Compressed Gases, Safe Practices.* Pamphlet 95, National Safety Council, 425 N. Michigan Ave., Chicago, Ill., 1957.
34. Feeley TW, Bancroft ML, Brooks RA, Hedley-Whyte J: Potential hazards of compressed gas cylinders: A review. *Anesthesiology* 48:72–74, 1978.
35. *Specification for Medical Gas Cylinders, Valves and Yoke Connections.* British Standard 1319. British Standards Institution, British Standards House, 2 Park St., London W.1A 2BS, 1976. (Available from the American Standards Institute, 1430 Broadway, New York, N.Y.)
36. Mead P: Hazard with cylinder yoke. *Anaesth Intensive Care* 9:79–80, 1981.
37. Czajka RJ: Cylinder caution: open slowly to minimize recompression heat. *Anesthesiology* 49:226, 1978.
38. Ito Y, Horikowa H, Ichiyanagi K: Fires and explosions with compressed gases: report of an accident. *Br J Anaesth* 37:140–141, 1965.
39. Garfield JM, Allen GW, Silverstein P, Mendenhall MK: Flash fire in a reducing valve. *Anesthesiology* 34:578–579, 1971.
40. Epstein RM, Rackow H, Lee ASJ, Papper EM: Prevention of accidental breathing of anoxic gas mixtures during anesthesia. *Anesthesiology* 23:1–4, 1962.
41. Cross A: Explosion of an "A" size gas cylinder. *Resp Care* 16:1–2, 1971.
42. Walter CW: Anesthetic explosions: a continuing threat. *Anesthesiology* 25:505–514, 1964.

CHAPTER 2

Medical Gas Piping Systems

The majority of hospitals today utilize a piping system to deliver nonflammable gases such as oxygen, nitrous oxide, air, carbon dioxide, nitrogen, and mixtures of these gases to operating rooms and other areas of the hospital where they are required. Gases such as nitrogen, air, and carbon dioxide, which may be needed only in certain areas, are sometimes piped from cylinders or, in the case of air, compressors set up in a room connected to the area where the gases will be used (1–3). In certain critical areas such as anesthetizing locations, the recovery room, intensive care unit and emergency room, emergency auxiliary systems for air and/or oxygen may be installed to supply these gases during a breakdown of the main system (4). This may also be done with a T-piece fitting or retrograde flow through a station outlet. However, retrograde flow through a station outlet may impose a severe flow rate limitation.

Usually central piping systems are installed by mechanical or plumbing contractors and maintained by the hospital engineering or maintenance department, with little input from the users. Not only does this system neglect a potentially valuable contribution, but, even more importantly, it leaves the persons ultimately responsible for directing the use of medical gases ignorant of how their system works, its strengths and weaknesses, its need for maintenance and repair, and, most critically how to fix it or get it fixed should a malfunction occur (5).

Anesthesiologists frequently have little knowledge of the piping system or the problems that can occur with it despite the fact that every day the lives of many of their patients may depend on it. Since most of the system is out of sight and usually functions well, it does not attract attention until a problem occurs. There may be a reluctance on the part of anesthesiologists to take an interest because of the implied legal responsibility.

This lack of familiarity with the design and operation of piping systems is most unfortunate, since it may compound an already serious problem if an emergency arises. Anesthesiologists and other hospital personnel who use the system should make an effort to acquaint themselves with the system and the problems that can occur. Circuit diagrams and maintenance procedures should be reviewed with the hospital engineers and gas suppliers to make certain they comply strictly with applicable codes.

When a new hospital or addition is being planned, the anesthesiologist should play a key role in designing the piping system. Physician input is important in determining the size of the system. The physician can tell where oxygen outlets should be placed (including remote parts of the hospital where patients are taken for diagnostic studies or various types of therapy) and can estimate the degree of use each outlet might receive. A little early planning will avoid expense and inconvenience at a later date. For example, extensions to existing pipeline installations may change the flow rates and render the resulting pipeline substandard unless adequate provision was made for the additional load in the original design. It has been suggested that it may be prudent to provide a spare pipeline extending from the central supply area to various sites in the hospital and capped at all points for installation of an additional piped gas in the future (6).

STANDARDS AND SOURCES OF INFORMATION

Current designs of medical gas systems in the United States are founded chiefly upon the principles set forth in the standards of the National Fire Protection Association (NFPA) and the Compressed Gas Association (CGA). These organizations publish a number of standards on safe practices (7–18). These have no legal force per se, but are incorporated into law in some states (19, 20). Compliance with these standards is one of the bases for accreditation by the Joint Commission on Accreditation of Hospitals. Unfortunately, there is no regulatory agency to inspect and certify these systems. In most instances compliance with standards is left to the gas supplier and the individual hospital. Lack of compliance with existing NFPA regulation is common (21).

The United Kingdom, Canada, and Australia have published codes of practice (6, 22–28) and there is an international standard in preparation.

In addition to national standards, there are many state and local codes that pre-empt, and sometimes exceed, national regulations.

SYSTEM COMPONENTS

A hospital piping system consists of the following: (a) a central supply system with control equipment; (b) a network of piping which delivers the gases to locations where they may be required, and (c) station outlets at each point of use. Hoses that extend from station outlets to the anesthesia machine or other equipment used in the treatment of patients, while not part of the piping system, will be discussed in this chapter because of their importance to anesthesiologists.

Central Supplies

The central supply consists of facilities for storage of gases, controls to deliver the gases to the piping system at the desired pressure and alarms and safety devices. Gases other than nitrogen are normally piped at a pressure of 50–55 psig (345–380 kPa). Nitrogen is normally delivered at 160–200 psig (1100–1400 kPa).

MEDICAL GAS SOURCES

Oxygen

Oxygen systems are of two sizes: bulk and smaller systems. A bulk oxygen system is defined as "an assembly of equipment . . . which has a storage capacity of more than 20,000 cu ft of gaseous oxygen including unconnected reserves on hand at the site." NFPA 50 (9) contains recommendations for the location, construction, and installation of bulk oxygen systems. NFPA 56F (8) and 56A (7) apply to both bulk oxygen systems and systems of lesser capacity.

Oxygen may be stored either as a liquid or a gas. When large quantities are required, liquid storage is usually preferred. Cylinder supplies are used for small hospitals, sections of hospitals

not completely piped for oxygen, and auxiliary systems. Central supplies may be located in the open air with the control panel protected from the weather or inside a specially constructed room. Access to the central supply area should be restricted to those individuals familiar with and responsible for adjustment of the system.

Gaseous Supply. The sources of gaseous oxygen are usually G or H cylinders that are transported between the gas distributor and the central supply area of the hospital or cylinders that are permanently fixed at the hospital site and refilled from a truck by the distributor.

A common type of gaseous oxygen supply is shown in Figure 2.1. Two banks (or units) of cylinders are provided. The number of cylinders in each bank is determined by the usage rate. Each bank must contain an average day's supply, with a minimum of two cylinders (8). Greater storage may be necessary in areas remote from suppliers. The cylinders are connected to a manifold (header) which converts them into one continuous supply. Check valves are placed in the lead between each cylinder and the manifold header. The primary (duty) supply is the portion actually supplying the system at any time. The secondary (standby) supply is the other bank of cylinders. Normal operating procedure is for the secondary bank to automatically switch in and supply the system when the primary bank becomes exhausted. The switchover is accomplished by a pressure-sensitive switch known as a manifold changeover device (29). The bank of exhausted cylinders may then be replaced with full ones and it becomes the standby supply. The primary and secondary banks constitute the operating supply. This is known as an alternating system since under normal operating conditions two sources alternately supply the system with gas.

Frequently a reserve supply is added to the supplies shown in Figure 2.1. It must contain at least three cylinders (8). It is automatically fed into the system when the main supply pressure reaches a preset value. It normally functions only in an emergency and its activation should trigger an alarm. An alarm signaling when the reserve supply is reduced to one average day's consumption may be required under some circumstances (8). The reserve supply may allow maintenance on the operating supply to be carried out.

Each bank of cylinders has a pressure regulator which reduces the pressure and maintains the pressure on the downstream side within

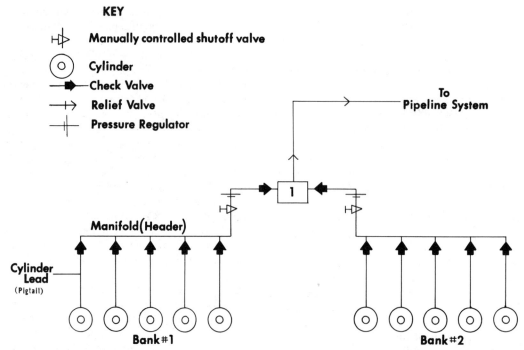

KEY

⊢▷ Manually controlled shutoff valve

(○) Cylinder

▬■▬ Check Valve

⟶▷ Relief Valve

⊣⊢ Pressure Regulator

Figure 2.1. Schematic drawing of central oxygen system without reserve supply. *1*, manifold changeover device. Check valves between each cylinder lead and the manifold prevent loss of gas from the manifolded cylinders in the event that the safety relief device on an individual cylinder functions or a cylinder lead leaks. Manual shutoff (ON-OFF) valves permit isolation of either bank. Check valves downstream of the regulators prevent the reversal of gas flow from either source. Filters may be installed upstream of the regulators. Each bank of cylinders must have its own pressure regulator. Fluctuations in the distribution pressure due to characteristics or settings of regulators in the central supply and the changeover between the primary and secondary supplies can be eliminated by reducing the pressure in two stages so a second regulator is installed in the outgoing pipe or further downstream in the piping network. A manual shutoff valve must be located upstream of each regulator and a shutoff or check valve must be located downstream. The changeover device ensures that the gas supply will automatically change over from a nearly empty bank of cylinders to a full bank. This may be accomplished by operating the regulators at different set pressures or by utilizing pressure-actuated valves. The operating alarm system provides a signal when a changeover from one portion of the operating supply to another portion occurs to let personnel know that empty cylinders require replacement. (Redrawn from *Standard for Nonflammable Medical Gas Systems.* NFPA 56F, 1970, p. 8.)

prescribed limits regardless of the pressure upstream.

Liquid Supply (30, 31). When large amounts of oxygen are required, it is less expensive and more convenient to store it as a liquid. One cubic foot of liquid oxygen at a temperature of −297°F yields 860 cu ft of gaseous oxygen at 70°F. A smaller storage space and less frequent deliveries to the hospital are required when liquid storage is used.

CGA pamphlets G-4 (12) and V-6 (15) deal with the shipping and storage of liquid oxygen. To prevent the liquid from evaporating, it must be kept at or below its boiling point (−297°F). This is accomplished by keeping it in special insulated containers (cisterns) under low pressure. The liquid oxygen is topped off at suitable intervals by pumping in liquid oxygen without interrupting the supply.

These containers are constructed using a principle similar to that of a thermos bottle, with outer and inner metal jackets separated by several layers of insulation and, usually, a layer of near vacuum, to retard external heat transfer into the cold liquid. The container should be provided with a contents indicator and alarm.

Because liquid oxygen vaporizes at low temperatures and a small quantity of liquid will produce a large volume of gas, it is important that liquid oxygen containers be provided with suitable safety relief devices (9) to allow some of the gas on top of the liquid to escape.

Although the insulation of such a tank is very good, it is not perfect and there is a small amount of heat absorbed continuously from the surroundings, causing evaporation of the liquefied gas. This amount of uncontrolled evaporation is usually considerably less than the daily oxygen demand from the tank. When there is no flow from the container to the pipeline the pressure in the container will slowly increase until the safety relief valve opens and oxygen is vented to atmosphere. If a liquid system is left standing unused for long periods of time, a significant amount of oxygen will be lost to the atmosphere. The use of liquid containers is economical only when there is a fairly constant high-volume demand. It is important to have the proper size container so that usage will approximate maximum vaporization rate and gas loss through venting will be minimized.

Liquid oxygen containers are equipped with vaporizers (evaporators, gasifiers), which supply heat to convert the liquid to gaseous form. An evaporator usually consists of an insulated pipe in the form of a coil, loop, or grill, which is exposed to atmosphere, utilizing heat from the atmosphere to accomplish conversion (32). The units can also be heated with electricity, steam, water, or water solutions that do not react with oxygen (32). When the pressure in the tank drops because of a lowering of the liquid level, a valve opens and liquid oxygen flows into the evaporator. This liquid absorbs heat and is returned to the top of the liquid tank as gas, increasing the gas pressure. The gaseous oxygen above the liquid is drawn off as required and passed through a superheater to bring it up to ambient temperature and thus raise its pressure (29).

Extreme caution must be exercised in handling liquid oxygen. The danger of fires is especially great. All components of a liquid oxygen system must be thoroughly cleansed of grease and oil before being put into service. Severe burns may result if the liquid or uninsulated pipe carrying the liquid comes in contact with human skin.

Liquid oxygen is most frequently supplied from fixed containers of large capacity that are refilled from supply trucks without interruption of service. When less capacity is required liquid oxygen containers that are transported between the supplier and the hospital can be used.

A typical liquid oxygen supply is shown in Figure 2.2. The reserve supply may consist of either a manifold of high pressure cylinders or another liquid oxygen container. This is known as a continuous type of system since under normal operating conditions one primary source (which is refilled periodically) always supplies the system with gas.

Nitrous Oxide

Central nitrous oxide supplies are covered in CGA pamphlet G-8.1 (13), NFPA 56F (8), and NFPA 56A (7). Most hospitals use high-pressure nitrous oxide cylinders manifolded together in banks, in an arrangement similar to that described for oxygen cylinders. One problem with nitrous oxide cylinders is that when they are located in a cold place the regulator may become so cold that it freezes. High use of gas can also cause a regulator to freeze (33). Nitrous oxide may also be stored as a liquid in specially designed insulated vessels.

Air

Compressed air is used for powering ventilators and surgical tools (34) and for supplying part of the inhaled mixture (especially in pediatrics). A number of anesthesia machines now include connections and flowmeters for air.

Compressed air piping systems are covered in NFPA 56F (8). The air may be supplied from manifolded cylinders containing air, from oxygen and nitrogen cylinders mixed by a proportioning device or, most commonly, by the use of motor-driven compressors. Air from cylinders is usually considered to be cleaner and of more exact composition than air from compressors, but is more expensive.

The vast majority of air piping systems employ two or more compressors, which are run alternately. Manifolded cylinders are frequently used as a standby source. Each compressor takes in ambient air and compresses it to above the working pressure. Each unit should be capable of meeting the average calculated demand. It must also be fitted with an automatic alternator and controls, so that the demand will be met even if the lead unit cannot maintain an adequate supply.

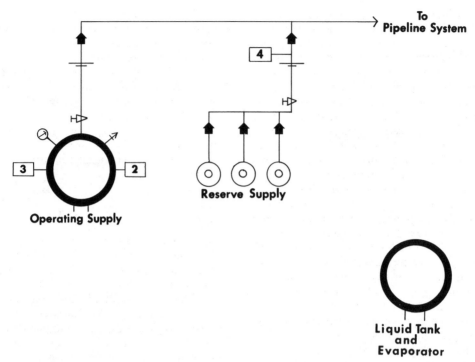

Figure 2.2. Liquid oxygen central supply system. *2*, liquid level alarm; *3*, contents indicator; *4* reserve-in-use alarm. The liquid tank is fitted with a pressure-relief device to prevent internal gas pressure from exceeding the safety point to which the vessel has been tested. The reserve supply could also be a liquid oxygen tank. If the check valves on the reserve supply are omitted, the reserve supply must be equipped with an alarm that signals when the reserve drops to one day's supply. The operating supply could include both primary and secondary liquid supplies, in which case an alarm should signal when a changeover from one portion of the operating supply to another has occurred. The reserve-in-use alarm warns that the reserve supply has been activated. It is activated when the pressure in the main supply line falls below 85 psig (586 kPa). (From *Standard for Nonflammable Medical Gas Systems.* NFPA 56F, 1970, p. 10.)

Each compressor incorporates one or more accumulators (reservoir tanks, storage receivers, reservoirs). These are tanks filled by the compressor from which air can be withdrawn as required. A receiver serves to buffer and even out the pressure peaks from the compressor and deliver a non-pulsatile air stream to the regulator. It also serves to reduce wear on the compressor.

The location of the compressor intake is important in ensuring that the air will be as free of contaminants as possible. It should be located outside the hospital at such a location as to suck in the cleanest possible air, free of dirt, fumes, and odors. Otherwise the piped air may contain significant amounts of substances such as carbon monoxide (35). The intake should be protected by a coarse mesh screen.

One or more filters should be installed be-tween the intake and the compressor to remove particulate matter. Devices to remove odors and oil are also installed downstream of the compressor but upstream of the final pressure control equipment, since most compressors are oil-lubricated and oil mist contamination can be a problem (36). Filters are also used, usually downstream of the dryer, to remove particulate contamination from the piping or compressor and/or fines from a dessicant dryer. Further purification of the air may be performed by devices that remove gaseous contaminants such as hydrocarbon vapors, carbon monoxide, nitrogen dioxide, etc. (37).

To render air suitable for medical use, its water content must be reduced. Atmospheric air contains variable amounts of water vapor and always more than is acceptable for medical air. After compression and subsequent cooling, the air stream is always saturated with water vapor. As it passes through the regulator and piping system it expands and cools. With cooling the moisture in the air condenses, leaving water in the piping system. This may damage surgical tools and some ventilators and can condense in low-lying parts of the piping system. Usually an aftercooler in which the air is cooled and the condensed moisture removed is installed downstream of each compressor. In addition, water may be removed by running the air through a drying chemical (29).

It should be noted that although medical air is usually very clean, it is not sterile. Some manufacturers of tools and some surgeons and other users specify that the air must be sterile at the point of delivery to the tool or apparatus. Some manufacturers advise that terminal point filters be used, and, in many instances, incorporate filters in their apparatus. Pre-sterilized disposable filters may be placed between the station outlet and the apparatus (29).

Nitrogen

Nitrogen piping systems have been installed in a number of hospitals to power certain tools and to mix with oxygen to provide artifical air. Central nitrogen supplies are covered by NFPA 56F (8). They usually consist of manifolded high-pressure cylinders. Liquid storage is also sometimes used.

Carbon Dioxide

Carbon dioxide is sometimes piped for use as an insufflating gas. The source consists of high-pressure cylinders and is covered by NFPA 56F (8).

ALARMS AND SAFETY DEVICES

Shutoff (isolating, isolator) and check (one-way) valves are important safety features of a central supply system. A manually operated shutoff valve is recommended upstream of each pressure regulator and a shutoff valve or check valve downstream.

Alarms are an important safety feature of the central supply system. NFPA standards require that they be designed to signal when a change-over from one portion of the operating supply to another portion has occurred, when the operating supply contents have dropped to a specified amount, or when the reserve supply goes into operation. Under certain circumstances, an alarm to indicate when the reserve supply is reduced to a specified amount is required. Alarms must also be installed in the nitrous oxide system to warn of malfunctions in thermal pressure control, and in the air system to warn of malfunction of one of the compressors or dryers, a rise in the moisture content of dried air above the permitted maximum, or problems with the proportioning system.

The locations of the alarm signal panels is of utmost importance. They should be located so as to ensure continuous visibility to responsible persons. There must be at least two master panels in separate locations. One should be in the office or principal working area of the individual responsible for the maintenance of the piping system. Another should be located where continuous responsible surveillance can be maintained, such as the telephone switchboard or security office.

Each alarm should be appropriately labeled for the gas and function it monitors. Alarm signals should be audible and visible and should continue until the fault has been remedied. Security measures should be taken to prevent accidental turning off of an alarm by someone unfamiliar with its purpose. Each alarm panel should contain a test mechanism to check the function of the alarm without interfering with its function and arrangements should be made to test the alarm periodically (see "Maintenance"). Alarms should be designed to function during power failures.

Sounding of the alarms should activate an organized, well-rehearsed series of events within the hospital. Clear, concise instructions should be given to the persons monitoring the alarms to ensure that they will take the proper action should an emergency arise. Cases have been reported where a hospital employee did not know what activation of an alarm signal meant (21).

The action to be taken in response to an alarm will depend upon the individual arrangements for each hospital and should be recorded in a procedure manual. This should be reviewed periodically and new employees given clear instructions regarding action to be taken when a signal is activated.

Pipeline Distribution System

PIPING

Recommendations for piping networks are covered in NFPA 56F (8) and 56A (7) and CGA

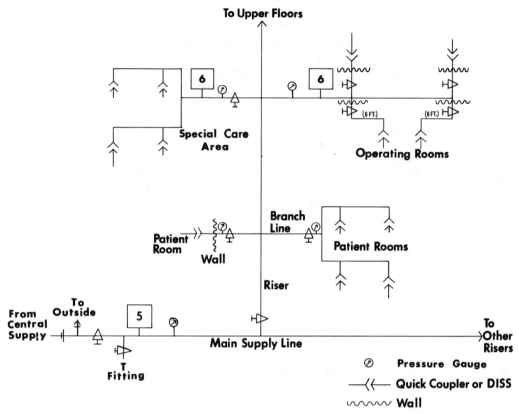

Figure 2.3. Pipeline network. *5,* main supply emergency alarm; *6,* area alarm system (local emergency alarm). The special "T" fitting downstream of the main supply line shutoff valve will allow connection of another supply in the event of damage to the usual central supply. The pressure relief valve in the main supply line is set at 50% above normal distribution pressure and is installed downstream from the regulator and upstream of the shutoff valve. The main supply line emergency alarm is activated by a 20% increase or decrease in line pressure. Special alarm systems should be installed in branch lines leading to intensive care units, recovery rooms, and operating rooms to monitor the pressure in the local supply line and signal if the pressure increases or decreases 20% from normal operating pressure. (Redrawn from *Standard for Nonflammable Medical Gas Systems.* NFPA 56F, 1970, p. 18.)

P-2.1 (38). Layouts of piping systems vary considerably. A typical one is shown in Figure 2.3. It consists of a main line, risers, and branch (lateral) lines. The main line comes from the central supply and runs on the same level. It connects the central source to the risers or branches or both. Risers are vertical pipes connecting the main line with the branch lines on various levels of the facility. Branch lines (laterals) are those portions of the piping system which serve a room or group of rooms on the same story of the facility.

Distribution pipes are made of copper or copper alloys. Identification of these pipes by labeling at frequent intervals (not more than 20 ft and at least once in every room and every story

traversed by the piping system) is important to ensure that those persons installing and maintaining a pipeline are fully aware of its gas content.

ALARMS AND SAFETY DEVICES

The main supply line must be equipped with a shutoff (stop) valve located near the entry of the gas source into the building. Its purpose is to allow the entire supply to the hospital to be shut off in case of emergency, routine maintenance, or modifications of the piping system. It should be installed outside the central supply area in a location well known and easily accessible to those responsible for maintenance of the piping system but where any attempt to tamper with it would be noticed.

Downstream of this valve it is desirable to place a valve with a T fitting, so that if the central supply is damaged or out of service for any reason, a temporary auxiliary supply can be connected at this point (5). Without such a T, restoration of flow to the pipeline can only be accomplished by "backfeeding" through terminal outlets, which is difficult, and a complete shutdown of the entire system may be necessary while repairs to the central system are made. On large sites, with many scattered buildings, it is sometimes considered necessary to provide standby oxygen manifold installations in each main block (6).

Each riser must be equipped with a shutoff (zone, on-off, isolating, section) valve adjacent to the riser connection. Each lateral branch line, except those supplying anesthetizing locations, is controlled by a shutoff valve located on the same story as the outlet stations it controls. The valve must be separated from these outlet stations by an intervening corridor wall. Anesthetizing locations are served with a lateral branch line fed directly from a riser with no intervening shutoff valve and a separate shutoff valve is required for each gas line entering an anesthetizing location. The valve is usually located just outside the room, but may be inside the room as long as it is at least 6 ft lateral to the station outlet.

These valves permit isolation of specific areas of the piping system in the event of a fire or other emergency and so that parts of the system can be isolated for maintenance or repair, periodic testing, or future expansions without the whole system having to be switched off. They should be located where they will be readily accessible in an emergency and unlikely to be obstructed by equipment. They should be housed in boxes or cabinets covered by easily breakable glass or an easily opened transparent door with a seal (Fig. 2.4). They should be clearly labeled in simple language with their function, the name of the gas controlled, and the area(s) affected by their operation. A line pressure gauge may be situated just downstream of the valve in the same box. This will facilitate testing the system for leaks. A pressure gauge must be provided downstream of each lateral branch line shutoff valve (8).

A pressure regulator is required in the main supply line, upstream of the main line shutoff valve (8). A second one is frequently installed to

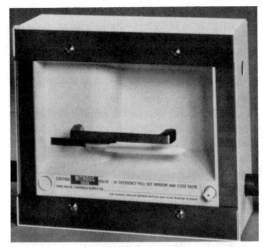

Figure 2.4. Wall mounted shutoff valve. The valve is mounted in a box with a clear plastic window to allow viewing. These valves should be readily accessible and labeled as to the gas and area they control. (Courtesy of Puritan-Bennett Corporation.)

provide reserve capability (30). With large piping systems, additional regulators may be located in the piping network to obtain a uniform pressure in the various areas. This permits use of smaller diameter pipes, since the gas can be piped at a higher distribution pressure. For example, the gas entering the hospital might be at 75 psig and each floor might have a regulator to reduce the pressure to 50 psig.

To provide for failure of a pressure regulator in the central supply, a pressure relief device set at 50% above normal line pressure is required downstream of the regulator(s), but upstream of the main line shutoff valve (8). The gas is vented outside the hospital. The valve should close automatically when the excessive pressure has been released.

All shutoff valves, regulators and relief valves should be permanently marked to indicate function and decrease the chance for operator error.

An alarm must be installed downstream of the main line shutoff valve to signal if the pressure in the main line increases or decreases 20% or more from the normal operating pressure. A rising pressure indicates a fault in the pressure regulator. A falling pressure may also indicate a regulator fault, but is more likely to be due to exhaustion of the central supply.

Special care areas such as the operating rooms, recovery rooms and intensive care units should each have a separate high/low area (local) alarm system and pressure gauges to monitor pressure in the local supply line. In anesthetizing locations the alarm will be upstream of the shutoff valves to the individual operating and delivery rooms. In other areas it will be downstream of the shutoff valve for the area. The area alarm signal panel should be located at the nurses' station or other suitable location where activation of the signal will be noticed immediately. Since alarms may monitor various functions at different points, it is important to properly label all alarms at each location.

Station Outlet (39) (Terminal Unit, Pipeline Outlet, Service Outlet, Terminal Outlet, Outlet Point, Outlet Station, Outlet Assembly)

The piping system terminates at the station outlet, which is connected permanently either to the fixed pipeline installation, or, in booms and hoses, to a distribution pressure hose. It is the first point at which the user normally makes connections and disconnections. Equipment may be connected to a station outlet either directly or by means of a flexible hose.

FEATURES

Face Plate

The face plate should be permanently labeled with the name and/or symbol of the gas it conveys. The identifying color may also be present. In some station outlets the face plate and primary valve are an integral unit.

Primary Valve (Automatic Shutoff Valve, Terminal Unit Valve, Self-Sealing Valve or Unit)

Each station outlet must contain a valve which opens and allows the gas to flow when the male probe is inserted and closes automatically when the connection is broken. This serves to prevent loss of gas when the nonfixed component is disconnected. This is sometimes called a check valve. However, it should be noted that this is *not* a unidirectional valve. It is not designed to prevent backflow once a connection is made to the outlet (40).

Secondary Valve Assembly (Shutoff Valve, Terminal Stop Valve, Maintenance Valve, Isolating Valve, Secondary Valve, Secondary Shutoff Valve)

The station outlet must incorporate a shutoff valve to permit repair or maintenance of other components of the station outlet without affecting the operation of other units. For hose booms and pendants incorporating hoses, this valve should be fitted at or near the end of the permanent pipework to permit maintenance of hoses as well as other components.

The secondary valve assembly is designed so that when the primary valve assembly is removed (e.g., for cleaning or seal replacement) the secondary valve assembly automatically closes to seal the remaining portion of the outlet station and prevent gas discharge.

Seals or O-rings are utilized between the secondary and primary valve assemblies to provide a gas-tight fit. Degradation of these seals or O-rings due to age results in leaky outlet stations, necessitating seal or O-ring replacement.

Generally the secondary valve assembly is factory-mounted to the outlet station box. This forms an integral unit which is mounted and connected to the gas system. The primary valve assembly and face plate (these may be integral) are installed to complete assembly of the outlet station. The primary and secondary valve assembly may be screwed together or held together by a separate flanged connection.

Retaining Device (Locking Device)

This is a device to hold the male and female connections securely together and guard against accidental ejection. A second locking device may be incorporated if it is anticipated that heavy equipment may be connected to the outlet.

Noninterchangeable Connection

Each station outlet must incorporate the fixed female component of a noninterchangeable connection, either a Diameter Index Safety System Connection or a quick coupler. The corresponding male component of the noninterchangeable connection is attached directly to the equipment to be used or to a flexible hose leading to the equipment.

The Diameter Index Safety System (41). The Diameter Index Safety System (DISS) was developed to provide threaded noninterchangeable connections for medical gas lines at pressures of 200 psig (1400 kPa) or less.

As shown in Figure 2.5, each DISS connection in the 1000 series consists of a body, nipple, and nut combination. The Safety System is based

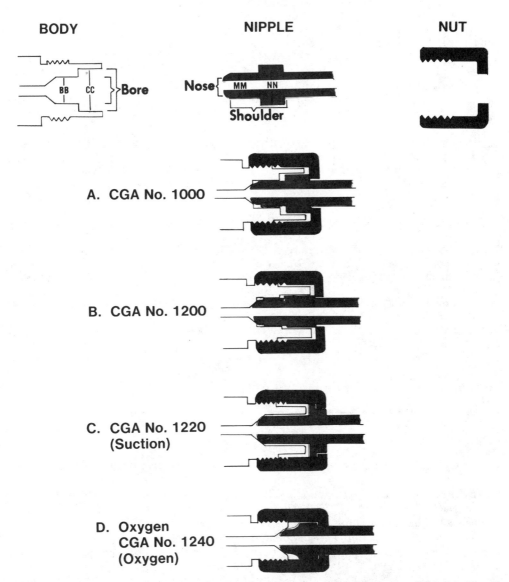

BODY   **NIPPLE**   **NUT**

Bore

Nose { MM   NN }

Shoulder

A. CGA No. 1000

B. CGA No. 1200

C. CGA No. 1220
   (Suction)

D. Oxygen
   CGA No. 1240
   (Oxygen)

Figure 2.5. Diameter Index Safety System (1000 Series). With increasing CGA number, the small shoulder of the nipple becomes larger and the large diameter smaller. Noninterchangeability of connections is assured, since either *MM* will be too large for *BB* or *NN* will be too large for *CC* if assembly of a nonmating body and nipple is attempted. (Redrawn courtesy of Compressed Gas Association.)

on having two concentric and specific bores in the body and two concentric and specific shoulders on the nipple. The small bore (BB) mates with the small shoulder (MM) and the large bore (CC) mates with the large shoulder (NN). The connection on the nut and body has 16 threads per inch and is ¾ inches in diameter.

To achieve noninterchangeability between different connections, the two diameters on each part vary in opposite directions, so that as one diameter increases, the other decreases. Table 2.1 gives the connection numbers and specifications for the diameters of the bores and shoulders. As shown in the table, with increasing connection number the small diameter becomes larger and the large diameter smaller. Connections not designed to mate will not fit together since either BB will be too small for MM or CC will be too small for NN.

Exceptions to these rules are made for oxygen

Table 2.1.
The Diameter Index Safety System

Gas	Connection No.	Small Bore (BB)	Large Bore (CC)	Small Shoulder (MM)	Large Shoulder (NN)
		inches	*inches*	*inches*	*inches*
Special mixture for limited experimental applications	1020, 1020A	0.299–0.302	0.539–0.542	0.296–0.293	0.536–0.533
Nitrous oxide	1040, 1040A	0.311–0.314	0.527–0.530	0.308–0.305	0.524–0.521
Helium, helium-oxygen ($O_2 < 19.5\%$)	1060, 1060A	0.323–0.326	0.515–0.518	0.320–0.317	0.512–0.509
Carbon dioxide, carbon dioxide-oxygen ($CO_2 > 7.5\%$)	1080, 1080A	0.335–0.338	0.503–0.506	0.332–0.329	0.550–0.497
Cyclopropane	1100, 1100A	0.347–0.350	0.491–0.494	0.344–0.341	0.488–0.485
Nitrogen	1120, 1120A	0.359–0.362	0.479–0.482	0.356–0.353	0.476–0.473
Ethylene	1140, 1140A	0.371–0.374	0.467–0.470	0.368–0.365	0.464–0.461
Air	1160, 1160A	0.383–0.386	0.455–0.458	0.380–0.377	0.452–0.449
Oxygen-helium (He ≤ 80.5%)	1180, 1180A	0.395–0.398	0.443–0.446	0.392–0.389	0.440–0.437
Oxygen-carbon dioxide ($CO_2 \le 7.5\%$)	1200, 1200A	0.407–0.410	0.431–0.434	0.404–0.401	0.428–0.425
Suction (vacuum)	1220	0.419–0.422	0.419–0.422	0.416–0.413	0.416–0.413
Oxygen	1240	—*	—*	—*	—*
		millimeters	*millimeters*	*millimeters*	*millimeters*
Nitrous oxide-oxygen mixtures (N_2O 47.5–52.5%)	1570	10.4–10.5	11.2–11.3	10.3–10.2	11.1–11.0

* Connection for oxygen does not conform to usual pattern (see text)

and suction. In the suction connection (Fig. 2.5C) BB = CC and MM = NN, forming single mating diameters for the body and nipple. The nipple of the suction connection has the largest nose diameter. This feature allows an extra large bore for better suction performance. For mechanical reasons it was necessary to make the suction nut ⅛ inch longer than the nuts used with other connections. In addition, the hole in the nut was enlarged to accommodate the larger diameter nipple.

Because of long-established use, oxygen (Fig. 2.5D) retains a ⁹/₁₆-inch, 18-thread connection on the body and nut. The oxygen nipple has a tapered nose and a single shoulder, in contrast to those for other gases.

In addition to the 1000 series, a series of connections named the 1000-A series was adopted in 1978. The purpose of this was to provide co-standards for the existing connections which are heavier so as to better support equipment which is sometimes connected by this means. The bodies in this new series are identical to those of the 1000 series, but the shoulder of the nipple has an increased shank diameter

and length (similar to the 1220 suction connection) and the suction nut is used for all connections except oxygen. Nuts and nipples of both the 1000 and 1000-A series will fit the same bodies.

There is an additional new series, the 1500 series, which provides eight new DISS connections. The 1500 series is similar in design to the 1000 and 1000-A series, but the dimensions are metric. The step arrangement is similar to that used with the 1000 and 1000-A series, but with slightly greater differences between the large and small diameters. Another difference from the 1000 and 1000-A series is that the nut on the 1500 series has a larger thread diameter so it will slip over the body thread on the 1000 and 1000-A series. Also the hole in the nut is enlarged so that a 1000 or 1000-A series nipple will fall through the nut. Thus nuts and nipples of the 1500 series cannot be used with the 1000 and 1000-A series bodies. As shown in Table 2.1, only one of the series 1500 connections has been assigned to date. A check valve may be added to the body portion of the connection (41).

Quick Couplers (Quick Connects). Because gases are frequently needed without delay, quick couplers have become popular. A quick coupler should allow the desired apparatus (hose, flowmeter, etc.) to be connected or disconnected from the station outlet by means of a single one-step motion using one hand.

Each quick coupler consists of male and female components which are noninterchangeable between gases. The male member is commonly called a plug, striker, probe, or jack. The female component is often called a socket. Insertion into an incorrect outlet is prevented by indexing—the use of different shapes for mating portions, different spacing of mating portions, or some combination of these (39).

LOCATION (6)

In general, station outlets should be placed in positions which will give the shortest routes for flexible hoses connecting them to apparatus. These routes should obstruct the movement of staff and equipment as little as possible. Hoses on the floor should be avoided because of the danger of tripping, the added wear and tear on the hose, the difficulty of keeping such hoses clean and the difficulty of maneuvering around them.

When a new operating room is being planned, it should be determined what the position of the operating room table will be most of the time and station outlets should be placed near the expected position of the head of the table and in line with it. An exception should be made for rooms to be used primarily for procedures on the eye, bronchoscopies, or craniotomies, in which the anesthesia machine is frequently at the side of the table.

In situations where it is undesirable or impossible to set up for all surgical procedures without changing the position of the operating table and anesthesia machine, a degree of flexibility can be obtained by installing two sets of station outlets on opposite sides of the room, by using a boom, or by installing columns or hoses on tracks (Figure 2.6) so they can be moved. If the position of the operating table is optional, and the room has a non-recirculating air conditioning system, consideration should be given to placing the station outlets near the outlet for the air conditioning system so that scavenging can be performed utilizing the air conditioning system. If an overhead location is chosen, it should be established that the station outlet will not interfere with movement of the operating

room light(s) under normal operating conditions.

In the recovery room station outlets should be placed to the side of the patient's head to facilitate access and minimize the chances of equipment falling on a patient.

The station outlet may be incorporated in a number of different devices in the operating room and recovery room. All have advantages and disadvantages.

Wall Outlets

These are mechanically simple, but have the disadvantage that the hoses to the machine frequently must be of considerable length and draped across the floor. It is strongly advised that at least two sets of wall outlets be placed in each room. It may be advantageous to mount a rail similar to a towel rack on the wall about 6 inches above floor level. The hoses can then be threaded behind the rail to bring them down to floor level.

Wall- or Ceiling-Mounted Swinging Boom (42)

An overhead boom carrying hoses terminating in the station outlets is mechanically simple, relatively cheap, and avoids cluttering the floor with hoses. When mounted on a side wall, it can serve an anesthesia machine at either end or one side of the table. In the event that some unusual placement of the operating table becomes necessary, the hoses can be temporarily unhooked from the boom. An effort should be made to keep the boom from passing over layouts of sterile equipment. Unfortunately, the outlets on a boom may be too high for small people to reach while tall people may hit their heads on the boom.

Rigid Column (43)

Columns mounted on the ceiling (Fig. 2.6) can provide connections for electrical outlets and monitoring channels as well as station outlets. This allows the majority of tubes and wires to approach the patient from one area, allowing greater mobility around the operating room table. They can be made movable by mounting them on overhead tracks. They can also be made retractable so that the column can be lower at the start of the case for attachment of the lines and then raised to keep it out of the way of tall people.

Disadvantages include the problem of people

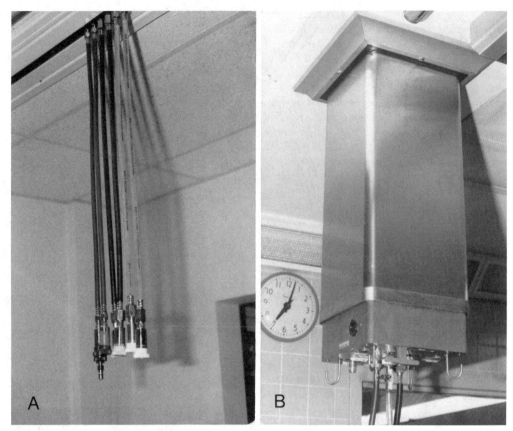

Figure 2.6. *A,* hoses are on tracks so that they can be moved from one end to the other. *B,* the rigid column can be made retractable and can be put on a track.

hitting their heads and the fact that the hoses inside the column are not easily checked for leaks.

Hoses (44)

A hose attached to the ceiling with the station outlet at its free end (Fig. 2.6) is simple, cheap, and less of a danger to heads than a rigid column. Its height should be low enough that short people will be able to make connections easily. Retractable hoses or hose reels are desirable in this respect. Since the hoses are out of reach, inspecting them for leaks is somewhat difficult. Hoses can be put on tracks but care must be taken when they are moved not to get dust on the sterile operating field.

THE NITROGEN PIPING STATION OUTLET

Since the pressure required for nitrogen-driven tools varies, a means of adjusting the pressure at the station outlet is necessary. An adjustable regulator of the type described in Chapter 3 is most often used. Two gauges are present in the station outlet, one indicating distribution pressure and the other reduced pressure. The regulator and gauges are incorporated into the wall (Fig. 2.7). The station outlet may be in the wall with the regulator and gauges or may be located on a hose or column.

Hoses (25, 28) (Droplines, Hose Assemblies, Low-Pressure Connecting Assemblies, Flexible Hose Assemblies)

Hoses are used to connect anesthesia machines and other apparatus to the fixed station outlet. Each end should have a permanently attached, noninterchangeable connector. The authors of this book recommended that the outlet connector (at the end of the hose which will be attached to the anesthesia machine) be DISS while the connectors at the end designed to connect to the station outlet be quick couplers.

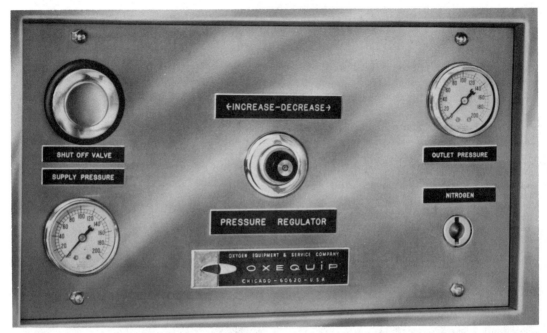

Figure 2.7. Termination of nitrogen piping system. Two gauges are present, one showing pipeline and one reduced pressure. The pressure regulator at the center varies the outlet pressure. A shutoff valve is in the upper left corner and the outlet for nitrogen is in the lower right corner. (Courtesy of Oxequip Company.)

This will encourage making connections and disconnections at the station outlet rather than the back of the machine, so that if there is a leak in the hose it will not leak when the apparatus is disconnected. If the hose is designed to go from the station outlet to a yoke block (see Chapter 3), the hose must be equipped with a backflow check valve to prevent flow of gas from the anesthesia machine into the hose and pipeline system or to air if the hose is not connected to the station outlet (7).

Having the name and/or chemical symbol of the contained gas on each connector is desirable. Color coding of the hose is also desirable. The hose should be resistant to occlusion by external forces under normal conditions of use. It must be conductive if used in an institution where flammable anesthetic agents are administered.

When an anesthesia machine is moved and a hose must be disconnected, it is recommended that this be done quickly and preferably without opening the valve of a cylinder on the machine since the cylinder may become depleted if the valve is not closed after the hose is reconnected. However, if it is necessary that the hose be disconnected for more than a few seconds, a cylinder should be opened and then closed as soon as the hose is reconnected.

The use of several extension hoses is undesirable. It is better to use one long hose, since resistance due to multiple connections may interfere with flow. Also since most leaks in hoses occur in the connectors or where the connector fits into the hose, one long hose is less likely to leak.

Hoses should be kept in good repair. They should be checked regularly for leaks, at least yearly. The hose should approach the anesthesia machine at a normal curve, especially when it comes from above. Acute angulations or full stretch should be avoided. Hoses should be connected securely so that the connection maintains its integrity when a force is applied to the hose.

TESTING AFTER INSTALLATION (6, 8, 23, 45–49)

Since problems with medical gas systems are most likely to occur with a new system or one that has been recently repaired or modified it is essential that such a system be thoroughly tested before being put into use. Testing should be repeated after any alterations are made to an existing system. Permanent records of tests should be maintained.

Responsibility for Testing

A major problem with hospital pipeline systems is that no formal system of inspection exists to assure that hospitals and gas suppliers comply with NFPA regulations.

Confusion concerning installation and testing of a medical gas system is compounded by a number of factors. There are usually a large number of people employed by different companies involved. Passage of time may require transfer of responsibility and information between a succession of individuals, each of whom is primarily concerned with his own area of involvement and less with whether the work before him has been performed according to specifications. Thus many workers at various stages of the enterprise only know what they themselves are to do and do not ask who is responsible for the rest or whether it was done properly.

There has been controversy over who should carry out the final (commissioning) tests. Responsibility for testing is usually poorly defined in building specifications (50). NFPA 56F states that the authority responsible for the facility will assure that the tests required by the NFPA will be successfully completed. The Canadian Standard (24) requires that the preoperational tests be made by a testing agency experienced in the field, independent of the contractor, gas and equipment suppliers, and the owner. It also requires that a member of the hospital staff and a representative of the installer be present to witness testing.

While he is not the person primarily responsible for testing the piping system, the anesthesiologist has an obligation to ensure that the piping system is properly designed and functions correctly. He should be encouraged to witness the tests performed, especially those for cross connections.

Testing Procedures (39)

TESTS OF ENTIRE SYSTEM

NFPA 56F calls for three levels of testing: pressure testing, cross-connection testing and final testing—purging and analyzing.

Pressure Testing

This should be performed to detect leaks and to make sure the piping system can withstand the designated working pressure.

Included are both an inspection of each joint in the entire system for leaks and a 24-hr standing pressure test with oil-free air or nitrogen at one and one-half times the maximum working pressure (but not less than 150 psig (1034 kPa)). These are performed before attachment of components such as alarms, pressure gauges, pressure-relief devices and completed station outlets. If any reductions in pressure (other than those due to changes in temperature) occur, the leaks must be located and eliminated.

The completed system with all components should then be subjected to a 24-hr standing pressure test at 20% above the normal operating line pressure. This permits testing without damaging system components or activating pressure-relief devices.

NFPA regulations require each segment of pipeline to be checked for pressure differentials indicating the presence of debris (21).

Testing for Cross-Connections
(Anti-Confusion Test, Continuity Test)

This is to determine that no cross-connection exists between piping systems for two gases.

One gas system is tested at a time. The first step is to turn off each gas (at the main supply line shutoff valve) except the one serving the pipeline to be checked. The pressure in all the piping systems is then reduced to atmospheric. The pipeline being tested is then filled with oil-free air or nitrogen at working pressure and each station outlet is tested to ensure that gas emerges only from the station outlets of the system under investigation. Each gas system should be tested in turn.

Purging

Purging is performed to remove test gases and reduce particulate and gaseous contamination. The proper gas should be connected to each respective system and the systems purged, starting with the outlets closest to the supply source. Satisfactory reduction of contamination by purging may require several days (47, 49).

Analyzing

After purging, each outlet should be checked with an appropriate analyzer for the specific content of the gas emerging from it.

Testing for particulate and gaseous impurities within a medical gas system is not easy. Work is proceeding on suitable devices to measure particulate contamination (45). In the past this has been done by such unsophisticated methods as holding a white cloth close to an outlet and looking for discoloration. Filters have been used on station outlets to detect particulate contamination (51). Smelling has been used, since gaseous contamination may cause odors. Recently used methods include mass spectroscopy (45, 47, 49), ultraviolet spectroscopy (49), and gas chromatography (45, 49). Gas supplied by the most remote terminal units in the system should be compared with gas obtained from the central source to make certain that the system is not adding impurities to the gas (6).

Standards exist for the maximum allowable concentration of contaminants such as carbon monoxide, carbon dioxide, water vapor, total volatile hydrocarbons, and a long list of halogenated hydrocarbons. If any contaminant is found to be above the limit the first attempted solution should be a purging program. If that fails, extensive troubleshooting may be necessary.

TESTS OF INDIVIDUAL COMPONENTS

In addition to the above tests, certain other tests are suggested by other national standards and the authors of this text.

Shutoff Valves

Shutoff valves should be checked for leakage to make certain that they control only those terminal units for which they are intended, and that they are properly labeled for the gas and zone controlled. The test for tightness is performed by closing the valve, releasing the pressure downstream, and monitoring this pressure for 30 min. If the pressure rises, the valve is not tight.

Station Outlets

Each station outlet should be checked for satisfactory mechanical operation by inserting appropriate equipment and checking that it locks into position and releases properly. It should be checked for proper labeling and to ensure that it accommodates only connections for the particular gas for which it was designed.

The pressure and flow rate at each terminal unit should be checked to ensure that the required flow can be delivered and there are no pressure differentials in the piping system. In the operating rooms, the oxygen outlet should be capable of delivering a minimum of 35 liters/min and nitrous oxide at least 10 liters/min.

Alarms

All alarms should be tested at the time of installation to make sure they function properly.

Pressure Relief Device Operation

Pressure relief devices should be tested to ensure that they discharge at the correct pressure and reseat when the excess pressure is released.

Central Supply

The central supply should be checked to ensure that the changeover devices, motor starters, and reserve supply function normally.

MAINTENANCE (23, 52)

The continued satisfactory performance of a piped medical gas system is dependent upon a routine maintenance program. Therefore inspection and testing of piping systems should be performed on a regular basis and the results recorded in a permanent log.

The installers of a piping system should be required to provide complete "as fitted" drawings, circuit diagrams, valve charts, and maintenance instructions, to be used as the foundation for the preventive maintenance program. These should be kept readily at hand in the offices of the department responsible for maintenance of the system.

It is recommended that pipeline pressure gauges be included on all new anesthesia machines that are purchased and that the pipeline pressures be checked before administration of anesthesia is begun. If the machines do not have pipeline pressure gauges, the pressure of the gases piped to the operating room should be checked on the area pressure gauge.

Alarms in the operating rooms and other critical care areas should be tested at least monthly by the use of test buttons and the results recorded in a permanent log.

At least annually, all hoses and station outlets in the operating room and recovery rooms should be checked for wear and damage and their performance checked. In addition the shutoff valves should be tested for tightness and the pipeline components downstream of the valve for leakage. This testing should be performed in conjunction with the hospital engineering department when no surgical procedures are in progress. To perform this test the valves on the cylinders of the anesthesia machines are closed, the zone valves outside each operating room are closed and gas released until the pipeline pressure gauges read 40 psig. This pressure is then monitored for 4 hr. It should remain at 40 psig. If the pressure rises, the shutoff valve is not working properly. If the pressure falls, there is a leak either in the pipe to the room, the station outlet or the hose to the anesthesia machine. (*Note:* This will not detect leakage in the primary valve in the station outlet. It is essential that the zone valves be reopened after this test has been performed.)

PROBLEMS (21, 30, 45, 51)

Problems in piping systems are due in large part to lack of awareness among hospital personnel, who have been lulled into believing that the piping system cannot fail and are not sufficiently familiar with the design, operation, and maintenance of a piping system to make emergency adjustments safely. Lack of proper communication between clinical and maintenance departments and commercial suppliers may also be a contributing factor (30). Finally, lack of adherence to existing codes is responsible for many hazards.

Inadequate Pressure

This is the most frequently reported malfunction (30). Loss of pressure may result in a flow rate insufficient to power a ventilator but sufficient to maintain adequate flow to the anesthesia machine.

CAUSES

Causes of inadequate pressure are numerous and include fires (45); vehicular accidents; theft of nitrous oxide tanks (21, 53); damage during construction (21); environmental forces (earthquakes, excessive cold, tornadoes (54), lightning (30)); human error (closure of central supply control valve (21), closure of a shutoff valve (4, 55–60), inappropriate adjustment of the main line pressure regulator (30)); and equipment failures (leaks, activation of the shutoff valve (60), regulator malfunction (61), problems with automatic switching gear (55), obstruction of the pipeline, frequently by debris left following installation (21), depletion of the supply with failure of the alarm mechanism, failure of a quick coupler to fit into a station outlet (62), quick couplers that appear connected but with no gas flowing (51, 58, 63–65), plugging of a connector with debris (66), detachment of a terminal unit (45), and kinking (67) or a break (68) in a hose). Deliberate tampering with a system is a possibility that cannot be overlooked.

EMERGENCY PLAN (30)

Because this is the most frequent dysfunction of a piping system and because the consequences can be so severe, each hospital should have a plan to deal with the sudden loss of piped gases, especially air or oxygen. The best alarm system is useless unless appropriate action is taken when it sounds an alarm.

Everyone directly involved in the patient support effort should be thoroughly familiar with what action is to be taken and these procedures should be included as part of the institution's disaster plan (30). Locations of shutoff valves should be known by the hospital staff, so that if the loss of pressure is due to a large leak in one area, the pipeline to that area can be isolated to prevent further loss of gas.

The organization of an effective response to the loss of a piped gas supply must include reliable communication pathways and individual responsibilities that take into account practical circumstances. The details of such a plan must be discussed and rehearsed in advance in the form of mock disaster drills if an effective response is to be expected during a real emergency.

The person discovering a fault in the piped air or oxygen supply should immediately inform the telephone operator who, in turn, should inform the maintenance department, respiratory therapy, the operating room, recovery room, obstetrics, the emergency room, special care units such as intensive care and nursery, the nursing supervisor, and the hospital administrator. If only the nitrous oxide supply is affected, only areas which use nitrous oxide plus the maintenance department need be alerted. Each department in turn should have carefully established procedures to deal with the emergency. These should be reviewed regularly, revised as necessary, and put in staff procedures manuals.

Since every anesthesia machine should have at least one emergency oxygen cylinder, there should be no acute threat to life in the operating rooms and immediate attention should be focused on the recovery room. It may be advantageous to move the anesthesia machines not in use into the recovery room to supply oxygen until other sources can be obtained. Alternately, patients in the recovery room can be wheeled back into the operating rooms. For patients on ventilators it will be necessary to use manual ventilation (using the breathing system in the operating room or a manual resuscitation bag in the recovery room). Attempts to use lower flows should be made.

The need for additional oxygen for the operating rooms and recovery room should be assessed, and elective surgery postponed until adequate supplies can be assured. Efforts should be coordinated with other departments, especially respiratory therapy, to determine the needs and the supplies on hand and with the maintenance department to determine how long the loss of piped gas will last.

EMERGENCY AUXILIARY SUPPLY

Because of the dangers associated with low pressures in piped oxygen and air systems, special areas such as intensive care units, recovery rooms, emergency rooms, etc., may have added an auxiliary oxygen and/or air supply (4). The areas selected must be capable of being isolated by means of a shutoff valve. When an emergency arises, the shutoff valve is turned off and the auxiliary source is connected to an outlet within the zone or by means of a specially installed "T". All outlets within the area can then operate from the auxiliary source.

Excessive Pressure (61)

This is also a relatively common problem (21). As shown in Figure 2.3, a pressure relief valve is required in the main supply line and this should offer some protection from excessive pressure, but this can be set improperly or can malfunction (46). Few anesthesia machines or ventilators have mechanisms to prevent damage from high pressures.

High pressures can result in damage to equipment, especially regulators (47, 61) and may cause barotrauma to patients. If the nitrous oxide flow were increased due to a higher pipeline pressure, a hypoxic mixture could be delivered to the breathing system (69). Some ventilators will not operate properly if the line pressure is too high.

The most common cause of high pressure is failure of the regulator. Nitrous oxide regulators may freeze due to cooling associated with the reduction in pressure (21). In humid atmospheres ice may form on the vaporizers in a liquid oxygen system. This will hamper heat transfer and may result in liquid oxygen passing into the

piping system with resultant damage to the regulator. This has also been reported after the addition of liquid oxygen to the main tank (47).

Other causes of high pressure include combustion of foreign material in a pipeline (21, 61) and deliberately increasing the pressure setting of the mainline regulator in an attempt to compensate for low pressure from the central system (61).

Whenever excessive pipeline pressure occurs it is best to disconnect the pipeline hoses and use cylinder gases until the problem is corrected.

Alarm Dysfunction

Failure or absence of an alarm is not uncommon (21, 70). The reserve alarm is frequently disconnected by the person who fills the liquid tanks because it annoys him and it may not be reconnected (56). An equally serious problem is that the alarm signal goes off but either the person who hears it does not know the proper course of action or fails to follow it (21, 30, 56).

False alarms are also a common problem. They may result from calibration drift in line pressure sensors (30). Repeated false alarms can cause complacency among personnel, which may have serious consequences if a real emergency occurs.

It is important that preventive maintenance be done on alarms and that they be tested periodically. When there is a personnel change in the hospital engineering department or departments where the alarm panels are placed, it is important that the new people be adequately instructed.

Crossover of Gases

The consequences of this are most grave and extremely costly. Most crossovers have occurred between nitrous oxide and oxygen, since they are the gases most frequently piped, but other combinations of crossed gases have been reported. Unfortunately, pipeline alarms indicate only pressure faults and give no signal if an incorrect agent is present.

Problems with cross-connection can be categorized according to the site at which the defect occurs.

CENTRAL SUPPLY

Cases have been reported in which oxygen tanks were filled with nitrogen (21, 70).

DISTRIBUTION SYSTEM

At least nine deaths may have been caused by a mixup in lines to the emergency room in a Canadian hospital and five deaths by a similar mixup at a hospital near Philadelphia. Several other cases have been reported (21, 71). One case has been reported where a fistula was created between air and nitrous oxide pipes during construction (49).

Flooding of an oxygen line with nitrogen has occurred when nitrogen was used to test for leaks after making repairs or extensions to an existing system and the shutoff valve to that area permitted backleak (45, 51, 55, 65). It is recommended that the section being modified be physically isolated from the sections in use.

STATION OUTLETS

One study showed that three wrong outlet panels were installed in a newly constructed hospital (49). A case has been reported where the female quick connectors for nitrous oxide and carbon dioxide located on the same station outlet were both able to receive a male nitrous oxide connector (72). In another case it was found that air plugs could be fitted into nitrous oxide and oxygen outlets (73). A case has been reported here in which the cover plates on station outlets could be installed incorrectly (74).

HOSES

Several cases have been reported where the wrong connector was put on one or more hoses (21, 75–77). Most of these cases have involved repairs to hoses performed by personnel in the hospital. Whenever a hose is altered or repaired, it should be checked carefully before it is put into service to make certain that the proper connectors are in each end. With extension hoses, this is easily performed by inserting one end of the hose into the other. The connections should fit as intended without undue force.

PERIPHERAL DEVICES

A case has been reported in which a defective check valve in a ventilator allowed oxygen to flow into the air pipeline (40).

A number of methods for detecting crossovers have been devised (51, 78–81). None are entirely satisfactory. Because the consequences are usually most severe when the crossover results in hypoxia, the authors of this text feel that a reliable oxygen analyzer should be included as a component of every anesthesia breathing system.

Contamination of Gases

PARTICULATE CONTAMINATION
(47, 51, 56)

Particulate contamination can be a serious problem, particularly when a new pipeline system is opened. Metallic and carbonaceous contaminants may be trapped inside and when gas is blown into the system these will be present in the gas coming from the station outlets. These particles can damage equipment, especially ventilators, and may be harmful to a patient if inhaled in large quantities.

During installation every effort should be made to keep the pipes, fittings, and valves as clean as possible. The majority of particles can be removed by purging and this may require several days (47), but it is doubtful whether particulate purging can ever be complete, especially in tall buildings (51).

GASEOUS CONTAMINATION

Inhalation of volatile hydrocarbons can be unpleasant and is potentially toxic (47, 82). Volatile hydrocarbons in the piped gas supplies may be due to materials left in the pipes during construction (49, 83), although the use of organic solvents to clean fittings and other components is prohibited. Contamination of the inlet of the hospital's air compressors is another source of contamination and one case has been reported in which a piped air system became contaminated when a filter was soaked in cleaning fluid and replaced without allowing it to dry (82). When gaseous contamination occurs, several days' purging may be necessary to lower the concentration to an acceptable level and it may be necessary to replace certain highly contaminated components (49).

BACTERIAL CONTAMINATION

Piped medical gases are not sterile and bacterial contamination has been documented (84–87). That this does not appear to be an important source of postoperative respiratory infections is indicated by recent studies (88, 89). An in-line filter has been demonstrated to be efficient in sterilization of gases (86). A case of hypoxia caused by cracks in such a filter in the oxygen line leading to a bubble oxygenator has been reported (87).

Fires (45)

Oxygen and, to a lesser extent, nitrous oxide pose the hazard of exacerbating any fire. Shutoff valves should be strategically located to allow isolation of the gas supply should a fire occur. Unfortunately, these are not always clearly labeled nor are their positions always known to the hospital staff.

Leaks

Leaks are also a common problem (21). They may occur anywhere in the piping system from the central supply to the hose.

They are probably most common in hoses, especially in the connectors and where the connectors fit into the hose. Service outlets all have valves which can, and eventually will, leak.

Leaks are expensive to the hospital in terms of lost gases and potentially hazardous if oxidizing gases are allowed to accumulate in closed spaces. Leaks of nitrous oxide may pose a health hazard to hospital personnel (see Chapter 9).

Extensive pressure testing after installation is recommended in NFPA 56F and other national standards. In addition, it is recommended that the test for leaks described under maintenance be performed at least yearly.

Depletion of the Reserve Supply (30)

Depletion of the reserve supply due to failures of connections, pressure imbalances, and leaks has been reported.

References

1. Conely JIM, Railton R, MacKenzie AI: Ventilator problems caused by humidity in the air supplied from simple compressors. *Br J Anaesth* 53:549–550, 1981.
2. Garg OP, Pande SK, Shah SK, Jha BK, Gattani SK, Chary VN: Use of compressed air in a continuous flow anaesthetic machine. *Br J Anaesth* 49:71–73, 1977.
3. Rogers RM: Considerations in constructing a respiratory intensive care unit. *Chest* 62:2S–9S, 1972.
4. Gjerde GE: Retrograde pressurization of a medical oxygen pipeline system: safety backup or hazard? *Crit Care Med* 8:219–221, 1980.
5. Eichhorn JH: In Lisbon A (ed): *Medical Gas Delivery Systems: Anesthetic Considerations in Setting Up a New Medical Facility*. Boston, Little, Brown, 1981.
6. *Piped Medical Gases, Medical Compressed Air and Medical Vacuum Installations*. Hospital Technical Memorandum 22, Department of Health and Social Security, 49 High Holborn, London WCIV6HB, England, 1972.
7. *Standard for the Use of Inhalation Anesthetics*. NFPA 56A, National Fire Protection Association, Batterymarch Park, Quincy, Mass. 02269, 1973.
8. *Nonflammable Medical Gas Systems*. NFPA 56F, National Fire Protection Association, Batterymarch Park, Quincy, Mass. 02269, 1977.
9. *Bulk Oxygen Systems at Consumer Sites*. NFPA 50, National Fire Protection Association, Batterymarch Park, Quincy, Mass. 02269, 1979.
10. *Inhalation Anesthetics in Ambulatory Care Facilities*. NFPA 56G, National Fire Protection Association, Batterymarch Park, Quincy, Mass. 02269, 1980.
11. *Respiratory Therapy*. NFPA 56B, National Fire Protection Association, Batterymarch Park, Quincy, Mass. 02269, 1976.
12. *Oxygen*. CGA G-4, Compressed Gas Association, Inc., 500 Fifth Ave., New York, N.Y. 10036, 1972.
13. *Standard for the Installation of Nitrous Oxide Systems at Consumer Sites*. CGA 8.1, Compressed Gas Association, Inc., 500 Fifth Ave., New York, N.Y. 10036, 1964.
14. *Commodity Specification for Air*. CGA G-7.1, Compressed Gas Association, Inc., 500 Fifth Ave., New York, N.Y. 10036, 1973.
15. *Standard Cryogenic Liquid Transfer Connections*. CGA V-6, Compressed Gas Association, Inc., 500 Fifth Ave., New York, N.Y. 10036, 1978.
16. *Compressed Air for Human Respiration*. CGA G-7, Compressed Gas Association, Inc., 500 Fifth Ave., New York, N.Y. 10036, 1976.
17. *Safe Handling of Compressed Gases in Containers*. CGA P-1, Compressed Gas Association, Inc., 500 Fifth Ave., New York, N.Y. 10036, 1974.
18. *Home Use of Respiratory Therapy*. NFPA 56HM, National Fire Protection Association, Batterymarch Park, Quincy, Mass. 02269, 1976.
19. McCormick JM: National fire protection codes 1968. *Anesth Analg* 47:538–547, 1968.
20. Dornette WL: Anesthesiologists, hospitals, and the National Fire Protection Association. *Anesth Analg* 51:271–276, 1972.
21. Feeley TW, Hedley-Whyte J: Bulk oxygen and nitrous oxide delivery systems: design and dangers. *Anesthesiology* 44:301–305, 1976.
22. *Pressure Regulators, Gauges, and Flow Metering Devices for Medical Gas Systems*. CSA Z305.3-M1979, Canadian Standards Association, 178 Rexdale Blvd., Rexdale, Ontario, Canada, M9W 1R3, 1979.
23. *Non-Flammable Medical Gas Piping Systems*. CSA Z305.1-1975, Canadian Standards Association, 178 Rexdale Blvd., Rexdale, Ontario, Canada, M9W 1R3, 1975.
24. *Qualification Requirements for Agencies Testing Non-Flammable Medical Gas Piping Systems*. CSA Z305.4-1977, Canadian Standards Association, 178 Rexdale Blvd., Rexdale, Ontario, Canada, M9W 1R3, 1977.
25. *Low-Pressure Connecting Assemblies for Medical Gas Systems*. CSA Z305.2-M1980, Canadian Standards Association, 178 Rexdale Blvd., Rexdale, Ontario, Canada, M9W 1R3, 1980.
26. *Piped Medical Gas Systems for Hospitals*. Hosplan,

Building Services Note, New South Wales Hospital Planning Advisory Centre 28-36, Foveaux St., Surry Hills, Australia, 1976.

27. *SAA Medical Agents and Gases Safety Code.* AS 1169, Standards Association of Australia, 80 Arthur St., N. Sydney NSW 2060, Australia, 1973.

28. *Medical Gas Pipeline Systems, Terminal Units, Hose Assemblies, and Connections to Medical Equipment.* British Standard 5682. British Standards Institution, British Standards House, 2 Park St., London WIA 2BS, 1978.

29. Howell RSC: Piped medical gas and vacuum systems. *Anaesthesia* 35:676–698, 1980.

30. Bancroft ML, du Moulin GC, Hedley-Whyte J: Hazards of hospital bulk oxygen delivery systems. *Anesthesiology* 52:504–510, 1980.

31. Glover DW: Liquid oxygen systems. *Resp Ther* 7:57–58, 77, 1977.

32. Grant WJ: *Medical Gases, Their Properties and Uses.* Chicago, Year Book Medical Publishers, 1978, pp 66–69, 114–116.

33. Fair JL: Canadian standards for piped gases. *Anesthesiology* 48:155, 1978.

34. Hall RM: Air powered surgical tools: a new approach to anesthetic safety. *Aorn J* 7:63–70, 1968.

35. Contaminated "medical" air. *Resp Care* 17:125, 1972.

36. Bushman JA, Clark PA: Oil mist hazard and piped air supplies. *Br Med J* 3:588–590, 1967.

37. Anonymous: Purification of compressed air. *South Hosp* 42:15, 1974.

38. *Standard for Medical-Surgical Vacuum Systems in Hospitals.* CGA 2.1, Compressed Gas Association, Inc., 500 Fifth Ave., New York, N.Y. 10036, 1967.

39. Anonymous: Modification of medical gas systems. *Health Devices* 9:181–185, 1980.

40. Bageant RA, Hoyt JW, Epstein RM: Error in a pipeline gas concentration: an unanticipated consequence of a defective check valve. *Anesthesiology* 54:166–169, 1981.

41. *Diameter-Index Safety System.* CGA V-5, Compressed Gas Association, Inc., 500 Fifth Ave., New York, N.Y. 10036, 1978.

42. Morris LE: An overhead boom for gas piping systems. *Anesthesiology* 14:412–413, 1953.

43. Wilder RJ, Williams GR: The ceiling-retractable service column. *JAMA* 246:1403–1404, 1981.

44. Zeller HR: Use of ceiling hose reels by anesthesiologists in the operating room. *Anesth Analg* 40:413–417, 1961.

45. Arrowsmith LWM: Medical gas pipelines. *Eng Med* 8:247–249, 1979.

46. Deas T: A preventable tragedy. *Items Topics* 23:6–7, 1977.

47. Eichhorn JH, Bancroft ML, Laasberg L, du Moulin GC, Saubermann AJ: Contamination of medical gas and water pipelines in a new hospital building. *Anesthesiology* 46:286–289, 1977.

48. Hedley-Whyte J: Medical gas line installations in hospitals. *Anesthesiology* 48:383, 1978.

49. Tingay MG, Ilsley AH, Willis RJ, Thompson MJ, Chalmers AH, Cousins MJ: Gas identity hazards and major contamination of the medical gas system of a new hospital. *Anaesth Intensive Care* 6:202–209, 1978.

50. LeBourdais E: Nine deaths linked to cross-contamination: Sudbury General inquest makes hospital history. *Dimens Health Serv* 51:10–12, 1974.

51. Dinnick OP: Medical gases-piping problems. *Eng Med* 8:243–247, 1979.

52. Elton V: Piped medical gases and vacuum. *Health Safety Executive* 29:4–30, 1976.

53. Stein DW: Anesthetic agent misuse reported. *ASA Newsletter* June 1978.

54. Johnson DL: Central oxygen supply verus mother nature. *Resp Care* 20:1043–1044, 1975.

55. Anonymous: Editorial. *Anaesthesia* 22:543–544, 1967.

56. Hedley-Whyte J: Mechanical failures leading to hypoxia. *Audio Digest* 19:14, July 18, 1977.

57. Eger EI, Epstein RM: Hazards of anesthetic equipment. *Anesthesiology* 25:490–504, 1966.

58. Newson AJ, Dyball LA: A visual monitor for piped oxygen supply systems to anaesthetic machines. *Anaesth Intensive Care* 6:146–148, 1978.

59. Gibson OB: Another hazardous pipeline isolator valve. *Anaesthesia* 34:213, 1979.

60. MacWhirter GI: An anesthetic pipe line hazard. *Anaesthesia* 33:639, 1978.

61. Feeley TW, McClelland KJ, Malhotra IV: The hazards of bulk oxygen delivery systems. *Lancet* 1:1416–1418, 1975.

62. Anonymous: Hospital negligent in supply of oxygen. *J Legal Med* 12–13, 1975.

63. Sniper W: Terminal fittings for medical gas pipelines. *Lancet* 1:457–458, 1975.

64. Eger EI, Epstein RM: Hazards of anesthetic equipment. *Anesthesiology* 25:490–504, 1964.

65. Ward DS: The prevention of accidents associated with anaesthetic apparatus. *Br J Anaesth* 40:692–701, 1968.

66. Janis KM: Sudden failure of ceiling oxygen connector. *Can Anaesth Soc J* 25:155, 1978.

67. Muir J, Davidson-Lamb R: Apparatus failure—cause for concern. *Br J Anaesth* 52:705–706, 1980.

68. Anderson EF: A potential ignition source in the operating room. *Anesth Analg* 55:217–218, 1976.

69. Finlay J, Pelton DA: Needed: error prevention. *Hospitals* 45:64–66, 1971.

70. Sprague DH, Archer GW: Intraoperative hypoxia from an erroneously filled liquid oxygen reservoir. *Anesthesiology* 42:360–362, 1975.

71. Anonymous: An accident in Edinburgh. *Lancet* 2:977, 1966.

72. Klein SL, Lilburn K: An unusual case of hypercarbia during general anesthesia. *Anesthesiology* 53:248–250, 1980.

73. Lane GA: Medical gas outlets—a hazard from interchangeable "quick connect" couplers. *Anesthesiology* 52:86–87, 1980.

74. Anonymous: Old-style Chemetron central gas outlets. *Health Devices* 10:222–223, 1981.

75. Anonymous: Nitrous oxide asphyxia. *Lancet* 1:848, 1974.

76. Anonymous: The Westminster inquiry. *Lancet* 2:175–176, 1977.

77. Mazze RI: Therapeutic misadventures with oxygen delivery systems: the need for continuous in-line oxygen monitors. *Anesth Analg* 51:787–792, 1972.

78. Allard MW, Findley IL, Conway CM: Monitoring gases supplied from pipelines. *Anaesthesia* 31:569–

570, 1976.

79. Wright M: Whistle discrimination for oxygen and nitrous oxide. Lancet 2:1008, 1977.

80. Allard MW, Findley IL, Conway CM: An assessment of the TM3 gas differentiator. *Anaesthesia* 32:170–173, 1977.

81. Marshall RD: The single hose or qualitative test and nitrous oxide cut-off device. *Anaesthesia* 33:639, 1978.

82. Lacklore LK, Perkins HM: Accidental narcosis. *JAMA* 211:1846, 1970.

83. Ford P, Hoodless DJ: Automatic electronic oxygen supply. *Br Med J* 1:548–551, 1971.

84. Hamel AJ, Deane RS, Paquette RD: Compressed air and oxygen supply lines as a source of contamination of respiratory therapy equipment. *Items Topics* 22:8–12, 1976.

85. Macpherson CR: Oxygen therapy—an unsuspected source of hospital infections? *JAMA* 167:1083–1086, 1958.

86. Mortensen JD, Hurd G, Hill G: Bacterial contamination of oxygen used clinically—importance and one method of control. *Dis Chest* 42:567–572, 1962.

87. Schwartz AJ, Howse J, Ellison N, et al: The gas line filter: a cause of hypoxia. *Anesth Analg* 59:617–618, 1980.

88. Garibaldi RA, Britt MR, Webster C, et al: Failure of bacterial filters to reduce the incidence of pneumonia after inhalation anesthesia. *Anesthesiology* 54:364–368, 1981.

89. Feeley TW, Hamilton WK, Xavier B, et al: Sterile anesthesia breathing circuits do not prevent postoperative pulmonary infection. *Anesthesiology* 54:369–372, 1981.

The Anesthesia Machine

The most important piece of equipment that the anesthesiologist uses is the anesthesia machine. The function of an anesthesia machine is to prepare a gas mixture of precisely known but variable composition (1). The gas mixture can then be delivered to a breathing system.

The first apparatus resembling an anesthesia machine appeared in 1905. Since then it has had a slow, relatively unstructured development on a component-by-component basis (2–4). It is quite possible that future anesthesia machines may differ radically from present models (5).

ANSI MACHINE STANDARD

In 1979, after many years of hard work, with input from both anesthesiologists and industry representatives, a standard for anesthesia machines was published by the American National Standards Institute (6). This document sets down basic performance and safety requirements for components of anesthesia machines. Reading of it is highly recommended. All American anesthesia machine manufacturers have agreed that machines sold after 1984 will comply with the standard. Most machines sold since 1979 already comply. Older machines that do not comply with all or part of the standard can still be serviced and there will be no time limitation on the sale of replacement parts for these machines.

The Canadian Standards Association has recently published two standards (7, 8) relating to anesthesia machines which set down requirements similar to those of the ANSI standard.

As shown in Figure 3.1, the anesthesia machine can be conveniently divided into three parts: the high-pressure system which receives gases at cylinder pressure, reduces the pressure, and makes it more constant; the intermediate pressure system which receives gases from the regulator or hospital pipeline and delivers them to the flowmeters or oxygen flush valve; and the low-pressure system which takes gases from the

flowmeters to the machine outlet. Vaporizers, which are found in the low-pressure system, will be considered in Chapter 4.

Connections of components inside the anesthesia machine are usually made using high-pressure metal tubing. To avoid accidents from incorrect connections inside the machine, the ANSI standard requires that either connections be made noninterchangeable or the piping be labeled at each junction.

THE HIGH-PRESSURE SYSTEM

The high-pressure system consists of all parts of the machine which receive gas at cylinder pressure. These include the following: (a) the hanger yoke which connects a cylinder to the machine; (b) the yoke block, used to connect cylinders larger than size E or pipeline hoses to the machine through the yoke; (c) the cylinder pressure gauge which indicates the gas pressure in the cylinder; and (d) the pressure regulator which converts a high, variable gas pressure into a lower, more constant pressure, suitable for use in the machine.

The Hanger Yoke Assembly (Connecting Yoke)

The hanger yoke orients and supports the cylinder, provides a gas-tight seal, and ensures a unidirectional flow of gases into the machine. It is composed of several parts: (a) the body, which is the principal framework and supporting structure; (b) the retaining screw which tightens the cylinder into the yoke and helps to establish a seal; (c) the nipple, through which gas enters the machine; (d) the index pins which prevent attachment of an incorrect cylinder to the yoke; (e) the washer, which also helps to form a seal between the cylinder and the yoke; (f) a filter to remove dirt from the cylinder contents; and (g) the check valve assembly, which ensures a unidirectional flow of gases through the yoke.

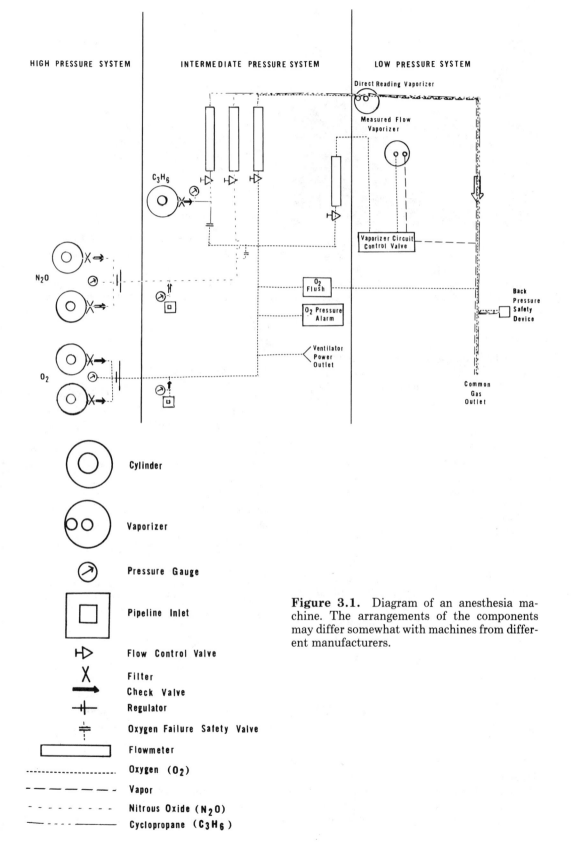

Figure 3.1. Diagram of an anesthesia machine. The arrangements of the components may differ somewhat with machines from different manufacturers.

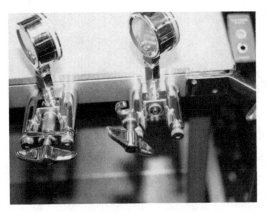

Figure 3.2. Machine with two single yokes. Each yoke has its own cylinder pressure gauge. The left yoke contains a yoke plug to protect against loss of gas and entry of particulate matter. The yokes are of the swivel gate type.

THE BODY

The body of the yoke is threaded into the frame of the machine and provides support for the cylinder. The body may be of one-piece construction as is found on most older machines, or of the swinging gate (toggle handle, swivel gate) type which has become popular. In the swinging gate type (Figure 3.2), one end of the distal part of the yoke is hinged while the other end fits over a pin. The retaining screw is in the middle of the gate.

The new machine standard requires that yokes be constructed so that the cylinder cannot be clamped unless the valve is securely fitted over the index pins and nipple. A properly constructed swinging gate type yoke meets this requirement, since the gate cannot be closed unless the cylinder valve is correctly in place (9).

THE RETAINING SCREW (CLAMPING DEVICE)

The retaining screw is threaded into the distal end of the yoke or the mid-portion of the gate. Tightening the screw presses the outlet of the cylinder valve against the washer and nipple so that a gas-tight fit is achieved. The cylinder is then supported by the retaining screw, the nipple of the yoke, and the index pins.

The point of the retaining screw must be tapered at an angle of 100–120 degrees and shaped to fit the conical depression of the cylinder valve (6). To prevent penetration of the safety relief device on the cylinder valve it is important that the point be rounded and not have an acute angle (10).

THE NIPPLE

The nipple is the part of the yoke through which the gas enters the machine. It projects from the proximal side of the yoke and fits into the port on the cylinder valve. If the nipple becomes damaged, it may not be possible to create a tight seal with the cylinder valve.

THE INDEX PINS

The index pins are mounted into holes of specific depth just below the nipple. The holes into which the pins are fitted should not extend too far into the body of the yoke. If they do it is possible to insert an incorrect cylinder into the yoke and in tightening it simply force the pins deeper into the yoke. This would bypass the safety of the Pin Index Safety System (11).

THE WASHER (GASKET)

A washer is used to effect a seal between the cylinder valve and the yoke. When a cylinder is fitted to a yoke, care should be taken to see that the washer is present and in good condition. A broken or curled washer should not be used, since a leak could result. An extra supply of washers should always be kept in case one becomes damaged. No more than one washer should ever be used. The use of two washers may prevent establishment of a tight seal or may nullify the Pin Index Safety System (11). Washers are generally supplied with a full cylinder and should only be used once. Some machine manufacturers supply long-life washers having a metal periphery and recommend discarding washers provided with cylinders.

THE FILTER

One or more filters must be installed between the cylinder and the regulator to prevent particulate matter from entering the machine where it could cause damage to the regulator or other components.

CHECK VALVE ASSEMBLY

The purpose of the check valve is to prevent retrograde flow of gases from the machine or from another cylinder to atmosphere when the yoke is not holding a cylinder. In the case of a double yoke or multiple yokes, the check valve prevents the transfer of gas from a cylinder at high pressure to one with a lower pressure. It also allows an empty cylinder to be exchanged for a full one while gas flow continues from the other cylinder into the machine with minimal loss of gas.

These check valves are not designed to act as permanent seals for empty yokes and may allow a small amount of gas to escape, especially if the pressure of the cylinder in use is low. To minimize such losses, yokes should not be left vacant for extended periods. As soon as the gas in a cylinder is exhausted, the cylinder valve should be closed and a full cylinder installed. If a full replacement cylinder is not available at the time of switchover, the exhausted cylinder should be turned off and left in the yoke. If, for some reason, a machine must be used with only one cylinder in a double yoke, a yoke plug should be placed in the empty yoke. A yoke plug (cylinder block or cylinder plug) (Figure 3.2) is a solid piece of metal or other material which has a conical depression on one end to fit the tip of the retaining screw and a hollowed out area at the other end to fit over the nipple. When in place, it forms a tight seal to prevent the escape of gases from the machine. It is sometimes chained to the machine. To prevent transfilling between paired cylinders due to a defective check valve, only one cylinder should be opened at a time.

There are two basic types of check valves. The most commonly used is the plunger type, shown in Figure 3.3. It consists of a plunger which slides away from the side of the greater pressure.

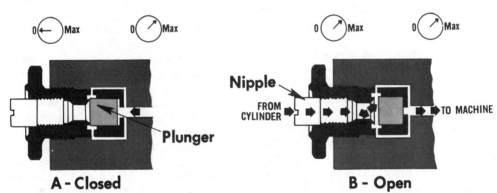

Figure 3.3. Yoke check valve—plunger type. *A*, when the pressure in the machine exceeds that in the cylinder, the plunger moves to the left, preventing escape of gas from the machine. *B*, when cylinder pressure exceeds machine pressure, the plunger moves to the right and gas flows into the machine. (From a drawing furnished by Ohio Medical Products, a division of Airco, Inc.)

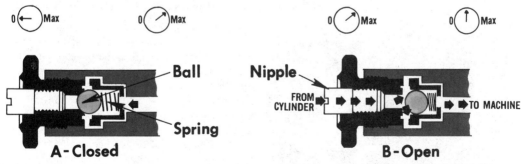

Figure 3.4. Yoke check valve—ball type. *A*, when the combined forces of the spring and the machine pressure acting on the ball exceeed that of the cylinder pressure, the ball is forced to the left, closing the valve. *B*, a higher cylinder pressure forces the ball to the right and gas flows into the machine. Note that the pressure of the gas is reduced. (From a drawing furnished by Ohio Medical Products, a division of Airco, Inc.)

When cylinder pressure exceeds the pressure on the machine side, the plunger moves to the right and gas passes into the machine. When machine pressure exceeds the cylinder pressure, the plunger moves to the left, blocking the flow of gases.

The other type of check valve is the spring-loaded ball type. As shown in Figure 3.4, it consists of a spring-loaded ball which is forced away from its seat by cylinder pressure. The spring and the pressure in the machine act to force the ball to the left. When the force of cylinder pressure pushing the ball to the right exceeds the combined forces of the spring and the pressure in the machine, the ball moves to the right and gas flows into the machine. When the forces are greater than the force of cylinder pressure on the ball, the ball moves to the left, shutting off the gas flow.

In addition to functioning as a unidirectional valve, this type of check valve also acts as a pressure-reducing valve. This is because the pressure from the cylinder must be significantly higher than that in the machine, since it must overcome the force of the spring in addition to moving the ball. This pressure reduction is important, since cyclopropane circuits often do not have a regulator. If the flow control valve is turned off but the cylinder valve left open and this type of check valve were not present, the pressure in the tubing between the flow control valve and the cylinder would be equal to the pressure in the cylinder. Liquid cyclopropane could then condense in the tubing, causing inaccurate flowmeter readings (12, 13).

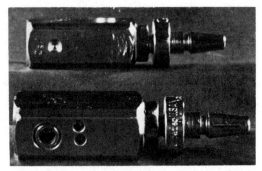

Figure 3.6. Front and back of a yoke block. A quick coupler is attached to the yoke block.

PLACING A CYLINDER IN A YOKE

The correct way to place a D or E cylinder in a yoke is first to retract the retaining screw as far as possible. With the gate type yoke the gate is swung open. The washer is placed over the nipple. The cylinder is then supported with the tip of the toe and raised into the yoke (Figure 3.5). The port is slid over the nipple and the index pins engaged into the appropriate holes. The gate is then closed. The retaining screw is advanced so that it contacts the conical depression on the cylinder valve and pushes the cylinder valve over the nipple and index pins. It is then hand-tightened. The cylinder valve should be opened to ensure that the cylinder is full and that there is no leak as evidenced by a hissing sound. It is important to ensure that the cylinder is correctly in place before tightening the retaining screw. Otherwise it may be tightened into the safety relief device on the cylinder (10) and could damage the pins on the yoke.

Yoke Block (Yoke Insert, Yoke Adapter)

A yoke block (Figure 3.6) is a piece of metal shaped like a cylinder valve that is pin indexed and has a port and conical depression to fit into a yoke. It has a connector that fits a connector on a flexible hose. It is used to connect cylinders larger than E to the machine or to connect the pipeline supply to machines which do not have pipeline connections. NFPA 56A requires a yoke block to have a backflow check-valve designed to function at pressures up to 2700 psig. The purpose of this is to prevent flow of gas from a cylinder attached to the same yoke and containing gas under high pressure into the hose attached to the yoke block should it be necessary to open the small cylinder in an emergency.

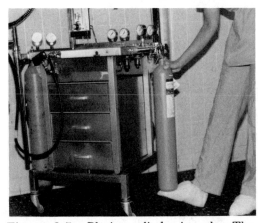

Figure 3.5. Placing cylinder in yoke. The cylinder is supported by the foot and guided into place manually.

This piece of equipment is associated with several hazards and its use should be discontinued. If it connects to a high-pressure cylinder without a regulator, the hose carrying gas at high pressure presents a danger to personnel should a leak or break occur (14). If it connects to a cylinder with a regulator or a pipeline source, it is far safer to equip the machine with pipeline inlet connections than use yoke blocks, since yoke blocks can be responsible for crossovers between gases in the anesthesia machine. Some yoke blocks do not have pin indexing holes and thus can be inserted in any yoke. Some others that do have pin indexing holes have a short top and can be inserted into the yoke upside down (1, 15). Also use of a yoke block may lead to fluctuations of the gas pressure supplied to the flow control valve, since the pressure regulators in the machine designed to accept gas at cylinder pressure may not function properly when supplied with gas at reduced pressure (7, 16). For these reasons use of yoke blocks should be discouraged and pipeline inlet connections be installed on machines when a source of supply other than D and E cylinders is to be used.

The Cylinder Pressure Gauge

The machine standard requires that each anesthesia machine be equipped with at least one cylinder pressure gauge for each gas supplied in cylinders. If there is more than one yoke for a gas, one gauge may be provided for each yoke or one gauge may be provided for a group of yokes. The gauge will indicate the pressure in a cylinder when the valve is opened.

These gauges are usually of the Bourdon tube (Bourdon spring) type, illustrated in Figure 3.7. A hollow metal tube is bent into a curve, sealed and linked to a clock-like mechanism. The other end is connected into the gas source and soldered into a socket. An increase in pressure of the gas inside the tube causes it to straighten. As the pressure falls, the tube resumes its curved shape. Since the open end is in a fixed position, the sealed end moves.

Through the clock-like mechanism these motions are transmitted to the indicator, which moves on a scale calibrated in units of pressure.

These gauges are constructed with a safety back and a heavy glass window so that if the Bourdon tube ruptures, the escaping gas will be vented out the back of the case rather than blowing out the window.

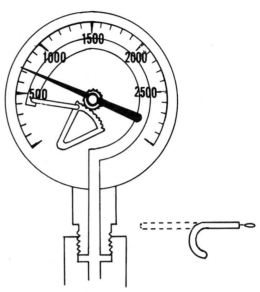

Figure 3.7. Bourdon pressure gauge. The flexible tube which is connected to the gas circuit straightens when pressure is applied. The attached clocklike mechanism moves the pointer. (From *Wright's Veterinary Anesthesia and Analgesia.* London, Bailliere, Tindall & Cassell, 1971.)

The machine standard requires that the full scale pressure indication be at least 33% greater than the maximum cylinder pressure. All cylinder gauges on a machine must have an equal span angle (between 180 and 280 degrees) from the lowest to the highest pressure indication, with the lowest indication between 6 and 9 on a clock face. The pointer must be shaped so that it will be immediately apparent to the user which is the indicator end. These requirements are designed to provide better resolution of the dial numbers and to facilitate recognition of the empty position on each gauge, which has been a problem in the past (17).

Cylinder pressure gauges must be identified by the name or symbol of the gas being measured and are frequently color-coded. They should be situated in a position where they can be easily seen and not covered by other items.

The Pressure Regulator

The pressure in a gas cylinder varies with the temperature and contents. In order to maintain constant flow with changing supply pressure, the anesthesia machine is fitted with pressure regulators. These devices reduce the high and variable storage pressure found in a cylinder to a lower more constant pressure suitable for use in an anesthesia machine.

INDICATIONS FOR USE (18, 19)

1. Before regulators were available, it was necessary for the anesthesiologist to readjust the flow control valve frequently to maintain a steady flow as the pressure in the cylinder declined (1). Since the regulator supplies gas at a relatively constant pressure, the need for repeated adjustments is eliminated.

2. When high pressure is supplied to a flowmeter, small adjustments in flow are difficult. With a lower supply pressure, the flow control valve can be constructed so that more rotations of the flow control valve are necessary to achieve the same change in flowmeter setting, enabling fine adjustments to be made more easily.

3. The pressure delivered from a cylinder is usually far too high to be used safely. Use of lower pressures reduces the possibility of a dangerous pressure buildup that could cause damage to the machine or harm to a patient.

PHYSICS

To understand the design of a regulator, a knowledge of the physics involved is essential. Pressure is defined as a force acting against a given area. One can increase force either by increasing the pressure or by increasing the area over which the pressure acts. To illustrate this, consider the simple balance shown in Figure 3.8.

A large pressure, Pc, acting on a small area, A1, is balanced by a smaller pressure, Pr, acting on a large area, A2. The force exerted by the higher pressure is

$$Pc \times A1$$

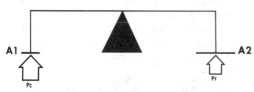

Figure 3.8. A large pressure acting over a small area is balanced by a smaller pressure acting over a large area. The relative sizes of the arrows represent the magnitudes of the pressures.

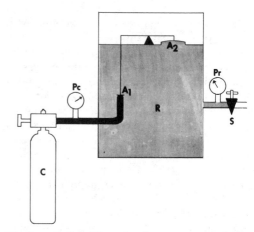

Figure 3.9. The simple pressure-reducing valve is represented in the closed state. See text for details.

This is balanced by the force on the right:

$$Pr \times A2$$

Since these forces are equal, it follows that

$$Pr \times A2 = Pc \times A1$$

Solving for Pr,

$$Pr = \frac{A1}{A2} \times Pc$$

In a pressure-reducing valve these same principles apply. In Figure 3.9 C is a cylinder of gas under a high pressure, Pc. R is the inside of a regulator containing gas under a reduced pressure, Pr. The opening between C and R is occluded by a seat of area A1. A2 is the area of a flexible diaphragm upon which Pr acts. When the stopcock (S) is closed, the forces are in balance. The seat seals the opening from the cylinder so that no gas flows into R.

In Figure 3.10, the stopcock is open and gas flows from R, causing the pressure, Pr, to drop. The forces are no longer balanced since Pc × A1 > Pr × A2.

The flexible diaphragm becomes flatter, the balance tips to the right and the seat no longer occludes the opening from the cylinder, so that gas flows from the cylinder into R. As long as the stopcock is open, the forces will be in balance and gas will continue to flow from the cylinder. This situation is analogous to opening the flow control valve on the anesthesia machine. When

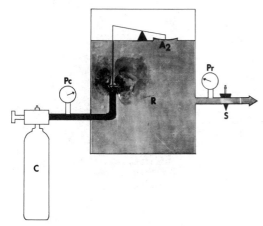

Figure 3.10. The simple pressure regulator is represented with the stopcock (*S*) open. An imbalance of forces is created, allowing gas to pass from the cylinder into the regulator. See text for details.

the stopcock is closed, gas will continue to flow briefly into *R*, until Pr increases to the point where a balance of forces is restored (Fig. 3.9). The small increase in Pr after the stopcock is closed is called the *static increment*.

The regulator shown in Figures 3.9 and 3.10 will yield a constant reduced pressure only if the supplied pressure, Pc, is constant. If Pc decreases, as when the cylinder pressure decays, Pr must decrease to preserve the balance of forces. With this type of regulator, the flowmeter would constantly need readjustment to compensate for the pressure drop.

To remedy this a main spring (*S1*) is added (Fig. 3.11). This spring exerts a downward force on the flexible diaphragm. The magnitude of this force depends on an adjusting screw which can be turned. Now the forces acting to push the diaphragm upward remain

$$Pr \times A2$$

Forces acting to push the diaphragm downward are:

$$(Pc \times A1) + F_{s1}$$

where F_{s1} is the force exerted by the spring. If the values for Pc, Pr, A1 and A2 remain unchanged, there would be an imbalance of forces, since the force of the main spring would be added to the force of Pc acting on A1. To compensate for this imbalance, A1 may be reduced,

A2 may be increased or both. At equilibrium,

$$(Pc \times A1) + F_{s1} = Pr \times A2$$

Solving this equation for Pr,

$$Pr = (F_{s1}/A2) + Pc(A1/A2) \tag{1}$$

The force exerted by Pr acting on the diaphragm, therefore, is opposed by two forces: a constant force from the spring ($F_{s1}/A2$) and a variable force from Pc acting on the seat, Pc(A1/A2). If the force exerted by the spring is large in comparison with the force exerted by Pc, large variations in Pc will cause only slight variations in Pr.

Example:

Suppose Pc initially is 100 and is then reduced to 50. If F_{s1} is small (20), A2 is 10 and A1 is 2. When Pc is 100,
  Pr = 20/10 + 100 (2/10)
  Pr = 2 + 20
  Pr = 22.
When Pc is reduced to 50.
  Pr = 20/10 + 50 (2/10)
  Pr = 2 + 10
  Pr = 12.
So the reduction in Pc is accompanied by a large change in Pr. However, if F_{s1} is large (1000) and A1 and A2 are adjusted appropriately (to 1 and 50 respectively),
  When Pc is 100,

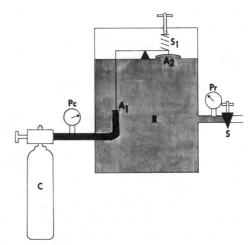

Figure 3.11. A mainspring (*S1*) and adjusting screw are added to the regulator. For details see text.

Pr = 1000/50 + 100 (1/50)
Pr = 20 + 2
Pr = 22.
When Pc is reduced to 50.
Pr = 1000/50 + 50 (1/50)
Pr = 20 + 1
Pr = 21.

A large change in Pc then has caused only a small change in Pr.

As seen in Equation 1, the value of Pr will depend upon F_{s1}. By means of the adjusting screw the tension in the spring can be varied and in this way Pr may be varied. For this reason the main spring is sometimes referred to as the adjusting spring.

One more addition to the regulator is necessary. In Figure 3.12 a sealing spring, or shutoff spring ($S2$) is added, which acts to force the seat against the opening from the cylinder. This prevents gas from flowing from C to R when the adjusting spring is completely relaxed and the stopcock open. Equation 1 then becomes

$$Pr = (F_{s1} - F_{s2})/A2 + Pc(A1/A2) \quad (2)$$

The value of F_{s2} is considerably smaller than F_{s1} so that $(F_{s1} - F_{s2})$ is large in comparison with Pc, and Pr will remain relatively constant in spite of variations in Pc.

There will, however, be some variations in Pr with variations in Pc. A change, ΔPc, in the cylinder pressure will produce a change, ΔPr, in the reduced pressure. From Equation 2,

$$\Delta Pr = \Delta Pc(A1/A2)$$

(see ref. 20)

As Pc decreases, Pr also decreases (*pressure-proportioned reduction*). The magnitude of the change in Pr is governed by the ratio of A1 to A2.

The significance of this lies in the effect it has on gas flow, particularly when oxygen is the gas under consideration. If one uses an E cylinder as the source of oxygen, a significant fall in primary oxygen pressure will occur during a prolonged case. If the flow control valve position remains unchanged, a decrease in oxygen flow will occur. This could be significant if the percentage of oxygen in the gas mixture being administered is close to the metabolic requirements of the patient.

The regulator illustrated in Figures 3.9 to 3.12 is an example of a *direct-acting* regulator. This is because the components are arranged so that the cylinder pressure tends to *open* the valve.

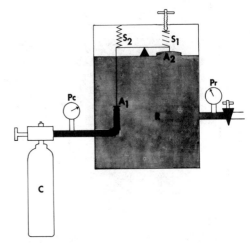

Figure 3.12.   A sealing spring has been added to complete the regulator. See text for details.

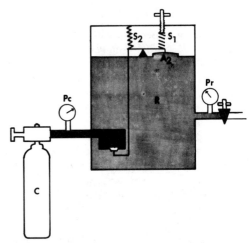

Figure 3.13.   Indirect-acting regulator. The components are arranged so that cylinder pressure tends to close the valve. See text for details.

An *indirect-acting regulator* is shown diagrammatically in Figure 3.13. In this case Pc acts to *close* the valve. Equation 2 then becomes

$$Pr = (F_{s1} - F_{s2})/A2 - Pc(A1/A2)$$

The variation in Pr with variation in Pc is given by the equation

$$\Delta Pr = \Delta Pc(A1/A2)$$

As Pc decreases, Pr increases (*pressure inversion*).

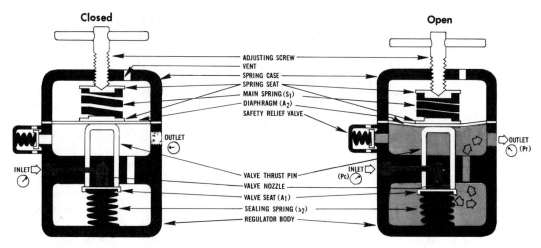

Figure 3.14. Direct-acting regulator. The *darker shades* are used for gas under high pressure while the *lighter shades* represent gas under reduced pressure. The *arrows* indicate the path of gas flow. The valve is opened by turning the adjusting screw. See text for details. (Redrawn courtesy of Ohio Medical Products, a division of Airco, Inc.)

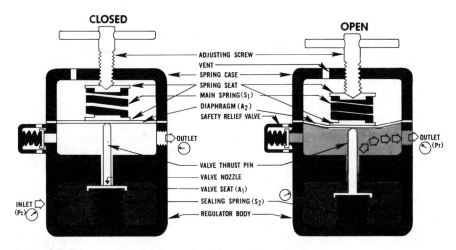

Figure 3.15. Indirect-acting regulator. In this case the cylinder pressure opposes the opening of the valve. As the adjusting screw is opened gas flows from the lower to the upper chamber along the valve thrust pin. (Redrawn courtesy of Ohio Medical Products, a division of Airco, Inc.)

THE MODERN REGULATOR

The modern regulator, depicted diagrammatically in Figures 3.14 and 3.15, functions on the same principles as the regulators shown in 3.12 and 3.13. All of the components shown in Figures 3.12 and 3.13 are present in the modern regulator, but their arrangement differs slightly.

The direct-acting regulator is shown in Figure 3.14. The valve's functioning is determined by a balance of forces acting to position the seat, A2. With the valve closed, the force of the sealing spring $(S2)$, pushing the seat up against the nozzle, is greater than the downward force exerted by the main spring $(S1)$ and the inlet pressure (Pc) against the seat. No gas flows from the inlet into the regulator. Pr is 0.

When the valve is opened by tightening the adjusting screw, the downward force of the main spring $(S1)$ is increased. This force is transmitted along the valve thrust pin to the seat and, in combination with the inlet pressure, overcomes the force of the sealing spring. Gas at reduced pressure (Pr) flows into the space under the diaphragm and exerts an upward force on the diaphragm (Pr × A2). Gas then flows on to the outlet. The forces are not in balance, but Pr will remain at a constant value, since a steady state is soon achieved. Gas will continue to flow until either the cylinder is exhausted or the gas flow is turned off at a point distal to the regulator. If it is turned off at a distal point, gas will continue briefly to flow into the space under the diaphragm. Here, its pressure will increase (static increment) until the force of the reduced gas on the diaphragm (Pr × A2) plus the force of the sealing spring, S2, balance the force of the cylinder pressure and the main spring (Pc × A2 + F_{s2}), as in Equation 2.

Figure 3.15 illustrates the indirect-acting regulator. With the valve closed, gas enters the space surrounding the sealing spring ($S2$) and the valve seat ($A1$). Its own pressure (Pc) tends to hold the valve seat against the nozzle. When the adjusting screw is turned so that the main spring exerts a downward force on the diaphragm (F_{s1}), the valve thrust pin moves downward, opening the seat, so that gas at reduced pressure (Pr) expands through the holes for the thrust pin and into the cavity under the diaphragm. When the gas flow is turned off distal to the regulator, the gas continues to flow into the space under the diaphragm. Here its pressure increases (static increment), pushing the diaphragm upward until the seat closes against the nozzle, stopping further flow.

Pressure regulators used in anesthesia machines are preset at the factory and should not be altered by the user. The machine standard requires that they be adjusted so that the machine uses only the gas supply from the pipeline when the pipeline inlet pressure is 50 psig or greater. This is to prevent the drawing of gas from the cylinder and pipeline supplies if a cylinder is left open while using the pipeline supplies.

If the machine is equipped with a power outlet for a ventilator the regulator for oxygen is usually set slightly below 50 psig. Machines not equipped with power outlets frequently have the oxygen regulators adjusted to a pressure between 37 and 42 psig. At least one modern machine is equipped with additional regulators downstream of both the pipeline inlets and the cylinder regulators. These reduce the pressure to approximately 12 psig. This minimizes bobbing of the flowmeter indicator resulting from pressure fluctuations in the pipeline inlets.

When pipeline supplies of gases are being used, cylinders should always be turned off. Decreases in the pipeline inlet pressure do occur (especially when a ventilator operated from the power outlet cycles) and the pressure may drop below that supplied by the cylinder regulator, especially if the regulator is set at a high pressure. If this occurs, and the cylinder valve is open, some gas will be withdrawn from the cylinder. Eventually the cylinder will be depleted. Another reason why cylinders should not be left open is that it may result in total use of cylinder supplies when the anesthesiologist, not recognizing that the pipeline supply is not connected or is not functioning, has the mistaken belief that he is using piped sources (21).

Most anesthesia machines use single-stage regulators such as those described. Some use two-stage regulators, which, as the name implies, are two single-stage regulators in series. The outlet of the first stage is the inlet of the second stage, so that the pressure reduction occurs in two steps instead of one. An advantage of this arrangement is reduced wear on the diaphragms, since their movement is reduced. A second advantage is that variations in Pr secondary to variations in Pc are reduced.

Regulators must be equipped with a relief valve or other mechanism to protect the rest of the machine from excessive pressure, as might occur with a problem in the hospital piping system (22). One case has been reported where impurities in the nitrous oxide damaged the diaphragm, causing it to rupture and transmit the high pressure to the reduced pressure side (23). The relief valve permitted the high pressure to be dissipated to outside air and protected the rest of the machine from damage. However, it should be noted that these requirements do not in themselves provide full protection against the delivery of gases at excessive pressures (7).

Regulators used in anesthesia machines are supplied for every gas except in some models, cyclopropane. Usually there is a regulator for every double or single yoke, but separate yokes for the same gas may be connected to one regulator. Cyclopropane yokes do not always have a regulator since the gas is supplied in the cylinder at a relatively low pressure. Also the spring-loaded check valve in the yoke may act to reduce the pressure during flow.

INTERMEDIATE PRESSURE SYSTEM

The intermediate pressure system (Fig. 3.1) includes the components of the machine which receive gases at reduced pressures (usually 37–55 psig). Pressures in this part of the machine are relatively constant. The intermediate pressure system includes the following parts: (a) the pipeline inlet connections which connect the machine to the hospital pipeline system; (b) the pipeline pressure gauges; (c) the ventilator power outlet which supplies driving gas to the ventilator; (d) oxygen pressure failure devices which either interrupt the flow of anesthetic gases or provide an alarm when the oxygen pressure fails; (e) the flowmeter assembly which provides control and metering of anesthetic gases and oxygen and (f) the oxygen flush which allows delivery of high flows of oxygen from the machine.

Pipeline Inlet Connections

All machines manufactured in the United States now provide as standard equipment pipeline inlet connections for oxygen and nitrous oxide. Suction and air inlets are available as options.

Pipeline inlets are fitted with male connectors of the Diameter Index Safety System (DISS). Noninterchangeable quick-connect fittings (Chapter 2) may be attached. The inlet must contain a check valve to prevent backflow of gas from the machine into the hospital piping system or to the atmosphere if no hose is connected. Some inlets contain filters.

The Pipeline Pressure Gauge (See Fig. 4.45)

Gauges to monitor the pipeline pressure to the machine are recommended, but not required, by the ANSI standard. They are usually of the Bourdon tube type.

On older machines, the pipeline pressure gauge may be attached either on the pipeline or the machine side of the check valve in the pipeline inlet. The machine standard requires that the gauge be on the pipeline side of the check valve. The position is important (24). If the gauge is on the pipeline side, it will monitor pipeline pressure only. If the pipeline is disconnected or improperly connected it will read 0.

If the gauge is on the machine side it registers not pipeline pressure, but rather the pressure within the machine. If a cylinder happens to be open and the pipeline supply fails, there may be little indication of such failure by the gauge until the cylinder is nearly empty (21). Thus this gauge will give a true indication of failure of the pipeline supply pressure only if the cylinders are turned off.

The relationship of the gauge to the check valve usually is not obvious on inspection of the machine. The user can ascertain the location of this connection by disconnecting the pipeline supply and turning on the cylinder supply. If the reading on the pipeline gauge remains zero, the gauge is connected on the pipeline side. If a reading is obtained, it is connected on the machine side.

It should be noted that even when the pipeline gauge indicates an adequate pressure it does not follow that gas is not being drawn from a cylinder. If for any reason the cylinder pressure exceeds that of the pipeline and a cylinder valve is open, gas will be drawn from the cylinder. It follows that cylinders should always remain closed when a pipeline supply is in use.

Pipeline pressure gauges should always be checked before the machine is used and should register between 45 and 55 psig (310–380 kPa). They should be observed repeatedly during use.

The Ventilator Power Outlet

Many machines are equipped with a power outlet connection to supply oxygen or air to power a ventilator. The power outlet is connected to the intermediate pressure oxygen system between the pipeline inlet and the flow control valve. It is fitted with a male DISS oxygen fitting. A quick coupler may be attached. A check valve should be present in the connection to prevent loss of gas when a ventilator is not attached.

On machines equipped with a power outlet the reduced pressure issuing from the cylinder regulator may be set just below 50 psig because some ventilators will not function properly at lower pressures. On some machines it is not possible to operate a ventilator from oxygen cylinders, but only from pipeline supplies.

Oxygen Pressure Failure Devices

Delivery of a hypoxic gas mixture due to a gradual or abrupt failure of the oxygen supply during an anesthetic procedure is a very serious problem. The prevention of such accidents has been the object of various inventions. Among the solutions offered have been devices which (a) cut off the supply of gases other than oxygen (oxygen failure safety valve) or (b) give an audible or visible warning (alarms) when oxygen pressure has fallen to a dangerous level.

DEVICES

Oxygen Failure Safety Valve (25) (Low-Pressure Guardian System, Oxygen Supply Pressure Failure Protection Device, Pressure Sensor Shutoff System, Safe-T-Lor, Fail Safe, Pressure Sensor System)

The ANSI machine standard requires that an anesthesia machine be equipped with a device such that a reduction in oxygen flow due to a drop in the oxygen supply pressure 50% below normal will result in the cessation of flow of all other gases, including compressed air, or will automatically produce a proportional drop in the flow of the other gases.

One such device is shown diagrammatically in Figure 3.16. It is similar to an indirect-acting pressure regulator with the adjusting spring replaced by oxygen pressure. The opening (B) is connected to the intermediate pressure oxygen system. Normal oxygen pressure will push the diaphragm and stem downward, opening the valve and allowing the anesthetic gas to pass around the seat and on to the outlet. When oxygen pressure drops, the combined force of the spring and the pressure of the anesthetic gas in the lower chamber will overcome the downward force from the oxygen and the valve will

close, stopping the flow of anesthetic gas. This valve, therefore, is a simple on-off valve.

There is a another type of oxygen failure safety device known as a gas-loaded regulator, which acts both as a regulator for an anesthetic gas and an oxygen failure safety valve. The second stage of the regulator is modified so that as the oxygen pressure falls, the reduced pressure of the anesthetic gas also falls. Eventually the oxygen pressure will become so low that the flow of anesthetic gas will cease. This differs from the previous type in that instead of the anesthetic gas flow being either on or off, the flow is gradually reduced as oxygen pressure falls.

As shown in Figure 3.1, the oxygen failure safety valves are located in the intermediate pressure lines upstream of the flow control valves of all gases except oxygen. Thus oxygen pressure acts as a control for all other gas systems. If the pressure is normal the flow of other gases will proceed to their respective flow control valves. When the oxygen pressure drops, these valves close and halt the delivery of all other gases.

Oxygen failure safety valves are now present on most anesthesia machines but may not be on older machines or may be present for only one

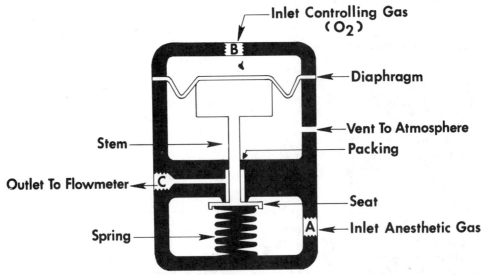

Figure 3.16. Oxygen failure safety valve. When oxygen pressure in the machine is normal, it will push the diaphragm and stem downward, opening the valve. The anesthetic gas then flows in at A, around the stem and out at C. When the oxygen pressure falls, the stem moves upward, closing the valve. The middle chamber is vented to atmosphere to prevent mixing of anesthetic gas and oxygen in the event that the diaphragm ruptures and the packing leaks. (Redrawn from a diagram furnished by Ohio Medical Products, a division of Airco, Inc.)

of several gases. To check an older machine to see if it has a properly functioning oxygen failure safety valve, open the cylinder valve on one oxygen and one other gas cylinder (or attach the pipeline inlet connections). Set a 4-liter/min flow on both the oxygen flowmeter and the flowmeter for the other gas. Close the oxygen cylinder valve (or disconnect the pipeline hose). Correct functioning of an oxygen failure safety valve will be indicated if the flowmeter indicator for the other gas falls to 0 after the oxygen in the machine circuit has been bled to atmosphere. Repeat this procedure for all gases on the machine. If the check reveals that the machine does not have an oxygen failure safety valve for all anesthetic gases and air, the manufacturer should be contacted and this added to the machine.

Alarms

Another approach to the loss of oxygen pressure has been to develop alarms which give an audible and/or visible warning of the loss of oxygen pressure.

Alarm devices are of two types: high-pressure and low-pressure (26). High-pressure alarms are sensitive to depletion of oxygen in cylinders attached to the machine. Low-pressure alarms are sensitive to a reduction in oxygen pressure in the intermediate pressure oxygen system. Since most anesthesia machines are now operated from pipeline supplies, low-pressure alarms are more common. In the past they have not been used much in the United States, although they have been popular in Europe. Recently, however, several American machine manufacturers have made alarms standard equipment on their new machines.

The machine standard recommends, but does not require, that an audible alarm which is activated when the oxygen pressure falls 50% below normal be fitted to an anesthesia machine. Such an alarm must sound for at least 7 sec if the machine is in use. The sole means of shutting off or resetting the alarm must be restoration of the oxygen pressure above the alarm point. On machines having a main on-off switch controlling the gas flows, turning the switch on usually activates the alarms present.

Alarms have been classified on the basis of what powers the alarm.

Oxygen Whistles. This type of alarm directs a stream of oxygen through a whistle when the oxygen pressure falls below a certain value (27–

34). This has the disadvantage that some of the already dwindling supply of oxygen will be lost through the whistle. If the loss of oxygen is rapid the whistle will sound for only a short time. Some manufacturers incorporate an oxygen reservoir to overcome these problems.

Nitrous Oxide Whistles (35–40). These divert a stream of nitrous oxide through a whistle when the oxygen pressure falls. These have the advantage over oxygen whistles of conserving oxygen. The main disadvantage is that with some of these devices the alarm will not function if the nitrous oxide supply becomes depleted prior to the oxygen supply or if it is not turned on. In addition, some, such as the Bosun, can be turned off (35, 40, 41).

Electronic Alarms. Electronic alarms incorporate a pressure-sensitive switch which initiates an audible or visible signal when the oxygen pressure falls below a preset value. These devices have the disadvantages that the batteries may wear out or the electrical contacts become corroded. Some require the user to turn them on.

LIMITATIONS (42, 43)

Problems have been reported with the oxygen pressure failure safety valves. In one case the diaphragm between the oxygen and nitrous oxide sections of the regulator developed a leak. Oxygen then diluted the nitrous oxide, causing awareness during anesthesia (44). Another case has been reported in which excessive oxygen pressure in the piping system damaged some gas-loaded nitrous oxide regulators.

The alarm devices, in addition to having the limitations listed above, may fail due to back pressure when used in conjunction with certain ventilators (45–49).

Of greater importance is the fact that any device that depends on pressure and not flow has limitations which may not be fully appreciated by the user. These devices do not in themselves offer total protection against a hypoxic mixture being delivered. They aid in preventing hypoxia due to some problems (such as disconnected oxygen hoses, low oxygen pressure in the pipeline, and depletion of oxygen cylinders) occurring upstream of them in the machine circuitry. They do not guard against accidents due to crossovers in the pipeline system or wrong contents in a gas cylinder. Equipment problems (such as leaks) or operation errors (such as closed or inadvertently downward adjusted oxygen flow control valves) that occur downstream of these devices are not prevented. Oxygen failure safety valves usually close the line at a pressure between 15 and 30 psig, depending on the manufacturer. If the machine is gas tight, the oxygen system may stay pressurized for weeks without even being connected to a source of oxygen. Thus anesthetic gas can be flowing with no flow of oxygen.

Fortunately, some new devices have been developed to overcome the problems of having anesthetic gases but no oxygen flowing. These will be discussed in association with flowmeters. Even these devices, however, do not guard against hypoxia due to the wrong gas coming through a flowmeter. The use of oxygen analyzers in the breathing system should be considered mandatory for safe anesthesia (50).

Flowmeter Assembly

The flowmeter assembly controls, measures, and indicates the rate of flow of a gas passing through it.

PHYSICAL PRINCIPLES (51)

The flowmeters used in modern anesthesia machines are of the variable orifice (variable area) type, also known as a Thorpe type. The Thorpe tube, shown in Figure 3.17, consists of a transparent tapered tube which has its smallest diameter at the bottom. It contains an indicator

or float which is free to move up and down inside the tube. When there is no flow of gas, the float rests at the bottom of the tube. As shown in Figure 3.17B, when the flow control valve is opened, gas enters at the bottom and flows up the tube, elevating the indicator. The gas passes through the annular opening between the float and the tube and on to the outlet at the top of the tube. The indicator floats freely in the tube at an equilibrium position where the downward force on it due to gravity equals the upward force due to the gas flow. As gas flow increases, the float rises. Since the tube is tapered, the size of the annular opening around the indicator increases with height. When the flow is decreased, gravity causes the indicator to settle to a lower level. A scale marked on or beside the tube indicates the gas flow.

The rate of gas flow through this tube will depend on three factors: the pressure drop across the constriction, the size of the annular opening, and the physical properties of the gas.

The Pressure Drop across the Constriction

As gas flows around the indicator, it encounters frictional resistance between the float and the wall of the tube. Also the flow becomes less laminar and more turbulent. There is a resultant loss of energy reflected in a pressure drop. This pressure drop is constant for all positions in the tube and is equal to the weight of the float divided by its cross-sectional area.

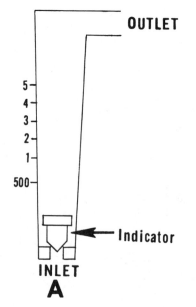
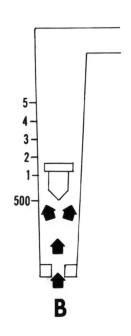

Figure 3.17. Variable orifice flowmeter. Gas enters at the base and flows through the tube, causing the float to rise. The gas passes through the annular opening around the float. The area of this annular space increases with the height of the indicator. Thus the height of the indicator is a measure of gas flow.

The Size of the Annular Opening

The larger the annular opening around the float, the greater will be the flow of gas. Since the pressure drop across the constriction is always balanced by the weight of the float, the increased or decreased area must be balanced by an increase or decrease in lifting force ($P = F/A$) caused by a change in the gas flow.

Physical Characteristics of the Gas

When low flows of gases are passing through the Thorpe tube, the annular opening between the float and the wall of the tube will be narrow. As flow increases, the annular opening becomes wider. The physical property that relates gas flow to the pressure difference on the two sides of the constriction varies with the form of constriction. With a longer and narrower constriction (low flow), flow is a function of the viscosity of the gas (Poiseuille's law). When the constriction is shorter and wider (high flow), flow depends on the density of the gas (Graham's law).

In the variable orifice flowmeter the annular cross-sectional area is varied and the pressure drop across the float remains constant for all positions in the tube. For this reason these flowmeters are often called constant pressure flowmeters. Increasing the flow does not increase the pressure drop but causes the float to rise to a higher position in the tube, thereby providing greater flow area for the gas. The elevation of the float is a measure of the annular area for flow and therefore of the flow itself.

Temperature and Pressure Effects

Flowmeters are calibrated at atmospheric pressure (760 torr) and room temperature (20°C). Temperature and pressure changes will affect both the viscosity and the density of a gas and so influence the accuracy of the indicated flowrate. Temperature changes as a rule are slight and do not induce significant changes.

With decreasing barometric pressure (as with increasing altitude), the increase in flowrate which occurs will depend on the flowmeter setting (52). At low indicated flowrates, there is no change in actual flow with increasing altitude; flow is laminar and depends on gas viscosity, which is independent of altitude. At higher indicated flowrates, as flow becomes more turbulent, the decrease in gas density with altitude will increase the actual flowrate.

CONVENTIONAL FLOWMETER BLOCKS

The majority of anesthesia machines currently in use have individual flow control valves for each gas. Proportioning devices will be discussed later.

Components

Flow Control Valve (Needle Valve, Pin Valve, Fine Adjustment Valve). The flow control valve controls the rate of flow of a gas through its associated flowmeter by manual adjustment of a variable orifice. Most flow control valves have both a control and an on-off function.

The Body. The body of the flow control valve is usually made of brass and screws into the base of the flowmeter.

Stem and Seat. The stem and seat are shown diagrammatically in Figure 3.18. The stem has fine threads which allow it to move only a short

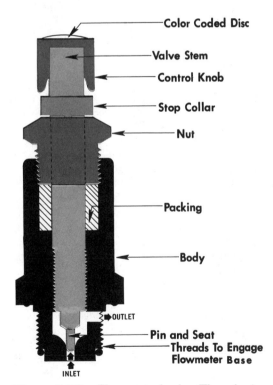

Figure 3.18. Flow control valve. The valve is shown in the closed position. Turning the stem creates a leak between the pin and seat so that gas flows to the outlet. The stop collar prevents overtightening of the pin in the seat. (Redrawn from a drawing furnished by Foregger Company, a division of Puritan-Bennett Corp.)

distance when a complete turn is made. The pin at the distal end of the stem is usually made of a durable metal such as stainless steel. It is conical and fits into a seat of metal or plastic. When the valve is closed, the pin fits into the seat and no gas can pass through the valve. When the stem is turned outward, an opening between the pin and the seat is created which allows gas to flow through the valve. By turning the screw one can increase or decrease the opening and thus control the flow of gas.

It is advantageous to have stops for the OFF and maximum flow positions (26). The stop for the OFF position avoids damage to the valve seat. The stop for the maximum flow position prevents the stem from becoming disengaged from the valve body.

The Control Knob. The control knob is joined to the stem. It should be large enough to be turned easily. The tips of the knobs are frequently color-coded and must be labeled as to the gas they control. A flow control knob for a flowmeter-controlled vaporizer is labeled with the name of the agent in the vaporizer. The standard for anesthesia machines requires that the knob for oxygen be touch-coded with a characteristic fluted profile (see Figs. 3.22 and 3.24). All other flow control knobs must be round with minimal serrations and they cannot have a larger diameter than the oxygen flow control knob.

The close proximity of the flow control knobs on some machines contributes greatly to the probability of errors (2). The machine standard requires a distance of at least 25 mm between knobs. In addition, the knobs must be designed so as to minimize their inadvertent change from a preset position. This can be accomplished by a shield, recess, guard, or other protective barrier to protect them, and by placing them high enough above the working surface to lessen the likelihood of contact with objects on those surfaces.

Knobs are turned counterclockwise to increase flow and clockwise to decrease flow. Some machines have a tension nut to vary the force needed to turn the knob. Flowmeter control knobs should be smooth and easy to adjust, yet stiff enough to resist unintentional changes from rotational or non-rotational forces. The machine standard requires that each flow control knob undergo at least a 90-degree rotation to move the indicator through the upper 90% of the flowmeter tube.

The flow control valve is a delicate piece of equipment and can be damaged by misuse. When the valve is closed, it should be turned only until the flow of gas ceases, as further tightening may result in damage to the pin or seat. This could cause an erratic flow of gas or extreme sensitivity of the flowmeter control (53). Some manufacturers provide a stop collar on the valve to prevent it from being closed too tightly. The stop, however, can be overridden or changed by an overturning of the knob.

Whenever a machine is not being used, the gas source (cylinder or pipeline) should be closed or disconnected. The flow control valves should be opened until the gas pressure is zero, then closed.

Before use of the machine is resumed, the flow control valves should be checked to see that they are closed. Sometimes the habit of leaving the flow control valves open after the gas is bled out to atmosphere develops. In addition, the flow control valves may be opened when the machine is cleaned or moved by people not in a position to understand the possible consequences. If the gas supply to an open flow control valve is restored and the associated flowmeter is not observed, the indicator may rise to the top of the tube where its presence may not be noticed by the operator for some time (54). Even if no harm to the patient results, the sudden rise of the indicator may damage it and impair the accuracy of the flowmeter.

Flowmeter Subassembly. The flowmeter subassembly consists of the tube through which the gas flows, the indicator, a stop at the top of the tube, and the scale which indicates the flow.

Components. TUBE. Flowmeter tubes are usually made of Pyrex. They may have either a single or a double taper. The single taper tube, shown in Figure 3.19 (right tubes), increases in diameter by a uniform amount from bottom to top. As seen in the figure, there is a compression of the intervals in the upper part of the tube. The reason for this is that the area of the annular space does not increase linearly as one moves up the tube but in steadily increasing increments. Consequently, gradations corresponding to equal increments in flowrate are closer together at the top of the tube.

To provide greater discrimination at low flowrates, the tube may have a double or "dual" taper, as shown in Figure 3.19 (left tubes). The taper of the lower part of the tube increases more slowly than the upper part.

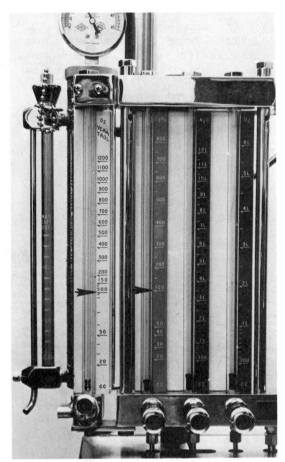

Figure 3.19. Flowmeter tubes. The two tubes on the *right* have single tapers and show the compression of intervals in the upper part of the tube. The two *left* flowmeter tubes have double tapers. The *arrows* point to the place where the taper changes.

In some flowmeters with ball indicators, rib guides are used. Rib guides are thickened bars running the length of the flowmeter tube, spaced equally around the circumference. Figure 3.20 shows sections at the upper and lower parts of the tube. The gas passes between the ball and the inner wall of the tube. Since the tube is tapered, this space increases from below upward. The area occupied by the rib guides varies with the height of the tube. Consequently, the compression of intervals usually seen in the upper part of the tube may not be present when rib guides are used.

INDICATOR. Rotameter. The rotameter consists of a rotating bobbin, or rotor, usually made of aluminum. As shown in Figure 3.21, the rotor has an upper rim whose diameter is larger than that of the body. Special slantwise grooves, or flutes, are cut into the rim. When gas passes between the rim of the bobbin and the wall of the tube, it impinges on the flutes, causing the bobbin to rotate. In the vertical position, the free spinning maintains the float in the center of the tube. This prevents fluctuations, reduces wear and tear, assists the passage of any small particles and improves accuracy by reducing errors due to friction between the tube and the float. When one sees the bobbin rotating one can be certain gas is flowing and the bobbin is not stuck. Deviations from the vertical position will result in the rotor striking the side of the tube, an indication that the flowmeter is not vertical.

Two types of rotameter bobbins are available: the plumb-bob float and the skirted float, shown in Figure 3.21. The skirted variety has the advantage of quicker recovery from mechanical disturbances (55). The reading is taken at the upper rim.

Nonrotating Floats. A second type of indicator, the nonrotating float, (Fig. 3.21) is similar to the rotameter except that it does not have

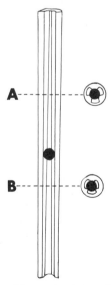

Figure 3.20. Flowmeter tube with rib guides, used with ball-type indicators. The triangular thickening of the inside of the tube keeps the ball centered. The area through which the gas flows increases with increasing height in the tube. (Redrawn courtesy of Fraser Harlake, Inc.)

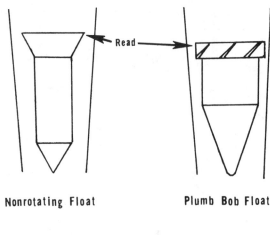

Nonrotating Float   **Plumb Bob Float**

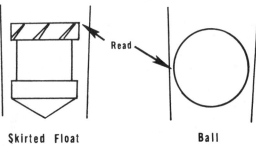

Skirted Float   **Ball**

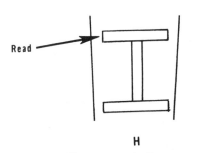

H

Figure 3.21. Flowmeter indicators. The plumb-bob and skirted floats are examples of rotameters which are kept centered in the tube by constant rotation. The reading is taken at the top. The ball indicator is held centered by rib guides. The reading is taken at the center. The nonrotating float and H float do not rotate and are kept centered by gas flow. (Redrawn partly from Binning R, Hodges EA: Flowmeters. Can they be improved? *Anaesthesia* 22: 643–646, 1967.)

flutes and hence does not rotate. The float is designed so that gas flows keeps it in the center of the tube if the tube is kept vertical. The reading is taken at the upper rim.

Ball Floats. A third type of indicator is the ball float (Fig. 3.21). This is made of a variety of materials, such as nickle and sapphire or glass. The reading is taken at the center of the ball. The ball is kept in the center of the tube by rib guides. The ball may rotate and sometimes has two colors so that the rotation can be more easily seen.

H Float. The "H" float or "I" (spool) float, shown in Figure 3.21, is a nonrotating float. The reading is taken at the upper rim.

STOP. The stop at the top of the flowmeter tube performs two functions. First, it prevents the indicator from ascending to the very top of the tube and plugging the outlet. Thus the stop ensures a continuous flow of gas whenever the flow control valve has been opened. It also prevents a rise in pressure in the tube arising from the indicator plugging the outlet.

The second function of the stop is to prevent the indicator from ascending to a point where it is hidden by the flowmeter head. This is dangerous because a flowmeter with the indicator hidden looks much like one which is turned off.

Stops have been known to break off and fall down into the flowmeter tube (56). If it descends far enough to rest on the indicator, it will cause the indicator to register less flow than is actually occurring. Care must be taken to assure that these parts are placed in the proper location after service or repair has been performed.

SCALE. The fourth component of the flowmeter subassembly is the scale. It should be color-coded for the gas it serves. The machine standard requires that the flowmeter scale either be marked on the tube (see Fig. 3.25), or, if separate, be located on the right side of the tube as viewed from the front (Figs. 3.19 and 3.22). On some older machines the scale may not be in this location, so care must always be taken to read the correct scale.

Most flowmeters are calibrated on the lowest accurate point and this is the first mark on the scale. Readings by extrapolation below this mark should not be attempted.

ON-OFF SWITCH. An on-off switch for flowmeters is sometimes fitted to a machine for safety convenience and economy (57). The switch must be turned on to obtain any flow through the flowmeters and sometimes flow through the oxygen flush valve. Turning on the switch usually activates other machine components, especially certain alarms.

Arrangement of Flowmeters. On an anesthesia machine a number of flowmeters for different gases are commonly grouped together side by side as an integral assembly. The part where the

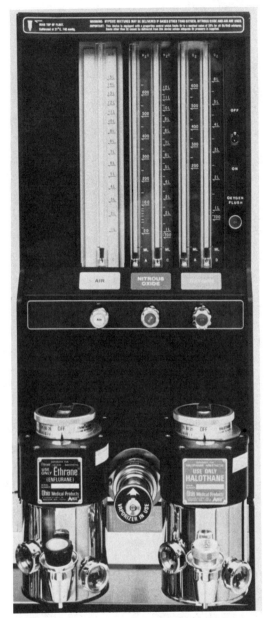

Figure 3.22. Flowmeters in series. Note the on-off switch and the touch-coded oxygen flow control valve knob with fluted profile. (Courtesy of Ohio Medical Products, a division of Airco, Inc.)

machine be equipped with only one flowmeter for each gas or flow-controlled vaporizer.

When there are two tubes for one gas the tubes may be arranged either in series or in parallel. The parallel arrangement features two complete flowmeter assemblies with two flow control valves. The total flow of that gas to the machine outlet is the sum of the flows on both flowmeters.

In the series arrangement (Fig. 3.22), there is one flow control valve for two flowmeter tubes. Gas from the flow control valve first passes through a flowmeter tube calibrated up to 1 liter/min total flow. The gas then passes to the base of a second flowmeter tube which is calibrated for higher flows. The total flow is not the sum of the two flowmeters but that shown on the higher flow flowmeter. For flows less than the maximum on the low flow scale, however, it is more accurate to read the low scale flowmeter.

Because accidental use of a low-flow oxygen flowmeter (when a high flow was intended) is a built-in hazard whenever two oxygen flow control knobs are fitted, the machine standard requires that only one flow control valve shall be provided for each gas. This requirement means that parallel flowmeters will not be provided in the future. When fine and coarse flowmeters are desired, the series arrangement fulfills the requirements of the standard.

Sequence of Flowmeters. Sequence of flowmeters is of great importance. It should be noted that the right hand location of the oxygen flowmeter is the standard in the United States and Canada but is in disagreement with the world draft standard. More countries have the oxygen flowmeter located at the left side. Eger and coworkers (58) demonstrated that improper flowmeter sequence could be a cause of hypoxia. Figure 3.23 shows four different arrangements for oxygen, nitrous oxide, and cyclopropane flowmeters. The normal gas flow is from bottom to top in each flowmeter and then from left to right at the top. A leak exists in the cyclopropane flowmeter (X in Fig. 3.23). Oxygen and nitrous oxide are flowing with the cyclopropane turned off. In arrangement A, oxygen exits both through the leak and through the normal outlet. The amount lost through the leak will depend on the size of the leak and the pressure in the flowmeter head. All of the nitrous oxide will exit through the normal outlet until all oxygen is directed through the leak. Until that time, a portion of the oxygen is flowing toward the normal outlet and this prevents any backward

various gas flows meet is called the flowmeter manifold. Sometimes there are two flowmeters for the same gas: one for low flows and one for high flows. Because use of more than one tube for the same gas has caused problems in the past, the anesthesia machine standard recommends, but does not require, that the anesthesia

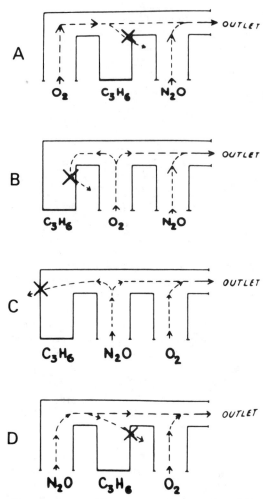

Figure 3.23. Flowmeter sequence. *A* and *B*, with the oxygen flowmeter upstream, a potentially dangerous situation arises if a leak should occur. *C* and *D*, with the oxygen entering downstream from the other gases, a safer situation is achieved. (From Eger EI, Hylton RR, Irwin RH, Guadagni N: Anesthetic flow meter sequence—a cause for hypoxia. *Anesthesiology* 24: 396–397, 1963.)

flow of nitrous oxide. The same situation holds in arrangement *B*, where the oxygen and cyclopropane flowmeters are interchanged. Several cases of hypoxia from this type of situation have been reported (59–62).

The hazard is remedied by using the flowmeter sequence shown in either *C* or *D*. By placing the oxygen flowmeter nearest the outlet a leak upstream from the oxygen results in a loss of anesthetic gas rather than oxygen. The anesthesia machine standard requires that when oxygen and other gases are delivered to a common man-

ifold, the oxygen must be delivered downstream of all other gases.

Prior to discovering that the sequence of flowmeters was important in preventing hypoxia, there was no consensus as to where the oxygen flowmeter should be in relation to flowmeters for other gases. Thus on older machines the oxygen flowmeter might be on the right, on the left or in the center of the flowmeter assembly (63). This was dangerous since an anesthesiologist unfamiliar with a particular anesthesia machine might instinctively reach for the site where he was used to finding his gas controls, but since their positions were reversed, cut off the oxygen supply rather than the nitrous oxide (64). In order to avoid such confusion the anesthesia machine standard requires that the oxygen flowmeter be placed on the right hand side of a group of flowmeters as viewed from the front. If a separate vaporizer flowmeter is placed to the right of the oxygen flowmeter it must be separated by at least 10 cm. The Canadian standards also requires that the oxygen flowmeter be placed on the right (64, 65).

Safety Devices. One of the most important hazards associated with flowmeters is the possibility that the operator will set the flows so that a hypoxic mixture will be delivered. Various devices have been developed to prevent this occurrence.

Touch-Coded Oxygen Flow Control Knobs (66). The anesthesia machine standard requires that the oxygen flow control knobs have a characteristic fluted profile (Figs. 3.22 and 3.24) and be as large or larger than all other flow control knobs. This tactile and visual identity should reduce the hazard of the oxygen flow control knob being confused with that of another gas and thereby unintentionally being turned off or adjusted to a lower setting.

Mandatory Minimum Oxygen Flow. On several anesthesia machines a minimum flow of oxygen is required before other gases will flow. This minimum flow is preset at the factory (sometimes to the customer's specifications). On some machines an alarm is activated if the oxygen flow goes below a certain minimum (even if no other gases are being administered).

This does not in itself prevent a hypoxic gas concentration from being delivered, since if the minimum flow of oxygen is set low a hypoxic gas mixture can be delivered with only modest anesthetic gas flows (67). If the fixed minimum flow of oxygen is set high, high total gas flows must be routinely used.

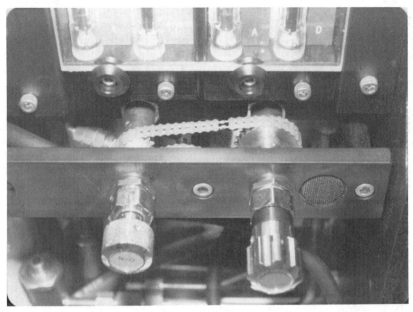

Figure 3.24. Linked oxygen and nitrous oxide flow control valves. Note the touch-coded oxygen flow control valve knob.

Minimum Oxygen Flow in Proportion to Total Gas Flow. Another method of ensuring that a hypoxic mixture will not be delivered is to equip the machine with devices that either deliver a minimum flow of oxygen in proportion to the total gas flow or provide an alarm that is set off if this proportion is too low.

ALARMS. Alarms are available on some machines to alert the operator when the oxygen/nitrous oxide flow rate has fallen below a preset value. Such an alarm may be linked to the main on-off switch (if present) so that it is activated whenever the switch is turned on.

DEVICES (68). Flow control valves can be linked mechanically (Fig. 3.24) or pneumatically in such a manner that the operator cannot set the oxygen/nitrous oxide flow ratio below a factory preset minimum (usually 25% or greater). This permits independent control of the gases as long as the percentage of oxygen flow is above the minimum. If the operator attempts to increase the nitrous oxide flow too much the oxygen flow is automatically increased. If the operator attempts to lower the oxygen flow too much, the flow of nitrous oxide is lowered proportionally. On some machines the minimum oxygen concentration is adjusted higher at low total gas flows to ensure adequate oxygen in the breathing system.

OXYGEN-NITROUS OXIDE PROPORTIONING DEVICES (69) (RATIOMETERS)

Proportioning devices offer an alternative to a block of conventional flowmeter tubes. They combine nitrous oxide and oxygen flowmeter assemblies so that the percentage of oxygen and the total fresh gas flow are dialed directly. In addition they have conventional flowmeter tubes so that the total gas flow and oxygen proportion can be confirmed visually.

The relative concentrations of nitrous oxide and oxygen are varied by adjusting the concentration dial which is usually calibrated between 30 and 100% oxygen. Adjustment of the second dial, the flow control dial, causes the flows of both nitrous oxide and oxygen to increase or decrease, but they remain in the proportion set on the concentration dial.

The Monitored Dial Mixer (70)

The Monitored Dial Mixer (MDM) was the first commercially available proportioning device. It is shown in Figure 3.25. It allows nitrous oxide and oxygen to be mixed in any proportion from 30% to 100% oxygen at total gas flow rates between 1 and 20 liters/min.

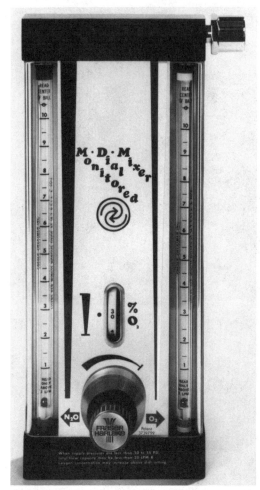

Figure 3.25. The Monitored Dial Mixer. (Courtesy of Fraser Harlake, Inc.)

Components. *Flow Control.* As shown in Figure 3.26, the flow control consists of two nitrous oxide supply regulators in series, one oxygen supply regulator and a flow control pressure regulator. These regulators are quite different and separate from the pressure regulators associated with the yokes. They prevent variations in the gas mixture due to gas supply pressure fluctuations by ensuring that the pressures of the nitrous oxide and oxygen presented to the mixture control dial are equal. They also ensure that if the oxygen pressure fails, the nitrous oxide flow will be cut off.

The oxygen and nitrous oxide supply regulators receive the oxygen and nitrous oxide at approximately 50 psig from either the pipeline inlets or the regulators associated with the yokes and transmit it at a lower pressure to the mix-

ture control dial. Each has a double movable diaphragm with an inner space vented to atmosphere. This inner space prevents internal gas mixing in the event of diaphragm leakage.

Oxygen flows into the flow control pressure regulator and enters the reference chamber. The flow control pressure regulator acts as an adjustable regulator, controlling the pressures of the gases presented to the mixture control dial. The pressure in the reference chamber is varied by adjusting the flow control dial. Changes in this pressure are transmitted to the oxygen and nitrous oxide supply regulators, causing the double diaphragms to move laterally or medially. This ensures that the pressures of both gases delivered to the mixture control dial will be equal.

An increase in the reference pressure moves the diaphragms laterally, causing a higher pressure in lateral chambers. The higher reference pressure at the mixture control valve will result in higher flows through it. When lower flows are desired, oxygen in the flow control pressure system is bled into the oxygen section of the mixture control valve through a control pressure vent orifice. The lower reference pressure causes the double diaphragms in the supply regulators to move medially, lowering the pressures (and hence the flows) of the gases at the mixture control dial.

If the nitrous oxide supply pressure drops, the oxygen flow is unaffected. Should the oxygen pressure fail, the diaphragms in the two nitrous oxide regulators will move to the right, cutting off the flow of nitrous oxide. Having two nitrous oxide supply regulators provides an additional safeguard in the event of oxygen supply failure.

Mixture Control. The mixture control receives nitrous oxide and oxygen at equal pressures from the nitrous oxide and oxygen supply regulators. The relative proportions of the two gases passing to the flowmeters are controlled by a differential needle valve which increases the concentration of one gas while decreasing the concentration of the other.

Flowmeters. Two conventional flowmeter assemblies with ball indicators allow the operator to confirm the percentage of oxygen in the mixture and to measure the total gas flow.

Evaluation. Heath and co-workers (70) investigated the performance of the MDM. He found that the two controls had negligible interaction and the delivered oxygen concentrations were sufficiently close to the mixture control setting for safety requirements over a wide range

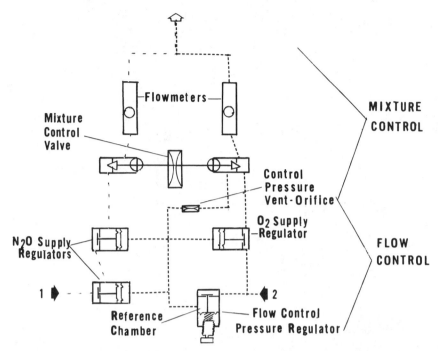

Figure 3.26. Diagram of Monitored Dial Mixer. (Redrawn from Heath JR, Anderson MM, Nunn JF: Performance of the Quantiflex monitored dial mixer. *Br J Anaesth* 45: 216–221, 1973.)

of conditions, including variations in gas input and outlet pressures and a wide range of flows and delivered concentrations.

Ohio 30/70 Proportioner

The Ohio 30/70 proportioning device is shown in Figure 3.27. An on-off valve is combined with the flow control knob, which allows a total gas flow from 3–16 liters/min. The concentration dial allows administration of oxygen concentrations from 30–100% in gradations of 10%.

The Ohio 30/70 proportioner device is shown diagrammatically in Figure 3.28. It has a number of interdependent components.

On-Off Valve. The on-off valve, which is mechanically linked to the total flow control valve, receives oxygen from the pipeline inlet or cylinder regulator and in the ON position routes it to the reference regulator. It has a vent which permits rapid depressurization when it is switched to the OFF position.

Reference Regulator. The reference regulator receives oxygen from the on-off valve at approximately 50 psig, reduces the pressure to 12 psig, and delivers it to the central control section of the proportioning regulator. A bleed orifice in the pressure line from the reference

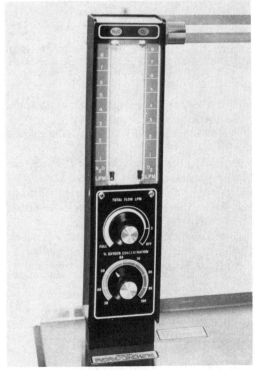

Figure 3.27. 30/70 proportioner machine. (Courtesy of Ohio Medical Products, Inc., a division of Airco, Inc.)

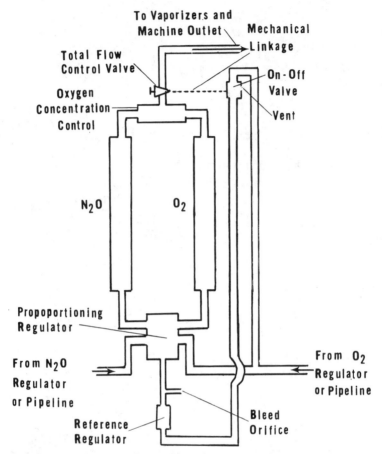

Figure 3.28. Ohio 30/70 proportioner machine. See text for details. (Redrawn from a diagram furnished by Ohio Medical Products, a division of Airco, Inc.)

regulator to the proportioning regulator permits a rapid reduction in the pressure when the on-off valve is turned OFF or when the oxygen pressure fails.

Proportioning Regulator. The proportioning regulator, shown diagrammatically in Figure 3.29, consists of three parts: a nitrous oxide section, an oxygen section, and the central control section. The central section is separated from the oxygen and nitrous oxide sections by flexible diaphragms which are connected to valve stems. These valve stems in turn contact throttling orifices.

Oxygen from the reference regulator enters the central control section and exerts pressure on the diaphragm. This causes the valve stems to move and open the orifices. Oxygen and nitrous oxide from pipeline inlets or cylinder regulators then flow into their respective sections of the proportioning regulator. When the pressure in either section becomes equal to the pressure in the central control section (12 psig) the diaphragm will be pushed toward the center, pulling the valve stem closing the orifice. Thus the proportioning regulator serves to maintain the pressures of both the nitrous oxide and oxygen sections at 12 psig. It also acts as an oxygen pressure failure device, since in the event the oxygen pressure fails, the central control section will depressurize and the flow of both oxygen and nitrous oxide to the flowmeters will cease.

Flowmeters. As shown in Figure 3.28, from the proportioning regulator the gases flow to standard flowmeter tubes which provide a visual indication of the rate at which the gases are flowing and the proportion of oxygen.

Oxygen Concentration Control. From the flowmeters the gases flow to the oxygen concentration control which consists of two inversely

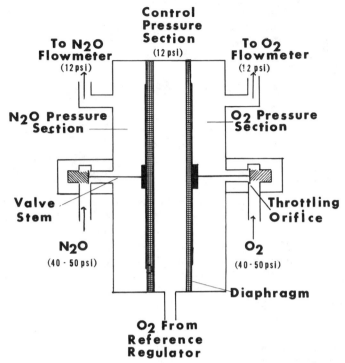

Figure 3.29. Proportioning regulator of Ohio 30/70 proportioner machine. The two flexible diaphragms separate the central control section from the oxygen and nitrous oxide sections. Movement of the valve stems opens and closes the throttling orifices, so that the outflow pressures of nitrous oxide and oxygen remain constant at 12 psi. (Redrawn from a diagram furnished by Ohio Medical Products, a division of Airco, Inc.)

coupled flow control valves. This means that as one is opened the other closes automatically. The control is designed to prevent the nitrous oxide from exceeding 70% of the total flow.

Total Flow Control Valve. The gases from the flowmeters flow through the needle valves into a common chamber where they are mixed and then to the total flow control valve. This valve is linked mechanically to the on-off valve so that when the on-off valve is in the OFF position, there will be no gas flow. Since the flow control valve is downstream of the flowmeters, they are back-pressure compensated (see section on problems with flowmeters), up to a pressure of 12 psig.

Advantages of Proportioning Devices

Convenience of Use. Since the oxygen concentration is dialed directly, it is not necessary to calculate it.

Inability to Deliver a Hypoxic Mixture. Since the concentration dial cannot be set below 30% oxygen, this adds an element of safety.

Disadvantages of Proportioning Devices

Inability to Obtain Low Fresh Gas Flows. These devices are difficult to use for low-flow or closed system anesthesia because there is a limit to how low a flow can be obtained.

A corollary is that leak testing is more difficult with these machines and requires a special device which must be supplied by the manufacturer.

Limit of Two Gases. Only two gases can be metered with a proportioning device.

PROBLEMS WITH FLOWMETERS

Inaccuracy

The importance of accuracy with regard to metering gas flows cannot be overemphasized. Studies of flowmeters in daily clinical use have shown that the percent of error increases as the rate of flow decreases and at flows below 1 liter/min it becomes clinically significant (71–74).

Inaccuracy at low flows is compounded by difficulties with reading. There may be compression of the scale. Most flowmeters are calibrated to the lowest accurate point and this is the first mark on the scale. Readings by extrapolation below this mark should not be attempted. Low flow tubes in series arrangements may help to provide better accuracy when low flows are required.

Inaccuracy can result from many causes.

Improper Assembly or Calibration. Routine maintenance by manufacturers may not include flowmeter calibration checks (71) and a new flowmeter cannot be assumed to be accurate (75).

The flowmeter tube, scale, and indicator are hand-calibrated as a unit under strict conditions for each gas. When any flowmeter parts are broken or damaged, the entire assembly must be replaced. A metal tube may be furnished by the manufacturer to put into the place of the broken tube until a new calibrated tube can be obtained.

Parts should never be interchanged. Reports have been made in which indicators were transposed (76) and in which the indicator and tube were placed next to the wrong scale (77, 78).

When flowmeters are cleaned, they should be removed one at a time and each one reinstalled before the next one is removed to avoid mixing components from different assemblies. A prototype pin indexing system to avoid transposition of tubes has been developed (63).

Dirt. Deposits in the flowmeter tube or on the float are most commonly seen with cyclopropane (12, 13) but occur with other gases. Flowmeters are sensitive to dirt, especially in the low flow range. If the dirt causes a decrease in the area around the indicator, the flowmeter will indicate higher than actual flow.

Dirt can also cause the indicator to stick, giving a reading either higher or lower than actual flow. Hypoxia due to a sticking indicator that showed oxygen flow when the oxygen cylinder was actually empty has been reported (79).

It may sometimes be possible to remove dirt by rapidly opening the flow control valve or by passing a high flow through the tube.

Back Pressure. Most flowmeters on anesthesia machines are not back-pressure compensated and are affected by pressure increases transmitted from the breathing system to the common gas outlet. Pressure increases are the result of use of the oxygen flush valve and from equipment mounted downstream of the flowmeters. These pressure increases cause the gas within the flowmeter tube above the float to be compressed. The lifting effect from gas flowing into the tube at the bottom is reduced and the float drops to a lower position so that it reads less than actual flow. The effect of these pressure fluctuations can be reduced by the use of certain devices near the common gas outlet.

The Thorpe tube flowmeters commonly used in respiratory therapy are back-pressure compensated. Their construction is similar to the uncompensated flowmeters used in anesthesia machines, except that the flow control valve is located downstream of the flowmeter tube. Thus the entire flowmeter up to the flow control valve is pressurized to approximately 50 psig. Restricting devices added at the outlet will cause back pressure, but as long as this pressure does not exceed 50 psig, gas will continue to flow into the flowmeter and the flowrate measurement will be accurate. At least one anesthesia machine, the 30/70 proportioner, is back-pressure compensated.

Improper Alignment. Flowmeters are designed to be kept in a vertical position. If the tube is not vertical the annular opening becomes asymmetrical and inaccuracy results. Also, sticking is more likely if the tubes are not vertical (49).

Static Electricity. Another possible source of flowmeter inaccuracy is sticking of the indicator due to static electricity (80–83). These charges may build up slowly over a period of days (80). It has been shown that as long as the indicator rotates in a normal manner there is no inaccuracy due to electrostatic charges (80). Indeed the first sign of inaccuracy often is when the indicator moves up and down in an irregular manner. In addition to flowmeter inaccuracy static electricity could pose an explosion threat if a flammable agent were being metered (80, 82).

Often a change of gas flow will redistribute the electrical charges so that the indicator becomes steady. Putting a moist fingertip on the flowmeter tube and the machine metal or use of antistatic sprays will remove charges from the outside of the tube. Charges inside the tube are more difficult to remove. Approaches include a radioactive pistol (82), incorporating an electrically conductive material into the tube wall (82, 84), coating the inside of the tube with such a material (80, 81) or application of a metal ring to the end of the tubes where they make contact with antitstatic material. The last two approaches appear to be effective (84, 85).

Float Damage. Float damage can result from the sudden projection of the indicator to the top of the tube when a cylinder is opened or a pipeline hose connected with the flow control valve open. Floats can become worn or distorted by handling, especially during cleaning (86).

Indicator at Top of Tube and Not Noticed

There have been several reports of hypercarbia which occurred because a carbon dioxide flowmeter indicator was at the top of a tube and not noticed (87–91). The bobbin can become impaled upon the stop at the top of the tube and stick in this position even if no gas is flowing (49).

Blockage of Outlet of Tube

The stop at the top of the tube may not be replaced after a flowmeter is cleaned or it may break off (56). This can result in the float closing the outlet so there is no flow, although the flowmeter will indicate a very high flow (92). A leak or rupture of the tube may result.

Flow Control Valve Knob Too Loose

If the flow control valve knob is too loose it may respond to a light touch or even accidental brushing (91). It then becomes dangerously easy to inadvertently alter the flow rates of gases.

Absence of Fine Control

Cases have been reported where only a small rotation of the control knob was required to achieve maximal flow. Cases of cardiovascular collapse (54) and severe hypercarbia (89) have resulted.

Reading of Wrong Flowmeter

It occasionally happens that an anesthesiologist in a moment of stress will reach for a flow control valve and turn it to increase or decrease the flow before he looks at the flowmeter. If he follows up by merely glancing at the flowmeter to make sure a float is at an elevation associated in his mind with the desired result and does not verify by inspection that it is the proper float, he may find that he has used the wrong flow control valve entirely. Deaths have occurred when an indicator was read beside an adjacent but inappropriate scale (1, 50).

Changes in Float Position

On some machines the level of the float may change after it is set (71). A change in the supply pressure (such as occurs when changing from pipelines to cylinders) will alter the float position.

Floats should be observed at frequent intervals, particularly soon after the first setting.

CARE AND CLEANING

Flowmeters should be protected by turning the flow control valve off when cylinder valves are opened or the pipeline hoses connected to the machine. This prevents a sudden rise of the indicator to the top of the tube, which might damage the indicator or allow it to remain unnoticed at the top of the flowmeter. In machines with an oxygen failure safety device the flowmeter for an anesthetic gas or oxygen will register zero when the oxygen pressure is low, even if the flow control valve is open. When the oxygen pressure is restored, there will be a sudden rush of anesthetic gas through the flowmeter, which may cause the indicator to rise abruptly to the top.

Flowmeter tubes may require cleaning from time to time. This is evidenced by the indicator not moving smoothly either up or down in the tube when the flow control valve is turned. Dirt can sometimes be removed by passing a high flow of gas through the tube. Cleaning of flowmeters is usually part of the manufacturer's servicing program and should not be carried out by the user unless so instructed in the service manual. With some machines the flowmeter modules are sealed and any tampering with them can be detected. Such tampering would place responsibility for any problems on the user.

Certain precautions must be observed when cleaning flowmeters. Only one flowmeter should be cleaned at a time. This is to prevent possible mixing of the indicator or tubes, which would result in inaccuracy. Care should be taken not to drop the indicator, as this can cause gross inaccuracies.

The Oxygen Flush Valve (O_2 Bypass)

The oxygen flush valve receives oxygen from the pipeline inlet or cylinder regulator and directs a high unmetered flow to the common gas outlet (Fig. 3.1). It enables the anesthesiologist to flood the breathing system with a high flow

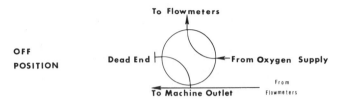

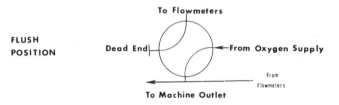

Figure 3.30. Type II flush valve. The oxygen flush is activated by turning a handle 90 degrees. Gas is then directed to the machine outlet.

of oxygen. The ANSI standard requires that the flow be between 35 and 75 liters/min. The standard also requires that concentration-calibrated vaporizers be located between the flowmeters and the common gas outlet so that a sudden high flow of oxygen will not be directed through them. There are three basic types of oxygen flush valves.

TYPE I

The type I oxygen flush valve is part of the type I vaporizer circuit control valve shown in Figure 3.32. When the oxygen flush is activated the oxygen flow to the vaporizer flowmeter is directed to atmosphere. The machine standard does not permit manufacture of oxygen flush valves of this design any longer.

TYPE II

The type II flush valve, shown in Figure 3.30, consists of a plastic cylinder with two channels. In the OFF position, the entire gas flow from the cylinder regulator or pipeline inlet passes through the valve and on to the flowmeters. When the valve is rotated 90 degrees to the ON position, the entire oxygen flow is directed to the machine outlet and the rest of the oxygen circuit is bypassed. Oxygen failure safety valves will then stop the flow of anesthetic gases, so that only oxygen is delivered to the machine outlet.

TYPE III

The type III flush valve is the type most commonly found in modern anesthesia machines. A typical type III flush valve is shown in Figure 3.31. It consists of a button and stem connected to a pin or ball. The pin or ball is in contact with the seat. When the button is depressed, the pin or ball is forced away from the seat, allowing the oxygen to flow to the machine outlet. A spring opposing the ball or pin will close the valve and hold it closed when the button is not manually depressed. The ANSI standard requires that the oxygen flush valve be of the self-closing type, but if requested by the user, it may be specially designed to lock in the open position.

The ANSI standard also stipulates that the flush valve be so situated or designed as to minimize inadvertent operation by equipment or personnel accidentally pressing against it. Barotrauma and cases of awareness (93) caused by this have been reported.

Depending on the machine, activation of the oxygen flush may or may not result in other gas flows being shut off. Activation of the oxygen flush may result in either a positive or negative pressure in the machine circuitry depending upon the design of the inlet of the flush line into the general fresh gas line. This pressure will be transmitted back to other structures in the machine such as flowmeters and vaporizers and may change the vaporizer output and the flowmeter readings. The effect of activation will

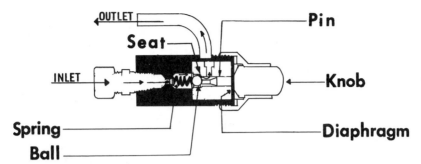

Figure 3.31. Type III oxygen flush valve. Depressing the knob causes the pin to push the ball away from the seat, allowing oxygen to pass directly to the machine outlet. (Redrawn from a diagram furnished by Ohio Medical Products, a division of Airco, Inc.)

depend on the pressure generated, the presence or absence of check valves in the machine, and the relationship of oxygen flush valve to other components.

LOW-PRESSURE SYSTEM

The low-pressure system (Figure 3.1) is the part of the machine downstream of the flowmeters in which the pressure is slightly above atmospheric. The components found in the low-pressure system are the following: (*a*) vaporizers, (*b*) vaporizer circuit control valves, (*c*) back pressure safety devices, and (*d*) the common gas outlet. Because of their complexity, vaporizers will be discussed in Chapter 4.

Vaporizer Circuit Control Valves (Vaporizer Selector Switch)

The vaporizer circuit control valve (VCCV) is used on machines with built-in, measured-flow vaporizers such as the Copper Kettle, Vaporator, or Verni-Trol. The purposes of this valve are to (*a*) direct a flow of carrier gas, oxygen, to the vaporizer when the vaporizer is in use; (*b*) direct the vapor-laden oxygen to the common gas outlet; and (*c*) isolate the vaporizer from the rest of the machine when it is not in use. With all vaporizer circuit control valves, it is important that they be placed in the bypass position when the vaporizer is not in use. If this is not the case, there may be leakage of vapor into the fresh gas line (94, 95).

TYPE I

Type I vaporizer circuit control valve is found on many older machines. It is not being produced any longer and will not be available in the future since it does not comply with the ANSI standard. It is included here because machines having this type of valve are still in widespread use and because there are some potentially very serious problems associated with it.

It is shown diagrammatically in Figure 3.32. There are three inlets: from the vaporizer flowmeter, from the vaporizer itself, and from the intermediate pressure oxygen supply. There are also three outlets: to the common gas outlet, to the vaporizer, and to atmosphere. There are three positions for the valve: VAPORIZER OFF, VAPORIZER ON, and OXYGEN FLUSH. Usually the valve is constructed so that the VAPORIZER OFF position is midway between the VAPORIZER ON and OXYGEN FLUSH positions and the lever is moved counterclockwise to open the vaporizer and clockwise to activate the oxygen flush. Usually the valve can be locked in the VAPORIZER ON or VAPORIZER OFF positions. A few machines allow the OXYGEN FLUSH position to be maintained, but on most the lever returns to the VAPORIZER OFF position when released. Machines which have two built-in vaporizers may have a double control valve, each complete with all three positions, with a selector switch to activate one or the other sets of positions.

A serious drawback of the type I vaporizer circuit control valve is that in the OFF position there will appear to be flow on the vaporizer flowmeter, but the oxygen will be directed to atmosphere and no vapor will be delivered to the common gas outlet. This is most likely to occur at the beginning of a case when the operator simply forgets to turn the valve to the

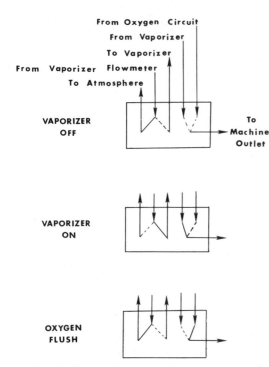

Figure 3.32. Type I vaporizer circuit control valve. The *solid lines* indicate a completed circuit while the *dotted lines* indicate an interrupted circuit. VAPORIZER OFF position, oxygen from the vaporizer flowmeter is directed to the atmosphere. VAPORIZER ON position, oxygen is directed to the vaporizer and returns to the valve carrying vapor and is directed to the machine outlet. OXYGEN FLUSH position, oxygen from the oxygen circuit goes directly to the machine outlet as a high flowrate. Oxygen from the vaporizer flowmeter is vented to atmosphere. (From Siker ES, Wolfson B, Wible LC: *Mechanical Hazards. Ventilators and Inhalation Therapy*, ed 2. Edited by AB Dobkin. Boston, Little, Brown, 1972.)

VAPORIZER ON position. Also it occasionally happens that during use of the vaporizer the need for a flush of oxygen arises and the operator turns the lever from the ON position through the OFF position to the OXYGEN FLUSH position and then after using the oxygen flush the valve is not returned back to ON, but is only moved to the OFF position. In this position, the valve is opened to atmosphere so that the flow registered on the vaporizer flowmeter is not delivered to the common gas outlet. If the vaporizer carrier gas is being used to provide part or all of the patient's metabolic oxygen require-

ments, serious hypoxia may result. Fatalities due to this have been reported. The consequences of not delivering the vapor to the common gas outlet are usually simply embarrassing, but are potentially quite serious.

The ANSI standard requires that all carrier gas flowing through a vaporizer flowmeter be delivered to the common outlet, thus eliminating the hypoxic hazard.

An explosion due to a problem with this type of shunt valve has been described (96). When the oxygen flush was utilized it was flushed into the vaporizer, which caused a rapid buildup of pressure that resulted in a blowout at the weakest point, the glass window in front.

TYPE II

The type II vaporizer circuit control valve is shown diagramatically in Figure 3.33. It consists of a cylinder into which two channels have been drilled. In the VAPORIZER ON position, oxygen flows from the vaporizer flowmeter through the vaporizer and, after returning to the vaporizer circuit control valve, on to the machine outlet. In the VAPORIZER OFF position, the vaporizer is isolated from the machine circuitry and the oxygen flowing through the vaporizer flowmeter is directed to the common gas outlet.

TYPE III

Figure 3.34 shows diagramatically the type III vaporizer circuit control valve. It consists of three parts: an on-off valve, a vaporizer inlet valve situated just upstream of the vaporizer flowmeter, and an outlet valve downstream of the vaporizer. Oxygen pressure from the intermediate pressure oxygen system of the machine controls the opening and closing of these valves through the on-off valve. In the OFF position the on-off valve does not transmit the oxygen pressure needed to open the inlet and outlet valves and the vaporizer is isolated from the machine circuitry. In the ON position, the oxygen pressure acting through the on-off valve causes the valves to open so that oxygen flows to the flowmeter and vaporizer and on to the machine outlet. When the OXYGEN FLUSH valve is activated, the on-off valve is depressurized, causing the inlet and outlet valves to close. All oxygen flow shown on the vaporizer flowmeter is directed to the common gas outlet.

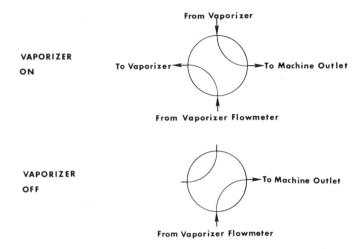

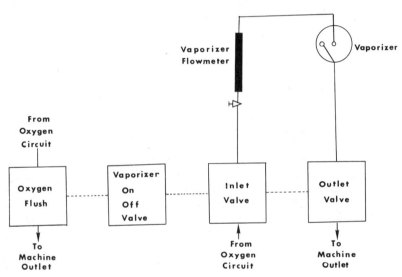

Figure 3.33. Type II vaporizer circuit control valve. In the VAPORIZER ON position, oxygen flows from the vaporizer flowmeter to the vaporizer and returns to the valve where it is directed to the machine outlet. By turning the valve 90 degrees the oxygen from the vaporizer flowmeter is directed to the machine outlet and the vaporizer circuit is isolated. (From Siker ES, Wolfson B, Wible LC: *Mechanical Hazards. Ventilators and Inhalation Therapy*, ed 2. Edited by AB Dobkin. Boston, Little, Brown, 1972.)

Figure 3.34. Type III vaporizer circuit control valve (pneumatic). The *dotted lines* indicate connections which transmit pressure, while the *solid lines* indicate connections where gas flow occurs. When the on-off valve is in the ON position, oxygen pressure from the oxygen flush valve is transmitted to the inlet and outlet valves opening these valves. This allows oxygen from the oxygen circuit to pass through the vaporizer flowmeter, the vaporizer and on to the machine outlet. Turning the oxygen flush valve to the FLUSH position eliminates the pressure needed to open the inlet and outlet valves so that these close and the vaporizer circuit is isolated. (Adapted from a drawing furnished by Dupaco, Inc.)

TYPE IV

The type IV vaporizer circuit control valve is found on only one current model anesthesia machine, the Ohio Modulus machine. When it is closed, oxygen flowing through the vaporizer flowmeter is directed to a measured-flow vaporizer and then on to the common gas outlet. When it is open, oxygen from the vaporizer flowmeter goes directly to the common gas outlet. Thus all gas registered on the vaporizer flowmeter is delivered to the common gas outlet.

The valve is closed automatically via a magnetic mechanism only when the following three conditions have been met: the selector-interlock valve control knob is rotated to select a vaporizer mounting location; a measured-flow vaporizer is mounted in the selected position; and that vaporizer is turned on.

Back Pressure Safety Devices

When ventilation is controlled or assisted, positive pressure from the breathing system is transmitted by the fresh gas line back to the machine. This increase in pressure has been shown to increase the concentration of volatile anesthetic agents issuing from vaporizers in the machine (97). It can also increase leaks and cause inaccurate flowmeter readings. Several devices have been used to minimize this problem.

PRESSURIZING VALVE

One method is to insert a resistance between the vaporizer and the anesthesia breathing system. This in effect acts as an obstruction to gas flow so that the pressure upstream of the valve increases. Small pressure variations in the breathing system then are of negligible effect. This has the disadvantage that it will tend to magnify leaks.

UNIDIRECTIONAL VALVE

Another approach is to insert a check valve between the anesthesia breathing system and the machine (98–100). This will lessen the pressure increase, but not prevent it, since gas must still flow from the flowmeters during inspiration. Such valves carry a potential danger. If a leak or disconnect occurs upstream of the check valve, the check valve will keep the breathing system tight and the problem may not be noticed immediately.

PRESSURE-RELIEF DEVICE

Some machines incorporate a pressure-relief valve near the machine outlet to prevent an excessively high pressure in the system from being transmitted back into the machine and to protect the patient from high pressures transmitted from the machine. This valve opens to atmosphere and releases fresh gas if a preset pressure is exceeded. Use of a pressure relief device in the breathing system just downstream of the common gas outlet has also been advocated (101).

If a direct-reading vaporizer with high resistance is placed downstream of such a pressure-relief valve the resistance of the vaporizer may result in a pressure in excess of the opening pressure of the valve, especially if high gas flows are used, such as when the oxygen flush is activated. The valve may open whenever the oxygen flush valve is used. Such vaporizers are better located between the flowmeters and the common gas outlet.

Common Gas Outlet

The common gas outlet receives all the gases and vapors from the machine. Most machines have an outlet with a 15-mm female slip-joint connection that will accept a standard tracheal tube connector, with a coaxial 22-mm male connection. They may also have a load-bearing fitting for secure attachment of accessory apparatus. Some machines have a locking device to prevent inadvertent disconnection of the fresh gas hose.

Some older anesthesia machines have two common gas outlets: one to a circle system and one to a non-rebreathing system. Multiple outlets pose a hazard in that confusion may arise as to which one is being used and connection to the wrong outlet may result in no gas flow to the proper system (102).

CABINETRY

Anesthesia machines have undergone some alterations in style. The trend now is to allow maximum versatility. Components are usually mounted on a chassis with wheels but may be attached to a wall or a portable stretcher. There are three types of cabinetry available.

Built-In Design

Anesthesia machines with a built-in design (Fig. 3.35) typically have a flowmeter assembly at the back and one or two built-in vaporizers. A significant drawback to these machines is that direct-reading vaporizers are not easily added. Although these machines were produced in great quantity in the past, only one manufacturer in the United States currently still produces them.

Back Bar Design

On this machine the flowmeters are on the left with the outlet on the upper right of the flowmeter assembly (Figure 3.36). The gases then pass directly to the direct-reading vaporizers, which are supported on a bar or rail. Measured-flow vaporizers may also be present.

Modular Design

The modular design machines are the newest generation. The components are separate mod-

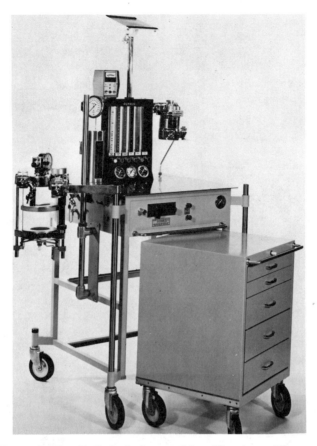

Figure 3.35. Built-in design machine. (Courtesy of Dupaco, Inc.)

ules that can be arranged in different ways within the framework of the machine. (Fig. 3.37). Placement of the components should be made in such a way as to promote more effective human engineering (103) and ease in adding components and making repairs.

SERVICING

Regular servicing is important to ensure that an anesthesia machine will perform reliably. Frequently a machine is not touched until a problem is noted and then it may be in the middle of a case. Servicing can reduce the frequency of such occurrences by replacing worn or damaged parts.

A frequently asked question is who should service a machine. Since many anesthesiologists are gadgeteers at heart, the temptation to modify the machine or make one's own repairs may be great. Servicing an anesthesia machine beyond the procedure described in Chapter 10 requires a detailed knowledge of the components, how

they function, and how they are fitted into the machine. In addition, it is necessary to have the proper replacement parts. It is recommended that the user not perform any service beyond those items which are in the manual that comes with the machine. Maintenance should not be attempted by hospital maintenance, respiratory therapy personnel, or biomedical engineers who have no particular training with anesthesia machines. Very serious hazards have resulted from repairs or alterations made to anesthesia machines by untrained personnel, and such actions will usually void any responsibility of the manufacturer.

Most companies provide service contracts for routine maintenance of their machines. With such a contract a service representative will inspect and perform routine maintenance (including testing, cleaning, lubrication, adjustments, and replacement of broken or damaged parts) on the machine at regular intervals, usually three or four times a year. There is great

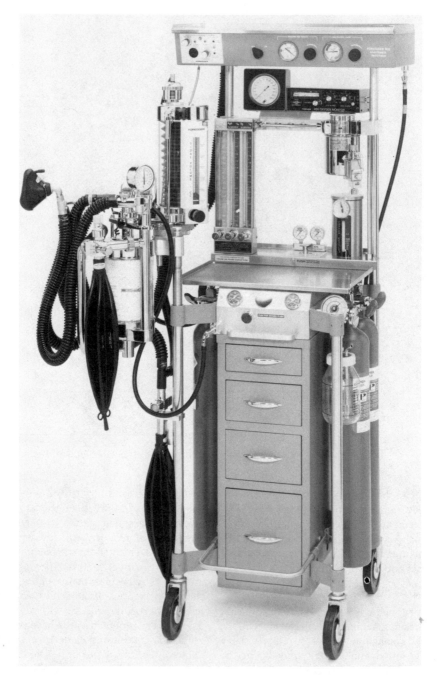

Figure 3.36. Machine with back bar design. (Courtesy of Foregger Company, a division of Puritan-Bennett Corp.)

variation in the quality of service representatives. It should not be taken for granted that servicing has been performed correctly. Whenever alterations have been made in a machine, it should be thoroughly checked before use.

There are important medico-legal implications in proper servicing. Should a problem occur with an anesthesia machine and a patient suffers harm, it is helpful to be able to show that proper servicing was performed. It should be

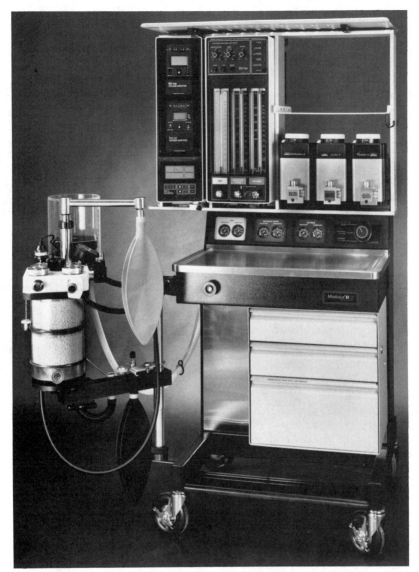

Figure 3.37. Modular type anesthesia machine. (Courtesy of Ohio Medical Products, a division of Airco, Inc.)

noted, however, that routine servicing does not relieve the user of the responsibility for checking the machine before each use and periodically in greater depth (see Chapter 10).

Record keeping is important. Records should be kept of each major piece of equipment including problems that occur, service performed, when it was performed, and by whom. Records on equipment are required by the Joint Commission on Hospital Accreditation, and they can be very helpful in the event of legal action.

CHOICE OF ANESTHESIA MACHINE

Only machines that meet all the requirements of the ANSI standard should be considered for purchase. At the time of the writing of this book, machines that meet this standard are manufactured by Chemetron, Dupaco, Foregger, Fraser Harlake, North American Drager, Ohio Medical Products, and Penlon.

Several things should be considered when

choosing which anesthesia machine best suits your particular requirements. A trial period with a model of a new machine is desirable.

Service

All machines which comply with the ANSI standard should perform well when new. All machines, however, will require servicing from time to time. The quality of that service varies among companies and from area to area within the same company. If you are receiving satisfactory service from one company it would make sense to consider newer models of this company's machines first. If this is not the case you should shop carefully, realizing that any sales representative will promise good service but you must determine which one will actually provide that service. One way is by inquiring into the experiences of colleagues in the same service areas. Determine whether they have long down times waiting for repairs, whether servicing is available locally, whether machines for loan are available, whether service contracts are honored, and the cost of servicing.

Size

Some manufacturers offer compact or wall-mounted machines for small operating rooms. If a machine needs to be transported to other departments outside the operating suite, a small machine will be easier to move. Larger machines usually offer more drawers and a larger table top which can be used as a work space.

Special Features and Accessory Equipment

Certain machines offer important safety features which may make them particularly desirable. Also, the ability to add additional equipment is important, since the practice of anesthesia can be expected to change over the lifetime of a machine. The chassis should be capable of accepting a wide variety of accessories.

References

1. Eger EI, Epstein RM: Hazards of anesthetic equipment. *Anesthesiology* 25:490–504, 1964.
2. Cooper JB, Newbower RS: The anesthesia machine: an accident waiting to happen. In Pickett and Triggs (eds): *Proceedings of NATO Symposium on Human Factors in Health Care.* Lexington, Mass., Lexington Books, 1975, pp 345–358.
3. Epstein HG, Hunter AR: Anaesthetic apparatus. *Br J Anaesth* 40:636–647, 1968.
4. Ream AK: New directions: the anesthesia machine and the practice of anesthesia. *Anesthesiology* 49:307–308, 1978.
5. Chang J, Larson CE, Bedger RC, Bleyaert AL: An unusual malfunction of an anesthetic machine. *Anesthesiology* 52:446–447, 1980.
6. *Minimum Performance and Safety Requirement for Components and Systems of Continuous Flow Anesthesia Machines for Human Use.* ANSI Z-79.8, American National Standards Institute, Inc., 1430 Broadway, New York, N.Y., 1979.
7. *Continuous-Flow Inhalation Anaesthetic Apparatus (Anaesthetic Machines) for Medical Use.* CSA Z168. 3-M1980, Canadian Standards Association, 178 Rexdale Blvd., Rexdale, Ontario, Canada, M9W 1R3.
8. *Pressure Regulators, Gauges, and Flow Metering Devices for Medical Gas Systems.* CSA Z305. 3-M1979, Canadian Standards Association, 178 Rexdale Blvd., Rexdale, Ontario, Canada, M9W 1R3.
9. Horn B: Correspondence. *Anesth Analg* 43:150–151, 1964.
10. Fox JWC, Fox EJ: An unusual occurrence with a cyclopropane cylinder. *Anesth Analg* 47:624–626, 1968.
11. Hogg CE: Pin-indexing failures. *Anesthesiology* 38:85–87, 1973.
12. Bracken A: Deposits in cyclopropane flowmeter tubes. *Br J Anaesth* 48:52, 1976.
13. Russell FR: Deposits in the cyclopropane flowmeter. *Br J Anaesth* 33:323, 1961.
14. Jones RJ: External vigilance. *Anesthesiology* 32:566, 1970.
15. Ranstron RE, McNeill TD: Pin index system. *Br J Anaesth* 34:591–592, 1962.
16. Collins VJ: *Principles of Anesthesiology.* Philadelphia, Lea & Febiger, 1966, pp 120–125.
17. Blum LL: Equipment design and human limitations. *Anesthesiology* 35:101–102, 1971.
18. Mushin WW, Epstein HG: The physics of the reducing valve. *Anaesthesia* 13:198–199, 1958.
19. Macintosh RR, Mushin WW, Epstein HG: *Physics for the Anaesthetist,* ed 3. Oxford, Blackwell Scientific Publications, 1963, pp 119–155.
20. Hill DW: *Physics Applied to Anesthesia.* London, Appleton-Century-Crofts, 1967, pp 37–43.
21. Newson AJ, Dyball LA: A visual monitor for piped oxygen supply systems to anaesthetic machines. *Anaesth Intensive Care* 6:146–148, 1978.
22. Eichhorn JH, Bancroft ML, Laasberg LH, duMoulin GC, Saubermann AJ: Contamination of medical gas and water pipelines in a new hospital building. *Anesthesiology* 46:286–289, 1977.
23. Hamelberg W, Mahaffey JS, Bond WE: Nitrous oxide impurities: a case report. *Anesth Analg* 40:408–411, 1961.
24. Dinnick OP: More problems with piped gases. *Anaesthesia* 31:790–792, 1976.
25. Epstein RM, Rackow H, Lee ASJ, Papper EM: Prevention of accidental breathing of anoxic gas mixtures during anesthesia. *Anesthesiology* 23:1–4, 1962.
26. Schreiber P: *Anaesthesia Equipment, Performance, Classification, and Safety.* New York, Sprin-

ger-Verlag, 1971.

27. Adler L, Burn N: A warning device for failure of the oxygen supply. *Anaesthesia* 22:156–159, 1967.

28. Dawkins M: Anaesthetic safety devices. *Br Med J* 3:299, 1973.

29. Davies RJ: Anaesthetic safety devices. *Br Med J* 4:299–300, 1973.

30. Holmes CM: An oxygen failure warning and patient protection system. The Howison unit. *Anaesth Intensive Care* 6:71–74, 1978.

31. Rosen M, Hillard EK: Oxygen fail-safe device for an anaesthetic apparatus. *Br J Anaesth* 43:103–106, 1971.

32. Ritchie JR: A simple and reliable warning device for failing oxygen pressure. *Br J Anaesth* 46:323, 1974.

33. Treloar EJ, Cornell R: Low pressure warning system with automatic transfer. *Can Anaesth Soc J* 17:83–87, 1970.

34. Ward CS: Oxygen warning device. *Br J Anaesth* 50:907–908, 1968.

35. Cartwright FF: Warning of an empty oxygen cylinder. *Lancet* 2:407, 1963.

36. Davenport HT, Wright BM: Simple oxygen-failure safety device. *Br Med J* 3:570–571, 1974.

37. Hill EF: Another warning device. *Br J Anaesth* 28:228–229, 1956.

38. Grogono AW: Warning device for oxygen cylinders. *Lancet* 1:144, 1965.

39. Scurlock JE: More fail-safes. *Anesthesiology* 42:226–228, 1975.

40. Anonymous: Doctors cleared of perjury. *Br Med J* 3:302–303, 1973.

41. Parfitt R: Anaesthetic safety devices. *Br Med J* 3:635, 1973.

42. Levin MJ, Balasaraswathi K: "Fail safe"? Unsafe! *Anesthesiology* 48:152–153, 1978.

43. Wright BM: Memorandum on oxygen supply pressure failure warning and protection devices. *Anaesthesia* 31:568, 1976.

44. Craig DB, Longmuir J: An unusual failure of an oxygen fail-safe device. *Can Anaesth Soc J* 18:576–577, 1971.

45. Fraser-Jones J, Jenkins AV, Thomas E: Intermittent positive pressure respirations and the "Bosun" oxygen warning device. *Anaesthesia* 20:95–96, 1965.

46. Fraser-Jones J, Jenkins AV, Thomas E: Dangerous anaesthetic device. *Br Med J* 4:1396, 1964.

47. Howells TH: Dangerous anaesthetic device. *Br Med J* 4:1659, 1964.

48. Hurter DJ, Williams D: The Bosun device. *Lancet* 2:480, 1964.

49. Ward CS: The prevention of accidents associated with anaesthetic apparatus. *Br J Anaesth* 40:692–701, 1968.

50. Mazze RI: Therapeutic misadventures with oxygen delivery systems: The need for continuous in-line oxygen monitors. *Anesth Analg* 51:787–792, 1972.

51. Foregger R: The rotameter in anesthesia. *Anesthesiology* 7:549–557, 1946.

52. Friedman J, Lightstone PJ: The effect of high altitude on flowmeter performance. *Anesthesiology* 55:A117, 1981.

53. Kopriva CJ, Lowenstein E: An anesthetic accident: cardiovascular collapse from liquid halothane delivery. *Anesthesiology* 30:246–247, 1969.

54. Lomanto C, Leeming M: A safety signal for detection of excessive anesthetic gas flows. *Anesthesiology* 33:663–664, 1970.

55. Binning R, Hodge EA: Flowmeters. Can they be improved? *Anaesthesia* 22:643–646, 1967.

56. Richardson JC: A potential danger. *Br J Anaesth* 44:610, 1972.

57. Seward EH: An on-off switch for flowmeters. *Anaesthesia* 33:647, 1978.

58. Eger EI, Hylton RR, Irwin RH, Guadagni N: Anesthetic flowmeter sequence—a cause for hypoxia. *Anesthesiology* 24:396–397, 1963.

59. Bishop C, Levick CH, Hodbson C: A design fault in the Boyle apparatus. *Br J Anaesth* 39:908, 1967.

60. Gupta BL, Varshneya AK: Anaesthetic accident caused by unusual leakage of rotameter. *Br J Anaesth* 47:805, 1975.

61. Katz D: Recurring cyanosis of intermittent mechanical origin in anesthetized patients. *Anesth Analg* 47:233–237, 1968.

62. Liew PC, Ganendran A: Oxygen failure: a potential danger with air-flowmeters in anaesthetic machines with remote control needle valves. *Br J Anaesth* 45: 1165–1168, 1973.

63. Rendell-Baker L: Some gas machine hazards and their elimination. *Anesth Analg* 55:26–33, 1976.

64. Wyant GM: Some dangers in anaesthesia. *Can Anaesth Soc J* 25:71–72, 1978.

65. Wyant GM: Anaesthetic machine standard. *Can Anaesth Soc J* 25:436–437, 1978.

66. Calverly RK: A safety feature for anaesthetic machines—touch identification of oxygen flow control. *Can Anaesth Soc J* 18:225–229, 1971.

67. Betts EK: Prevention of hypoxic gas concentrations. *Anesthesiology* 50:75, 1979.

68. Davenport HT, Wright BM: Simple oxygen-failure safety device. *Br Med J* 4:407, 1974.

69. Lundsgaard JS, Einer-Jensen H, Juhl B: High precision mixing of anesthetic gases based on a new principle. *Acta Anaesth Scand* 21:308–313, 1977.

70. Heath JR, Anderson MM, Nunn JF: Performance of the quantiflex monitored dial mixer. *Br J Anaesth* 45:216–221, 1973.

71. Sadove MS, Thomason RD, Thomason CL, Ries M: An evaluation of flowmeters. *J Am Assoc Nurse Anesthetists* 44:162–165, 1976.

72. Saunders RJ, Calkins JM, Gooden TM: Accuracy in rotameters and linear flowmeters. *Anesthesiology* 55:A116, 1981.

73. Waaben J, Stokke DB, Brinklov MM: Accuracy of gas flowmeters determined by the bubble meter methods. *Br J Anaesth* 50:1256, 1978.

74. Waaben J, Brinklov MM, Stokke DB: Accuracy of new gas flowmeters. *Br J Anaesth* 52:97–100, 1980.

75. Kelley JM, Gabel RA: The improperly calibrated flowmeter—another hazard. *Anesthesiology* 33:467–468, 1970.

76. Slater EM: Transposition of rotameter bobbins. *Anesthesiology* 41:101, 1974.

77. Chadwick DA: Transposition of rotameter tubes. *Anesthesiology* 40:102, 1974.

78. Walts LF, Inglove H: Malfunction of a new anesthetic machine. *Anesthesiology* 25:867, 1964.
79. Mazzia VDB, Mark LC, Binder LS, Crawford EJ, Gade H, Henry EL, Marx GF, Schrier RI: Oxygen and the anesthesia machine. *NY State J Med* 62:2845–2846, 1962.
80. Clutton-Brock J: Static electricity and rotameters. *Br J Anaesth* 44:86–90, 1972.
81. Clutton-Brock J: Static electricity and rotameters. *Br J Anaesth* 45:304, 1973.
82. Hagelsten J, Larsen OS: Static electricity in anaesthetic flowmeters eliminated by radioactive pistol. *Br J Anaesth* 37:799–800, 1965.
83. Hagelsten JO, Larsen OS: Inaccuracy of anaesthetic flowmeters caused by static electricity. *Br J Anaesth* 37:637–641, 1965.
84. Dobb G: Electrical conductivity of flowmeter tubes. *Br J Anaesth* 50:1270, 1978.
85. Greenbaum R, Hesse GE: Electrical conductivity of flowmeter tubes. *Br J Anaesth* 50:408, 1978.
86. Hodge EA: Accuracy of anaesthetic gas flowmeters. *Br J Anaesth* 51:907, 1979.
87. Dinnick OP: Accidental severe hypercapnia during anaesthesia. *Br J Anaesth* 40:36–45, 1968.
88. Edwards G, Morton HJV, Park ER, Wylie WD: Deaths associated with anaesthesia. *Anaesthesia* 11:194–220, 1956.
89. Prys-Roberts C, Smith WDA, Nunn JF: Accidental severe hypercapnia during anaesthesia. *Br J Anaesth* 39:257–267, 1967.
90. Ross EDT: Accidental hypercapnia and rotameter bobbins. *Br J Anaesth* 40:45, 1968.
91. Trubuhovitch RV: Carbon dioxide cylinders on anaesthetic machines. *Br J Anaesth* 39:607–608, 1967.
92. Prickett GL: A potential danger. *Br J Anaesth* 44:1335, 1972.
93. Dodd KW: Inadvertent administration of 100% oxygen during anaesthesia. *Br J Anaesth* 51:573, 1979.
94. Cook TL, Eger EI, Behl RS: Is your vaporizer off? *Anesth Analg* 56:793–800, 1977.
95. Greenhow DE, Barth RL: Oxygen flushing delivers anesthetic vapor—a hazard with a new machine. *Anesthesiology* 38:409–410, 1973.
96. Cohen DD, Gorveman JE: "Explosion" in an anesthesia vaporizer. *Anesthesiology* 27:331, 1966.
97. Hill DW, Lowe HJ: Comparison of concentration of halothane in closed and semiclosed circuits during controlled ventilation. *Anesthesiology* 23:291–298, 1962.
98. Keet JE, Valentine GW, Riccio JS: An arrangement to prevent pressure effect on the Verni-Trol vaporizer. *Anesthesiology* 24:734–737, 1963.
99. Keenan RL: Prevention of increased pressures in anesthetic vaporizers with a unidirectional valve. *Anesthesiology* 24:732–734, 1963.
100. Karl WF: Valve and bag assembly for halothane vaporizer. *Anesthesiology* 23:584–585, 1962.
101. Norry HT: A pressure limiting valve for anaesthetic and respirator circuits. *Can Anaesth Soc J* 19:583–588, 1972.
102. Longmuir J, Craig DB: Misadventure with a Boyle's gas machine. *Can Anaesth Soc J* 23:671–673, 1976.
103. Boquet G, Bushman JA, Davenport HT: The anaesthetic machine—a study of function and design. *Br J Anaesth* 52:61–67, 1980.

CHAPTER 4

Vaporizers

Most of the general anesthetic agents in use today are liquids under normal conditions and must be converted into vapors before use. A vapor is the gaseous phase of an agent which is normally a liquid at room temperature and atmospheric pressure. A vaporizer is an instrument designed to facilitate the change of a liquid anesthetic into its vapor and add a controlled amount of this vapor to the flow of gases going to the patient.

PHYSICS

A knowledge of the physics of heat and vaporization is essential to an understanding of vaporizers. The following subjects will be considered: vapor pressure, boiling point, concentrations of gases, heat of vaporization, specific heat and thermal conductivity.

Vapor Pressure

Figure 4.1A shows a volatile liquid inside a container closed to the atmosphere. Molecules of liquid break away from the surface and enter the space above, forming a vapor. If the container is kept at a constant temperature, an equilibrium is formed between the liquid and vapor phases so that the number of molecules in the vapor phase remains constant. These molecules bombard the walls of the container, creating a pressure. This is called the vapor pressure and is represented by the density of the dots above the liquid.

If heat is supplied to the container (Fig. 4.1B), the equilibrium will be shifted so that more molecules enter the vapor phase. The vapor pressure will, therefore, be higher. If heat is taken away from the system (Fig. 4.1C), more molecules will enter the liquid state and the vapor pressure will be lower. It is meaningless, therefore, to talk about vapor pressure of a liquid without specifying the temperature. Vapor pressures of the commonly used anesthetic agents at different temperatures are shown in Figure 4.2 and Table 4.1.

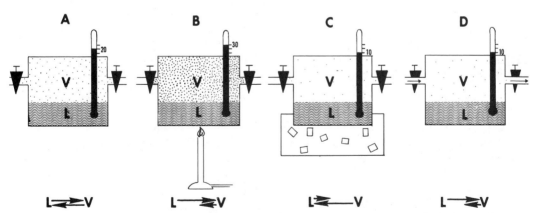

Figure 4.1. *A* to *C*, vapor pressure changes with varying temperature. *A*, the liquid and vapor are in equilibrium. *B*, the application of heat causes the equilibrium to shift so that more molecules enter the vapor phase, as illustrated by the increased density of dots above the liquid. *C*, lowering the temperature causes a shift toward the liquid phase and a decrease in vapor pressure. *D*, effect of carrier gas flow. Passing a carrier gas over the liquid shifts the equilibrium toward the vapor phase because vapor is carried away from the system. The temperature falls as heat is lost during vaporization.

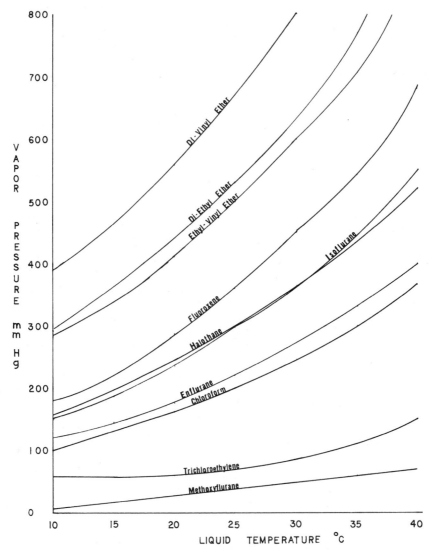

Figure 4.2. Vapor pressure curves of the commonly used anesthetic agents in the clinically useful temperature range.

Vapor pressure depends only on the liquid and the temperature. It does not depend on the barometric pressure within the range of pressures encountered in anesthesia.

Boiling Point

The boiling point of a liquid is that temperature at which the vapor pressure is equal to the atmospheric pressure. The lower the atmospheric pressure, the lower the boiling point. The boiling points for some commonly used anesthetic agents at sea level (760 mm Hg) are shown in Table 4.1.

Concentration of Gases

Two methods are commonly used to express the concentration of a gas or vapor: partial pressure and volumes percent.

PARTIAL PRESSURE

A mixture of gases in a closed container will exert a pressure on the walls of the container. The part of the total pressure due to any one gas in the mixture is called the partial pressure of that gas. The total pressure of the mixture is the sum of the partial pressures of the constit-

Table 4.1.
Properties of Common Anesthetic Agents

Agent	Trade Name	Formula	Molecular Weight	Boiling Point °C, 760 mm Hg	Vapor Pressure at 20°C torr	Density of Liquid g/cc, 20°C	Heat of Vaporization cal/g, 20°C	Heat of Vaporization cal/cc, 20°C	Specific Heat of Liquid cal/g	Specific Heat of Liquid cal/cc	Rubber Gas*	MAC in O₂† %
Diethyl ether	Ether	$C_2H_5OC_2H_5$	74.12	34.6	440	0.71	87	62	0.53	0.38	58.0	1.92
Halothane	Fluothane	$CF_3CClBrH$	197	50.2	243	1.86	35	65	0.19	0.35	121	0.75
Methoxyflurane	Penthrane	$CCl_2HCF_2OCH_3$	165	104.65	23	1.42	58.6	83.7	0.289	0.413	630.0	0.16
Enflurane	Ethrane	$CF_2H{-}O{-}CF_2CFHCl$	184.5	56.5	175	1.517 (25°C)	42 (25°C)	63 (25°C)			74.0	1.68
Isoflurane	Forane	$CF_2H{-}O{-}CHClCF_3$	184.5	48.5	238	1.496 (25°C)	41 (25°C)	62 (25°C)			62.0	1.15

* From Titel JH, Lowe HG: Rubber-gas partition coefficients. *Anesthesiology* 29:1215–1216, 1968.
† MAC, minimum anesthetic concentration. From Quasha AL, Eger EI, Tinker JH: Determination and applications of MAC. *Anesthesiology* 53:315–334, 1980.

uent gases. Under the usual conditions of vaporization, the total pressure will be equal to atmospheric pressure. The partial pressure exerted by the vapor of a liquid is unaffected by the total pressure above the liquid. The highest partial pressure of a gas that can be achieved at a given temperature is its vapor pressure.

VOLUMES PERCENT

The concentration of a gas in a mixture can also be expressed in terms of its percentage of the total volume. The term volumes percent is defined as the number of units of volume of a gas in relationship to a total of 100 units of volume for the total gas mixture. In a mixture of gases, each constituent gas exerts the same proportion of the total pressure as its volume is of the total volume. In other words, volumes percent expresses the relative ratio of gas molecules in a mixture, while partial pressure expresses an absolute value.

Although gas and vapor concentrations are most commonly expressed in volumes percent, patient uptake and the level of anesthesia are directly related to partial pressure, but only indirectly to volumes percent (1). While a certain partial pressure represents the same anesthetic potency under various barometric pressures, this is not the case with volumes percent.

$$\frac{\text{Partial pressure}}{\text{Total pressure}} = \frac{\text{Volumes percent}}{100} \quad (1)$$

Heat of Vaporization

It takes energy for the molecules in a liquid to break away and enter the gaseous phase. The heat of vaporization of a liquid is the number of calories necessary to convert 1 g of liquid into a vapor. Heat of vaporization can also be expressed as the number of calories necessary to convert 1 cc of liquid into a vapor (2). The two values can be converted by use of the following formula:

$$\frac{\text{Heat of vaporization}}{\text{gram}} \times \text{Density}$$

$$= \frac{\text{Heat of vaporization}}{\text{cc}} \quad (2)$$

The heats of vaporization of the commonly used anesthetic agents are shown in Table 4.1.

The heat of vaporization is a function of the temperature of the liquid (2). The colder the liquid, the greater the quantity of heat needed to convert a given amount of liquid into vapor.

The heat required for vaporization usually is supplied in part from the remaining anesthetic liquid. This causes a drop in temperature of the liquid. This is illustrated in Figure 4.3, *left*. The data was obtained by bubbling oxygen through liquid ether. The graph plots the decrease in the temperature of the liquid with time. As the temperature falls below that of the surroundings, a temperature gradient is created so that heat flows from the surroundings to the liquid. The lower the temperature, the greater the temperature gradient and the greater the flow of heat from the surroundings. Eventually an equilibrium is established so that the heat lost to vaporization is matched by the heat supplied from the surroundings. At this point the temperature ceases to drop.

The importance of heat of vaporization is illustrated in Figures 4.1*D* and 4.3, *right*. In Figure 4.1*D* a flow of gas (carrier gas) is passed through the container and molecules of vapor are carried away with it. This causes the equilibrium to shift so that more molecules from the liquid enter the vapor phase. Unless some means of supplying heat is available, the liquid will cool. As the temperature drops, so does the vapor pressure of the liquid and fewer molecules will be picked up by the carrier gas. This results in a decrease in vaporizer output as shown in Figure 4.3, *right*.

Specific Heat

The specific heat of a substance is defined as the quantity of heat required to raise the temperature of 1 g of the substance 1°C (2). The higher the specific heat, the more heat required to raise the temperature of a given quantity of that substance. A slightly different definition of specific heat, more useful to the anesthesiologist, is the amount of heat required to raise the temperature of 1 cc of the substance 1°C (2). Conversion from one quantity to the other may be made by use of the following formula:

$$\frac{\text{Specific heat}}{\text{gram}} \times \text{Density} = \frac{\text{Specific heat}}{\text{cc}} \quad (3)$$

Water is the standard with a specific heat of 1 cal/g/°C or 1 cal/cc/°C.

Specific heat of anesthetic liquids is important when considering the amount of heat which must be supplied to a liquid to maintain a stable temperature when heat is lost through vaporization. Values of specific heats for some common liquid anesthetics are given in Table 4.1.

Specific heat is also important in the choice of material from which a vaporizer is constructed. A substance with a high specific heat will change temperature more slowly than one with a low specific heat. Thus, a container con-

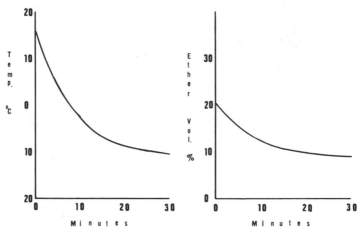

Figure 4.3. Changes in temperature and vaporizer output concentration with vaporization. *Left*, as vaporization proceeds, heat is lost and the remaining anesthetic liquid cools. *Right*, cooling of liquid results in a lower vapor pressure and lower output concentration. (From Macintosh R, Mushin WW, Epstein HG: *Physics for the Anaesthetist.* Oxford, Blackwell Scientific Publications, 1963, p 37.)

Table 4.2.
Materials Used in Construction of Vaporizers

Material	Specific Heat	Thermal Conductivity
	$cal/°C/g$	$\dfrac{cal/sec}{cm^2 \times C°/cm}$
Copper	0.1	0.92
Aluminum	0.214	0.504
Glass	0.16	0.0025
Air	0.0003	0.000057
Steel	0.107	0.115
Brass	0.0917	0.260

structed from a material with a high specific heat will provide a more stable temperature than one constructed of a material of low specific heat, if the masses are the same. The specific heats of some substances used in the construction of vaporizers are given in Table 4.2.

Thermal Conductivity

Another consideration in choosing material from which to construct a vaporizer is the thermal conductivity of the material. Heat flows from an area of higher temperature to one of lower temperature. The thermal conductivity is a measure of speed with which heat flows through a substance (3). The higher the thermal conductivity, the better the substance conducts heat. The thermal conductivity of some common substances used in vaporizers is shown in Table 4.2. Metal transports heat well but glass and air transmit heat poorly.

As seen in Table 4.2, copper has a moderate specific heat and a high thermal conductivity. For these reasons it has been used extensively in vaporizers.

CLASSIFICATION OF VAPORIZERS

Many authors have attempted to classify vaporizers on the basis of a single physical or mechanical characteristic. The wide variety of vaporizers available makes any single method of classification difficult and incomplete. The classifications shown in Table 4.3 list five aspects which describe most of the important points about each vaporizer.

Method of Regulating Output Concentration

The vapor pressures of most anesthetic agents at room temperature are much greater than the partial pressure required to produce clinical anesthesia. A vaporizer must bring about dilution of the saturated carrier gas in a controlled fashion (4). This can be accomplished in one of two ways.

1. The total flow from the machine goes through the vaporizer and is divided into two parts: some passes through the vaporizing chamber (the part of the vaporizer containing the liquid anesthetic agent) and the remainder through a bypass to the vaporizer outlet. This is known as a variable bypass vaporizer.

2. A measured amount of gas is supplied to the vaporizer and all of the gas passes through the vaporizing chamber. It is then diluted by additional flow from the machine. This is known as a measured-flow vaporizer.

VARIABLE BYPASS (DIRECT-READING, CONCENTRATION-CALIBRATED, DIAL-CONTROLLED, AUTOMATIC PLENUM, VAPORIZER CHAMBER BYPASS ARRANGEMENT, PERCENTAGE TYPE)

These vaporizers accept the total gas flow from the anesthesia machine flowmeters and in turn deliver the gas flow, along with a predictable concentration of vapor, to the common gas outlet. The American National Standards Institute (ANSI) machine standard (5) requires that such vaporizers be capable of accepting a gas flow of 15 liters/min.

Table 4.3.
Classification of Vaporizers

A. Method for regulating output concentration
   1. Variable bypass
   2. Measured flow
B. Method of vaporization
   1. Flow-over
      a. With wick
      b. Without wick
   2. Bubble-through
   3. Flow-over or bubble-through
C. Location
   1. Outside the breathing system
   2. Inside the breathing system
D. Temperature compensation
   1. None
   2. By supplied heat
   3. By flow alteration
E. Specificity
   1. Agent specific
   2. Multiple agent

Control of the vapor concentration is provided by a single calibrated knob or dial that is an integral part of the vaporizer. This is usually calibrated in volumes percent. The ANSI standard requires that this control knob open counterclockwise and that a means be provided to lock the control knob in the OFF position.

Figure 4.4 shows a vaporizer with a variable bypass. In the OFF position, the bypass mechanism (*dark squares*) occludes the inlet and outlet of the vaporizing chamber. Gas flows through the bypass to the outlet. In the half ON position, the incoming gas flow is divided into two portions: one part going through the bypass and the other to the vaporizing chamber, where it is enriched or saturated with the vapor of the liquid anesthetic agent. The portion going to the vaporizing chamber is called the carrier gas. Both gas flows rejoin downstream. In the MAX position, the entire inflow of fresh gas may be directed through the vaporizing chamber. In some vaporizers, however, the full on position means only that the maximum amount of gas that the vaporizer will allow goes through the vaporizing chamber. The ratio of gas flowing through the bypass to that flowing through the vaporizing chamber depends upon the ratio of resistances in these two pathways. This in turn

depends on the variable orifices in these pathways. The adjustable orifice in the line through the vaporizing chamber may be in the inlet or outlet line. In most modern vaporizers, it is in the outlet line (6).

The ratio of flows through the bypass and vaporizing chambers also will depend on the composition and flowrate of the gases entering the vaporizer (7–16). The machine standard (5) requires that manufacturers supply diagrams or tables to determine vaporizer output at different gas flows. Also the effect of carrier gas composition on vaporizer output should be supplied. These effects will be discussed in the section on individual vaporizers.

MEASURED-FLOW VAPORIZERS (KETTLE TYPE, FLOWMETERED VAPORIZERS, FLOWMETER-CONTROLLED VAPORIZER SYSTEMS)

This type of vaporizer utilizes a measured flow of carrier gas, usually oxygen, to pick up anesthetic vapor. Each vaporizer system consists of three parts. (*a*) A vaporizer. The ANSI machine standard requires that this be equipped with a thermometer to indicate the average temperature within the vaporizer. (*b*) A flowmeter as-

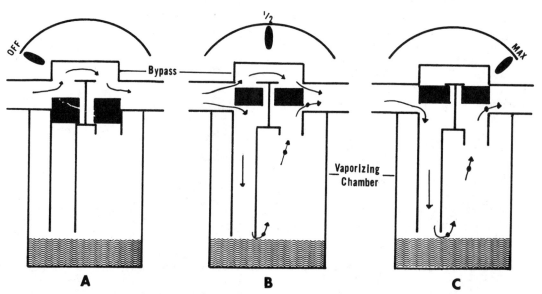

Figure 4.4. Variable bypass vaporizer. *A,* in the OFF position, all of the inflowing gas is directed through the bypass. *B,* in the ½ position, gas flow is divided between the bypass and the vaporizing chamber. *C,* in the MAX position, all of the gas flow goes to the vaporizing chamber.

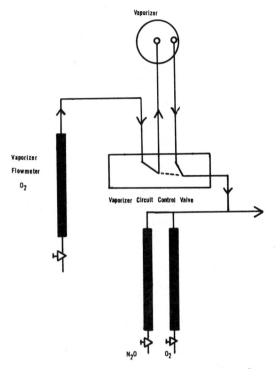

Figure 4.5. Measured flow vaporizer. Gas from the vaporizer flowmeter flows to the vaporizer circuit control valve. In the VAPORIZER ON position, the gas is directed to the vaporizer and returns to the vaporizer circuit control valve. It then joins the diluent flow from the oxygen and nitrous oxide flowmeters and flows to the machine outlet. See Chapter 3 for further details.

sembly. The flowmeter may be calibrated either for the flow of gas acting as a vehicle or for the flow of vapor. (c) A vaporizer circuit control valve. Figure 4.5 shows this type of vaporizer incorporated into the anesthesia machine. A measured amount of carrier gas flows through a flowmeter and on to the vaporizer circuit control valve (see Chapter 3). In the ON position, the vaporizer circuit control valve directs the carrier gas to the vaporizer where it becomes saturated with anesthetic vapor. The vapor-laden gas is returned to the vaporizer circuit control valve. After passing through the valve, it is diluted by gases from the other flowmeters and the resulting mixture flows to the machine outlet.

To calculate the vaporizer output one must know the vapor pressure of the agent, the atmospheric pressure, the total flow of gases and the flow to the vaporizer. The formula is

% concentration

$$= \frac{\text{Vaporizer output of anesthetic}}{\text{Total flow}}$$

$$\times 100 \quad (4)$$

or

% concentration

$$= \frac{(VF)(V_{pa})}{AP(VF + DF) - (V_{pa})(DF)}$$

$$\times 100 \quad (5)$$

where
DF = diluent flow
VF = flow to the vaporizer
V_{pa} = vapor pressure of the liquid anesthetic
AP = atmospheric pressure (see ref. 17)

By using this formula and making periodic adjustments for temperature changes, a vaporizer of this type can be used accurately with a number of different anesthetic agents.

Calculators have been produced to facilitate calculations in these situations.

When calculating the concentration of gases in the outflow from a machine when using a measured-flow vaporizer, it is important that the oxygen going through the vaporizer flowmeter be counted as additional to that metered on the other flowmeters (unless the oxygen on the vaporizer flowmeter has already gone through one of the other flowmeters, as on the Ohio DM 5000). It is important not to turn on a measured-flow vaporizer until the flows on other flowmeters have been set in order to reduce the possibility of a lethal concentration of anesthetic vapor from being delivered.

Method of Vaporization

The method of vaporization refers to the pathway followed by the carrier gas as it travels through the vaporizing chamber. The amount of vapor picked up by a given flow of carrier gas will depend on two factors: the vapor pressure of the liquid and the efficiency of vaporization.

The higher the vapor pressure, the more molecules of anesthetic which will be in the vapor phase and hence the more will be carried away by the carrier gas.

The amount of vapor picked up will depend also on the efficiency of vaporization. Vaporization may be considered 100% efficient if the gas leaving the vaporizing chamber is saturated with anesthetic vapor at the temperature of the liquid.*

FLOW-OVER VAPORIZERS

In a flow-over vaporizer a stream of carrier gas passes over the surface of a volatile liquid and removes vapor. The efficiency of vaporization will depend on three factors: the area of the gas-liquid interface, the velocity of carrier gas flow and the height of gas flow above the liquid.

Area of the Gas-Liquid Interface

The efficiency of vaporization can be improved by increasing the area of the carrier gas-liquid interface. One method is to employ baffles or spiral tracks to lengthen the pathway of the gas over the liquid (18). The method most frequently used today employs wicks which have their bases in the liquid. The liquid moves up the wick by capillary action.

Velocity of Carrier Gas Flow

The speed with which the gas passes over the liquid will influence the vapor output (19). Time is required to establish equilibrium between the liquid and its vapor. If the flow of carrier gas is too fast to allow such an equilibrium to be attained, the vapor output will be lowered.

Height of the Gas Flow above the Liquid

A gas passing just above the surface of a liquid will pick up a given amount of vapor. If the same amount of gas passes high over the liquid, less vapor is carried away (18).

---

* The term "efficiency" as applied to vaporizers has been given a variety of meanings which include accuracy, dependability, and ease of operation.

In this book efficiency of a vaporizer means the ability of a vaporizer to saturate the carrier gas passing into the vaporizing chamber at the temperature of the liquid. To illustrate, a calibrated vaporizer may deliver up to 5% halothane. Inasmuch as a saturated vapor would contain 32% halothane (at room temperature), this might be considered to be an inefficient vaporizer. However, if the internal construction of the vaporizer is examined, only $\frac{1}{6}$ to $\frac{1}{7}$ of the total gas flow passes through the vaporizing chamber, the rest goes through the bypass. The part which passes through the vaporizing chamber becomes fully saturated and is diluted with bypass gas. By our definition, therefore, this would be considered a 100% efficient vaporizer.

BUBBLE-THROUGH VAPORIZERS

Another means of providing contact between the carrier gas and the volatile liquid is to bubble the gas through the liquid. Efficiency of vaporization will be influenced by the size of the bubbles, the depth of the liquid and the velocity of the carrier gas flow.

Size of the Bubbles

The smaller the bubbles, the greater the surface area in proportion to the amount of gas in the bubbles and the more quickly equilibrium will be attained. If the bubbles are small enough, saturation will occur almost immediately (20, 21).

Depth of the Liquid

The deeper the liquid, the more time required for the bubbles to rise to the surface and the greater the opportunity for an equilibrium to be established.

Velocity of Carrier Gas Flow

The faster the flow of bubbles, the less time there will be to establish an equilibrium between the bubbles and the liquid so that saturation of the carrier gas may be incomplete. Bubble-through vaporizers present the danger of foaming (see hazards section), which is not a problem with flow-over vaporizers (22, 23).

BUBBLE-THROUGH OR FLOW-OVER VAPORIZERS

A few older vaporizers could be adapted to either flow-over or bubble-through.

Location

There are two possible locations for a vaporizer: inside or outside of the breathing system.

OUT-OF-SYSTEM VAPORIZERS

Dedicated Circuit

All measured-flow vaporizers are located out of system. They have their own flowmeter assembly and other connections to the system (Fig. 4.5). The circuit is connected to the diluent gas flow at a place upstream of the common gas outlet.

In the Main Gas Stream between the Flowmeters and the Common Gas Outlet

The preferred location for variable bypass vaporizers is between the flowmeters and the common gas outlet. This is the location recommended by the machine standard. In many machines the vaporizers are mounted on a trolley bar to the right of the flowmeter head.

Between the Common Gas Outlet and Breathing System

Vaporizers connected in this location are located in the delivery hose. If a department has a limited number of vaporizers for a specific agent, it might be more convenient to place a vaporizer in this location and move it from machine to machine than to mount it onto one machine and move the entire machine from location to location. The machine standard recognizes this as a possible location for vaporizers and requires that such vaporizers permit the use of flows of up to 70 liters/min.

There are at least three problems associated with using this position for vaporizers. First, it is essential that a vaporizer in this location be properly secured to prevent it from being tipped.

Second, as noted in Chapter 3, some machines have a relief valve in the low pressure part of the machine near the common gas outlet. This vents gas to the atmosphere if a certain pressure is exceeded. If a vaporizer is inserted downstream of such a valve, the resistance of the vaporizer will cause an increase in pressure, especially with use of the oxygen flush. If the pressure exceeds the opening pressure of the relief valve, the result will be the loss of an undetermined volume of fresh gas and a decrease in flow with the oxygen flush.

The third potential problem is incorrect connection. Since the vaporizers are usually connected with slip-on connections between the hose and the vaporizer, it is possible that the flow of carrier gas could be opposite to proper flow through the vaporizer. If the vaporizer were a bubble-through design, retrograde flow of gas through the vaporizer could push liquid agent into the delivery hose. In other vaporizers the output would be unpredictable and possibly dangerously high.

The machine standard (5) requires that variable bypass vaporizers not suitable for use in the breathing system be made available with 23-mm size fittings. The inlet of the vaporizer must be male and the outlet female. The direction of gas flow must be marked with arrows. A manufacturer may make the vaporizer available with other fittings also, but the standard 22- or 15-mm male or female fittings cannot be used. This is to prevent the vaporizer from being fitted into the breathing system.

IN-SYSTEM VAPORIZERS

The machine standard (5) requires that vaporizers suitable for use in the breathing system have standard male and female 22-mm fittings or standard screw-threaded weight-bearing fittings. The inlet and outlet ports must be marked and the direction of gas flow indicated by arrows.

In-system vaporizers may be used in inside the circle system or as inhalers.

In-Circle Vaporizers

The circle system will be discussed in more detail in Chapter 8. It consists of a carbon dioxide absorber, unidirectional valves, fresh gas input source and tubings which form the rough configuration of a circle. Movement of gas inside the circle is determined by the rate and depth of ventilation. A vaporizer may be located on either the inspiratory or expiratory side of the circle.

Inhalers

An inhaler is a vaporizer designed to be used in a breathing system in which air (the carrier gas) is drawn through the vaporizer by the patient's respiration. An anesthesia machine is not necessary. Usually it is used with the patient breathing spontaneously. However, some systems incorporate a means for assisting or controlling ventilation. With some inhalers it is possible to add supplemental oxygen.

COMPARISON OF IN-SYSTEM AND OUT-OF-SYSTEM VAPORIZERS

There are three points of comparison to be made between vaporizers in and out of system: resistance, determinants of vaporizer output, and capability of the vaporizer.

Resistance

A low resistance is more important with an in-system than an out-of-system vaporizer. With an out-of-system vaporizer, resistance is overcome by the pressure of the fresh gas. In-system vaporizers, however, must have a low resistance, because the patient must breathe through them.

Determinants of Vaporizer Output

The term "vaporizer output" refers to the concentration of vapor at the outlet of a vaporizer. The term "vaporizer concentration" denotes the concentration delivered by a vaporizer when fresh gas containing no vapor passes through it (24). In the case of out-of-system vaporizers, vaporizer output and vaporizer concentration are equal. In the case of in-circle vaporizers, the vaporizer receives, in addition to the fresh gas flow, gas containing anesthetic not taken up by the patient. Thus vaporizer concentration and vaporizer output are likely to differ.

This discrepancy between vaporizer output and vaporizer concentration with in-circle vaporizers has implications for safety (24). Certain vaporizers have been alleged to be inherently safe because when calibrated with a continuous fresh gas flow they cannot deliver a high concentration of anesthetic. However, when such a vaporizer is placed in a circle system with a low fresh gas flow, the vaporizer output may rise to a dangerous level.

Capability of the Vaporizer

Capability of the vaporizer refers to the maximum concentration that can be delivered by a vaporizer at the highest setting of the concentration dial. An out-of-system vaporizer or an in-system vaporizer used in a non-rebreathing system must have a high capability because no more anesthetic will be added to the gas going to the patient. The in-circle vaporizer, on the other hand, need not necessarily be capable of delivering high concentrations because the gas may circulate through the vaporizer many times, each time picking up additional vapor.

In-system vaporizers must possess easy access for washing and drying, since water vapor from the patient's expired gases readily condenses on the container.

Temperature Compensation

As a liquid is vaporized, energy is lost in the form of heat. As the temperature of the liquid decreases, so does the vapor pressure. In order to maintain a constant vapor output in the face of this heat loss, two general means have been employed. One is to supply heat and the other is to alter the flow of carrier gas to compensate for heat loss.

SUPPLIED HEAT

Various methods have been employed to supply heat to keep the temperature of the anesthetic liquid stable. One is to use a large mass of copper in the construction of the vaporizer to conduct heat from the atmosphere to the vaporizer (20, 25–27). Because of its high specific heat and thermal conductivity, copper maintains a more nearly constant temperature than glass or other metals. Copper vaporizers may be attached to a copper machine top for even better heat transfer.

In vaporizers containing wicks it is important that the wicks be in direct contact with a metal part so that they can replace the heat lost due to vaporization.

In the past water was sometimes used as the heat source by placing a water jacket around the vaporizing chamber or setting the vaporizer in a pan of water, but this proved to be rather inefficient.

Another method of supplying heat uses an electric heater inside the vaporizer. This adds problems which make its practical use complicated so that no vaporizers with this feature are currently being produced.

FLOW COMPENSATION

Another means for compensating for the decrease in vapor pressure from the lowering of temperature is to increase the percentage of the carrier gas that is directed through the vaporizing chamber. Most variable bypass vaporizers automatically adjust flow by a thermostatic mechanism which opens and closes the point of exit of the gas from the vaporizing chamber. In other vaporizers temperature compensation must be made manually by adjusting the flow. Such vaporizers must have reliable thermometers.

Specificity

Some vaporizers are designed to be used with a single agent whereas others may be used with a variety of agents. This is not necessarily related to the accuracy of the vaporizer because some all-purpose vaporizers are quite accurate whereas many agent-specific vaporizers are quite inaccurate. What makes a vaporizer specific for an agent may be a type of flow device or temperature-compensating device which is geared to the vapor pressure or concentration range of the specific agent. Some older vaporizers had interchangeable parts so that they could be adapted to a variety of agents.

It is important that a vaporizer always be labeled as to its contents. If a measured-flow vaporizer is specific for an agent, the flow control knob for the vaporizer must be labeled with the name of that agent. The use of various agents in the same vaporizer is not advisable, since it may lead to a mixture of different agents in the vaporizer with an undetermined effect.

If two agents have similar vapor pressures, the concentration delivered by a vaporizer designed for one agent should give concentrations close to those on the dial. One study found that when isoflurane was used in vaporizers designed for halothane, the concentrations delivered were acceptably predictable and relatively consistent over a wide range of commonly encountered conditions (28). Another study found that using isoflurane in a vaporizer designed for halothane could result in delivery of excessive isoflurane concentration by as much as 25% (29). When halothane was placed in a vaporizer designed for isoflurane, low concentrations of halothane were delivered. After exposure to a non-specified agent, each vaporizer delivered a lower concentration of the specific agent than before exposure.

EFFECTS OF ALTERED BAROMETRIC PRESSURE

Inasmuch as vaporizers are sometimes taken into hyperbaric chambers or to high altitudes where atmospheric pressure is low, it is important to have some knowledge of how they will perform when the barometric pressure is changed. The ANSI machine standard requires that the effects of changes in ambient pressure on vaporizer performance be stated in catalogs and operation manuals.

Lowered Atmospheric Pressure

VARIABLE BYPASS VAPORIZERS

Most vaporizers of this type will deliver the same partial pressure with decreases in barometric pressure, but will deliver increasing concentrations measured as volumes percent (1). Since partial pressure is the important factor in achieving depth of anesthesia, the clinical effect

of a given setting will be independent of atmospheric pressure. The effect of a change in barometric pressure on the volumes percent output of this type of vaporizer may be calculated as follows:

$$c' = c(p/p')$$

where c′ is the output concentration at a different barometric pressure in volumes percent

c is the dial setting of the vaporizer in volumes percent

p is the barometric pressure for which the vaporizer is calibrated

p′ is the barometric pressure for which c′ is being established.

MEASURED-FLOW VAPORIZERS

With this type of vaporizer the delivered partial pressure as well as the volumes percent changes (1). Partial pressure increases and volumes percent increases even more if the surrounding pressure is lowered. How much depends on the barometric pressure and on the vapor pressure of the agent, and thus on the temperature. The closer the vapor pressure is to the barometric pressure, the more of a percentage-wise effect is created (1).

Speer (30) analyzed the effects of high altitudes on delivered and alveolar partial pressures and total anesthetic depth and found that, as expected, the delivered and alveolar concentrations of volatile anesthetics were greater at high altitude than at sea level using the same flowmeter settings. The total anesthetic depth achieved was the same when 50% nitrous oxide was included in the inspired mixture. This was explained by the fact that the increased partial pressure of the potent agent was offset by the decreased alveolar partial pressure of the nitrous oxide.

High Atmospheric Pressures

VARIABLE BYPASS VAPORIZERS

It might be predicted that the partial pressure delivered by this type of vaporizer would be independent of barometric pressure, while volumes percent would increase. McDowall (31) found that the Fluotec Mark 2 vaporizer delivered the same partial pressure at 2 atm as at normal atmosphere at settings above 2%, but more halothane than predicted at settings of 2% and below. Prins and co-workers (10) suggested that these results were due to changes in density in the gases and that the bypass flow resistance in this vaporizer is more density-dependent (i.e., turbulent) than vaporizer chamber resistance.

MEASURED-FLOW VAPORIZERS

On theoretical grounds it would be predicted that a measured-flow vaporizer should deliver a lower concentration, expressed either as partial pressure or volumes percent, when atmospheric pressure is increased.

In a hyperbaric chamber, as the pressure is increased, liquid anesthetic may be pushed back into the vaporizer inlet (32). This can be avoided if a low flow of oxygen is maintained while the pressure is increased, by filling the vaporizer after the pressure is increased or by opening the inflow line to atmosphere. If a check valve is present to prevent back pressure effects it will prevent equilibration of pressures in the vaporizer. This can be avoided by opening the filling port of the vaporizer or by maintaining a low flow of oxygen. Finally, vaporizers which close off both the inflow and outflow ports in the OFF position may collapse during compression.

EFFECTS OF INTERMITTENT BACK PRESSURE

A factor of great significance when using out-of-system vaporizers is the effect of pressure fluctuations in the anesthesia breathing system machine on the vaporizer output. Numerous investigators have shown that when assisted or controlled ventilation is used, the positive pressure generated during inspiration is transmitted from the breathing system back along the delivery tube to the vaporizer (33–37). Another source of back pressure is the oxygen flush valve. On many machines the output from the oxygen flush valve enters the machine circuitry downstream of the vaporizers. Greenhow and Barth (38) found that activating the oxygen flush valve produced pressures between 94 and 112 torr in the circuit.

This intermittent back pressure may either increase the vaporizer output (pumping effect) or decrease it (pressurizing effect).

The Pumping Effect

FACTORS

Hill and Lowe (34) investigated concentrations of anesthetic delivered by a calibrated va-

porizer during free flow to atmosphere and when used with a circle system employing controlled or assisted respirations. They found that concentrations delivered by the vaporizer during controlled or assisted respiration were considerably higher than when the vaporizer was used with free flow. The following factors affect the magnitude of the observed increase in vaporizer concentration: the magnitude of the pressure fluctuations, the flow of carrier gas and the dial setting of the vaporizer.

The Magnitude of the Back Pressure

Increasing the transmitted pressure increases the vaporizer concentration. Hill and Lowe (34) found that the maximal effect occurred when a mean circle pressure of 20 cm of water was reached. Increasing the pressure further produced little change in the vaporizer concentration.

Flow of Carrier Gas

Hill and Lowe (34) found that the increase in vaporizer concentration was greatest at low gas flows. This was confirmed by Lowe (36) (Fig. 4.6).

Dial Setting of the Vaporizer

The lower the dial setting of the vaporizer, the greater the relative increase in vaporizer output (Fig. 4.6).

MECHANISM OF THE PUMPING EFFECT

Variable Bypass Vaporizers

The proposed mechanism for the pumping effect for variable bypass vaporizers is shown in Figure 4.7a, b, and c. Figure 4.7a shows the vaporizer during exhalation. The flows to the bypass and the vaporizing chamber are determined by the relative resistances of the outlets (3 and 4). Note that the ratio of flows through 3 and 4 corresponds to the flows into the bypass and into the vaporizing chamber.

Figure 4.7b shows the inspiratory phase. The positive pressure at C prevents the outflow of gases and vapor. The pressure is transmitted to A and B. This results in compression of gas in the vaporizing chamber and bypass. Inasmuch as the bypass has a smaller volume than the vaporizing chamber, more molecules go to the vaporizing chamber. The normal ratio between

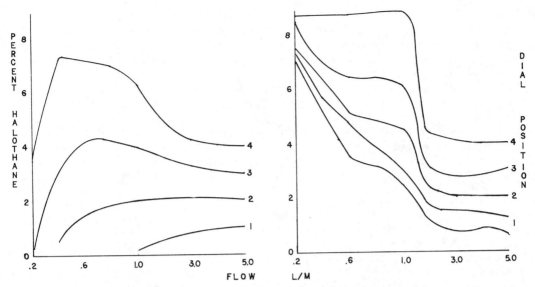

Figure 4.6. Effects of back pressure on the Fluotec Mark II. *Left*, output at free flow; *right*, effects of IPPB. Note that increase in vaporizer output is greater at low flows and low dial settings. (Redrawn from Lowe HJ, Beckman LM, Han YH, Evers JL: Vaporizer performance. Closed circuit fluothane anesthesia. *Anesth Analg* 41:746, 1962.)

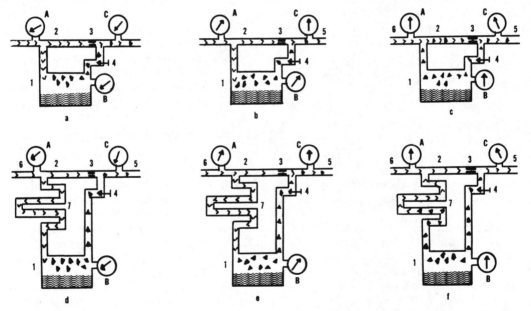

Figure 4.7. The pumping effect in a variable bypass vaporizer. *a, b,* and *c,* during exhalation gas containing anesthetic vapor flows into the bypass, increasing the vaporizer output. *d, e,* and *f,* the long spiral tube prevents vapor-laden gas from reaching the bypass. (From Hill DW: The design and calibration of vaporizers for volatile anaesthetic agents. *Br J Anaesth* 40:656, 1968.)

the flow to the vaporizing chamber and the flow through the bypass is disturbed. There is, in effect, an increased flow to the vaporizing chamber, which then picks up anesthetic vapor.

Figure 4.7c shows the situation just after the beginning of exhalation. The pressure at C falls rapidly and gas flows suddenly from the vaporizing chamber and the bypass into the outlet.

Because the bypass has less resistance than the vaporizing chamber outlet, the pressure in the bypass falls more quickly than that in the vaporizing chamber and gas containing anesthetic vapor flows from the vaporizing chamber into the bypass. Because the gas in the bypass (which dilutes the gas from the vaporizing chamber) now carries anesthetic vapor and the gas flowing from the vaporizing chamber is still saturated, the vaporizer concentration is increased.

Measured Flow Vaporizers

Inasmuch as measured flow vaporizers do not have a bypass, a different mechanism must be postulated for the increase in vapor output with back pressure fluctuations.

As discussed previously, the gas flow to these vaporizers becomes saturated with anesthetic vapor and is joined by gas from other flowmeters which dilutes its concentration. When back pressure is applied, there is a retrograde flow of gas so that the diluted gas mixture is forced back into the vaporizer. Because this gas is not saturated it will then pick up anesthetic vapor. The result is an increase in flow of gas to the vaporizer and an increase in vaporizer concentration.

MODIFICATIONS TO MINIMIZE THE PUMPING EFFECT

Alterations in the Variable Bypass Vaporizer

Changing the Relative Volumes of the Vaporizing Chamber and the Bypass. The increase in vaporizer output from back pressure in variable bypass vaporizers is related to the relative sizes of the space above the liquid in the vaporizing chamber and the space in the bypass. By keeping the size of the vaporizing chamber to a minimum or by increasing the size of the bypass, the effects of back pressure can be decreased.

Preventing Extra Gas Flow to the Vaporizing Chamber from Picking up Anesthetic Vapor. This can be accomplished in several ways. One method is to employ a long spiral or large diameter tube leading to the vaporizing chamber (Fig. 4.7*d*, *e*, and *f*). The extra gas forced into this tube and subsequently returned to the bypass does not reach the vaporizing chamber, so it does not contain anesthetic vapor.

Another method is to exclude wicks from the area where the inlet tube joins the vaporizing chamber.

Special Alterations. A pressurizing valve has been developed for the Fluotec Mark II (39). It is inserted in the gas line just distal to the vaporizer. It incorporates a diaphragm to which is attached a disc held onto a seat by a spring. The area of the disc is smaller than that of the diaphragm. The arrangement is such that the gas flowing out of the vaporizer pushes against the entire diaphragm and opens the valve, allowing gas to flow from the vaporizer. Back pressure from the system, however, acts only on the area of the disc. So pressure fluctuations at the vaporizer are less than the fluctuations in the system and gas continues to flow through the vaporizer through the entire respiratory cycle.

Alterations in the Measured Flow Vaporizer

Decreasing the Size of the Vaporizing Chamber. If the vaporizing chamber is kept small, less unsaturated gas will be forced back into the chamber.

Increasing the Size of the Outlet Tube. The longer the outlet tube, the farther the unsaturated gas will have to pass before picking up anesthetic vapor.

Special Modifications. Some of these vaporizers have a relief valve at the outlet to limit the pressure. Others have a check valve to prevent backward flow of gas. The ANSI machine standard (5) requires a measured-flow vaporizer to have a shutoff valve or check valve, or both.

Alterations in the Anesthesia Machine

These devices (pressurizing valve, unidirectional valve, pressure-relief device) were discussed more fully in Chapter 3. A check valve at the machine outlet offers incomplete protection from the pumping effect, in contrast to a check valve at the outlet of a measured-flow vaporizer, which will eliminate the pumping effect (40, 41).

The ANSI machine standard requires that the line from the oxygen flush valve to the common gas outlet be designed so as to minimize pressure fluctuations that may produce a pumping effect. It also requires the manufacturers to state in catalogs and operations manuals the extent to which back pressure affects a vaporizer's performance. It also requires that the concentration delivered by a vaporizer not change by more than 20% with typical intermittent back pressures.

With these requirements the pumping effect should be a significant problem only with older equipment.

The Pressurizing Effect

FACTORS

Cole (33) investigated the vaporizer concentrations of a Fluotec Mark II used in conjunction with certain systems incorporating automatic ventilators and found that vaporizer concentrations were lower with the breathing system than during free flow to atmosphere. The following factors affected the decrease in vaporizer output: the magnitude of the pressure fluctuations, the flow-rate, and the vaporizer dial setting. The effect on vaporizer output was greater with high flowrates, large pressure fluctuations and low vaporizer settings.

MECHANISM OF THE PRESSURIZING EFFECT

The explanation for the pressurizing effect is shown in Figure 4.8A and B. A shows a vaporizer flowing free to atmosphere. The pressure in the vaporizing chamber and the bypass is P. As the gas flows to the outlet, the pressure is reduced to R. The number of molecules of anesthetic agent picked up by each cubic centimeter of carrier gas depends on the density of the anes-

thetic vapor molecules in the vaporizing chamber. This, in turn, depends on the vapor pressure of the agent. The vapor pressure depends solely on the temperature and is not affected by alterations in the atmospheric pressure. (See section on vapor pressure at the beginning of this chapter.)

B shows the situation when an increased pressure, p′ is applied to the vaporizer outlet and transmitted to the vaporizing chamber (p). The increased pressure in the vaporizer will compress the carrier gas so there will be more molecules per cubic centimeter. The number of molecules of anesthetic vapor in the vaporizing chamber will not be increased, however, since this depends on the saturated vapor pressure of the anesthetic and not on the atmospheric pressure. The net result is a decrease in the concentration of anesthetic in the vaporizing chamber and the vaporizer outlet.

Interplay of Pressurizing and Pumping Effects

Whenever a vaporizer is placed in the fresh gas flow between the flowmeters and the anes-

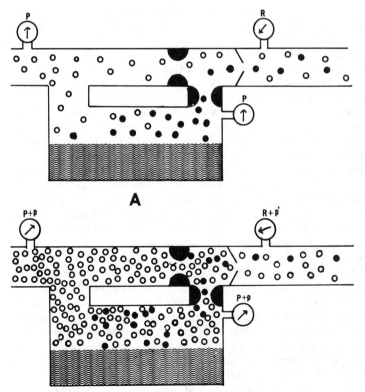

Figure 4.8. The pressurizing effect. An increase in pressure (p′) causes an increase in pressure (p) inside the vaporizer. The vapor pressure of the volatile anesthetic is unaffected by changes in the total pressure of the gas mixture above it. As a result, the concentration is reduced.

thesia system without a device to prevent back pressure effects, the resulting vaporizer concentration will be an interplay between the pressurizing and the pumping effects.

The changes in vaporizer output caused by the pumping effect usually are greater in magnitude than those associated with the pressurizing effect. The pressurizing effect is seen with high gas flow and the pumping effect at low flows. Inasmuch as one is usually more concerned with an increase in vaporizer output than a decrease, the pumping effect probably has more clinical significance.

SPECIFIC VAPORIZERS
Copper Kettle

MANUFACTURER

Foregger Company, Division of Puritan-Bennett.

CLASSIFICATIONS

Measured-flow, bubble-through, out of system, temperature compensation by supplied heat and manual flow alteration and multiple agent.

CONSTRUCTION

The Copper Kettle is designed to be used in the system described in Figure 4.5. Each Copper Kettle is supplied with a vaporizer circuit control valve (see Chapter 3) and a flowmeter assembly. The reader is referred to the sections on the vaporizer circuit control valve in Chapter 3.

The internal construction of the Copper Kettle is illustrated in Figure 4.9. Copper is used in the construction because of its high heat capacity and thermal conductivity. Further thermostability may be added by attaching it to a metal tabletop (19, 20–26, 4).

Gas enters the vaporizer from the vaporizer flowmeter and passes upward through the center tube to enter the surge chamber or loving cup. The loving cup is designed to lessen the effect of a sudden surge of gas into the vaporizer. The gas then passes downward around the center tube and enters the diffuser at the base of the vaporizer. At the top of the diffuser is a sintered bronze (Porex) disc. The disc conducts heat to the gas-liquid interface so that less heat is taken from the liquid itself and less cooling occurs (19, 21, 26, 42). As the gas penetrates the disc, bubbles are formed which rise through the liquid, becoming saturated with anesthetic vapor. The saturated vapor then rises to the top of the kettle and passes out through the discharge tube.

A Copper Kettle is shown in Figures 4.9 and 4.45. A thermometer is present to indicate the temperature of the vaporizer. In front is a window through which the liquid level can be seen. To one side of the window is a scale indicating the number of cubic centimeters of liquid present in the vaporizer. The vaporizer is filled through a filling port at the back. Older models were filled from the top and could be overfilled. Older models should be replaced by new versions.

There are two basic models of the Copper Kettle, differing only in size. The 400-cc model is furnished with a flowmeter which can supply large volumes of oxygen (up to 3 liters/min). The other model has a capacity of 160 cc. It is joined to a flowmeter which provides low volumes of oxygen (up to 400 cc/min).

EVALUATION AND USE

This vaporizer is designed to be permanently mounted on the anesthesia machine and is not portable. This was the first device where precision vaporization was possible (19, 20).

The accuracy of two 1½-year-old Copper Kettles taken from clinical use with no special maintenance was reported by Noble (43) during free flow to atmosphere. His results indicate that vaporizer output corresponds well with the calculated concentration but with a slight tendency toward the low side. One of the vaporizers delivered 0.1% halothane in the OFF position.

Cook and colleagues (44) studied six copper kettle vaporizers and found that none delivered any anesthetic in the OFF position. However, when the on-off valve was turned to the ON position, even with no flow through the vaporizer, appreciable (up to 3300 ppm halothane) and variable concentrations were delivered.

Gartner and co-workers (45) found that Copper Kettle vaporizers delivered concentrations near predicted values over a wide range of vaporizer flows. They also found that the Copper Kettle had the ability to rapidly change delivered concentrations with alterations in the vaporizer flow. They felt the only major disadvantage was incomplete temperature compensation.

Hill and Lowe (34) demonstrated higher than expected concentrations with intermittent positive pressure breathing (IPPB). The effects of intermittent back pressure on the Copper Kettle were investigated further by Lowe and co-work-

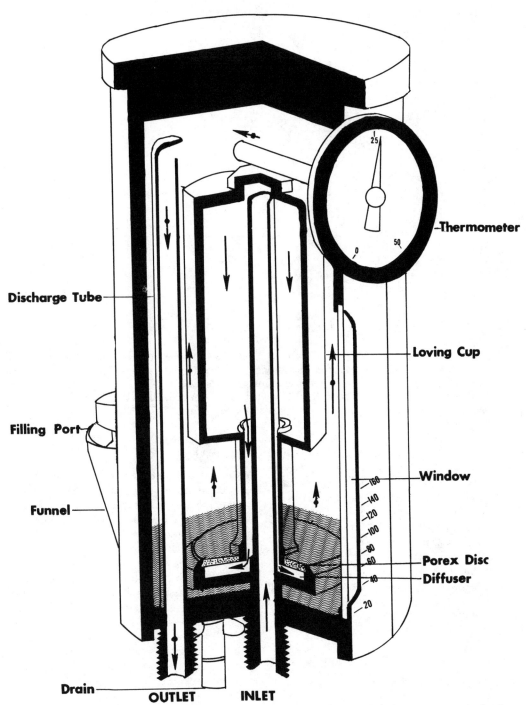

Figure 4.9. Copper Kettle vaporizer. The redesigned version with the filling port at the back to prevent overfilling. See text for details. (Redrawn courtesy of Foregger, Division of Puritan-Bennett Corporation.)

ers (36). The kettle used in their investigations had an internal volume of 950 cc. With a flow to the kettle of 18 ml oxygen/min and a diluent flow of 500 cc, a 1.8% concentration of halothane was delivered during free flow to atmosphere. With IPPB pressures of 20 cm of water and 14

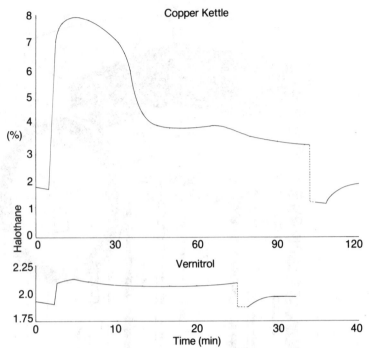

Figure 4.10. Effects of back pressure on the Copper Kettle and sidearm Verni-Trol. With the discontinuation of IPPB, the vapor output drops below calculated value before returning to the expected value. In most newer machines, back pressure check valves eliminate or reduce the effects of back pressure on output. (Redrawn from Lowe HJ, Beckham LM, Han HH, Evens JL: Vaporizer performance. Closed circuit fluothane anesthesia. *Anesth Analg* 41:747, 1962.)

respirations/min, the output of halothane increased to nearly 8%, but gradually dropped to around 4% after 30 min and remained constant until the IPPB was discontinued (Fig. 4.10). At this point the output dropped to 1.1% and gradually returned to the original value after 30 min. The authors attributed much of the fluctuation to the large size kettle being used.

To counteract the effects of back pressure, a back pressure check valve in the Copper Kettle outlet is present on newer machines. For older machines produced before 1968, a check valve may be installed by the manufacturer.

CARE AND CLEANING

Care and cleaning of the vaporizer are important, but it must be remembered that its function is also dependent on a clean vaporizer flowmeter and a properly functioning flow control valve. Periodic inspection and maintenance of these and the vaporizer circuit control valve are essential to the accuracy of the kettle. If halothane is used, the kettle should be drained periodically to prevent the buildup of thymol.

HAZARDS

Most of the problems in the use of Copper Kettle stem from incorrect use. Errors in calculation of the vapor output can be made. It is not uncommon for the operator to neglect to turn the vaporizer circuit control valve to the VAPORIZER ON position.

Older models of the Copper Kettle are filled from the top (Fig. 4.45) and it is possible to overfill the vaporizing chamber. This is most likely to occur if the room is not brightly lit and the liquid level in the kettle is difficult to see. Overfilling may result in spillage of liquid anesthetic into the discharge tube. When the vaporizer flowmeter is turned on, this liquid may be forced into the delivery tube to the system. Newer models are fitted with a side-pour funnel to prevent this hazard (46). Anyone having an older model should replace it with a newer model to eliminate this hazard.

"Tec" Vaporizer (Older Model)

These include the Fluotec Mark II and the Pentec Mark I.

MANUFACTURER

Cyprane Limited, England. Serviced by Fraser Harlake, Orchard Park, N. Y.

CLASSIFICATION

Variable bypass, flow-over with wick, out of system, temperature compensation by automatic flow alteration, and agent-specific (halothane or methoxyflurane).

CONSTRUCTION

The internal construction of the Fluotec Mark II is shown in Figure 4.11. The vaporizing chamber is round and contains a series of concentric wicks. It is provided with a filling tap at the side, a drain at the bottom, and a window on the side to allow observation of the liquid level in the chamber.

The temperature compensation mechanism consists of a bimetallic strip which is located at the outlet of the vaporizing chamber and which regulates the amount of gas that passes through the chamber. This is in contrast to most other variable bypass vaporizers (including the Fluotec Mark III) in which the temperature compensation element is located in the bypass.

The flow of gas through the vaporizing chamber is also controlled by a spindle which moves to the right and rotates as higher concentrations are dialed. In the OFF position the vaporizing chamber is isolated from the bypass and all the fresh gas flows directly to the outlet. When the spindle is pulled toward the operator and rotated counterclockwise, the inlet and outlet ports of the vaporizing chamber are opened while more resistance is offered to gas passing through the bypass. This causes more gas to pass through the vaporizing chamber and less through the bypass.

The vaporizer is pictured in Figure 4.12. The

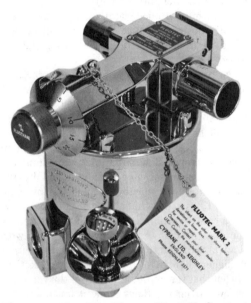

Figure 4.12. The Fluotec Mark II. See text for details. (Courtesy of Fraser Harlake.)

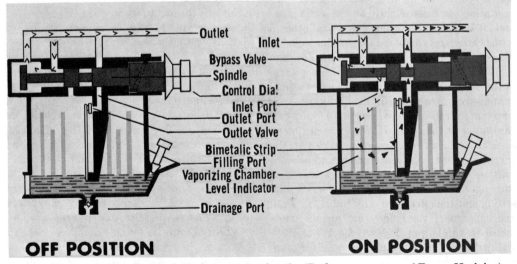

OFF POSITION   **ON POSITION**

Figure 4.11. Fluotec Mark II. See text for details. (Redrawn courtesy of Fraser Harlake.)

control dial must be pulled forward prior to being turned on by counterclockwise rotation.

The Pentec Mark I differs from the Fluotec Mark II in that there are more wicks, the sizes of the openings in the bypass and vaporizing chamber are different, and the temperature compensation device is different.

EVALUATION AND USE

The Fluotec Mark II was the first common concentration-calibrated vaporizers. It is perhaps the most studied vaporizer. Although these vaporizers are no longer being manufactured, there are thousands still in use throughout the world.

Performance data given by the manufacturer are shown in Figure 4.13. It is not accurate at flows below 4 liters/min. A number of authors have calibrated the Fluotec Mark II and found variable accuracy (8, 13, 42, 47, 48).

Lin (8) investigated the Fluotec Mark II in low carrier gas flow situations and found the performance much like that supplied by the manufacturer. At flowrates of 2000 ml/min and dial settings of less than 2%, the vaporizer delivers a concentration less than that indicated by the dial. At dial settings above 2%, and with flow rates of less than 2000 ml/min, the output is higher than that shown by the dial setting. He felt that the unpredictability of the vaporizer at low carrier gas flows made it unsuitable for use in this situation.

The influence of carrier gas composition on vaporizer output has been investigated by several authors with varying results. Stoelting (11) demonstrated that the delivered halothane concentration increased slightly at dial settings below 1.0% when 60% nitrous oxide was included in the carrier gas compared to oxygen alone, but did not find this at concentrations greater than 1%, Diaz (49) found that the output was greater at the 0.5 and 1% dial setting and lower at dial settings from 2 to 4% with nitrous oxide as the carrier gas. Prins and co-workers (10) found that the output of the Mark II was increased at all settings when nitrous oxide was added to the carrier gas flow. Lin (8) found that addition of nitrous oxide to the carrier gas flow increased the vaporizer output slightly at the 1% dial setting, but the effect was only transient. Knill and colleagues (12) found that nitrous oxide increased the output at both the 1% and 3% settings, and these changes persisted for more than 1 hr.

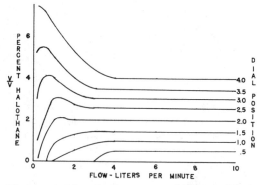

Figure 4.13. Performance of Fluotec Mark II. (Redrawn courtesy of Fraser Harlake, Orchard Park, NY)

Murray and Flemming (50) studied the output of the Fluotec Mark II at positions between OFF and 0.5% at a flow rate of 6 liters/min, and found that the output did not decrease linearly to 0. The lowest concentration delivered with the dial nearly off was 0.44%. When the dial was turned below 0.5%, there was very little decrease in concentration until the OFF position was reached.

Latto (13) also investigated the Fluotec Mark II in the 0–0.5% dial setting range and found that the output was governed mainly by the fresh gas flow (increasing as fresh gas flow increased) and was affected minimally by the dial setting. With the slide pulled out but the dial in the 0 setting, the mean output of five vaporizers was 0.55% with an 8-liter/min flow of 50% oxygen and 50% nitrous oxide. When the dial was halfway back, the concentration delivered was 0. Turning the dial to the 0.5% setting increased the mean output to 0.7%. When a single Fluotec Mark II was investigated using the same fresh gas mixture but varying the flow, the vaporizer output fell with fresh gas flow, so that at a 2-liter/min flow the output was less than 0.1% at a dial setting of 0.5%.

Back pressure plays an important role in the performance of the Fluotec Mark II, particularly at low fresh gas flows (8, 34, 36). A graph showing the results of one investigator is given in Figure 4.6. At fresh gas flows over 2 liters/min the effects of back pressure were insignificant.

Cole (33) used the Fluotec with a circle system and different ventilators. At high fresh gas flows (8–12 liters/min) he found a small decrease in the concentration of halothane in the outflow, which was attributed to the pressurizing effect.

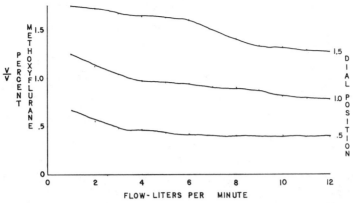

Figure 4.14. Performance of Pentec Mark I. Temperature 21°C. (Redrawn from a graph furnished by Fraser Harlake.)

Cook (44) and Robinson and co-workers (51) found that the Fluotec Mark II in the OFF position could leak small amounts of vapor into the bypass.

Manufacturer's data for vapor output of the Pentec Mark I plotted against fresh gas flow is given in Figure 4.14. At low fresh gas flows the vapor output may be considerably higher than the vaporizer setting.

North and Stephen (52) investigated eight new Pentec Mark I vaporizers and found considerable variation among them at the same dial setting. Stoelting (11) demonstrated that the output concentration of methyoxyflurane varied if the composition of the carrier gas was altered. An increase in the output at the 0.1% setting was observed when nitrous oxide was added to oxygen in the carrier gas. This effect of nitrous oxide was not seen at the 0.3% setting.

CARE AND CLEANING

The manufacturer recommends that both the Fluotec Mark II and the Pentec Mark I be returned to an authorized service facility yearly for servicing.

Halothane contains a preservative which is not vaporized during normal use and will accumulate in the vaporizer. For this reason, the manufacturer recommends that the vaporizer be drained every two weeks and the drained agent be discarded.

HAZARDS

Hazards related to this vaporizer are common to vaporizers of this type and are discussed in the section on hazards.

Cyprane "Tec" Vaporizer (Newer Model)

This includes the Fluotec Mark III, the Pentec Mark II, the Enfluratec, and the Fortec.

Manufacture of these vaporizers has been discontinued with the introduction of the Tec 4 vaporizers.

MANUFACTURER

Cyprane Limited, England. Serviced by Fraser Harlake, Orchard Park, N.Y.

CLASSIFICATION

Variable bypass, flow-over with wick, out of system, temperature compensation by automatic flow alteration and agent-specific (halothane, methoxflurane, enflurane, and isoflurane).

CONSTRUCTION

The Fluotec Mark III, Pentec Mark II, Enfluratec, and Fortec are essentially the same vaporizer with minor modifications for the different agents. They are completely different from the older model "Tec" vaporizers described in the preceding section.

The vaporizer is shown in Figure 4.15. It consists of two sections: a lower vaporizing chamber and an upper duct and valve system. Control of the concentration delivered by the vaporizer is achieved by the rotation of the single control dial. Movement of this dial opens and closes appropriate ports and thus regulates the proportion of gas passing through the vaporizing chamber.

In the OFF position (Fig. 4.15, *left*), gas enters

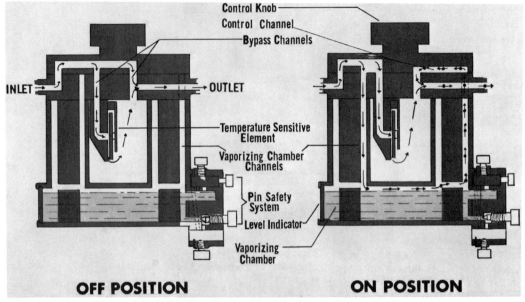

Figure 4.15. Fluotec Mark III. The filter at the inlet is not shown. (Redrawn courtesy of Fraser Harlake.)

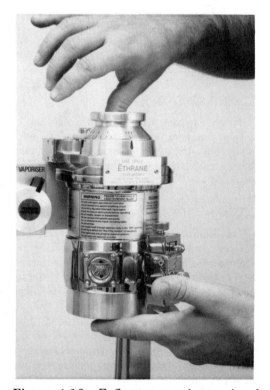

Figure 4.16. Enfluratec vaporizer equipped with agent-specific filling device. The locking lever is at the left of the concentration dial. This vaporizer has an extender ring which extends the base below the filler block. This allows the vaporizer to be placed upright on a flat surface.

at the inlet and passes through a filter to the outlet via two bypass channels. One of these channels directs a small stream of gas past a bimetallic temperature-sensitive element. This element is located concentrically within the vaporizing chamber so that its temperature is close to that of the anesthetic agent (53). The inlet and outlet of the vaporizing chamber are closed to the gas stream.

In the ON position (Fig. 4.15, *right*) the top bypass channel is closed and the two vaporizing chamber channels and the control channel are open. Gas travels down the vaporizing chamber channels and over the liquid, by the wicks (where it becomes saturated with vapor), and out of the chamber by way of the vaporizing chamber channel. The gas then enters the control channel. This channel is long and wide in relation to its depth. Rotation of the control dial increases its depth. Gas still flows past the temperature-sensitive element in the lower bypass channel.

Cooling causes increased resistance to flow in the bypass, so that more gas flows through the vaporizing chamber. The delivered concentration is determined by the resistances to flow of

A selector valve is to the left of the vaporizer. Note the front drain screw and filler plug chained to the agent-specific filling device. (Courtesy of Fraser Harlake.)

both the temperature-sensitive element and the control channel.

Compared to the older models, this model has a larger bypass. The tube leading to the vaporizing chamber is longer and has an expansion area. Wicks are excluded from the area of the vaporizing chamber near the inlet. These changes help to reduce the effects of intermittent back pressure on vaporizer output.

The external design of the newer "tec" models is similar and is shown in Figure 4.16. The concentration dial is turned on by counterclockwise rotation. At the left of the concentration dial is a locking lever which must be depressed to turn the vaporizer on. On the Enfluratec the locking lever must also be depressed to increase the concentration above 5%. On the Pentec Mark II, it is necessary to depress the lever to increase the concentration above 2%. There is a sight window on the left to allow observation of the liquid level and a filling mechanism at the bottom right.

EVALUATION AND USE

The manufacturer's performance data are given in Figure 4.17A, B, and C. Data for the Fortec are given in Figure 4.17D. All are quite accurate with lower dial settings. At higher dial settings, most put out higher-than-expected concentrations at low flowrates and lower-than-expected concentrations at high flowrates.

Paterson and co-workers (53) evaluated the Fluotec Mark III. Their findings of vapor output agreed closely with the manufacturer's data. Noble (42) found also that the Fluotec Mark III was quite accurate. Lin (8) investigated the Fluotec Mark III and the Enfluratec in low-flow situations and found the output agreed closely with the manufacturer's data. He found that abrupt increases or decreases in carrier gas flow, intermittent back pressure, and upstream oxygen flushing had negligible effect on vaporizer output. Another evaluation found the Fluotec III and Enfluratec reasonably accurate (54).

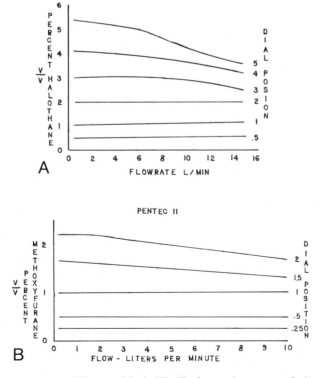

Figure 4.17. *A,* performance of Fluotec Mark III. (Redrawn from a graph furnished by Fraser Harlake.) *B,* performance of Pentec Mark II vaporizer. (Redrawn from a graph furnished by Fraser Harlake.)

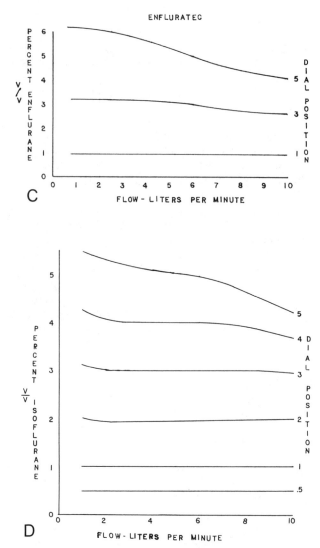

Figure 4.17. *C*, performance of Enfluratec vaporizer. (Redrawn from a graph furnished by Fraser Harlake.) *D*, performance of Fortec vaporizer. (Redrawn from a graph furnished by Fraser Harlake.)

Paterson and colleagues (53) found that nitrous oxide in the carrier gas had little effect on output. This was also determined by Prins (10) for both the Fluotec Mark III and the Enfluratec. Lin (8, 14) found slight decreases in the Enfluratec and Fluotec Mark III outputs when nitrous oxide was added to the carrier gas. Stoelting and co-workers (16) also found a slight decrease in the Enfluratec output with nitrous oxide added to the carrier gas flow.

Latto (13) investigated the performance of the Fluotec Mark III in the 0–0.5% dial setting range and found that, unlike the older model, the output was governed mainly by the position of the concentration dial and was little affected by the fresh gas flow. For approximately the first half of the rotation of the dial from the OFF to the 0.5% position, the output was 0. In the second half of the distance there was an almost linear increase in output to approximately 0.6% at a dial setting of 0.5%. Altering the flow of fresh gas affected the vaporizer output only slightly.

Manufacturer's data indicated no effect on vaporizer output from intermittent back pressure. This was confirmed by Patterson and colleagues (53) for the Fluotec Mark III and by Lin (8) for the Fluotec Mark III and the Enfluratec.

Steffey (28) found that with a Fortec or when isoflurane was put in a Fluotec Mark III peak intermittent pressures of less than 12 torr caused little effect on vaporizer output. Pressures of 48 torr did increase the output. Two authors found that the Fluotec Mark III leaked small amounts of vapor into the bypass in the OFF position (44, 51).

CARE AND CLEANING

To assure continued satisfactory performance from the vaporizer, the manufacturer recommends that annual preventive maintenance be performed.

HAZARDS

These vaporizers are subject to most of the hazards discussed in the hazards section.

Three reports have been made of a faulty vaporizer of this type in which the device which limits the movement of the control dial failed, making it possible to turn the dial beyond the OFF position (55–57). In two of the cases, both involving Enfluratecs, a clinically significant amount of enflurane was delivered. In the other case, involving a Fluotec Mark III, the dial was rotated 180 degrees and there was difficulty in obtaining a satisfactory vapor output.

Another case report has been made in which a damaged compression gasket in a Fluotec Mark III caused a leak that allowed half the fresh gas flow to exit around the top of the vaporizer when the control dial was at a setting other than 0 (22).

Tec 4 Vaporizer

These include the Fluotec 4, Enfluratec 4, and the Fortec 4.

MANUFACTURER

Cyprane Limited, England. Serviced by Fraser Harlake, Orchard Park, N.Y.

CLASSIFICATION

Variable bypass flow-over with wick, out of system, temperature compensation by automatic flow alteration (variation of bypass flow) and agent-specific (halothane, enflurane, or isoflurane).

CONSTRUCTION

The Tec 4 vaporizers are modified versions of the Tec 3 vaporizers discussed previously. They are designed to be attached to the back bar of the anesthesia machine by means of the Select-a-Tec manifold system which allows for easy removal and exchange of vaporizers.

The Fortec 4 is shown in Figure 4.18. On top is a control dial that is turned counterclockwise to increase the concentration. A release button is located to the left of the control dial. This must be depressed before the vaporizer can be turned on. To the rear of the control dial is a locking lever. This is connected with the control dial so that the vaporizer cannot be turned on until it is locked on the manifold.

Before mounting a vaporizer, any adjacent vaporizer must be turned off and the control dial must be in the OFF position. The vaporizer

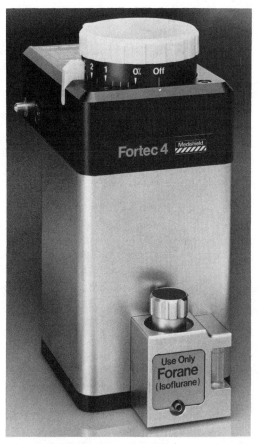

Figure 4.18. Fortec 4 vaporizer. (Courtesy of Fraser Harlake.)

is fitted onto the manifold and the locking lever turned clockwise to the LOCKED position.

When the vaporizer is turned on, two plungers within the vaporizer operate to open the valve ports in the back bar, connecting the vaporizer into the fresh gas stream. These cause the vaporizer to be isolated from the fresh gas flow when the vaporizer is turned off. Also, when the vaporizer is turned on, two extension rods are extended and locked. These prevent operation of any adjacent vaporizer.

To remove a vaporizer from the manifold, the control dial is turned to OFF and the locking lever is turned to the UNLOCK position. The vaporizer can then be lifted off the manifold.

The vaporizer is available with either of two filling mechanisms. One is a screw cap, shown in Figure 4.18. Below the cap is a drain plug which extends into the center of the cap. This plug is unscrewed to drain the vaporizer. The other filling device is a keyed filling system that differs from the filling system previously offered in that there is a single port for filling and emptying. To fill, the adaptor attached to the bottle is inserted into the port with the bottle downward and the clamp screw is tightened. The bottle is then lifted up and a valve on the top of the filler unit opened. After the desired level of liquid has been reached (as seen through the sight tube on the side), the valve on the top is closed, the bottle lowered, the screw clamp loosened, and the bottle removed. The same procedure is used to drain the vaporizer, except that the bottle is always held below the level of the vaporizer.

A diagram of the internal construction of the vaporizer is shown in Figure 4.19. When the vaporizer is in the OFF position, incoming gas flows from the inlet, through the bypass, and on to the outlet. When the vaporizer is turned to ON, the incoming stream of gas is split into two streams by the rotary valve attached to the concentration setting dial. One stream is directed through the vaporizing chamber. That gas first enters one of two chambers which surround the bypass chamber. After passing from this chamber it is directed over two concentric wicks along the sides of the vaporizer. The wicks enclose a copper helix which convert this space into a long spiral outlet channel. The wicks dip into the liquid and assure maximum contact between the carrier gas and the anesthetic agent. The vapor-laden gas leaves via the second chamber surrounding the bypass chamber, past the rotary valve to the outlet.

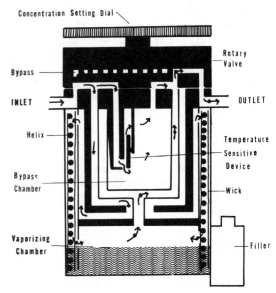

Figure 4.19. Diagram of Tec 4 vaporizer. See text for details. (Redrawn from a diagram furnished by Fraser Harlake.)

The balance of the fresh gas flow to the vaporizer passes through the bypass chamber. Inside this chamber is a temperature-sensitive element which causes more gas to flow into the vaporizing chamber as the vapor cools.

The internal construction of the vaporizer is designed so that liquid agent cannot reach the valve mechanism after tilting or even inversion.

EVALUATION AND USE

The manufacturer's performance data for the Fluotec 4 and Enfluratec 4 are given in Figures 4.20A and B. Steady back pressure will reduce the vapor output. Under normal clinical circumstances the effect is of such small magnitude that it can be ignored.

Pressures in excess of approximately 400 mm Hg should not be imposed on the vaporizer, since these may overcome the loads imposed by internal thrust springs. The effects of these excess pressures cannot be predicted but will most likely cause a reduction in output concentration.

Fluctuating back pressures can increase the concentration by intermittently altering the flow distribution within the vaporizer. The greatest effects are observed with low flowrates, low dial settings, and large and frequent pressure fluctuations. This vaporizer is designed to comply with specifications in the ANSI anesthesia machine standard so that output will not be

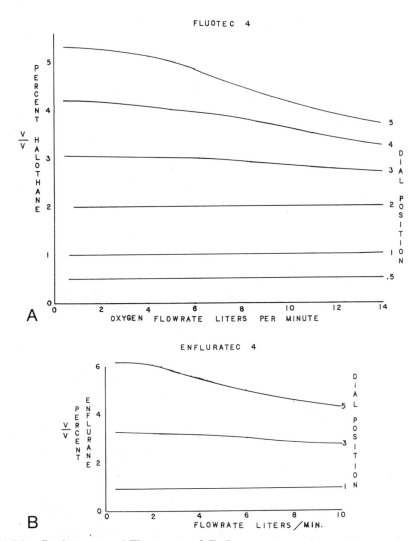

Figure 4.20. Performance of Fluotec 4 and Enfluratec 4 vaporizers at various flowrates and vaporizer settings. (Redrawn from graphs furnished by Fraser Harlake.)

affected by fluctuating back pressures that occur under normal clinical conditions.

Carrier gas composition affects the output of the vaporizer. Variations in output with carrier gas composition are normally less than 10% of setting. The usual effect is that the output is slightly depressed when nitrous oxide is employed compared with when oxygen is the carrier gas.

The vaporizer should be filled and used in an upright position. Small deviations from the upright position will not affect the output or the safety of the vaporizer, but may give a misleading impression of the amount of agent in the vaporizer.

CARE AND CLEANING

The manufacturer recommends that the vaporizer be returned for servicing annually. In-field calibration is not a satisfactory substitute for this servicing.

When the liquid level is low, it is good practice to drain the vaporizer of residual anaesthetic agent and discard the small amount of liquid. This will preserve drug purity by removing oxidized impurities, accumulated stabilizers and contaminants.

At intervals—ideally not exceeding two weeks—when the liquid is low, the vaporizers should be drained into an appropriately marked container and the liquid discarded. Less frequent intervals may be used if the anesthetic agent does not contain additives or stabilizing agents.

Foregger "Matic" Direct-Reading Vaporizers

These include the Fluomatic, Pentomatic, Ethermatic, Enfluramatic, and the Isofluromatic.

MANUFACTURER

Foregger Company, Division of Puritan Bennett Corporation.

CLASSIFICATION

Variable bypass, flow-over with wick, out of system, temperature compensation by automatic flow alteration, and agent-specific (diethyl ether, halothane, methoxyflurane, enflurane, isoflurane).

CONSTRUCTION

The Foregger direct-reading vaporizer for halothane is shown in Figure 4.21. In the ON position, the gas enters the vaporizer through the inlet and is divided into two streams. One stream passes through a bypass resistance to the vaporizer outlet. The second stream passes through a long spiral tube to the vaporizing chamber. In the vaporizing chamber, the carrier gas passes over the liquid and around the wicks to the outlet. The control valve regulates the size of the outlet of the vaporizing chamber. It consists of two resistance elements in series attached through a stem to the control dial. The variable resistance, which is composed of a specially treated Teflon, is tapered so that as the concentration on the dial is increased, the opening becomes larger and more gas passes through the chamber. As the temperature changes, the plastic expands or contracts, allowing more or less gas to pass through. The variable resistance is so designed that it does not come into contact with its seat even in the OFF position. This reduces wear which might impair the accuracy of the vaporizer. The second or fixed resistance is composed of Teflon and operates in series with the first element to achieve temperature compensation.

The vapor-laden gas then joins the main stream of gas from the bypass and travels to the vaporizer outlet. An additional feature is a relief valve which allows a sudden surge of gas (such as occurs when the oxygen flush valve is used) to flow through the bypass instead of the vaporizing chamber. It opens at 3–4 psi.

When the vaporizer control dial is turned

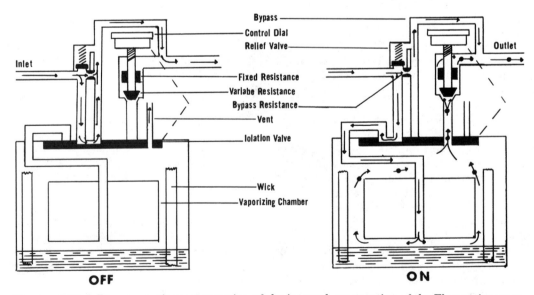

Figure 4.21. Diagrammatic representation of the internal construction of the Fluomatic vaporizer in both ON and OFF positions. (Redrawn courtesy of Foregger, Division of Puritan-Bennett Corporation.)

below the lowest setting a resistance can be felt because of the movement of the isolation valve to the right, as shown in Figure 4.21, *left*. In the OFF position the isolation valve diverts the stream of gas from the tube leading to the vaporizing chamber around the bypass resistance to the vaporizer outlet. The outlet from the vaporizing chamber is also blocked.

The external construction of the Foregger vaporizers is shown in Figures 4.22 and 4.45. The original model (Fig. 4.45) has a top-mounted dial which was turned in a clockwise direction to increase the concentration. This direction of turning does not conform to the new machine standard which requires control dials to be turned on in the counterclockwise direction. A front-mounted version has been developed which conforms to this standard. It is shown in Figure 4.22. The control dial is the outer ring which when turned counterclockwise increases the concentration. The arrow on the ring points to the concentration. The internal construction of the vaporizer is unchanged from the top-dial model.

There is a sight window at the base of the vaporizer. This is at the bottom left on funnel filled models (see Figs. 4.22 and 4.45) and incorporated into the filler block on models so equipped.

EVALUATION AND USE

The manufacturer's performance characteristics for the Fluomatic and the Pentomatic are given in Figures 4.23 and 4.24. Accuracy is greatest at flows less than 5 liters/min. and at lower

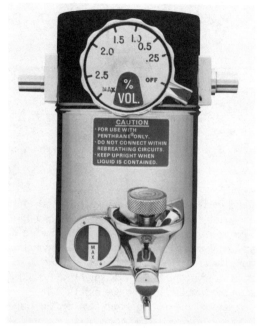

Figure 4.22. Foregger DRV with front face control knob. (Courtesy of Foregger, Division of Puritan-Bennett Corporation.)

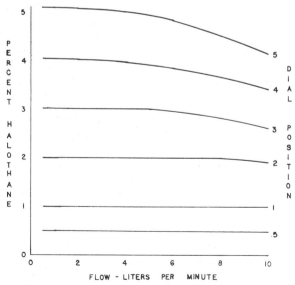

Figure 4.23. Fluomatic performance. Temperature 21°C. (Redrawn courtesy of Foregger, Division of Puritan-Bennett Corporation.)

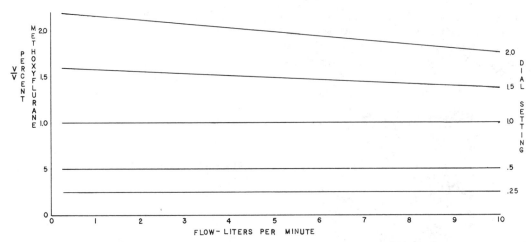

Figure 4.24. Performance of Pentomatic vaporizer. Temperature 70°F. (Redrawn courtesy of Foregger, Division of Puritan-Bennett Corporation.)

concentrations. Bluth (47) investigated the Flu-omatic and found it performed well. Lin (8) investigated the Fluomatic and Enfluramatic and judged them acceptable for use with low flows, although upstream oxygen flushing increased the output concentration more than 10%.

The vaporizer is back pressure compensated. This is accomplished primarily with the long spiral tube inlet to the vaporizing chamber. Lin (8) found no demonstrable effects from intermittent back pressure. Steffey (28) found when pressures of 48 torr were used, there was a decrease in the concentration of isoflurane delivered by a Fluomatic.

The outputs of the Fluomatic and Enfluramatic decrease when nitrous oxide is added to the carrier gas (8, 49). Cook and co-workers (44) found that the Fluomatic did leak small amounts of vapor into the bypass gas when in the OFF position.

CARE AND CLEANING

As with any piece of precision equipment, it must receive periodic maintenance. It should be serviced once a year by the manufacturer.

HAZARDS

In addition to the hazards listed in the hazards section, two possible problems should be kept in mind with the older model vaporizers. It is possible to inadvertently turn the dial when the vaporizer is mounted in certain positions. The position on the back bar of certain machines puts the vaporizer high enough that assistants may grab the dial when moving the machine. This may cause inadvertent administration of an agent or increase or decrease the concentration. If the vaporizer is mounted low and to the front of a machine, the dial might be turned if someone brushed against the dial.

It should be kept in mind that on the older model vaporizers the concentration dial is turned clockwise (looking at it from the top) to increase the concentration. This could cause confusion as in the future most vaporizers will require turning in the other direction to increase the output.

A case has been reported in which the plastic piece which makes the clicking sounds as the concentration is changed broke off (58). This jammed the dial at the 1.2% position, preventing the vaporizer from being turned off.

Ohio Calibrated Vaporizer

MANUFACTURER

Ohio Medical Products, Madison, Wis.

CLASSIFICATION

Variable bypass, flow-over with wick, out of system, temperature compensation by flow alteration, agent-specific (halothane, enflurane, or isoflurane).

CONSTRUCTION

A schematic drawing of the Ohio calibrated vaporizer is shown in Figure 4.25. The carrier

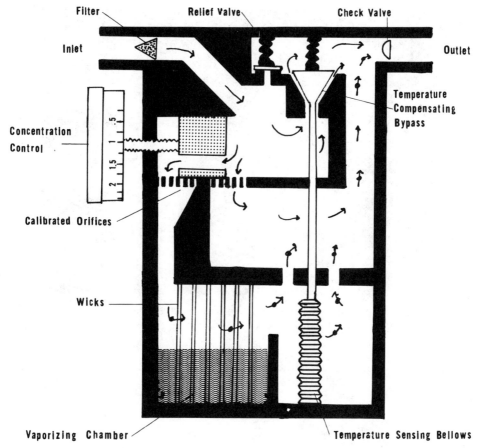

Figure 4.25. Schematic drawing of Ohio calibrated vaporizer. For the purpose of illustration the concentration control dial is shown at the left when it is actually at the top. (Redrawn from a drawing furnished by Ohio Medical Products, a division of Airco, Inc.)

gases from the anesthesia machine enter the vaporizer and pass through a filter in the vaporizer inlet. There are three possible paths for these gases to follow. The first channel is through the relief valve at the top, which opens when the pressure rises above normal, as, for example, when the oxygen flush is used.

During normal operation, the gas flow entering the first chamber of the vaporizer splits into two. Most of the gas flows directly to the vaporizer outlet via the temperature-compensating bypass. This is designed to compensate for the changes in agent volatility with temperature. The temperature of the gas leaving the vaporizing chamber is detected by the temperature-sensing bellows. When the vapor is warm, the bellows expands, increasing the size of the opening around the bypass so that more of the incoming gas goes directly to the vaporizer outlet. As

the vapor cools, the bellows contracts and partially closes the valve. This action will force a greater proportion of the incoming gas through the vaporization chamber, bringing the concentration back up to the selected setting.

The remaining gas flows to the two sets of calibrated orifices where it is split. The flow through one set of orifices is directed to the vaporizer outlet. The flow through the other set of orifices is directed to the vaporizing chamber. The ratio between gas diverted to the outlet and the gas diverted to the vaporizing chamber is determined by the setting of the concentration control valve. Turning the concentration control valve simultaneously opens one set of orifices while closing the other set.

Carrier gas entering the vaporizing chamber flows around a series of wicks where it becomes saturated with vapor. It then leaves the vapor-

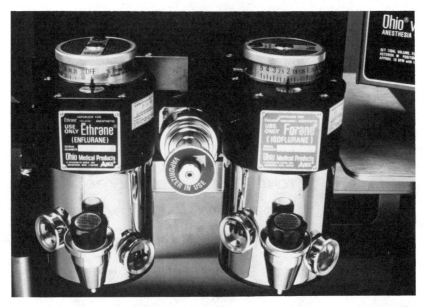

Figure 4.26. Ohio calibrated vaporizers. Note selector valve between vaporizers. (Picture courtesy of Ohio Medical Products, a division of Airco, Inc.)

izing chamber, flows around the temperature-sensing bellows and on to the the vaporizer outlet.

The vaporizer is shown in Figure 4.26. There are two sight glass windows: one with a FULL and one with an EMPTY indicator. The filling port can be either of the funnel type or of the pin index block. The concentration dial is at the top. Concentrations are increased by rotating the dial counterclockwise. There are clicks at each increment on the dial. There is a locking button at the top rear which must be depressed before the dial can be turned on. On the enflurane vaporizer the dial relocks at the 5% position and the locking button must be depressed to dial a concentration greater than 5%.

EVALUATION AND USE

Figures 4.27 and 4.28 show the manufacturer's data for enflurane and halothane at different flows. It is accurate between 16 and 32°C (60 and 90°F). The vaporizers are designed for accuracy at fresh gas flows of from 300 ml to 10 liters/min.

Lin (8) evaluated the ethrane and halothane vaporizers at fresh gas flows from 100 to 5000 ml/min and found they performed satisfactorily. Considerable change in output did occur when the fresh gas flow was lowered suddenly. Intermittent downstream pressure fluctuations did

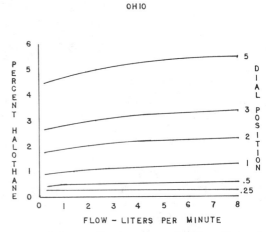

Figure 4.27. Performance of Ohio calibrated vaporizer (halothane). (Redrawn courtesy of Ohio Medical Products, a division of Airco, Inc.)

affect vaporizer output, but mean output did not change when compared to free flow to atmosphere. Upstream oxygen flushing increased the output more than 10%. Another evaluation showed these vaporizers to be reasonably accurate (54).

The manufacturer's product literature indicates that the addition of nitrous oxide to the carrier gas will lower the output. Several authors (8, 10, 12, 14, 16) found this true at settings

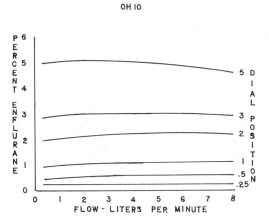

OH IO

PERCENT ENFLURANE

FLOW - LITERS PER MINUTE

DIAL POSITION

Figure 4.28. Performance of Ohio calibrated vaporizer (enflurane). (Redrawn courtesy of Ohio Medical Products, a division of Airco, Inc.)

below 3%. Stoelting (16) found a slight increase in vapor pressure at a dial setting of 4% and Prins and co-workers (10) found an increase at a 3% setting.

CARE AND CLEANING

The vaporizer should be drained periodically and the liquid discarded. The manufacturer recommends that the vaporizer be returned to its service center yearly for cleaning and calibration.

HAZARDS

Hazards associated with these vaporizers are similar to others of this type. When the anesthesia machine is in use and the vaporizer control knob is turned to OFF, a small amount of vapor can diffuse from the vaporizing chamber into the bypass circuit. Although the amount of vapor is small, it could be significant to someone sensitive to the agent. To avoid delivering this small amount of vapor, prior to administering an anesthetic the fresh gas hose should be disconnected from the breathing system and a 5-liter/min flow turned on for a minute to allow the accumulated vapor to be diluted to atmosphere. The vaporizer should be in the OFF position.

These vaporizers can be tilted up to 20 degrees from the upright position even when fully charged without a problem. If not in use, they can be tilted up to 45 degrees without any effect on their operation. If tilted more than these

amounts, especially if fully charged, liquid may enter the control head and a higher-than-expected concentration will be delivered, even after it is restored to an upright position.

Ohio Number 8 Bottle

MANUFACTURER

Ohio Medical Products, Madison, Wis.

CLASSIFICATION

Variable bypass, flow-over with wick, in-system, no temperature compensation, and multiple agent.

CONSTRUCTION

The Ohio Number 8 bottle vaporizer is pictured in Figure 4.29. It consists of an upper head with a control lever and a lower glass jar into which the liquid is poured. The glass jar contains a wick.

Inside the head is a mechanism which splits the flow of gas entering the vaporizer into two paths. With the control lever in the OFF position, all the flow through the vaporizer passes through the bypass. When the control lever is turned on, the inlet and outlet of the vaporizing chamber are opened. As the lever is opened further, increasing amounts of gas are allowed to pass through the glass jar. At the full ON

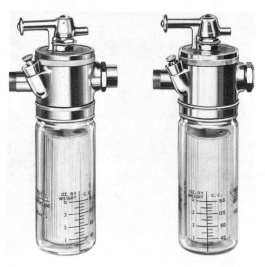

Figure 4.29. Ohio No. 8 vaporizer. (Courtesy of Ohio Medical Products, a division of Airco, Inc.)

position, all of the gas passes through the glass jar. A scale on the side of the glass indicates the amount of liquid contained in the jar. The maximum safe level is shown. There is a filling port near the control lever at the head.

EVALUATION AND USE

This vaporizer was designed to be placed inside the circle breathing system. It has been used most frequently for diethyl ether, and, less often, methoxyflurane. In some anesthesia departments, this vaporizer is filled with water and turned to ON to increase humidification of the inspired gases. Because of the many variables associated with an in-system vaporizer, it is not possible to give performance data.

CARE AND CLEANING

When in use, the efficiency of this vaporizer is decreased by water condensing on the wick. An extra wick should always be readily available for quick substitution to allow water to evaporate from a wick used for several hours. The wick should be removed from the jar and the jar emptied when not in use.

The vaporizer should be serviced regularly by the manufacturer.

HAZARDS

It is important that the vaporizer be empty when not in use, to avoid potential leak of agent into the breathing system and thus inadvertent administration of agent. A case has been reported where a corroded washer in the bypass mechanism allowed anesthesia vapor to pass into the breathing system when the vaporizer was in the OFF position (59).

If the jar is broken or removed for emptying and cleaning, it should be replaced immediately. If the bottle is not present and the control lever is accidentally turned on, a leak in the breathing system will result.

Ohio DM 5000 Electrically Heated Vaporizer

MANUFACTURER

Ohio Medical Products, Madison, Wis. Production of this vaporizer has been discontinued.

CLASSIFICATION

Measured-flow, bubble-through, out of system, temperature compensation by supplied heat (electric), and agent-specific (halothane, methoxyflurane, diethyl ether, isoflurane, enflurane).

CONSTRUCTION

This vaporizer is built into the Ohio DM 5000 anesthesia machine and is diagrammed in Figure 4.30. An on-off valve controls the inlet and outlet of the vaporizing chamber. In the OFF position, the inlet and outlet are closed so that no gas flows to the vaporizer. In the ON position, gas flows through the flowmeter to the inlet of the vaporizer. A check valve prevents liquid from backing up into the flowmeter. The gas then passes down a tube below the level of the liquid. The tube has a series of 12 slots. This creates small bubbles that rise through the liquid. Vapor-laden gas then passes out through a tube located at the top of the vaporizing chamber

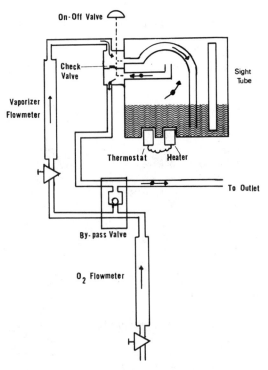

Figure 4.30. Schematic diagram of Ohio 5000 vaporizer. (By approval of Ohio Medical Products, a division of Airco, Inc.)

and through the vaporizer outlet where it is joined by gas from the other flowmeters.

Temperature compensation is by means of an electric heater which keeps the temperature between 74 and 76°F. A back pressure regulator located near the machine outlet keeps the internal parts of the machine at 800 torr.

On the back of the machine are the filler funnels and drain cocks. On either side of the drains are lights that indicate when power is available to the vaporizer and when the heater is operating.

EVALUATION AND USE

The vaporizer flowmeters on this machine differ from the ones for the Verni-Trol and Copper Kettle vaporizers in that they are calibrated in millimeters of anesthetic vapor rather than carrier gas. The flow to the vaporizer is gas which has already passed through the oxygen flowmeter. The concentration of anesthetic delivered to the machine outlet is determined by dividing the millimeters registered on the vaporizer flowmeter by the sums of flows of diluent gases and anesthetic vapor and multiplying by 100 (60).

Although the vaporizer is pressurized to prevent pressure fluctuations in the breathing system from affecting its performance, activation of the oxygen flush valve with the on-off valve in the ON position has been reported to cause a significant amount of agent to be delivered (38).

CARE AND CLEANING

Diethyl ether should be drained at the end of the day because it may become oxidized. Other vaporizers should be periodically drained and rinsed with agent. The vaporizer should be serviced regularly.

HAZARDS

A case has been reported in which a leak in the outlet tube of the vaporizer allowed liquid anesthetic to be delivered to the fresh gas line of the machine when the vaporizer was filled (61).

The filling funnels are arranged in a row on the back of the machine. Although they are labeled it is a situation where the incorrect agent could easily be placed in a vaporizer (60).

Another problem with this vaporizer is caused

by the increased internal pressure. Because of this any leak in the machine will be magnified. If the vaporizer filler cap is not tight a large leak of gas will occur (62). Placement of the funnels on the back of the machine makes them susceptible to brushing by people passing by.

Vapor

These include the halothane Vapor, methoxyflurane Vapor, and enflurane Vapor. These vaporizers are no longer being produced.

MANUFACTURER

Drägerwerk AG, Lübeck, West Germany. Distributed in the United States by North American Drager, Telford, Pa.

CLASSIFICATION

Variable bypass, flow-over with wick, out of system, temperature compensation by flow alteration (manual), and agent-specific (halothane, enflurane, methoxyflurane).

CONSTRUCTION

A diagram of the halothane and enflurane models is shown in Figure 4.31. Gas enters the inlet and flows to the bypass valve. This consists of male and female cones designed to produce laminar flow. Fresh gas which does not pass through the bypass flows to the on-off valve. In the OFF position, the on-off slide is moved to the left. Gas is prevented from passing into the vaporizing chamber and the chamber is vented to atmosphere. In the ON position, the on-off slide moves to the right and the fresh gas passes through the spiral inlet tube to the vaporizing chamber. Here the gas passes around some wicks and up a center tube to a valve constructed similar to the bypass valve. The male cone of the valve is connected to the concentration dial by a shaft. Altering the concentration dial causes axial displacement of the male cone, changing the flow from the vaporizing chamber. Vapor-laden gas flows from this valve to the bypass where it joins the diluent gas and passes to the outlet.

Temperature compensation is accomplished in two ways. The vaporizing chamber is constructed of a heavy copper block to add thermostability. Secondly, there is a thermometer

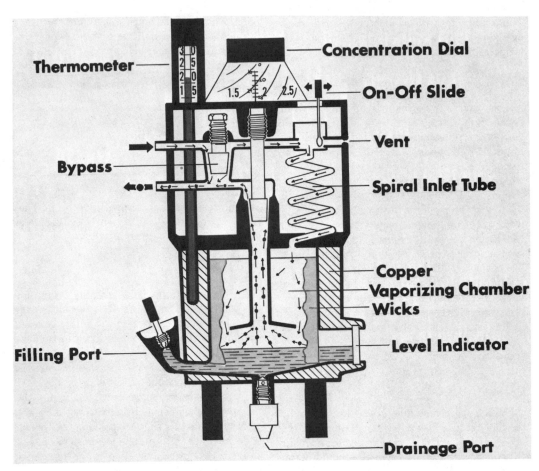

Figure 4.31. Halothane Vapor. See text for details. (Courtesy of Drägerwerk AG, Lübeck, West Germany.)

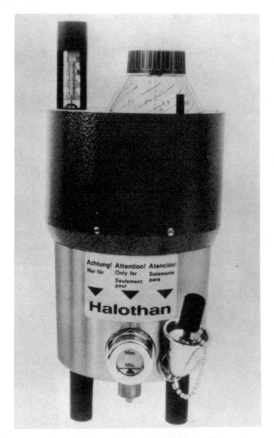

embedded in the copper block. By reading the temperature from the thermometer, the concentration knob can be altered manually so that additional gas flows from the vaporizing chamber as cooling takes place.

The methoxyflurane model differs in that the bypass is not fixed, but is connected to the concentration dial shaft in such a way that as the concentration is increased, the bypass is decreased. This design allows maximal flow through the vaporizing chamber when high concentrations are desired.

The Vapor is pictured in Figure 4.32. The concentration dial consists of a series of slanted lines, each of which represents a different concentration of agent in volumes percent. On a clear plastic overlay is a temperature scale. To provide a certain concentration, the appropriate line is aligned so that it crosses the temperature registered on the thermometer on the overlay.

The filling port is located at the bottom right of the vaporizer. To the left of this is a window where the liquid level in the vaporizing chamber can be seen. A drainage port is at the bottom of the vaporizer.

EVALUATION AND USE

Figure 4.32. Halothane Vapor. (Courtesy of North American Drager.)

The manufacturer's data for halothane is given in Figure 4.33. This vaporizer has been

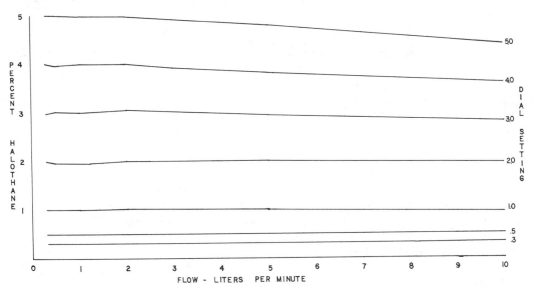

Figure 4.33. Halothane Vapor performance. Room temperature 16–28°C. (Redrawn courtesy of Drägerwerk AG, Lübeck, West Germany.)

evaluated frequently in the literature (8, 42, 63–65) and found to be quite accurate.

Lin (8) investigated the halothane model in both high and low flows and found it performed quite well. There was no demonstrable pumping or pressurizing effect. There was a greater than 10% increase in halothane concentration caused by upstream oxygen flushing at low initial fresh gas flows. Abrupt changes in fresh gas flow from high to low caused minimal changes in output concentration. Another evaluation found the halothane and enflurane versions to be accurate (54).

The vaporizer is installed between the flowmeters and the machine outlet. Because of its high resistance, it should not be placed downstream of the oxygen flush valve. If more than one vaporizer is installed on the same machine, a selector valve should be used to direct gas to only one vaporizer, since the combined resistance of more than one vaporizer would be dangerously high.

The Vapor is accurate when used with IPPB, largely because of the spiral inlet tube (8, 63, 64). However, Steffey (28) found that very high peak inspiratory pressures did decrease the concentration of isoflurane delivered by a halothane Vapor.

The composition of the carrier gas does affect the vaporizer. When nitrous oxide is added to the carrier gas, the output decreases (8, 49).

Cook and co-workers (44) found that with the on-off lever in the ON position and the concentration dial on, substantial amounts of vapor were found in the bypass gas. Robinson and colleagues (51) found that with the on-off valve in the OFF position and the concentration dial in the "1" position, halothane leakage as high as 0.1% could be detected. Both authors found that with the concentration dial on "0", leakage of vapor was similar to other vaporizers of this type.

CARE AND CLEANING

The halothane Vapor should be drained periodically and the contents discarded to remove thymol. The thermometer is one of the most vulnerable parts of the vaporizer and care should be taken to protect it from damage. Servicing should be carried out by an authorized service agent.

HAZARDS

The vaporizer is quite heavy and should be made a permanent part of the anesthesia machine. If dropped, it could injure operating room personnel.

One of the principal reasons for its discontinuation was that the control dial turned on in the opposite way from that required in the new ANSI machine standard. This could pose a problem in departments in which there are vaporizers that turn the other way.

Vapor 19.1

Manufacturer: Drägerwerk AG, Lübeck, West Germany. Distributed by North American Drager, Telford, Pa.

CLASSIFICATION

Variable bypass, flow-over with wick, out of system, temperature compensation by flow alteration (automatic), and agent-specific (halothane, enflurane, isoflurane).

CONSTRUCTION

The Vapor 19.1 is the successor to the Vapor. It is essentially a new vaporizer. Compared to the Vapor it is more compact and lighter in weight. The concentration dial turns on in a counterclockwise direction and the temperature compensation is automatic rather than manual. The vaporizing chamber is isolated in the OFF position so that there is no leakage of anesthetic agent into the fresh gas line. The Vapor 19.1 is the newest model and differs from the Vapor 19 in that it has a lock for the "0" position.

The Vapor 19.1 is shown schematically in Figure 4.34. There is an on-off control which is activated by the concentration knob. In the OFF position the inlet and outlet from the vaporizing chamber are interconnected and vented externally. This prevents anesthetic from entering the fresh gas unintentionally. Fresh gas passes directly through a bypass in the vaporizer with practically no resistance.

In the ON position (Fig. 4.34), the fresh gas flow is diverted to the lower vaporizing section of the vaporizer. Part of the fresh gas will become saturated with anesthetic agent while the balance traverses the bypass. The desired vapor concentration is achieved by varying the position of the control cone at the vaporizing chamber outlet. Gases from the bypass and the vaporizing chamber meet in the mixing chamber then pass on to the outlet.

Temperature compensation is accomplished by an expansion member which extends into the

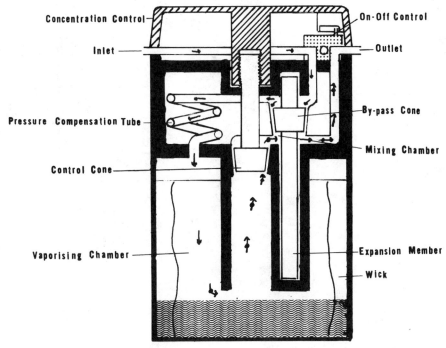

Figure 4.34. Vapor 19.1. ON position. See text for details. (Redrawn from a drawing furnished by North American Drager.)

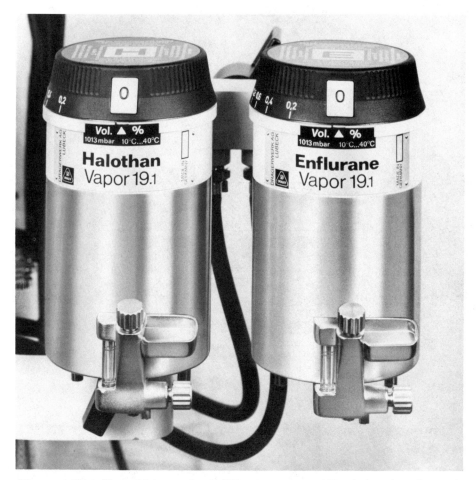

Figure 4.35.   Vapor 19.1 vaporizers. (Picture courtesy of North American Drager.)

vaporizing chamber. A change in temperature will cause a change in the gas flow to the vaporizing chamber by altering the vaporizing chamber bypass cone.

The Vapor 19.1 is shown in Figure 4.35. The concentration dial is at the top and is turned counterclockwise to increase the concentration. The "0" must be depressed to unlock the concentration dial before it can be turned. A filling spout, sight glass, and drain are located at the bottom front of the vaporizer. The concentration knob must be set at "0 Vol. %" for the vaporizer to be filled.

There are two models of both the halothane and enflurane Vapor 19.1. One halothane model is calibrated up to 4%. A special type is calibrated up to 5%. One enflurane model is calibrated to 5% and a special model is calibrated to 7%.

EVALUATION AND USE

The manufacturer's data for the halothane Vapor 19.1 is shown in Figure 4.36. It is accurate in the range of 0.3–15 liters/min. The vaporizer is designed to operate from 10–40°C with a deviation from the set concentration of ±10%. At temperatures outside this range, however, temperature compensation is not sufficient to maintain this degree of accuracy.

Lin (8) investigated the Enflurane Vapor 19.1 with high and low fresh gas flows and found it performed accurately.

Pressure fluctuations in the vaporizer are minimized by incorporation of a compensation device so that the vaporizer meets the ANSI machine standard requirements and can be operated safely in conjunction with all well-known anesthesia machines and ventilators.

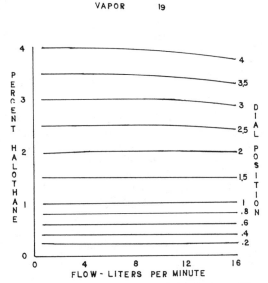

VAPOR 19

Figure 4.36. Performance of halothane Vapor 19.1 vaporizer. Ambient temperature 22°C. (Redrawn from a graph furnished by North American Drager.)

The concentration delivered depends upon the composition of the fresh gas. The Vapor 19.1 is calibrated using air. When operated on pure oxygen, the delivered concentration is 5–10% higher than the set concentration. When operated with 30% oxygen and 70% nitrous oxide, the concentration is 5–10% lower.

CARE AND CLEANING

Thymol may build up in the halothane Vapor 19.1. This is evidenced by a yellow discoloration. The flow control unit may gum up, leading to lower delivered concentrations. The manufacturer recommends that every four weeks the vaporizer be drained following a gentle shake to loosen the thymol accumulations. If the yellowish color is still present the thymol residues may be dissolved by gently rotating the vaporizer filled with fresh halothane for about one hour. This procedure should be repeated until the drained halothane shows no more yellow discoloration.

Following cleaning, the halothane Vapor 19.1 should be flushed with 10 liters/min of fresh gas for 10 min with the vaporizer empty and the concentration knob set at 4%.

The above procedures need not be carried out with the Enflurane and Forane Vapor 19.1s because these agents do not contain any stabilizer.

The manufacturer recommends inspection twice yearly by a trained specialist. When there is an extensive accumulation of dirt in the Vapor 19.1, the wick must be changed by an authorized service representative.

HAZARDS

Hazards with this vaporizer are similar to other vaporizers of this type.

If a Vapor 19.1 filled with anesthetic agent is inclined more than 45 degrees, liquid anesthetic can spill into the control device. This can result in either an increased or lowered delivered concentration. Should the vaporizer be tipped more than 45 degrees, it should be flushed with a flow of 10 liters/min at a dial setting of 4% for at least 1 min. If a filled vaporizer is in the horizontal position for an unknown period of time, it should be flushed for 10 min after the vaporizer is emptied.

Verni-Trol

The machines on which this vaporizer was supplied are no longer being produced.

MANUFACTURER

Ohio Medical Products, Madison, Wis.

CLASSIFICATION

Measured-flow, bubble-through, out of system, temperature compensation by supplied heat and manual flow adjustment, and multiple agent.

CONSTRUCTION

A diagram of the internal construction of the vaporizer is given in Figure 4.37. The main body is composed of silicon bronze for thermostability. Oxygen from the Verni-Trol flowmeter enters at the bottom, ascends through the inner inlet tube, descends in the outer tube and bubbles through the liquid in the vaporizing chamber. It then flows to the outlet tube.

The vaporizer is mounted behind the flowmeters on certain anesthesia machines. A glass tube (sight glass) that indicates the liquid level inside the vaporizer is located to the right of the vaporizer. A drain is at the base of the sight glass. The filling port is at the top of the vaporizer.

The vaporizer is supplied with a flowmeter

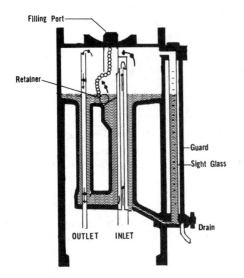

Figure 4.37. The Verni-Trol vaporizer. See text for details. (Redrawn courtesy of Ohio Medical Products, a division of Airco, Inc.)

and type I vaporizer circuit control valve (see Chapter 3). Some machines have parallel flowmeters to supply high or low flows.

EVALUATION AND USE

The output of the Verni-Trol is calculated by using the principles discussed in the section on measured flow. The manufacturer has a calculator available which allows rapid determination of the vaporizer flow needed to achieve a given concentration.

The vaporizer output is affected by intermittent back pressure and may be augmented considerably by the pumping effect (40). This can be completely eliminated by installation of a check valve at the vaporizer outlet or partially eliminated by a check valve at the machine outlet.

Cook and co-workers (44) found that if the on-off valve was in the OFF position, there was no leakage of vapor into the fresh gas line. If the switch was in the ON position with no flow through the vaporizer, 5–331 ppm of halothane could be detected in the outflow from the machine.

CARE AND CLEANING

If halothane is used in this vaporizer it should be drained periodically and the contents discarded to prevent the buildup of thymol.

The Verni-Trol should receive regular servicing by an authorized service repairman.

HAZARDS

An anesthetic accident has been reported in which liquid halothane was delivered to the patient because of a damaged seat on the flow control valve (66). Inspection of five machines revealed that two were capable of delivering liquid halothane when the flowmeter indicator was at the top of the scale and if the vaporizer were more than ¾ full. A limiting valve can be installed to prevent this hazard (67).

It is possible to overfill the Verni-Trol. If this occurs liquid agent can flow into the outlet.

Certain machines equipped with this vaporizer did not have a pressure-relief valve installed (68). With these machines, there have been instances where the machine outlet was blocked and liquid anesthetic flowed backward into the flowmeter tube or was released into the delivery line. To prevent these problems a relief valve set to relieve at 150 mm Hg should always be present on machines with this vaporizer.

The most common problems with the Verni-Trol are associated with improper use. Failure to turn on the vaporizer circuit control valve is common, as is incorrect calculation of the delivered concentration. When there are flowmeters in parallel, care must be taken that the fine and coarse flowmeters are not confused.

Sidearm Verni-Trol

MANUFACTURER

Ohio Medical Products, Madison, Wis.

CLASSIFICATION

Measured-flow, bubble-through, out of system, temperature compensation by supplied heat and manual flow adjustment, multiple agent.

CONSTRUCTION

The sidearm Verni-Trol is designed as an add-on unit for certain anesthesia machines. It has its own flowmeter assembly and an on-off valve. There is no vaporizer circuit control valve associated with it.

A diagram of the complete vaporizer unit is shown in Figure 4.38. It consists of a thick-walled brass container for thermostability. Ox-

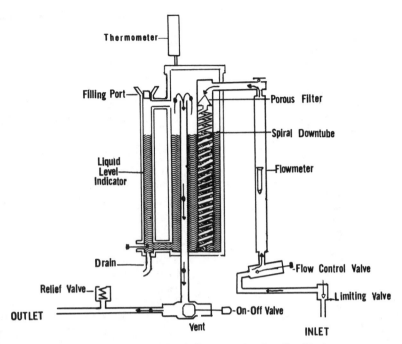

Figure 4.38. Older model sidearm Verni-Trol. See text for details. (Redrawn courtesy of Ohio Medical Products, a division of Airco, Inc.)

ygen enters at the inlet and passes through a limiting valve. This is set to restrict oxygen flow to slightly beyond the range of the vaporizer flowmeter. Its purpose is to prevent the delivery of excessive unmetered quantities of oxygen and anesthetic vapor to the vaporizer outlet and to avoid damage to the vaporizer.

The oxygen next passes through the flowmeter assembly. Flowmeter tubes are available with varying maximum calibrations, depending on the agents to be used. The oxygen then enters the top of the vaporizer, passes through a porous filter and descends in a spiral downtube to the bottom of the vaporizing chamber. It bubbles up through the liquid and leaves through the outlet tube.

At the base of the Verni-Trol is an on-off valve which directs the flow of the vapor-laden gas either to the machine or to a vent to atmosphere. When the ring handle is pulled toward the operator and turned in either direction, it is locked in the ON position On some machines with a back bar, this on-off valve is located to the right of the flowmeter assembly head and the ring is pulled down. The vapor-laden gas then passes a relief valve and flows into the machine where it is diluted by the gases from other flowmeters. The relief valve limits the

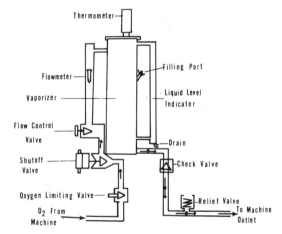

Figure 4.39. Newer model sidearm Verni-Trol vaporizer. See text for details. (Redrawn courtesy of Ohio Medical Products, a division of Airco, Inc.)

pressure in the flowmeter and vaporizer and prevents reverse flow of agent into the flowmeter tube or discharge of liquid anesthetic into the vaporizer outlet.

A glass tube at the left of the vaporizer indicates the liquid level. The filling port is at the

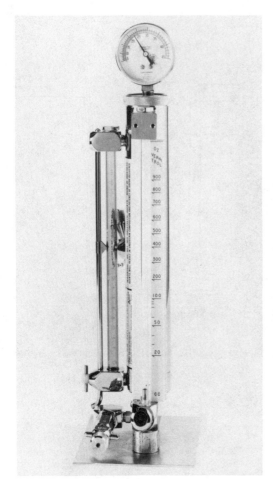

Figure 4.40. Sidearm Verni-Trol vaporizer. Newer version. Note that the filling funnel is at the side rather than the top to prevent overfilling. Also the on-off valve at the base has been changed. (Courtesy of Ohio Medical Products, a division of Airco, Inc.)

top and a drain is at the bottom. There is a thermometer connected to the top.

Newer versions of this vaporizer, one of which is diagrammed in Figure 4.39 and pictured in Figure 4.40, have a knob which is pulled out and turned 90 degrees to turn the vaporizer on. It is marked as to whether it is on or off. This is located upstream of the flowmeter assembly rather than downstream as in older models. Oxygen will not flow through the flowmeter unless the on-off valve is in the ON position. On newer models, the filling port is at the side of the brass body at the height of the maximum safe level to prevent overfilling. Finally, on

newer models there is a check valve upstream of the relief valve to minimize loss of gases from the rest of the machine through the vaporizer (69), and to prevent intermittent back pressure from affecting vaporizer output or liquid anesthetic from being discharged into the flowmeter tube. Consideration should be given to replacing older models with the newer versions.

EVALUATION AND USE

Vaporizer output can be determined using the equation in the section on measured-flow vaporizers or by using the calculator supplied by the manufacturer.

Lowe and colleagues (36) studied the effects of back pressure on the older sidearm Verni-Trol and found the output was increased by the pumping effect (Fig. 4.10). The addition of the check valve should eliminate this, however.

Cook and co-workers (44) found that if the on-off valve was in the OFF position, there was no leakage of vapor into the fresh gas line. If the switch was in the ON position but there was no flow through the vaporizer, halothane concentrations from 2–16 ppm could be detected in the machine outflow.

CARE AND CLEANING

Refer to the section on the Verni-Trol vaporizer.

HAZARDS

Most of the hazards discussed with the Verni-Trol apply to the sidearm model. Overdose stemming from a defective flow control valve has been reported (70).

There is a report of liquid anesthetic backing up into the flowmeter tube due to a loose cap at the top of the flowmeter (71). This is not an immediate hazard to the patient. However, residue remaining in the tube can cause the indicator to stick and become inaccurate. If this occurs, the flowmeter should be cleaned by an authorized service representative.

As with other measured-flow vaporizers, errors in calculating output can be made. Another common problem is forgetting to turn the on-off valve to the ON position.

It should be noted that although there is no vaporizer circuit control valve, the danger discussed in Chapter 3 with the type I vaporizer circuit control valve exists. If metabolic oxygen is metered through the older model sidearm Verni-Trol and the on-off valve is in the OFF position, a hypoxic mixture may be delivered to the patient.

Modulus Verni-Trol

MANUFACTURER

Ohio Medical Products, Madison, Wis.

CLASSIFICATION

Measured-flow, bubble-through, out of system, temperature compensation by supplied heat and manual adjustment, multiple agent.

CONSTRUCTION

The Modulus Verni-Trol is designed for installation only on the Ohio Modulus anesthesia machine. The vaporizer can only be installed if the machine has an appropriate vaporizer flowmeter assembly, a type IV vaporizer circuit control valve, plus a selector-interlock valve. Two Verni-Trol vaporizers may be installed on a machine, but only one vaporizer flowmeter assembly will be present.

The vaporizer itself is shown in Figure 4.41. It is cylindrical in shape. At the top is a flanged on-off control knob which requires a 90-degree rotation to go from OFF to ON. At the front of the vaporizer is a filler funnel. Sight windows (FULL and REFILL) are to either side of the funnel. A plastic skirt surrounds the bottom of the vaporizer. This enables the vaporizer to remain upright when placed on a level horizontal surface. The drain spigot is located under the plastic skirt. A dial thermometer which registers the temperature of the agent within the vaporizer is at the bottom right. The vaporizer inlet, vaporizer oxygen inlet and vaporizer outlet are located at the rear. The mounting bracket is also at the rear.

The vaporizer flowmeter is calibrated from 20 ml/min to 1 liter/min. A limiting device on the flow control valve restricts flow to no greater than 1300 ml/min so that excessive unmetered quantities of oxygen and anesthetic vapor will not be delivered.

Oxygen from the vaporizer flowmeter enters the vaporizer, descends in an inlet tube, and bubbles up through the liquid anesthetic. The walls of the vaporizing chamber are made of brass for thermostability.

Manifold caps are supplied to be placed over

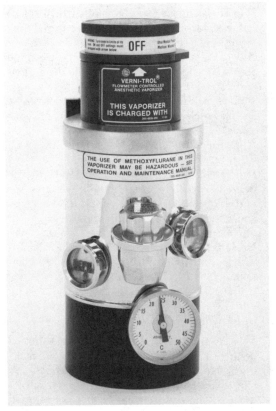

Figure 4.41. Modulus Verni-Trol vaporizer. (Courtesy of Ohio Medical Products, a division of Airco, Inc.)

the vaporizer mounting location if there is no vaporizer in place. A cap must be installed in the absence of a vaporizer or all gas flow may be vented to atmosphere. The caps are chained to the machine. When not in use, they are stored under the vaporizer mounting location behind the vaporizer.

Between the vaporizer flowmeter assembly and each vaporizer is a check valve to prevent backflow of gases if there is an obstruction downstream of the selector interlock valve. These machines are equipped with a check valve near the common gas outlet to minimize effects of intermittent back pressure on the vaporizer.

EVALUATION AND USE

To use this vaporizer one must first be familiar with the use of the Modulus anesthesia machine. The metered flow of vaporizer oxygen must be considered as additional to the flow registered on the other flowmeters.

In addition, one must be familiar with calculation of vaporizer output with a measured-flow vaporizer. The manufacturer has available a flow calculator which can be used to determine the vaporizer flow needed to provide the desired concentration.

Since this is a multiple-agent vaporizer, it should be clearly labeled as to the agent contained.

To use the vaporizer the selector-interlock valve on the machine must be pulled forward and rotated so that the arrow points to the desired Verni-Trol vaporizer. For effective vaporizer operation, the liquid agent level must be above the sight window refill line.

When not in use, the vaporizer and its flowmeter should be turned to OFF and the selector-interlock valve returned to the BYPASS position.

CARE AND CLEANING

To clean the vaporizer the agent must first be drained. The vaporizer is then filled to its maximum level with 95–100% ethyl alcohol and allowed to stand for 20 min. The alcohol is then drained. The vaporizer should then be mounted onto the machine and a flow of 200 ml/min of oxygen allowed to pass through it for 30 min or until no alcohol can be detected in the gas flow.

HAZARDS

Hazards are those generally associated with any vaporizer of this type. The vaporizer should never be tipped more than 45 degrees while it contains liquid anesthetic agent. Use after such tilting may cause dangerously high concentrations of vapor to be delivered to the patient. If it is suspected that the vaporizer has been tilted more than 45 degrees, the vaporizer should be turned on and a flow of 500 cc/min set on the vaporizer flowmeter and allowed to flow for at least 10 min.

The vaporizer control knob should never be left in a position between ON and OFF. Such a setting could cause unwanted anesthetic vapor to be delivered to the patient.

Since this is a bubble-through type vaporizer, it is of utmost importance that materials containing silicone not be used around the vaporizer. Should the vaporizer inadvertently become contaminated with such a material it should be returned to an authorized service center.

AGENT-SPECIFIC FILLING DEVICE (72) KEYED FILLER SYSTEM, KEYED FILLING DEVICE, PIN SAFETY SYSTEM

The ANSI machine standard recommends, but does not require, that a vaporizer designed for use with a single agent be fitted with a permanently attached, agent-specific device to prevent accidental fillings with the wrong agent.

Presently the Keyed Filling System is the device being used to fulfill this recommendation. This system was developed with the cooperation of vaporizer manufacturers and producers of volatile liquid anesthetic agents.

Components

The system is composed of a keyed bottle collar, an adaptor tube, and a vaporizer filler receptacle. The adaptor tube is keyed at both ends so that it will fit only the bottle and the vaporizer filler receptacle for which it was designed.

KEYED BOTTLE COLLAR

Each bottle of liquid anesthetic has a specially designed and colored collar attached securely at the shoulder. Each collar has two projections, one thicker than the other, which are designed to mate with corresponding indentations on the bottle cap of the adaptor. The colors for the commonly used agents are: green (methoxyflurane), red (halothane), orange (enflurane), and purple (isoflurane). The colors are also used on the bottle labels.

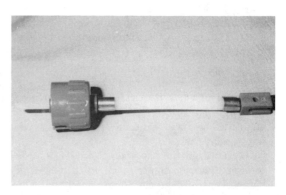

Figure 4.42. Adaptor tube. The bottle cap is at left and the filler block at right. Note the groove (slot) in the side and the two holes on the flat surface of the filler block.

ADAPTOR TUBE (BOTTLE ADAPTOR)

The adaptor tube is shown in Figure 4.42. At one end is a bottle cap which has a screw thread to match the thread on the bottle and a skirt which extends beyond the screw threads and conforms to the collar on the bottle. This is color-coded and keyed so that it fits only a bottle of the agent for which it was designed. A short length of tubing with passages inside for both air and liquid connects the bottle end to the vaporizer end. The tubing allows the bottle to be held higher or lower than the level of the vaporizer receptacle. The other end of the adaptor tube has a male fitting called a filler block (tube block) which is designed to fit into the vaporizer receptacle. It consists of a rectangular piece of plastic with a groove on one side and two holes on the flat surface (Fig. 4.42). The groove is designed to prevent the adaptor of one agent from being placed in an incorrect vaporizer. The larger hole is for the agent to enter or leave the vaporizer and the smaller hole is for air.

VAPORIZER FILLER RECEPTACLE (FILLER SOCKET, VAPORIZER FILLER UNIT, FILL AND DRAIN SYSTEM)

The vaporizer filler receptacle is attached to the front or side of the vaporizer. It contains two sockets (tunnels), two retaining screws (on the top and bottom of the receptacle), and one or two screws on the front (Fig. 4.43). If there is

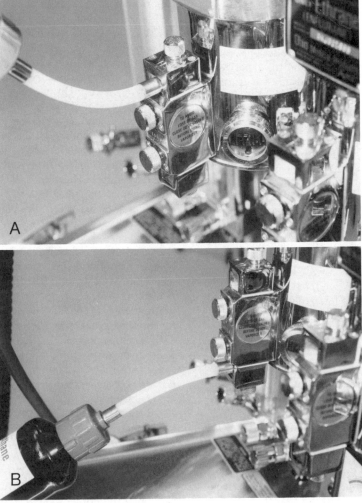

Figure 4.43. Keyed filling device with two front screws. *A*, filling the vaporizer; *B*, draining the vaporizer.

only one front screw (Fig. 4.16) a filler plug will be present, often chained to the receptacle. The upper socket is for filling the vaporizer and the lower for draining it. Each socket has a bead or pin inside to stop all filter blocks except the one that has been slotted, i.e., indexed, for it.

The filler plug is tightened and loosened by turning the retaining screw at the top of the receptacle. This stays in the top socket when the vaporizer is not being filled or drained.

The front screws control openings to the vaporizing chamber. They are opened by turning counterclockwise. When a top front filling screw is present, it must be opened before the vaporizer can be filled. The bottom drain screw must be opened to drain the vaporizer.

Use

FILLING

When it is desired to fill a vaporizer, the cap from the appropriate bottle is removed and the adaptor tube screwed to the collar until airtight. If the connection is not tight, the vaporizer may be overfilled. The vaporizer must be turned off before proceeding further. The filler plug, if present, is removed by loosening the top retaining screw and pulling out the plug. The filler block is then inserted with the holes pointing down (Fig.4.43, *top*) During insertion the tube should be bent slightly so that the bottle is below the inlet level to prevent spilling. After the filler block is inserted, the top retaining screw is tightened. The upper front valve is opened. The bottle is then held higher than the filler socket (avoiding kinking of the tube) and the liquid agent allowed to run into the vaporizer. Gentle up-and-down motion will clear air bubbles and facilitate filling. When the liquid is at the FULL mark, the bottle is lowered, the retaining screw loosened and the filler block removed. The plug is then reinserted and the retaining screw tightened or the front valve closed. This last step is especially important to prevent a leak when the vaporizer is turned on.

DRAINING

To drain the vaporizer, the adaptor is attached to an appropriate bottle. The filler block is inserted similar to filling except that the bottom socket is used and the two holes face up. To facilitate draining, the filler plug is removed (or the top screw opened). The bottle is then held below the receptacle without kinking the tube (Fig.4.43, *bottom*). The drain valve on the front is opened. After the vaporizer is drained, the drain valve is closed, the bottom retaining screw loosened and the adaptor tube removed. The filler plug should be reinserted or the filling screw closed.

Evaluation

This system performs a useful function in that it helps prevent placement of an incorrect agent in an agent-specific vaporizer. In addition, it may result in less pollution of operating room air by volatile anesthetic agents, since spilling is reduced.

It does present difficulties. If the holes do not align properly it may be difficult to fill the vaporizer. Filling usually takes more time than with a conventional filling funnel. If the filling device is lost it will be almost impossible to fill the vaporizer.

The filler receptacle extends below the base of the vaporizer and will prevent the vaporizer from being set upright on a flat surface so it is necessary to set it at the ends of the surface with the block extending over the edge. This increases the possibility of the vaporizer being knocked to the floor. A useful addition in this case is a ring which is fitted to the base of the vaporizer and which extends the base below the projection of the filler block (Fig. 4.16). This ring allows the vaporizer to be placed upright on a flat surface.

This device should be regarded as a backup to the basic safety rule that labels should always be read before use. One case has been reported where the bead was too small to prevent incorrect filling (73). Another case has been reported where the bottle cap for one agent fitted a bottle for another agent which did not have a collar (74). All suppliers of volatile liquid anesthetics will, on request, supply their agents in bottles fitted with index collars (75). Anesthesiologists are urged to insist that their hospital's purchasing department specify that these collars be fitted when they place their orders.

Another disadvantage of having this system on a vaporizer is that if the liquid level is low and the vaporizer screw or filler plug loose, this leak will be more difficult to detect than with a conventional filling device in which liquid will well up in the funnel when a leak is present.

ARRANGEMENT OF VAPORIZERS

Since it is usually desired to have more than one vaporizer on an anesthesia machine the arrangement of these vaporizers assumes some importance. The ANSI machine standard states that vaporizers must be connected so that gas never passes through the vaporizing chamber of one vaporizer and then through that of another. Note that this does not outlaw using vaporizers in series.

Series Arrangement

A large number of machines in common use have vaporizers in series. The number of vaporizers that can be used is limited only by the space available for mounting.

A hazard with this arrangement is that agent from the upstream vaporizer may be deposited in the downstream vaporizer if the vaporizers are accidentally or purposely turned on simultaneously (76–78). This will result in changes in both the upstream and downstream agent concentrations. During subsequent use the output of the downstream vaporizer will be contaminated with agent from the upstream vaporizer and the effect of the resulting mixture will be indeterminant and could be toxic (79).

If it is necessary to use vaporizers in series, then it is important to prevent cross-contamination. Only one vaporizer should be turned on at a time. The sequence of connection should be such that the agent with the lowest vapor pressure and potency is upstream. The arrangement of methoxyflurane-enflurane-isoflurane-halothane (from upstream to downstream) minimizes the potential for vaporizer contamination from considerations of vapor pressure (volatility) and potency (MAC).

Since this type of arrangement will not meet the machine standard requirement, mechanisms have been devised to satisfy it. Conversion to one of these may involve some changes in the vaporizer as well as the machine. Also additional effort on the part of the user may be required.

Interlock Devices

These are applied to the control dial of the vaporizer so that only one can be turned on at a time (Figs. 4.44 and 4.45). These can be used with vaporizers in series or may be combined with a selector valve (see below) so that a va-porizer can be turned on only if the selector valve is directing flow to it. Cross-contamination caused by diffusion of agent can still occur.

Selector Valve (Exclusion Device)

A selector valve directs the gas flow to one vaporizer while isolating all other vaproizers from the machine circuitry.

There is considerable variety in the selector valves commercially available. Some have a by-pass position in which all vaporizers are isolated (Fig. 4.26). In others (Fig. 4.16), the flow is always directed to one vaporizer. A selector valve may be combined with an interlock device or a physical disconnection device. Some selector valves block either the gas flow to or the gas flow from the vaporizers in the OFF position. Others control both the inlet and outlet of the vaporizers. With the first type, a diffusion pathway may permit trace concentrations to enter the fresh gas line. With the latter type, there should be no diffusion pathway.

Unless a selector valve is combined with an interlock device, the operator may dial a concentration on a vaporizer which is not connected to the fresh gas line and the expected concentration is not delivered.

There is one case report where malfunction of a selector valve allowed delivery of vapor from two vaporizers (59).

Physical Disconnection Devices

With this method when it is desired to change from one vaporizer to another, the inlet and/or outlet connections are switched (Fig. 4.46) or the vaporizer is removed from its mounting position and another vaporizer put in its place. With some arrangements all vaporizers may be excluded, while with others one vaporizer will always be "in line." If the vaporizer itself is changed there will be no limit to the number of vaporizers that can be used. When the connections are changed, the number of vaporizers will be limited only by the space available for mounting. These may be combined with a selector valve.

Problems can occur with these. If the connections are changed, the possibility of leaks is increased. If the vaporizers are changed, the danger of tipping increases.

Leakage of anesthetic vapor into the fresh gas line from a vaporizer can be eliminated by a

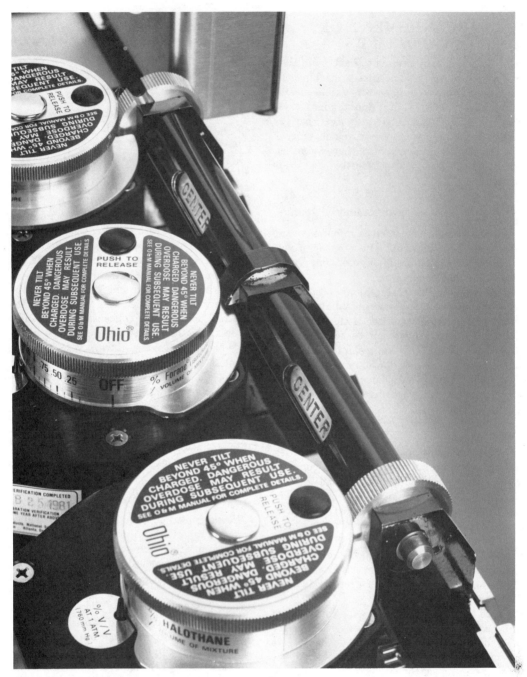

Figure 4.44. Interlock device. The concentration dials of the left and right vaporizers cannot be turned on while the center one is in use. (Courtesy of Ohio Medical Products, a division of Airco, Inc.)

physical disconnection device that prevents any vaporizer from being "in line."

Regardless of the circuit arrangement, the anesthesiologist should always be aware of the vaporizer setting and whether there is gas flow to it. If a selector valve has a bypass position, it should be returned to this when a vaporizer is not in use. With physical disconnection devices all vaporizers should be excluded if possible, except when one is in use.

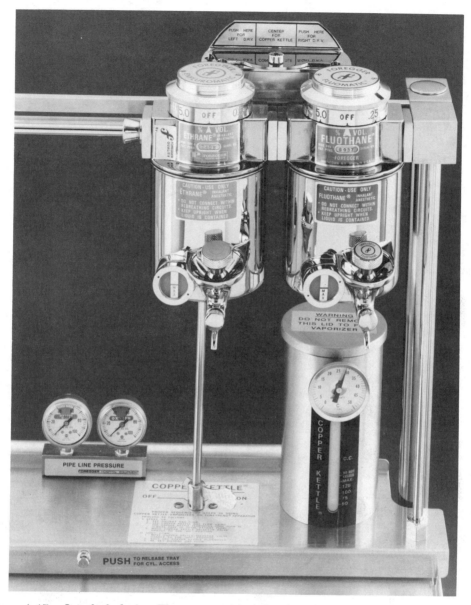

Figure 4.45. Interlock device. There are positions for three vaporizers. (Courtesy of Foregger, Division of Puritan-Bennett Corporation.)

HAZARDS OF VAPORIZERS

Incorrect Agent

As discussed previously, some vaporizers are specific for one agent, whereas others can accept a variety of agents. A common hazard involves filling an agent-specific vaporizer with an agent other than the one for which it was designed (60, 73). If a vaporizer designed for a highly volatile agent is inadvertently filled with an agent of low volatility, the result will be a patient who remains awake. The reverse of this situation may be irreversible overdose. This problem can be avoided by using a keyed filler system (see previous section).

In multiple-agent vaporizers, confusion can arise as to which agent is in the vaporizer (45, 80). Such vaporizers should always be clearly marked for the agent contained.

Agents should never be mixed in a vaporizer.

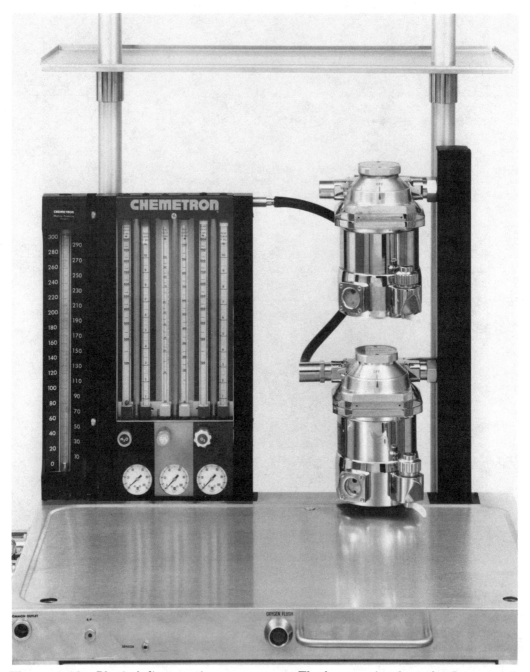

Figure 4.46. Physical disconnection arrangement. The hose coming from the flowmeters is attached to the vaporizer to be used. (Courtesy of Chemetron Medical Division, Allied Healthcare Products, Inc.)

The vapor delivered could have an adverse effect on the patient. Mixing of agents could result in an unpredictable chemical reaction.

A vaporizer should always be drained into a container labeled with the name of the drained agent and never into an unmarked container.

Smelling will give no assurance as to the agent in a vaporizer since the smell of a small amount of one agent can completely mask the odor of a less pungent agent, even if the second agent is present in much higher concentration (81).

If it is desired to change agents in a vaporizer, or if it is filled with the wrong agent, it must be completely drained and gas flowed through it until no agent can be detected in the outflow before it is refilled. Draining cannot be relied upon to completely empty a vaporizer, especially if it contains wicks.

Tipping

As can be seen from the drawings and discussions of individual vaporizers, if most vaporizers are tipped sufficiently, liquid from the vaporizing chamber can get into the bypass of the vaporizer outlet (82, 83). If this occurs, a high concentration of agent will be delivered when the vaporizer is again put into use.

Tipping can be avoided by mounting vaporizers securely in the erect position and handling them with care when they are not mounted. Unless specifically designed to be transported with liquid in the vaporizing chamber, a vaporizer should be drained before being transported.

Should tipping occur, a high flow of gas should be run through the vaporizer for 20 min with the vaporizer set at a low concentration.

Foaming

Foaming also creates the possibility of liquid anesthetic passing into the outlet of a vaporizer with anesthetic overdosage as a result. It has been found to occur in bubble-through vaporizers (23, 84, 85) and has been traced to the presence of silicone lubricants and sealants used in parts of the vaporizer and the vaporizer circuit control valve. Another source is bubble-forming solutions used to test for leaks. Foaming has been a problem, especially with methoxyflurane. As little as 17 ppm of silicone in methoxyflurane will cause foaming (86).

The machine standard requires that a vaporizer incorporate a means to prevent the displacement of foam from the vaporizer to the common outlet under normal operating conditions.

Because there is no way to assure that foaming cannot occur with any agent, silicones should not be used as lubricants or sealants in vaporizers or elsewhere in the gas piping system of the machine and leak-detection fluids should not be used around vaporizers.

Overfilling

An important step in the checking procedure of an anesthesia machine is to confirm that a vaporizer contains the correct amount of liquid agent. If a vaporizer is overfilled, liquid agent may enter the fresh gas line. If this occurs, lethal concentrations may be delivered to the patient. This has been a problem mainly with vaporizers that are filled from the top (46, 86, 87). A clear sight glass may make the liquid level hard to see so that an overfilled vaporizer looks like an empty one.

The machine standard requires that all vaporizers be equipped with a liquid-level indicator and be designed so that they cannot be overfilled. Most vaporizers now have the filling port on the side at the maximum safe level so that a vaporizer cannot be overfilled. Liquid will pour over the edge of the funnel before the liquid level inside the vaporizer rises to a dangerous level. Newer models of both the Copper Kettle and sidearm Verni-Trols have the filling port located on the side. Older models that have the top filling port should be updated. Some models with side filling funnels can be overfilled if they are tipped.

Agent-specific filling devices prevent overfilling of the vaporizer by a connection of the air intake in the agent bottle to the inside of the vaporizer chamber. The filling process is interrupted by blocking the air intake to the bottle. Many users of keyed filling devices have found that by slightly unscrewing the filling device from the bottle during the filling process, air from atmosphere can enter the bottle and the speed of filling is increased. Turning the concentration dial of the vaporizer on during filling will accomplish the same end. Such practices override the safety features in the filler system which prevent overfilling (88).

Discharge of Liquid Agent into Delivery Line

Displacement of liquid from a vaporizer to its outlet tubing can be a cause of gross overdosage because not only vaporizer flow but total carrier gas flow then vaporizes the liquid in an uncontrolled manner (89, 90). This can be caused by overfilling or tipping. It has also occurred with certain measured-flow vaporizers when the vaporizer is turned on with the flow control valve open. If the fresh gas line becomes occluded and is suddenly opened, the sudden release of pressure may create sufficient turbulence so that liquid anesthetic is released into the delivery line (68). This has also occurred when the flow through the vaporizer was too high (66, 70). The machine standard requires that each vaporizer incorporate a means that prevents the displacement of liquid from the vaporizer in the event of high flows or with occlusion and opening of the common gas outlet.

One case has been reported where a leak inside a built-in vaporizer allowed liquid to get into the delivery line when the vaporizer was filled (61).

Reversed Flow

Connecting a free-standing vaporizer between the common gas outlet and the breathing system backwards is easily done and easily overlooked. Although the machine standard requires that the inlet of the vaporizer be male and the outlet female, the direction of gas flow be marked and the inlet and outlet parts be labeled, it is quite easy to connect the fresh gas delivery line of the anesthesia machine to the outlet side of the vaporizer and the delivery tube to the breathing system to the inlet side of the vaporizer.

In bubble-through vaporizers, the inlet tube extends below the surface of the liquid. If flow were reversed through the vaporizer, gas entering the outlet tube would enter above the liquid. The pressure increase would push liquid up the inlet tube and into the delivery hose.

Marks and co-workers (91) investigated the effect of reversed flow with the Fluotec Mark II and III vaporizers and the Ethranetec. They found that reversed flow resulted in approximately double the output indicated on the vaporizer dial. In addition, back pressure compensation will be adversely affected (92).

With some in-system vaporizers, reversal of the direction of flow may push liquid out of the vaporizing chamber. With these it is important to incorporate safety valves that will stop the gas and liquid from moving in the wrong direction.

Concentration Dial Turned Wrong Way

Another hazard associated with vaporizers stems from the lack of a standard direction of rotation for controls (86, 93). Some vaporizers are turned on in the clockwise and others in the counterclockwise direction. This is dangerous, especially if both are on the same machine. The anesthesiologist accustomed to increasing or decreasing the concentration by turning in a certain direction, when confronted with a different vaporizer, might turn the dial the wrong way. The error of turning a vaporizer full on when intending to turn it off might be disastrous. The new machine standard requires that all vaporizer control knobs will turn off with a clockwise twist and shall open counterclockwise (which is the same as the flow control knobs).

Concentration Dial in Wrong Position

It is not unusual that the previous use of an anesthesia machine by a colleague results in a vaporizer concentration dial being left on (94). For this reason checking vaporizer control dials as well as contents should be part of the preanesthetic checking procedure.

The concentration dial may be changed during a case without the operator's knowledge, especially if the vaporizer has the concentration dial at the top. Operating room personnel, when moving a machine or simply passing by, may grab the concentration dial and change the setting.

Reflux of Liquid Anesthetic into Vaporizer Flowmeter (Fig. 4.47)

This has occasionally been a problem with measured flow vaporizers when the on-off valve is left in the ON position and there is occlusion of the fresh gas line (68, 71). This does not jeopardize the patient, but may require substitution of a different machine and necessitates a service call to clean the flowmeter. The machine standard states that a vaporizer must incorporate means to prevent the displacement of liquid from the vaporizer to its flowmeter in the event of occlusion of the common gas outlet.

Leaks in Vaporizers

A leak in the gas and/or vapor circuitry of an anesthesia machine may result in partial or complete loss of anesthetizing agents, oxygen, or both. With a leak in a vaporizer, the machine will function normally until the vaporizer (or the vaporizer circuit control valve on a measured-flow vaporizer) is turned on. At this point the flow from the machine will be reduced and may contain little or no anesthetic vapor. In addition to affecting fresh gas composition and flow, leaks cause pollution of operating room air with anesthetic agents.

Leaks may occur in any location in the machine, but are frequently found in vaporizers.

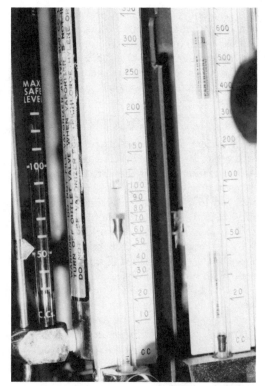

Figure 4.47. Reflux of liquid anesthetic into a vaporizer flowmeter.

The consequences of such a leak will depend on the size of the leak, its location, and whether or not there is a check valve at the vaporizer outlet. Most measured-flow vaporizers and some direct-reading vaporizers have such check valves. These will minimize the loss of gas should there be a leak inside or upstream of a vaporizer (69), although anesthetic vapor delivery will be less than expected.

Leaks are especially a problem with the Ohio DM 5000 machine. This machine has a pressurizing valve which maintains the pressure inside the machine at approximately 800 torr so that leaks are accentuated.

Probably the most common cause of a leak is failure to replace the vaporizer filler cap or to tighten it adequately (95, 96).

On the DM 5000 machine the filler caps are at the back of the machine, out of the operator's view, and project out from the machine, making them susceptible to accidental disturbance by passersby.

One case has been reported where the vaporizer filler plug was incorrectly threaded and would not seat properly (62).

Personnel responsible for filling vaporizers should be instructed to always close filler caps (or the filler plug or filling screw if a keyed filling system is present) tightly. It is a good idea to make sure these are tight when the machine is checked prior to use.

Other locations for leaks include the vaporizer circuit control valve (69, 97, 99), a relief valve (97) and various parts of direct-reading vaporizers (22, 99). The tubing connecting to the inlet or outlet of a vaporizer mounted downstream of the common gas outlet may become loose (100). The metal-to-metal fitting between a vaporizer and its inlet or outlet connection may also become loose. Some manufacturers supply a clamping device to avoid this problem.

Leaks should be suspected if a vaporizer appears to require filling with unusual frequency (99). With vaporizers that have a funnel filling device, if the filling cap is not tight, spattering of the liquid from the port will be observed when fresh gas goes through the vaporizer. This telltale sputtering may not be seen if a keyed filling device is in place and the filler plug or the filling screw on the front is loose. The only obvious sign of a leak in this case may be the odor of the agent in the operating suite. If there is a high turnover of air, even this signal may be lost.

Leaks in a vaporizer can be detected when the anesthesia machine is tested prior to use if each vaporizer is turned on (see Chapter 10). With measured-flow vaporizers it is necessary to turn the on-off switch to the ON position.

Leaks may be avoided by regular servicing of vaporizers (22). Leak testing is normally included in servicing and replacement of worn or damaged parts may prevent a leak. When vaporizers are mounted, the connections should be made tight by tapping lightly with a soft hammer.

Vapor Leak into the Fresh Gas Line

One assumes that when a vaporizer is turned off that it does not deliver anesthetic, but this is not always the case. Cook and co-workers (44) and Robinson and colleagues (51) found that most direct-reading vaporizers leaked small amounts of vapor into the bypass when turned off. When measured-flow vaporizers were examined no leaks were found if the on-off valve was in the OFF position. If it was turned to the ON position, with no flow through the vaporizer, vapor could be detected in the machine outflow. The output from a measured-flow vaporizer may be accentuated by intermittent back pressure (38).

While the amounts delivered were for the most part too small to produce a clinical effect, in a few cases they were as high as 0.33% halothane. Even a small leak might cause a "sensitized" individual to be exposed to a halogenated agent and could possibly trigger malignant hyperthermia in a sensitive patient (51, 101).

This apparently results from diffusion from the vaporizing chamber. While the machine is not in use anesthetic vapor will accumulate in the bypass of a variable bypass vaporizer, so that initially when the fresh gas flow is turned on, a bolus of vapor will be swept out. The same would be true for a measured-flow vaporizer whose on-off valve were left in the ON position. After the initial bolus is swept out, a very small amount of vapor will continuously enter the outlet circuit.

The extent of such contamination will depend on the ambient temperature (and hence the vapor pressure of the liquid) as well as the size and configuration of the internal ports, tubing, etc.

This small vapor diffusion is inherent in most direct-reading vaporizers, but can be reduced considerably by the use of well-designed bypass units (51) and regular servicing. A vaporizer should not be turned from its OFF to 0 setting unless it is to be used. With measured-flow vaporizers, it is important to leave the on-off valve in the OFF position when the vaporizer is not in use.

The machine standard states that controls should be provided on direct-reading vaporizers to minimize the escape of vapor from the vaporizing chamber to the fresh gas line when the vaporizer is in the OFF position. Measured-flow vaporizers are required to have a shutoff valve or check valve or both.

Another possible source of leakage of vapor into the fresh gas line is vaporizer malfunction. Cases have been reported in which a malfunction prevented a vaporizer from being turned off (59, 102). Two cases have been reported in which it was possible to turn the concentration dial past the OFF position. At this position, the vaporizer delivered concentrations of vapor high enough to produce clinical effects (55, 57). Such a problem may be suspected if, when filling a vaporizer in the OFF position, liquid pours out the filling port while flow is going through the bypass.

Interlock devices will not prevent this problem if the vaporizers are connected in series. Robinson and colleagues (51) found that a selector valve would not prevent it since there is still a diffusion pathway via the selector valve. Physical disconnection devices will avoid this problem.

SERVICING

Vaporizers are precise instruments and, as with other mechanical devices, require regular, skillful maintenance if they are to remain reliable and precise. Moving parts in vaporizers are designed to require a minimum of lubricants. Some cleaning and lubrication is needed periodically to keep them in good working order. Misuse of vaporizers is difficult to control. For these reasons it is in the interest of safety that vaporizers be serviced regularly.

It should be remembered that when an anesthesia machine is serviced by an authorized representative he may not necessarily check the vaporizers, especially if they are manufactured by another company.

The machine standard requires that manufacturers' manuals should state the intervals at which vaporizers shall be serviced. Most manufacturers recommend that vaporizers be returned to them yearly or any time improper calibration or operation is suspected. Servicing includes checking for proper operation, calibration, cleaning, changing filters, as well as checking for leaks and for damaged or worn parts. By replacing damaged or worn parts problems such as leaks may be prevented.

Manufacturers occasionally carry out minor design changes even on products that are quite reliable. It is sometimes the practice to incorporate these changes into a vaporizer at the time of annual service (103).

Since the number of facilities servicing vaporizers is limited, most vaporizers must be sent long distances. It is important to have at least one extra agent-specific vaporizer for each agent used, so that servicing will result in a minimum of inconvenience. Some companies will provide the loan of a vaporizer during servicing.

CHOICE OF VAPORIZER

Which vaporizers should be purchased will depend on the needs of a department. Today the direct-reading vaporizers are popular because they are accurate and easy to use.

It is desirable to have in each department at

least one anesthesia machine with a multiple-agent vaporizer. As agents come and go, the anesthesiologist may wish to evaluate them. This may not justify the expense of an agent-specific vaporizer for every machine. If the agent stands the test of clinical use, purchase of agent-specific vaporizers may be justified.

The question arises as to whether a department should have one type of vaporizer or a large variety. Unquestionably, having one type of vaporizer simplifies interchange and servicing procedures. Safety will be enhanced if all direct-reading vaporizers have concentration dials that turn in the same direction.

References

1. Schreiber P: Effects of barometric pressure on anesthesia equipment. *Audio Digest* 17, No. 14, 1975.
2. Macintosh R, Mushin WW, Epstein HG: *Physics for the Anaesthetist*. Oxford, Blackwell Scientific Publications, 1963.
3. Blackwood O, Kelly W: *General Physics*. New York, John Wiley & Sons, 1955.
4. Hill DW: The design and calibration of vaporizers for volatile anaesthetic agents. *Br J Anaesth* 40:648–659, 1968.
5. *Minimum Performance and Safety Requirements for Components and Systems of Continuous Flow Anesthesia Machines for Human Use*. ANSI 2-79.8, American National Standards Institute, Inc., 1430 Broadway, New York, N.Y., 1979.
6. Schreiber P: Questions and answers. *Audio Digest* 17: No. 14, 1975.
7. Cowan SL, Scott RD, Suffolk SF: The Oxford vaporizer No 2. *Lancet* 2:64–66, 1941.
8. Lin C: Assessment of vaporizer performance in low-flow and closed-circuit anesthesia. *Anesth Analg* 59:359–366, 1980.
9. Nawaf K, Stoelting RK: Nitrous oxide increases enflurane concentration delivered by enflurane vaporizers. *Surv Anesth* 23:363, 1979.
10. Prins L, Strupat J, Clement J, Knill RL: An evaluation of gas density dependence of anaesthetic vaporizers. *Can Anaesth Soc J* 27:106–110, 1980.
11. Stoelting RK: The effect of nitrous oxide on halothane output from Fluotec Mark 2 vaporizers. *Anesthesiology* 35:215–218, 1971.
12. Knill R, Prins L, Strupat J, Clement J: Nitrous oxide and vaporizer outputs: transient or continuous effect? *Anesth Analg* 59:808–809, 1980.
13. Latto IP: Administration of halothane in the 0–0.5% concentration range with the Fluotec Mark 2 and Mark 3 vaporizers. *Br J Anaesth* 45:563–569, 1973.
14. Lin C: Enflurane vaporizer accuracy with nitrous oxide mixtures. *Anesth Analg* 58:440–441, 1979.
15. Nawaf K, Stoelting RK: Nitrous oxide increases enflurane concentrations delivered by enflurane vaporizers. *Anesth Analg* 58:30–32, 1979.
16. Stoelting RK, Nawaf K: Enflurane vaporizer ac-

17. Schreiber P: *Anesthesia Equipment. Performance, Classification, and Safety*. New York, Springer-Verlag, 1972.
18. Epstein HG: Principles of inhalers for volatile anaesthetics. *Br Med Bull* 14:18–26, 1958.
19. Morris LE, Feldman SA: Considerations in the design and function of anesthetic vaporizers. *Anesthesiology* 19:642–649, 1958.
20. Feldman SA, Morris LE: Vaporization of halothane and ether in the copper kettle. *Anesthesiology* 19:650–655, 1958.
21. Morris LE: Questions and answers. *Anesth Analg* 43:210–211, 1964.
22. Rosenberg M, Solod E, Bourke DL: Gas leak through a Fluotec Mark III vaporizer. *Anesth Analg* 58:239–240, 1979.
23. Sweatman F: Foaming of methoxyflurane contaminated with silicone. *Anesthesiology* 38:407, 1973.
24. Mapleson WW: The concentration of anaesthetics in closed circuits with special reference to halothane. I. Theoretical study. *Br J Anaesth* 32:298–309, 1960.
25. Hill DW: Physics applied to anaesthesia. IV. Heat. *Br J Anaesth* 38:219–222, 1966.
26. Morris LE: A new vaporizer for liquid anesthetic agents. *Anesthesiology* 13:587–593, 1952.
27. Hill DW, Jackson DC: Recent developments in vaporizers. *Anaesthesia* 19:191–205, 1964.
28. Steffey EP: Isoflurane concentrations delivered by isoflurane and halothane specific vaporizers. *Anesthesiology* 53:S19, 1980.
29. Shih A, Wu W: Potential hazard in using halothane-specific vaporizers for isoflurane and vice versa. *Anesthesiology* 55:A115, 1981.
30. Speer DL: Vaporization of anesthetic agents at high altitude. In Aldrete JA, Lowe HJ, Virtue RW (eds): *Low Flow and Closed System Anesthesia*. New York, Grune & Stratton, 1979, pp 235–250.
31. McDowall DG: Anaesthesia in a pressure chamber. *Anaesthesia* 19:321–336, 1964.
32. National Academy of Science-Federal Reserve Council: Hyperbaric oxygenation: anesthesia and drug effect. *Anesthesiology* 26:812–824, 1965.
33. Cole JR: The use of ventilators and vaporizer performance. *Br J Anaesth* 38:646–651, 1966.
34. Hill DW, Lowe HJ: Comparison of concentration of halothane in closed and semiclosed circuits during controlled ventilation. *Anesthesiology* 23:291–298, 1962.
35. Andreesen IH, Bay J: Halothane concentrations obtained by the combined use of the Manley ventilator and the Fluotec vaporizer. *Br J Anaesth* 38:641–645, 1966.
36. Lowe HJ, Beckham LM, Han YH, Evers JL: Vaporizer performance: closed circuit fluothane anesthesia. *Anesth Analg* 41:742–754, 1962.
37. Gordh T, Hallen B, Okmian L, Wahlen A, Stern B: The concentration of halothane by the combined use of Fluotec vaporizer and Engstrom respirator. *Acta Anaesthesiol Scand* 8:97–105, 1964.
38. Greenhow DE, Barth RL: Oxygen flushing deliv-

curacy with nitrous oxide mixtures. *Anesth Analg* 58:441, 1979.

ers anesthetic vapor—a hazard with a new machine. *Anesthesiology* 38:409–410, 1973.

39. Edmondson W, Hill DW: A pressurizing valve for the Fluotec vaporizer. *Br J Anaesth* 34:741–745, 1962.

40. Keet JE, Valentine GW, Riccio JS: An arrangement to prevent pressure effect on the Verni-Trol vaporizer. *Anesthesiology* 24:734–737, 1963.

41. Morris LE: Problems in the performance of anesthesia vaporizers. *Int Anesthesiol Clin* 12:199–219, 1974.

42. Morris LE: Copper Kettle. *Anesthesiology* 17:21–28, 1962.

43. Noble WH: Accuracy of halothane vaporizers in clinical use. *Can Anaesth Soc J* 17:135–143, 1970.

44. Cook TL, Eger EI, Behl RS: Is your vaporizer off? *Anesth Analg* 56:793–800, 1977.

45. Gartner J, Stoelting RK: A laboratory comparison of Copper Kettle, Fluotec Mark 2, and Pentec vaporizers. *Anesth Analg* 53:187–190, 1974.

46. Marx LC, Marx GF, Erlanger H, Joffe S, Kepes ER, Ravin MB: Improper filling of kettle-type vaporizers. *NY State J Med* 65:1151–1152, 1965.

47. Bluth M, Gelb EJ, Steen SN: A new concept for the continuous monitoring of anesthetic gases. *Anesthesiology* 33:449–451, 1970.

48. Morgan M, Lumley J: Reliability of halothane vaporizers. *Anaesthesia* 23:440–445, 1968.

49. Diaz PM: The influence of carrier gas on the output of automatic plenum vaporizers. *Br J Anaesth* 48:387–391, 1976.

50. Murray WJ, Fleming P: Fluotec Mark 2 halothane output: nonlinearity from "off" to 0.5 percent dial settings. *Anesthesiology* 36:180–181, 1972.

51. Robinson JS, Thompson JM, Barratt RS: Inadvertent contamination of anaesthetic circuits with halothane. *Br J Anaesth* 49:745–753, 1977.

52. North WC, Stephen CR: Pentec vaporizer for administering methoxyflurane anesthesia. *South Med J* 58:158–162, 1965.

53. Paterson GM, Hulands GH, Nunn JF: Evaluation of a new halothane vaporizer: the Cyprane Fluotec Mark 3. *Br J Anaesth* 41:109–119, 1969.

54. Anonymous: Evaluation: anesthesia units. *Health Devices* 10:31–51, 1980.

55. Davies JR: Enfluratec vaporizer. *Br J Anaesth* 52:356–357, 1980.

56. Novack GD, Ursillo RC: Malfunctioning halothane vaporizer. *Anesth Analg* 60:121, 1981.

57. Miller JM, Cascorbi HF: Yet another vaporizer hazard. *Anesth Analg* 59:805, 1980.

58. Bjoraker DG: Inability to shut off a halothane vaporizer. *Anesthesiology* 50:53–54, 1979.

59. Lewis JJ, Hicks RG: Malfunction of vaporizers. *Anesthesiology* 27:324–325, 1966.

60. Munson ES: Hazards of agent-specific vaporizers. *Anesthesiology* 34:393, 1971.

61. Personal communication: Lutheran General Hospital, Park Ridge, Ill., 1980.

62. Dolan PF: Vaporizer leak. *Anesthesiology* 49:302, 1978.

63. Hill EF: Percentages of fluothane vapour delivered from a Trilene bottle. *Br J Anaesth* 29:12–16, 1957.

64. Hill DW: Der Drager-Verdunster "Vapor." *Anaesthesist* 12:11–15, 1964.

65. Theilman NC: Design and safety of vaporizers. In *Proceedings of the Third Asian and Australian Congress of Anesthesiology*. London, Butterworth, 1970, pp 179–183.

66. Kopriva CJ, Lowenstein E: An anesthetic accident: cardiovascular collapse from liquid halothane delivery. *Anesthesiology* 30:246–247, 1969.

67. Rendell-Baker L, Milliken RA: Vaporizer overflow, a preventable hazard. *Anesthesiology* 50:478, 1979.

68. Medical device alert. Ohio Medical Products, 3030 Airco Drive, Madison, Wis. 53701, Feb 13, 1976.

69. Anonymous: Medical alert: shut-off valve of side arm Verni-Trol vaporizers. *Item Topics* 12: 1976.

70. Sharrock NE, Gabel RA: Inadvertent anesthetic overdose obscured by scavenging. *Anesthesiology* 49:138, 1978.

71. Gabel RA, Danielsen JB: Backflow of liquid halothane into a flowmeter. *Anesthesiology* 34:492–493, 1971.

72. *Keyed Filling Devices Applied to Anaesthetic Equipment*. CSA Z168.4-1975, Canadian Standards Association, 178 Rexdale Blvd., Rexdale, Ontario, Canada M9W 1R3.

73. McBurney R: Letters to the Editor. *Can Anaesth Soc J* 24:417–418, 1977.

74. Klein SL, Camenzind T: Hazards of bottle adaptors for vaporizers. *Anesth Analg* 57:596–597, 1978.

75. Rendell-Baker L: Bottle adaptors for vaporizers. *Anesth Analg* 58:156, 1979.

76. Dorsch SE, Dorsch JA: Chemical cross-contamination between vaporizers in series. *Anesth Analg* 52:176–180, 1973.

77. Murray WJ, Zsigmond EK, Fleming P: Contamination of in-series vaporizers with halothane-methoxyflurane. *Anesthesiology* 38:487–489, 1973.

78. Wickett RE, Jenkins LC, Root LS: Downstream contamination of in-series vapourizers. *Can Anaesth Soc J* 21:114–116, 1974.

79. Corssen G: Effects of halogenated anesthetic agents on human embryonic kidney cells. *Anesth Analg* 48:858, 1969.

80. Anonymous: Accidental use of trichlorethylene (Trilene, Trimar) in a closed system. *Anesth Analg* 43:740–743, 1964.

81. Paull JD, Sleeman KW: An anaesthetic hazard. *Br J Anaesth* 3:1202, 1971.

82. Munson WM: Cardiac arrest: Hazard of tipping a vaporizer. *Anesthesiology* 26:235, 1965.

83. Long GJ, Marsh HM: A danger—insecure positioning of anaesthetic vaporizers. *Med J Aust* 1:1108, 1969.

84. Larsen ER: Foaming in halogenated anaesthetics—the chemistry of modern inhalation anaesthetics. In Chenoweth HR (ed): *Modern Inhalation Anaesthetics*. New York, Springer-Verlag, 1972, p 29.

85. DeGuzman CM, Cascorbi HF: An unusual hazard of methoxyflurane. *Anesthesiology* 36:305, 1972.

86. Rendell-Baker L: Equipment standards in anesthesia practice—elimination of the hazards. *Clin Trends Anesthesiol* 7 (No 2): May–June, 1977.

87. Safar P, Galla SJ: Overdose with Ohio halothane vaporizer. *Anesthesiology* 23:715–716, 1962.

88. Personal communication: Peter Schreiber.
89. Epstein RM: Guest discussion. *Anesth Analg* 56:798–800, 1977.
90. Kaufman MJ: Vaporizer malfunction. *J Am Assoc Nurse Anesthetists* 39:56–57, 1971.
91. Marks WE, Bullard JR: Another hazard of free-standing vaporizers, increased anesthetic concentration with reversed flow of vaporizing gas. *Anesthesiology* 45:445–446, 1976.
92. Personal communication: Chalmers Goodyear.
93. Wyant GM: Some dangers in anaesthesia. *Can Anaesth Soc J* 25:71–72, 1978.
94. Austin TR: A warning device for the "Fluotec" Mark II and III. *Anaesthesia* 26:368, 1971.
95. Anonymous: Medical equipment alert: gas leaks in anesthesia machine circuitry. *Items Topics*, April, 1973, p 8.
96. Mullin RA: Letter to the Editor. *Can Anaesth Soc J* 25:248–249, 1978.
97. Eldrup-Jorgensen S, Sprissler GT: Gas leaks in anesthesia machines. *Anesthesiology* 46:439, 1977.
98. Mulroy M, Ham J, Eger EI: Inflowing gas leak, a potential source of hypoxia. *Anesthesiology* 45:102–104, 1976.
99. Hunter L: Leaking halothane vaporizers. *Med J Aust* 2:716, 1974.
100. Capan L, Ramanathan S, Chalon J, O'Meara JB, Turndorf H: A possible hazard with use of the Ohio ethrane vaporizer. *Anesth Analg* 59:65–68, 1980.
101. Ellis FR, Clarks IMC, Modgill EM, Appleyard TN, Dinsdale RCW: New causes of malignant hyperthermia. *Br Med J* 1:575, 1975.
102. Bahl CP: A cause of inaccuracy in vaporizer delivery. *Anaesthesia* 32:1037, 1977.
103. Carter RW: Enfluratec vaporizer. *Br J Anaesth* 52:356–357, 1980.

The Breathing System. I. General Considerations

The breathing system is an assembly of components from or through which the patient breathes. It allows the anesthesiologist to take an anesthetic mixture from the anesthesia machine and present this mixture to the patient. In this way anesthetics are conveyed to and from the patient and normal exchange of oxygen and carbon dioxide can occur. There are several types in common use today. They will be discussed in a series of four chapters. Chapter 5 will discuss general principles, common components and classifications. Chapter 6 will deal with the Mapleson systems and their variants. Chapter 7 is concerned with systems containing non-rebreathing valves. Chapter 8 will consider the circle system.

PRINCIPLES OF BREATHING SYSTEMS

Resistance

PHYSICS

When gas passes through a tube, a pressure gradient can be observed between the ends of the tube. This gradient is a measure of the resistance to the passage of the gas through the tube (1). Resistance varies with the volume of gas passing through per unit of time. Therefore, flowrate must be stated when a specific resistance is mentioned.

The nature of the gas flow is important in determining resistance. Gas flow may be either laminar or turbulent. In clinical practice flow is often a mixture of laminar and turbulent.

Laminar Flow

Figure 5.1A shows a laminar flow of gas through a tube. The flow is smooth and orderly and the lines of flow are parallel to the walls of the tube. Flow is fastest in the center of the tube where there is less friction.

When flow is laminar, the Hagen-Poiseuille law applies. This law states that

$$\Delta P = \frac{L \times v \times V}{D} \qquad (1)$$

where D is the diameter of the tube
ΔP is the pressure gradient across the tube (resistance)
L is the length of the tube
v is the viscosity of the gas
V is the volume flowrate.

The resistance is directly proportional to the flowrate with laminar flow.

Turbulent Flow

Figure 5.1B shows a turbulent flow of gas through a tube. The lines of flow are no longer parallel. Eddies, composed of fluid particles moving across or opposite the general direction of flow, are present. The flowrate is the same across the diameter of the tube.

For turbulent flow the Fanning equation (2) is used. This can be expressed as follows:

$$\Delta P = \frac{V^2 \times L \times K}{D^5} \qquad (2)$$

where K is a constant including such factors as gravity, friction and gas density. Resistance is proportional to the *square* of the flowrate with turbulent flow.

Turbulent flow can be generalized or localized.

Generalized Turbulent Flow. When the flow of gas through a tube exceeds a certain value, called the critical flowrate, generalized turbulent flow results. The critical flowrate varies directly with the internal diameter of the tube. It is also influenced by the ratio of the density to the viscosity of the gas (1).

Localized Turbulent Flow. As seen in Fig-

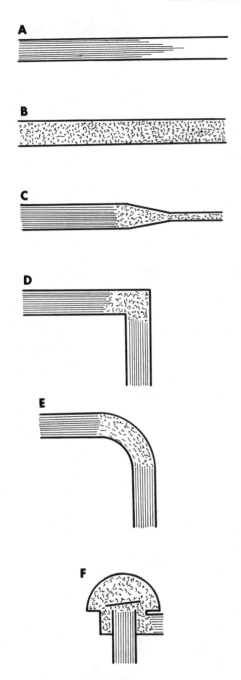

ure 5.1, *C* to *E*, when gas flow is below the critical flowrate but encounters constrictions, sharp curves, valves or other irregularities, an area of localized turbulence occurs. The increase in resistance will depend on the type and number of obstructions encountered.

Minimal apparatus resistance, therefore, dictates that gas-conducting pathways be of minimal length, maximal internal diameter and without sharp bends or sudden variations in diameter.

In general, the resistance offered by the breathing system is small compared to that introduced by endotracheal tubes and their connections (3, 4).

EFFECTS OF INCREASED RESISTANCE

Much has been written about the effects of resistance in anesthesia apparatus upon the patient (3, 5–14). A full discussion is beyond the scope of this book. There is lack of agreement about what level of resistance should be considered excessive (6, 7, 15–17). However, it would seem wise for the anesthesiologist to know how much resistance items of equipment offer and to employ, as far as possible, those items offering the least resistance.

For certain patients, a degree of increased expiratory resistance may be desirable. It is suggested that this be achieved by use of special devices designed for this purpose.

Rebreathing

Rebreathe means literally to breathe again. This includes any gas which has been previously exhaled from which carbon dioxide may or may not have been removed. There is a tendency to associate the word "rebreathing" with carbon dioxide accumulation. This is unfortunate because while it is true that rebreathing can result in higher carbon dioxide concentrations than are normally present in the inspired air, it is possible to employ partial or total rebreathing without an increase in carbon dioxide concentration. Breathing systems should prevent accumulation of carbon dioxide but prevention of rebreathing is not necessarily desirable.

FACTORS INFLUENCING REBREATHING

The amount of rebreathing will depend on three factors: the fresh gas flow, the mechanical

Figure 5.1. Laminar and turbulent flow. *A*, laminar flow: the lines of flow are parallel and are slower near the sides of the tube. This is due to resistance caused by friction with the sides of the tube. *B*, generalized turbulent flow: this occurs when the critical flowrate is exceeded. The lines of flow are not parallel and eddies occur. *C* to *F*, localized turbulence: this occurs when gas changes direction or passes through constrictions.

dead space and the design of the breathing system.

Fresh Gas Flow

The amount of rebreathing varies inversely with the total fresh gas flow. If the total volume of fresh gas supplied per minute is equal to or greater than the patient's minute volume, there will be no rebreathing, provided provision is made for unimpeded expiration to atmosphere or a scavenging system at a point close to the patient's respiratory tract (18). If the total volume of gas supplied per minute is less than the minute volume, a certain proportion of the exhaled atmosphere must be rebreathed to make up the required volume (assuming no air dilution).

Mechanical Dead Space

The mechanical dead space is the space in a breathing system occupied by gases which are rebreathed without any change in composition. The minimum volume of gas that can be rebreathed is equal to the mechanical dead space. Any increase in dead space therefore increases rebreathing. Apparatus dead space may be minimized most effectively by separating inspiratory and expiratory gas streams as close to the patient as possible (19). The volume of rebreathed gas may exceed the mechanical dead space volume.

The mechanical dead space should be distinguished from the physiological dead space which includes (a) anatomical dead space consisting of the conducting airway of the patient down to the alveoli and (b) alveolar dead space, which is the volume of alveoli which are ventilated but not perfused. The mechanical dead space may be considered a simple extension of the patient's physiological dead space except that it is usually near room temperature and less moist.

The composition of the gas in the mechanical dead space will vary according to whether it is occupied by anatomical dead space gas, alveolar gas or mixed expired gas. Gas exhaled from the anatomical dead space has a composition similar to inspired gas, but is saturated with water vapor and at a temperature of approximately 32°C (9). Alveolar gas is saturated with water vapor at body temperature and has less oxygen and more carbon dioxide than inspired gas. Also the concentration of anesthetic gases will differ from the inspired gas. Mixed expired gas will have a composition intermediate between dead space and alveolar gas.

Design of the Breathing System

In addition to the above factors, the various components of a breathing system may be arranged so that there is more or less rebreathing. This will be discussed more fully under the individual systems.

EFFECTS OF REBREATHING

With no rebreathing, the inspired gas is identical to the fresh gas mixture delivered by the anesthesia machine. With rebreathing the inspired gas is composed partly of fresh gas and partly of rebreathed gas.

Retention of Heat and Water

Fresh gas from the anesthesia machine is anhydrous and at room temperature. Exhaled gases are warm and saturated with water. Hence rebreathing reduces heat and water loss from the patient. In most breathing systems heat is rapidly lost to atmosphere and the gas which is reinhaled has a lower temperature and water content than exhaled gas (20).

Alteration of Inspired Gas Tensions

The effects of rebreathing on inspired gas tensions will depend on what parts of the exhaled gases are reinhaled and whether these pass to the alveoli (and so influence gas exchange) or only to the anatomical dead space of the patient (20).

Oxygen. Rebreathing of alveolar gas will cause a reduction in the inspired oxygen tension. This is due to several factors: patient uptake of oxygen, and the addition of nitrogen, carbon dioxide, and water vapor to the gas.

Anesthetic Gases. The rebreathing of alveolar gas exerts a "cushioning" effect on changes in inspired gas composition with changes in the fresh gas composition. During induction, when alveolar tensions are lower than those in the fresh gas flow, the rebreathing of alveolar gas will reduce the inspired tension and prolong induction. During recovery, the alveolar tension exceeds that of the inspired gases. Rebreathing maintains a higher alveolar tension and slows the elimination of anesthetic gas.

Carbon Dioxide. Rebreathing of alveolar gas will cause an increase in inspired carbon dioxide tension unless the gas passes through an absorber before being rebreathed.

The efficiency with which carbon dioxide is eliminated from a breathing system without an absorber varies. This is because carbon dioxide is concentrated in the alveolar portion of the expired gas. If the design of the circuit is such that this part is preferentially eliminated through the relief valve, carbon dioxide retention will be minimal, even with a low fresh gas flow. Circuits that do not maintain the separation between fresh gas, dead space gas and alveolar gas tend to be inefficient and require high gas flows to eliminate carbon dioxide.

Carbon dioxide retention is generally considered undesirable with spontaneous respiration. While a patient can compensate by increasing minute volume, a price must be paid in terms of increased work of breathing and, in some cases, the compensation may not be adequate. It is possible that in the spontaneously breathing patient under anesthesia some hyperventilation may be desirable (21).

During controlled ventilation, rebreathing can be turned to advantage. An increase in dead space will allow normocarbia to be maintained with hyperventilation. Thus hypocarbia can be avoided and heat and moisture retained while using large tidal volumes to keep the lungs well expanded.

Discrepancy between Inspired and Delivered Concentrations

The composition of the gas mixture which issues from the machine outlet may be modified by the breathing system so that the mixture the patient inspires differs considerably from that delivered to the system. There are several contributing factors.

REBREATHING

The effect of rebreathing will depend on the volume of the rebreathed gas and its composition. This will depend on the factors discussed previously.

AIR DILUTION

If the fresh gas supplied per respiration is less than the tidal volume and the inspiratory limb is open to atmosphere, the patient may inhale air while breathing spontaneously. The amount of air dilution will depend on the presence or absence of reservoirs in the system, the respiratory pattern and the total fresh gas flow.

Air dilution makes it difficult to maintain a stable anesthetic state. When it occurs, the concentration of anesthetic in the inspired mixture falls. This results in lighter anesthesia with attendant stimulation of ventilation. The increased ventilation causes more air dilution. The opposite also is true. Deepening anesthesia depresses ventilation. Depression of respiration decreases air dilution and thereby increases the inspired concentration of anesthetic. This in turn leads to further depression of respiration. Fortunately, depression of respiration limits the rise in alveolar concentration and apnea usually supervenes before lethal concentrations are reached in the lungs.

LEAKS

When a leak occurs, positive pressure in the system will force gas out of the system. The composition and amount of the gas lost will depend on the location of the leak, the size of the leak, the pressure in the system, and the compliance and resistance of both the system and the patient.

UPTAKE OF ANESTHETIC AGENT BY THE SYSTEM

Uptake of anesthetic agents in rubber, plastics, metal, and carbon dioxide absorbent can produce a lower inspired concentration at the beginning of a case and can contribute anesthetic agent to the system when the concentration in the system falls.

The uptake of anesthetic by the system components will be directly proportional to: (a) the gradient between the gas and the components, (b) the partition coefficient, (c) the surface area, (d) the diffusion coefficient, and (e) the square root of time.

The diffusion coefficients and partition coefficients are constant for any anesthetic agent. Some partition coefficients are shown in Table 4.1. The surface area will depend on the system used and must include the delivery hose from the machine. Concentration and time will vary. It is difficult to predict the uptake of agent by the breathing system with any precision.

RELEASE OF ANESTHETIC AGENT FROM THE SYSTEM

Elimination of anesthetic agent from the breathing system will depend on the same factors as uptake. Of some clinical significance is the fact that with some anesthetics the system may function as a low output vaporizer for many hours after the primary vaporizer has been turned off (22–24) even if the rubber goods and absorbent are changed. Thus, the possibility exists for unplanned exposure of a patient to an agent. This may have great significance if "sensitization" is a mechanism for anesthetic-induced hepatotoxicity. It is also of significance for patients susceptible to malignant hyperpyrexia.

Heat and Humidity

PHYSICS

Humidity

Humidity refers to the amount of water vapor in a unit volume of gas at a given temperature. Three terms are commonly used to express it: absolute humidity, relative humidity, and water vapor partial pressure.

Absolute humidity is defined as the weight of water vapor in a unit volume of gas. It is usually expressed in milligrams per liter.

Relative humidity, or percent saturation, is the water vapor actually present in a volume of gas stated as a percentage of the highest possible vapor content for the gas. In other words,

Relative humidity

$$= \frac{\text{Absolute humidity of the gas sample}}{\text{Absolute humidity of saturated gas sample}}$$

In order to calculate relative humidity it is necessary to know the amount of water vapor that can be held by a volume of gas at that temperature. This will vary with the temperature. Table 5.1 shows the absolute water content of saturated gas at various temperatures.

If a gas saturated with water vapor is heated, it can hold more water. Its relative humidity falls, but its absolute humidity remains unchanged. Conversely, if a gas saturated with water vapor is cooled, it will rain out (condense) the amount of water vapor it held at the original temperature less the amount it can hold at the lower temperature. Absolute humidity will fall, but relative humidity will remain at 100%. Using relative humidity as a measure of humidification of gases can be misleading, since the relative

Table 5.1.
Absolute Water Contents and Partial Pressures of Saturated Gas

Temperature	Water Vapor Partial Pressure*	Absolute Humidity†
°C	mmHg	mg/liter
10	9.2	9.3
11	9.8	9.9
12	10.5	10.6
13	11.2	11.3
14	11.9	12.0
15	12.7	12.7
16	13.6	13.5
17	14.5	14.3
18	15.4	15.2
19	16.4	16.1
20	17.5	17.1
21	18.6	18.1
22	19.8	19.2
23	21.0	20.3
24	22.3	21.5
25	23.7	22.8
26	25.2	24.1
27	26.7	25.5
28	28.3	26.9
29	30.4	28.5
30	31.8	30.0
31	33.6	31.7
32	35.6	33.5
33	37.7	35.3
34	39.8	37.2
35	42.1	39.2
36	44.5	42.1
37	47.0	45.5

* From Chalon J, Ali M, Turndorf H, Fischgrund GK: *Humidification of Anesthetic Gases.* Springfield, Ill., Charles C Thomas, 1981.
† From Kaye GWC, Laby TH: *Tables of Physical and Chemical Constants and Some Mathematical Functions*, ed 12. New York, Longmans, 1959.

humidity of gases delivered at room temperature falls when the gases attain body temperature.

Humidity may also be expressed as the pressure exerted by water vapor in a gas mixture. Table 5.1 shows the water vapor pressure of saturated gas at various temperatures.

Specific Heat

Specific heat was discussed in Chapter 4. The specific heats of gases are low. As a consequence, they quickly assume the temperature of the surrounding environment. Inhaled gases quickly approach body temperature and gases in corrugated tubes rapidly approach room temperature.

Heat of Vaporization

The heat of vaporization of water is relatively high (580 cal/g). Hence, vaporization of water requires considerably more heat than warming of gases. Conversely, condensation of water produces more heat than cooling of gases. There is little difference in heat loss or gain from a patient whether hot or cold gases are inhaled, if they are dry.

CLINICAL CONSIDERATIONS

Water is intentionally removed from all medical gases—piped or from cylinders—to prevent clogging of regulators and valves. Gases emerging from the anesthesia machine are dry and at room temperature. Anesthesia breathing systems presently in use contribute a wide range of humidity and heat to the inspired gas mixture. With most anesthesia circuits, the inspired gas is at a lower temperature and humidity than alveolar gas.

In its passage to the alveoli, inspired gas is brought to body temperature (either by heating or cooling) and 100% relative humidity (either by evaporation or condensation). In the unintubated patient the upper respiratory tract (especially the nose) functions as the principal heat and moisture exchanger. Endotracheal intubation or tracheostomy bypasses the upper airway, modifying the pattern of heat and moisture exchange, so that the tracheobronchial mucosa must assume more of the burden of heating and humidifying arid gases before they reach the alveoli. Dery and co-workers (25) have shown that the endotracheal tube to a considerable extent performs the function of the upper airway in alternately condensing expired moisture and adding it to the inhaled gases. In addition, apparatus deadspace functions as a heat and moisture exchanger, but of rather low efficiency.

Sources of humidity in a breathing system include the following: (a) water intentionally added to the system; (b) water contributed by carbon dioxide absorbents; (c) moisture exhaled by patients into the system. This includes patients on whom the system has been previously used.

Means of adding moisture to the breathing system will be discussed later in this chapter. Contributions by carbon dioxide absorbents will be discussed in the chapter on circle systems.

In systems which allow rebreathing, the humidity and temperature of inspired gases depend upon the relative proportions of fresh gases and expired gases reinhaled. As fresh gas flow increases, the temperature and humidity of inspired gases are reduced by dilution (26, 27).

Previous use of a system on other patients can significantly affect inspired humidity. Water condensed in tubing (including the ventilator hose) and other parts of a system that are not changed between cases can contribute significantly to the initial inspired humidity.

There are a number of clinical effects that have been suggested to result from the use of dry anesthetic gases: (a) Impairment of ciliary function (28–30). (b) Increased loss of body heat (31–36). This is especially important in pediatric patients who are susceptible to heat loss. The incidence of postanesthetic shivering increases as humidity is decreased (37). (c) Decreased water content of mucus and accumulation of viscid secretions. This could lead to plugging of the endotracheal tube. (d) Damage to the tracheal and bronchial mucosa (30, 38–42).

Several studies show a significant decrease in postoperative pulmonary complications when gases are humidified (36, 43–45) but one study showed no difference (46).

There is no agreement as to what level of humidity is necessary to prevent pathophysiological changes. Recommendations range from saturation at 20–30°C (47) to greater than 90% saturation at 37°C, with many intermediate values also recommended (25, 28, 39). The duration of exposure must always be considered. It is unlikely that very brief exposure of the tracheobronchial tree to dry inspired gases will result in damage, but as exposure time increases the likelihood of a significant effect rises.

There are a number of dangers associated with artificial humidification. Infection is always a risk where water is present. Humidification systems capable of delivering high volumes of water (especially nebulizers) can produce a positive water balance and possible overhydration, especially in infants, if used for a prolonged period of time (30, 48). An increased postanesthetic incidence of severe bronchopneumonia has been demonstrated using ultrasonic nebulizers (49).

Some humidification devices have a high resistance so that when they are interposed into the fresh gas line significant back pressure is created, making flowmeter and vaporizer readings inaccurate (34).

Dead space and resistance may be increased with the addition of apparatus between the breathing system and the endotracheal tube.

This can be a significant problem in the small infant. Resistance of bacterial filters may be increased by humidity (37).

Other equipment problems include sticking valves (50), leaks (51), and disconnections. The accuracy of some oxygen analyzers may be affected if condensate forms on the sensor. If the gases must pass from a heated source through unheated tubing to the patient, condensation can be a formidable problem, causing noise that hinders monitoring and even occlusion to flow.

Heating of the water source and/or the inspiratory limb can result in hyperthermia (52) or tracheitis (53) unless the temperature is carefully regulated. There is evidence that at least one anesthetic agent is altered by passage through a heated humidifier (54). Electric heating devices add the dangers of fires, electrical shocks, and inhalation of noxious fumes due to combustion of plastic containers. They cannot be used with flammable anesthetic agents.

To summarize, the importance of humidification in anesthesia remains uncertain. It is probably of more significance in pediatric patients, in procedures of long duration, and in those involving patients at increased risk of developing pulmonary complications. The benefits of deliberately increasing humidification must be weighed against its hazards. Clearly, this is an area which is important to those administering anesthesia and one which warrants further investigation.

COMMON COMPONENTS

Certain pieces of equipment are found in only one type of breathing system. These will be discussed under the individual systems. However, other components are common to more than one system so that their discussion in a general chapter such as this is indicated. The following will be discussed: bushings, sleeves, connectors and adaptors, reservoir bags, breathing tubes, and relief valve assemblies.

Bushings (Mounts)

A bushing is an adaptor which alters the internal diameter. Most often it has a cylindrical form and is inserted into and becomes part of a pliable component, such as a reservoir bag or a corrugated tube.

Sleeves

A sleeve is an adaptor which alters the external diameter of a component.

Connectors and Adaptors

DEFINITION OF TERMS

The terms "connector" and "adaptor" have been used more or less interchangeably. According to International Standards Organization terminology, a connector is a fitting intended to join together two or more components, whereas an adaptor is a specialized connector that establishes functional continuity between otherwise disparate or incompatible components.

An adaptor or connector may be distinguished by: (a) shape (straight, right-angled, Y-piece); (b) component(s) to which it is attached; (c) added features (with nipple, with pop-off) and (d) size and type of fitting at either end (15-mm male, 22-mm female).

An adaptor of special importance is the mask/endotracheal tube connector. Almost all anesthesia systems terminate at the patient end by connecting to a mask or endotracheal tube connector. By convention, all modern masks, both adult and pediatric, have a 22-mm female opening and all endotracheal and tracheostomy tube connectors have a 15-mm male fitting at the machine end. To facilitate the change from mask to endotracheal tube and vice versa, a mask/endotracheal tube adaptor having a 22-mm male fitting with a concentric 15-mm female opening to fit both a mask and an endotracheal tube is used in most systems.

Connectors and adaptors are most commonly used to join a tracheal tube connector or a mask to the breathing system. They serve several purposes: (a) to extend the distance between the tracheal tube and the breathing system. This is especially important in head and neck surgery where the presence of the breathing system near the head may make it inaccessible to the anesthesiologist and/or interfere with the surgical field. (b) to change the angle of connection between the tracheal tube and the breathing system. When a straight tracheal tube connector is used it will be vertical unless the patient's head is turned to the side. The breathing system is usually horizontal so that a connector is necessary. (c) to allow a more flexible and/or less kinkable connection between the tracheal tube and the breathing system and (d) to increase the dead space. This is most often desirable when prolonged mechanical ventilation is being used.

There are a large number and variety of connectors available commercially (Fig. 5.2) and many more have been described in the literature.

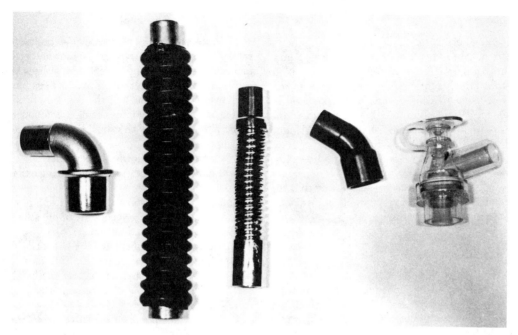

Figure 5.2. Typical connectors. The left connector connects the breathing system to either a mask or endotracheal tube connector. Thus, the change from mask to endotracheal tube is easily made. The second connector is a flexible rubber connector with metal fittings at either end. It can be kinked only by an extreme 180-degree turn. The third connector is a flexible metal connector. It will hold its shape once bent. The next connector is curved 45 degrees. The connector on the right is a swivel connector with a suction port.

Connectors should have a 15-mm male (OD) fitting at the machine end and either a 22-mm male/15-mm female fitting for connection to either a tracheal tube connector or a mask or simply a 15-mm female fitting for connection to a tracheal tube connector.

In selecting a connector, several principles should be kept in mind.

1. Resistance increases markedly with sharp curves and rough sidewalls.

2. Connectors add dead space. In the average adult patient this may not be of much significance. However, in infants any increase in dead space may be excessive. The need for connectors should always be carefully considered in these cases.

3. Use of connector(s) increases the possible locations at which disconnection can take place. Disconnection between two tube components is an ever-present and dangerous problem. The anesthesiologist must always be alert for such an occurrence. It is best avoided by making sure connections are tight and are not under traction. In addition, a number of devices have been described to prevent this problem (see Chapter 10).

SIZE AND SEQUENCE OF CONNECTORS

A source of great frustration for the anesthesiologist and hazard to the patient in the past has been the existence of many different sizes of fittings on the components of anesthesia systems. This unhappy situation resulted from the fact that there were many different equipment companies, each manufacturing its own sized fittings, necessitating many adaptors to fit one company's components to another's.

In recent years, progress has been made toward a standardized set of sizes and fitting sequences for components of breathing systems. The Compressed Gas Association has published standards for the size and sequence of connectors of components (55). Breathing system components conforming to it are compatible with essentially all anesthesia breathing system components manufactured in the United States in recent years.

Sequence

Connectors forming a part of components such as absorbers, vaporizers, Y-pieces, non-rebreathing valves, etc., whose purpose is to permit attachment of these components to reservoir bags, breathing tubes, or masks shall be male and "rigid." The breathing tube, mask and reservoir bag connectors shall be female and non-rigid (resilient).

The standard also requires that all breathing system components in which the direction of gas flow is critical be marked in such a way that the intended direction of gas flow is immediately apparent to the operator.

Size

All connectors in the modern adult system are 22 mm. The component which is designed to connect to an endotracheal tube connector should have a coaxial 15-mm female fitting at the patient end.

All fittings of the pediatric system are 15 mm. The component designed to fit into a mask must have a coaxial 22-mm male fitting.

Reservoir Bag

The reservoir bag is also known as the respiratory bag, breathing bag, or, somewhat erroneously, the rebreathing bag (56). Most bags are composed of rubber, although plastic bags have been available. The neck of the bag may terminate in a fitting which joins the next component or may be supplied with a bushing (bag holder or adaptor).

The bag has the following functions:

1. It allows accumulation of gas during exhalation so that a reservoir of gas is available for the patient's next inspiration. This permits rebreathing, allows greater economy of anesthetic gases and prevents air dilution.

2. It provides a means whereby the anesthesiologist may assist or control respirations.

3. It can serve through visual and tactile observation as a monitor of a patient's spontaneous respirations.

4. It acts as a built-in safety valve, protecting the patient from excessive pressure in the breathing system (57–59).

Parmley and co-workers (57) studied the pressure-volume characteristics of rubber bags. Their results are shown in Figure 5.3. Initially

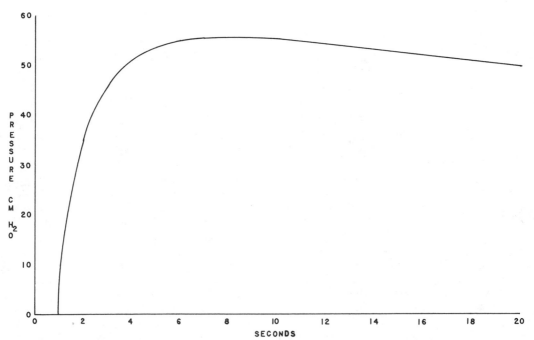

Figure 5.3. Pressure-volume characteristics of a reservoir bag. Flowrate 50 liters/min. (Redrawn from Parmley JB, Tahir AN, Dascomb HE, et al: Disposable versus reusable rebreathing circuits: advantages, disadvantages, hazards and bacteriologic studies. *Anesth Analg* 51: 890, 1972.)

adding volume to a bag causes a negligible rise in pressure until the nominal capacity of the bag is reached. As more volume is added, the pressure rises rapidly to a peak and attains a plateau. As the bag distends further, the pressure falls slightly. The peak pressure is of particular interest as this represents the maximal pressure that will develop in a breathing system. The American Standard for anesthetic reservoir bags requires that with a bag distended to four times its nominal capacity, the pressure not exceed 50 cm H_2O (60). Stone and colleagues (59) found this pressure was often exceeded, especially if the bag was new and there was a high inflow rate.

New bags develop greater pressures when first overinflated than bags which have been overinflated several times or prestretched (57, 59, 61). It is good practice to overinflate or stretch each new bag a few times before it is used. This will not limit the anesthesiologist's ability to produce higher airway pressures by squeezing and will increase the margin of safety.

Disposable plastic bags are inelastic and do not stretch after full inflation. Excessively high pressure may develop within seconds when these units are inadvertently overfilled with gases (57, 62). They should not be used.

The size of the bag that should be used will depend on the patient, the system in which it is used, and the anesthesiologist's preference. Too large a bag may be difficult to squeeze and will make monitoring of the patient's respirations more difficult because the bag excursions will be smaller. A small bag, on the other hand, provides less of a safety factor for distention and may not provide a large enough reservoir.

A spare bag should always be kept immediately available. A bag may rupture at any time or become lost while a ventilator is in use. If a spare bag is not immediately available, the anesthesiologist may be confronted with the problem of ventilating an apneic patient. This may be accomplished by occluding the bag attachment point while the oxygen flush is activated. The hand is removed for exhalation. This is a somewhat dangerous method and will not keep the patient anesthetized.

Breathing Tubes

Large bore, non-rigid breathing tubes, composed of rubber or plastic and usually corrugated, are found in most breathing systems. The wrinkles in corrugated tubes prevent kinking from causing obstruction. At the same time, they lend flexibility. Plastic tubes allow visualization of the tube's interior. In addition, they are lightweight, causing less "drag" on the endotracheal tube or mask. Inadvertent extubation and/or disconnection may be less likely with their use. They absorb less of the halogenated agents than rubber tubes and they have a lower compliance.

Most breathing tubes are of unit construction, terminating in integrally attached fittings that mate with the next component. Some are supplied with bushings (breathing tube adaptors). The ANSI standard (63) requires that both ends have 22-mm female connectors. Some disposable circle breathing systems have the Y-piece integrally attached to the tubings, in which case the Y must have a standard coaxial 22-mm outside diameter and a 15-mm internal diameter. Some tubes have a loop near the end for hanging.

Breathing tubes have two functions. One is to act as a reservoir in certain systems. A second function is to provide a flexible, low-resistance, lightweight connection from one part of the system to another. The resistance of corrugated tubes is small compared to the resistance of equipment to which they are attached (11, 64).

Breathing tubes have some distensibility but not enough to prevent excessive pressures from developing in the system (62). Circuits vary in their compressible volume but generally fall between 1 and 4 ml/cm H_2O (65, 66). During spontaneous ventilation, breathing tubes tend to collapse on inspiration and bulge on exhalation. This may cause some rebreathing and is referred to as "backlash." During controlled and assisted ventilation, the tubes tend to bulge on inspiration and return to a resting position on exhalation. This is referred to as "wasted ventilation" since it results in less volume entering the patient than leaves the ventilator or reservoir bag. This assumes some importance when a respirometer is used to measure tidal volumes. Unless the respirometer is between the tubes and the patient, part of the volume measured will be expended in distending the tubes and compressing the gases and the patient will actually receive less than that measured. The rigidity of plastic tubes is an asset, since the lower distensibility minimizes backlash and wasted ventilation.

Disposable breathing systems are used in large numbers today. Most are supplied clean, but not sterile. Sterile disposable breathing systems are available. Unfortunately, quality control is sometimes lacking. New circuits may be kinked, indented, fractured, or separated at the Y or swivel (67). Disposable systems, especially those with swivel adapters, are more likely to leak than nondisposable ones (68).

A number of tubing supports have been devised to elevate the tubes from the patient's face and reduce the likelihood of dislodgement of the endotracheal tube (69–71).

Relief Valve Assembly (Overspill Valve, Pop-off Valve, Overflow Valve, Dump Valve, Blow-off Valve, Safety Relief Valve, Adjustable Pressure-Limiting Valve, Spill Valve, Exhaust Valve, Expiratory Valve, Excess Gas Valve, Pressure Release Valve, Release Valve)

Any breathing system in which the input of gases is greater than the uptake by the patient and breathing system will need to have some mechanism to relieve the system of excess gases and release them either to atmosphere or to the collection device of a scavenging system. A hole in the tail of the reservoir bag sometimes serves this purpose, but more commonly a relief valve is used.

There are two general types of relief valves: high-pressure and low-pressure.

HIGH-PRESSURE RELIEF VALVES

These are the more commonly used. They are designed to relieve gas to atmosphere or a scavenging system when the pressure in the breathing system reaches a certain level.

Construction

Control Part. The control part serves to control the pressure at which the valve relieves. Several types of control parts are used.

Spring-Loaded Disc. The most commonly used relief valve utilizes a disc held onto a seat by a coiled spring (Fig. 5.4). A threaded screw cap over the spring allows the pressure exerted by the spring to be varied. When the cap is fully tightened, the disc will prevent any gas from escaping from the system. As the cap is rotated and moves upward the tension on the spring is less and the pressure required to raise the disc from the seat falls. Most relief valves are built so that rotating the cap clockwise increases

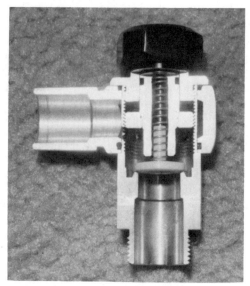

Figure 5.4. Relief valve with spring-loaded disc. Gas from the breathing system enters at the base and passes into the collection device at the *left.* Turning the screw cap varies the tension in the spring and the pressure necessary to lift the disc off its seat.

spring tension and counterclockwise rotation decreases it.

When the pressure in the breathing system increases, it exerts an upward force on the disc. When this force exceeds the downward force exerted by the spring, the disc rises and gas flows out of the system. When the pressure in the system falls, the disc returns to its seat. When the cap is at its maximum upward position, there will be no pressure exerted by the spring. The weight of the disc will ensure that the reservoir bag will fill before the disc rises.

Stem and Seat. Another control part employed in relief valves is the stem and seat (Fig. 5.5). This is similar to the flow control valve in that a threaded stem allows variable contact with a seat. As the valve is opened, the opening at the seat becomes larger and more gas is allowed to escape. There is a device (ball, disc, etc.) that must be moved to open the valve. This will ensure that there will be sufficient pressure in the system to fill the reservoir bag before the valve opens.

Movable Plates. Another type of relief valve utilizes a mechanism in which there are parallel plates, one above the other (Fig. 5.6). The top plate, which has an annular orifice, is movable.

The lower plate has a round hole. As the annular orifice is moved over the round hole, the size of the pathway for gases escaping from the breathing system increases. A disc at the base of the valve prevents gases from being drawn into the system and allows the reservoir bag to fill before the valve opens.

With each of these relief valves negative pressure from the scavenging system could cause evacuation of gases from the breathing system.

Diaphragm. A diaphragm valve is shown in Figure 5.7. It works in a manner similar to the disc valve except that the cap and spring push a diaphragm rather than a disc onto the seat. Increased pressure in the breathing system will

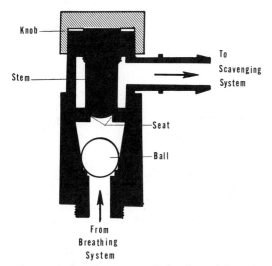

Figure 5.5. Pressure relief valve with stem and seat. Rotation of the control knob at the top causes the opening between the stem and seat to vary. The ball ensures that the reservoir bag will fill before the valve opens. (Redrawn from a drawing furnished by Boehringer Laboratories.)

push the diaphragm off its seat. Increasing or decreasing the tension of the spring on the diaphragm controls the amount of gas which will escape through the valve.

With the diaphragm valve, if negative pressure occurs in the scavenging system, the diaphragm is pulled onto the seat and the negative pressure is not transmitted to the breathing system.

There is a danger associated with this type of relief valve. If the diaphragm is closed by negative pressure and gas continues to flow into the breathing system it cannot escape unless the pressure inside the system exceeds the negative pressure which has closed the diaphragm. Thus there will be increased resistance to exhalation through the valve. The only quick way to relieve pressure in the breathing system would be to disconnect the scavenging system at some point until the source of the negative pressure in the scavenging system has been corrected.

Collection Device. Almost all relief valves are now fitted with collection devices which collect all the gases that are vented and direct them to a scavenging system.

Use

Spontaneous Respiration. With spontaneous respiration excess gas escapes when the relief valve's opening pressure is exceeded during exhalation, while it remains closed during inspiration. The opening of the relief valve determines the effort required by the patient to exhale through it. It should be closed only enough that the pressure for gas to escape is higher than the collapsing pressure of the reservoir bag. Otherwise the bag will not function as a reservoir. Usually this means the valve is fully open.

With spontaneous respiration, the anethesiol-

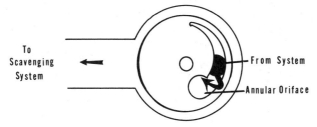

Figure 5.6. Relief valve with movable plates (viewed from the top). Moving one plate over the other causes the opening from the breathing system to increase or decrease. (Redrawn from a drawing furnished by Dupaco, Inc.)

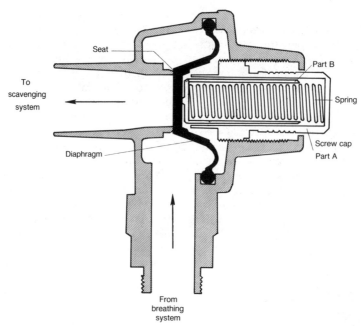

Figure 5.7.   Relief valve with diaphragm. Turning the screw cap varies the tension in the spring and thus controls the amount of gas that is vented through the valve. Negative pressure in the scavenging system will pull the diaphragm onto its seat. (Redrawn from a drawing furnished by Ohio Medical Products, a division of Airco, Inc.)

ogist must be constantly aware of the amount of bag inflation. If his attention is diverted, the bag may collapse or become overdistended. Relief valves are not always dependable because of sticking and various other mechanical difficulties. Negative pressure transmitted from the scavenging system may result in either a closure of the relief valve or evacuation of gases from the system. An obstruction in the scavenging system may result in the bag becoming overdistended and the patient unable to exhale.

There is considerable variation in the resistance of relief valves when fully open (72–76). These valves should be checked periodically.

Manual Controlled or Assisted Ventilation. During controlled or assisted manual ventilation, the valve is usually left partially open. During inspiration, the bag is squeezed and pressure is developed until the preset "pop-off" pressure is reached. Before this point, the patient receives all of the gas displaced from the bag (less a small amount due to compression of the gas and expansion of the tubes). Once the relief valve opens, the additional volume the patient receives is determined by the relative resistances to flow into the patient and through the relief valve. Careful and frequent adjustments of the

valve are necessary to achieve the desired level of ventilation and maintain adequate filling of the reservoir bag. If compliance of the lungs and thorax falls, the relief valve must be tightened in order to maintain the desired tidal volume. Adjustment should be made on the basis of chest movements and/or exhaled volume measurements. A further help is to evaluate the resistance felt during bag compression. This, however, does not give true information on the magnitude of the inspired volume, as this depends on the relative resistance to inflation of the lungs and the resistance to flow through the valve. An increase in resistance to ventilating the patient will result in more gas being lost through the relief valve unless the valve setting is changed. Dependence on the "educated hand" is totally unreliable (77, 78).

An alternative method is to close the valve completely and open it periodically to release excess gas or set the fresh gas flow so low that it equals uptake by the patient and the system. This can only be done safely with the circle system.

Mechanical Ventilation. When a ventilator is used the relief valve should be closed completely. Gas will be vented from the ventilator during expiration. If the relief valve is left open and gas vented from the system during inspiration, inconsistent ventilation will result, since changes in the dynamics of the system will result in changes in the amount of gas vented through the relief valve (79).

Selector valves (bag/ventilator valves) which facilitate the change from manual to automatic ventilation are available and are discussed in Chapter 8. Some of these automatically isolate the relief valve when the selector valve is turned to automatic ventilation.

LOW-PRESSURE RELIEF VALVES (PRESSURE-LIMITING VALVE OR DEVICE

This type of relief valve is designed to distinguish between the rapid rise of pressure during assisted or controlled ventilation and the relatively slow rise which occurs when fresh gas flow is greater than the patient's uptake. When the pressure in the system is low, the valve will be open and excess gases will escape to atmosphere. Enough pressure is maintained in the system, however, to prevent the reservoir bag from deflating. A sudden increase in pressure within the system, as from squeezing the bag, will close the valve, allowing respiration to be assisted or controlled. Any volume of gas squeezed out of the bag goes into the patient. Excess gas is vented from the circuit during exhalation.

This type of valve may be used in place of or in addition to a high-pressure relief valve. In situations where respirations are being controlled or assisted manually and it becomes necessary for the anesthesiologist to perform another task, it is not necessary to readjust the relief valve. Pressure will not build up in the system.

They are also useful in systems employing non-rebreathing valves, for preventing a dangerous pressure buildup when the fresh gas flow exceeds minute volume ventilation (80, 81) and in the Magill system during controlled ventilation to improved economy of the fresh gases (82). Finally, they may provide a safety factor in that the discrepancy between the amount of gas squeezed from the bag and the amount entering the patient is very small, since little gas is lost through the relief valve during bag squeezing. Thus the user is supplied with additional information about the adequacy of ventilation.

The Georgia Valve (83)

The Georgia valve is shown in Figure 5.8. It consists of a piston contained within a cylinder-

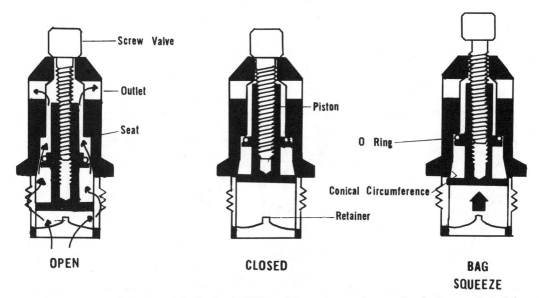

Figure 5.8. The Georgia valve. In the OPEN position, gas travels past the O-ring portion of the piston and escapes through the outlet. In the CLOSED position, the O-ring seals against the seat and no gas can escape. When a sudden increase in pressure in the system occurs, the screw valve is thrust upward and the O-ring seals against the seat. No gas can escape from the system. (Redrawn from a drawing furnished by Ohio Medical Products, a division of Airco, Inc.)

shaped valve body. A screw valve is connected to the piston. The screw and piston together are free to move vertically within the body as a unit. Upward movement is limited by a seat in the midplane of the valve. The base of the valve communicates with the breathing system. A retainer at the base prevents the piston from dropping into the system.

In the OPEN position, the piston rests on the retainer under the influence of gravity. Gas enters at the base, flows around the piston and through a narrow opening between the valve body and the O-ring of the piston. Gas exits at the outlet near the top of the valve. By turning the screw valve the piston is raised or lowered and the area of the opening between the valve body and the O-ring is changed. Turning the screw valve counterclockwise lowers the piston and increases the opening. The screw valve should be adjusted so that the bag is inflated to a volume convenient for the hand of the anesthesiologist prior to being squeezed, but there is minimal resistance to exhalation.

When the screw valve is turned fully clockwise (Fig. 5.8, *center*) the piston is drawn upward. The O-ring seals against the seat. Gas cannot overflow the valve at any pressure. This position is used for closed circuit anesthesia.

Figure 5.8, *right*, shows the valve closed in response to a sudden increase in pressure in the system, as from squeezing the bag. The piston and screw valve are thrust upward and the O-ring seals at the seat. Approximately 4 mm Hg is required to close the valve.

Since the valve is dependent upon gravity for its successful operation, it needs to be kept vertical. It is possible for a patient's exhalation, inadvertent pressure on the bag, or even a high fresh gas flow to inadvertently close the valve. If this occurs, light pressure by the anesthesiologist's finger on the screw will open the valve and allow excess gas to be vented. Conversely, the valve can be held closed to hasten filling of the bag by pulling firmly on the screw valve.

A gas evacuation kit can be attached to the Georgia valve for venting to a scavenging system.

Pressure-Equalizing Valve (80, 81, 84) (Steen Valve)

The pressure-equalizing valve is shown in Figure 5.9. It contains a flapper valve which moves between seats A and B. A spring holds it against the lower seat. A toggle handle at the top controls a metal rod that projects downward.

In the OPEN position (Fig. 5.9, *left*), the toggle handle is up. Excess gas entering at the base tilts the flapper valve off seat A and gas escapes at the outlet. Approximately 1.5 cm H_2O is

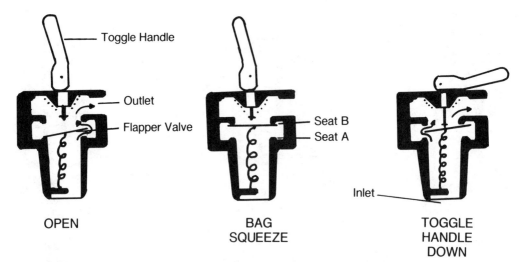

Figure 5.9. Pressure-equalizing valve. The base of the valve communicates with the breathing system. *A*, with the toggle handle up, a low pressure in the system opens the flapper valve and gas escapes to atmosphere. *B*, a rapid increase in pressure closes the flapper valve for controlled or assisted ventilation. *C*, with the toggle handle down, the flapper valve cannot close. (Redrawn from Steen SN, Lee ASJ: Prevention of inadvertent excess pressure in closed systems. *Anesth Analg* 39:264–266, 1960.)

needed to overcome the force of the spring holding the flapper valve onto seat A (80, 81, 84). This should be sufficient to allow the reservoir bag to fill.

Figure 5.9, *center*, shows the effect of squeezing the bag. The pressure pushes the flapper valve against seat B, closing the valve. No gas can escape. In contrast to the Georgia valve, the pressure-equalizing valve is either open or closed and the pressure at which overflow occurs cannot be varied.

In Figure 5.9, *right*, the toggle handle is depressed. This causes the metal rod to protrude below the level of seat B. This prevents the flapper valve from sealing against seat B. Thus if the flapper valve should seal off seat B inadvertently, it can be corrected by depressing the toggle handle until the excess gas is vented. With the lever in this position it is not possible to inflate the lungs.

This valve is portable and can be used in a position other than vertical by replacing the flapper valve with a valve spring-loaded against seat A (80).

VIGILANCE AIDS

Probably the greatest advance in anesthesia equipment in recent years has been the development and use of vigilance aids. These provide separate, often confirming, information about the functioning of equipment. Some also give early warning of problems with the patient. With their use, anesthesia is changing from an art into a science with greater patient safety as the primary benefit.

The use of vigilance aids has some similarity to the use of seat belts in automobiles. While their routine use may be inconvenient and appear unnecessary, studies indicate that on rare occasions they can prevent a catastrophe.

Vigilance aids should not be regarded as a substitute for an alert anesthesiologist, but as a tool to make his watchfulness more effective.

Oxygen Analyzers (Oxygen Monitors)

The functions of an oxygen analyzer are to continuously measure and indicate the concentration of oxygen in the breathing system and to signal when that concentration varies from the desired level. The importance of this should be obvious to anyone administering anesthesia. An oxygen analyzer is the last line of defense against the inadvertent delivery of a hypoxic mixture. Its use allows greater confidence in the employment of low-flow techniques. It may also be useful in providing early warning of a problem with the patient (such as malignant hyperthermia).

An oxygen analyzer may also detect an unexpected increase in oxygen concentration due to equipment problems (85–87) or exhaustion of the nitrous oxide supply, offering protection from patient awareness, damage to the lungs and development of retrolental fibroplasia.

Continuous monitoring of the oxygen concentration in the breathing system is considered by many, including the authors of this book, essential for patient safety during inhalation anesthesia. Many professional liability insurance companies require their use. While some expense is involved in their purchase and use, this can be offset to some extent by use of low-flow or closed system anesthesia.

In the past, paramagnetic oxygen analyzers were sometimes used for intermittent sampling during anesthesia. Today electrochemical analyzers, which allow continuous measurement, are most useful in anesthesia, while mass spectrometers are finding increasing application.

TYPES

Amperometric

An electrochemical oxygen analyzer is shown schematically in Figure 5.10. It consists of a sensor which is exposed to the gas to be sampled and the analyzer box, which contains the electric circuitry, meter, and alarms. A gain control allows the analyzer to be calibrated with gas containing a known partial pressure of oxygen.

Current flow from the sensor is proportional to the partial pressure of oxygen in the sample gas. For convenience, however, the meter scale is usually marked in percentage oxygen concentration. The meter reading on an oxygen analyzer may be seen to fluctuate during the respiratory cycle in proportion to the pressure in the breathing system. As pressure builds up, the partial pressure of the oxygen increases proportionally and the meter reading likewise increases; the percentage of oxygen has not changed, however. This fluctuation may not be apparent if the oxygen analyzer has a slow response time.

The sensor is an electrochemical cell that consumes a small amount of oxygen. It contains two electrodes, a cathode and an anode, surrounded by electrolyte gel. The electrolyte is

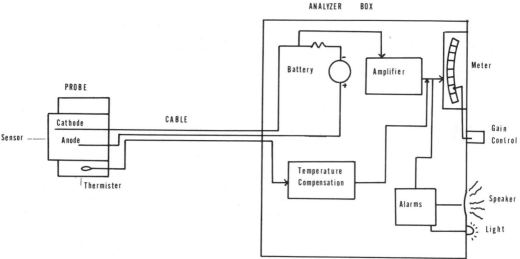

Figure 5.10. Representative diagram of electrochemical oxygen analyzer. The sensor is connected by a cable to the analyzer box, which contains the meter, alarms, and gain control. A thermistor compensates for changes in oxygen diffusion due to temperature. An amplifier is present in the polarographic, but not the galvanic, cell analyzer, and temperature compensation is usually designed into the amplifier in the polarographic cell analyzer.

required for the electrochemical reaction. Both the cathode and the anode are separated from the gas by an oxygen-permeable membrane. The membrane is permeable to gases such as oxygen but is nonpermeable to liquids. The membrane is necessary to make the current from the sensor a linear function of oxygen partial pressure. It also acts as a barrier to keep the electrolyte from evaporating.

Because temperature affects the rate of diffusion of oxygen into the sensor and hence the partial pressure of oxygen seen by the sensor, a thermistor (an electrical element whose resistance changes with temperature) is incorporated in the sensor housing (probe) to compensate for temperature changes.

There are two basic types of sensors: the polarographic and the galvanic cells. The polarographic cell, the most commonly used, requires an external power source to generate a polarizing potential. The galvanic cell utilizes a spontaneous reaction.

Galvanic Cell (Fuel Cell, Microfuel Cell)

A galvanic cell sensor is shown in Figure 5.11. Oxygen diffuses through the membrane and electrolyte to the cathode where it reacts, absorbing electrons and forming hydroxide ions. By simple diffusion the hydroxide ions travel to the lead anode, where they oxidize to form lead oxide and water, liberating electrons. An electron flow between anode and cathode is thus generated which is directly proportional to the oxygen level seen by the sensor. This current is displayed directly on a meter.

Since the sensor current is strong enough to operate the meter directly, a separate power source is not required and failure of the power source does not affect meter readout. However, a separate power source (either battery or wall current) is required for alarms.

The sensor must be replaced when the fuel cell becomes exhausted. It cannot be restored. Its useful life is cited in percent hours, which is defined as the product of hours of exposure and oxygen percentage. The more frequently the sensor is exposed to higher oxygen concentrations, the shorter its life. Different sensors have different life expectancies. The sensor comes packaged in a container from which oxygen has been removed and its limited life begins when the package is opened.

Polarographic Cell (Clark Electrode)

A polarographic sensor is shown in Figure 5.12. The anode and cathode are separated by the electrolyte solution, which is held in place by the membrane. There is a mechanism (usu-

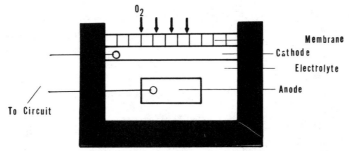

Figure 5.11. Galvanic cell sensor. The membrane is permeable to gases but nonpermeable to liquids. At the cathode oxygen molecules are reduced to hydroxide ions. At the anode hydroxide ions give up electrons. An electron flow between the anode and cathode is generated, which is directly proportional to the partial pressure of oxygen in the sample gas. (Redrawn from a drawing furnished by Biomarine Industries, Inc.)

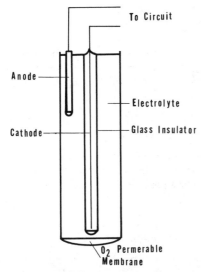

Figure 5.12. Polarographic cell oxygen analyzer sensor. The tip of the cathode is exposed to a thin layer of electrolyte. Oxygen diffuses through the membrane and electrolyte to the tip of the cathode. When a polarizing voltage is applied to the cathode the oxygen molecules are reduced to hydroxide ions. The current flow between cathode and anode will be proportional to the partial pressure of oxygen. (Redrawn from Bageant RA: Oxygen analyzers. *Resp Care* 21:415, 1976.)

ally a battery) for inducing a negative potential of approximately 0.75 V between the anode and the cathode.

Oxygen diffuses through the membrane to the electrolyte. When a polarizing voltage is applied to the cathode, electrons combine with the oxygen molecules at the cathode and reduce them to hydroxide ions. A current flows between the anode and cathode which is proportional to the partial pressure of oxygen in the sample. This current is much weaker than that of a galvanic cell and must be amplified to be displayed on a meter.

DESIRABLE FEATURES (89, 90)

There are a number of oxygen analyzers on the market for use in anesthesia. One should not be considered unless it meets the requirements of the ANSI standard for oxygen analyzers (91). Among other requirements, oxygen analyzers must be accurate to within 3% and interference from anesthetic agents must not exceed 4%.

Care should be taken in choosing an instrument. The following points should be considered.

Alarms

An analyzer should not be considered for purchase if it is not equipped with a low-level alarm. It should not be possible to set this alarm below 20%. A high-level alarm is desirable to prevent the occurrence of awareness and other problems due to high inspired oxygen concentrations.

Warning signals should be both audible and visible. Visual alarms alone are not sufficient, since they may be missed if the anesthesiologist is preoccupied (92). When an audible alarm sounds, a visual alarm is useful in helping to quickly identify the source.

It should not be possible to deactivate an audio alarm permanently. An audible alarm that can be *temporarily* deactivated can avoid aggravation; a continuous audible signal can be a significant irritation during the time the user is attempting to correct the condition. When an override (reset) mechanism exists, the visual alarm should stay on until the alarming condition has been corrected (90).

Reliability

In the past the most frequent complaint has been that the unit failed within a short time after being put into use. Widespread experience has now confirmed that current models are fairly reliable. While it is true that they require more care and effort than most other equipment used by the anesthesiologist, the analyzers presently being produced perform quite reliably with minimal care. Before purchasing an instrument it would be wise to check with colleagues who already have these instruments and select a model with a good reputation for dependability.

Ease of Calibration

Galvanic cell sensors do not require a warm-up time, while most polarographic sensors do. The warm-up time is usually longer after the batteries are changed. The amount of time required for calibration will also depend on the response time (the time required for the electrode output to change to 97% of the final value for a change in oxygen tension). Most polarographic sensors have a faster response time than galvanic cells (89). Response time increases with the age of the sensor (89).

Lack of Electrosurgical Unit Interference

Under certain conditions, high-frequency interference from electrosurgical units has caused erratic readings of the analyzer meter with activation of alarms (93). This has been largely suppressed in newer models (94). It is suggested that the analyzer be evaluated under clinical conditions before purchase.

Ease of Use in the Breathing System

Rugged adaptors for mounting the sensor in the breathing system(s) expected to be used in the department should be available. The cable to connect the sensor with the analyzer box should be of sufficient length to prevent stress at points of connection under conditions of normal use. It should be possible to mount the monitor in an accessible location where it can be seen easily by the operator.

Cost

This must include initial cost plus servicing. In most cases analyzers with polarographic sensors are more expensive but the operating costs will be lower than those utilizing a galvanic cell sensor (90).

Use with Explosive Anesthetics

Most analyzers are not officially approved for use with flammable anesthetic agents. If flammable agents are to be used an analyzer certified for use in such an atmosphere is required.

Ease of Servicing

Some analyzers require less frequent servicing and are easier to service than others. Analyzers with polarographic sensors require membrane and electrolyte changes. Sensors, membranes, and electrolyte should be easy to replace. Batteries should be readily obtainable and easy to change.

Ease of Disinfection

It should be possible to disinfect or sterilize the sensor. The manufacturer's instructions should be consulted for the methods that can be used.

Effects of Humidity

Most oxygen analyzers are not affected by humidity unless excessive condensate forms on the sensor, in which case erroneously low readings may result (90, 95, 96). Most have an efficient water-repelling membrane over the basic polymeric membrane to minimize the problem of water condensation.

The manufacturer's instructions should be consulted to see if the analyzer is affected if the atmosphere contains particulate water or when condensation would tend to form on the sensor. Some analyzers have special adaptors or heating assemblies to prevent condensation on the membrane. An effort should be made to place the analyzer where the humidity will be lowest. See following section on use.

USE

Oxygen analyzers are generally accurate, but must be used with logic and caution.

Calibration

The calibration procedure should be performed daily, preferably before each case. Most analyzers will remain accurate for 8 hr after calibration. However, as often as it is deemed necessary, calibration can be checked by removing the sensor from the breathing system temporarily and verifying that it indicates approximately 21% oxygen.

Since the calibration procedure will vary with each analyzer, the manufacturer's instructions should be read carefully. The following are the procedures to be followed for most analyzers.

Galvanic Sensors. No warm-up time is required. The sensor should be exposed to 100% oxygen and adjusted so that the meter reads correctly. It is not easy to obtain 100% oxygen in a breathing circuit and repeated flushing is required. The probe may be removed from its adaptor and exposed to 100% oxygen from the fresh gas line. The sensor should then be exposed to room air and the meter should read approximately 21%. If the sensor will not calibrate, the connection with the analyzer box should be checked. If this is not at fault, the sensor should be replaced. If changing the sensor does not allow the sensor to be calibrated, the analyzer should be returned to the manufacturer.

Polarographic Sensors. (*a*) With the function switch in the OFF position, the meter should be checked to see that it reads 0. If it does not, it should be adjusted to 0 by turning the appropriate control. Failure may be due to a loosely connected or nonfunctioning sensor. (*b*) Batteries should be checked and replaced if indicated. (*c*) The analyzer is then turned to the ON position. Sufficient time should be allowed for the sensor to warm up. This will vary with the analyzer. The sensor should then be calibrated as described for the galvanic sensor.

If the unit cannot be calibrated, a loosely connected sensor probe should be checked for. If this is not the problem, the electrolyte should be changed. If this fails to correct the situation, the membrane should be changed. (With many oxygen analyzers the entire sensor is disposable and it is not possible to change the electrolyte or membrane. If so, these two steps should be omitted.) If the unit will still not calibrate, the sensor should be changed. If all these measures fail, the analyzer should be returned to the manufacturer.

Checking the Alarms

It is essential that the alarms be checked each day. In some oxygen analyzers there are three batteries: two for operating the sensor and one for the alarms (97). Checking the batteries for operation of the meter may not check the battery for the alarm, which must be checked independently.

The sensor should be put in room air and the low alarm set above 21%. The visual alarm should flash and the audio alarm sound. If the unit has a high alarm the alarm dial should be moved below 21% and checked for visual and audio signals.

If the lamp(s) fail to light or if the audio alarm is weak, the batteries should be replaced and the alarms rechecked. If this fails to remedy the situation, the unit should be returned to the manufacturer for servicing or replacement.

Location in the Breathing System

The tip of the sensor of an oxygen analyzer is usually placed in a T-adaptor which is either in the fresh gas line or inside the breathing system.

Insertion near the patient is sometimes recommended because this is the most frequent site for disconnections, but it should be emphasized that an oxygen analyzer is not a reliable disconnect alarm. Placing it between the mask or endotracheal tube connector and the breathing system will increase dead space, and the increased weight and bulk in this position may pose problems.

The sensor should be upright or tilted slightly to prevent water from accumulating on the membrane. Unless it is unaffected by humidity, it is preferable to place the analyzer where humidity will be lowest. This will usually be in the inspiratory limb unless a humidifier is in use, in which case it is best to place the analyzer upstream of the humidifier or in the expiratory limb. The recommended position will be discussed more fully under the sections on individual breathing systems.

Setting the Alarms

The alarms should be set according to the patient's disease and surgery. The low alarm should be set just below the minimum and the high alarm just above the maximum acceptable concentration.

There should be a place on the anesthesia record for recording the alarm limits and the oxygen percentages.

Maintenance

With galvanic sensors no membrane or electrolyte replacement is necessary. Sensors must be replaced when they become exhausted.

With some polarographic sensors, the electrolyte gel must be changed routinely, at monthly to quarterly intervals. It is not necessary to replace the membrane each time the electrolyte is changed, but the membrane must be changed periodically. Some polarographic sensors have a disposable cartridge that changes easily, eliminating the need for handling the membrane and electrolyte solutions.

The manufacturer's instructions should be consulted as to the frequency with which electrolyte, membranes, or sensors should be changed.

Pressure Alarm (Ventilator or Respiratory Monitor or Alarm, Pressure Monitor, Pressure Alarm System, Anesthesia Circuit Monitor)

Pressure alarms are more important in anesthesia now than formerly because the use of mechanical ventilators has increased, scavenging systems have been added to most breathing systems, and the breathing systems themselves have become more complex.

When ventilation is manually controlled, the feel of the bag provides a very effective monitor of ventilation. With use of a mechanical ventilator this advantage is lost. Some ventilators react to a disconnect or other pressure problem with a different sound or a collapsed bellows, but the anesthesiologist may not notice these immediately. With some ventilators there is no change in sound and function will appear normal in the face of a problem. Mortality or morbidity can result if a dangerous condition remains unnoticed.

Monitoring of breath sounds with a precordial or esophageal stethoscope and observation of chest wall movements and the pressures on the breathing system manometer are valuable, but frequently these activities must be intermittent because attention to other aspects of patient care is required.

Most pressure alarms are fairly low in cost and require little maintenance. Their use is highly recommended whenever general anesthesia is administered. A mechanical ventilator should never be used without at least a low-pressure alarm.

Pressure alarms may be free standing or incorporated into a ventilator and/or anesthesia machine. Free-standing devices can be mounted to almost any ventilator or anesthesia machine. Most of the newer anesthesia ventilators have at least a low-pressure alarm as standard equipment. Add-on alarms are available for many older ventilators.

In order to be effective, an alarm should be automatically ready to perform its functions when needed. Many free-standing pressure alarms can be interfaced with a ventilator so that the alarm is activated when the ventilator is turned on. It is strongly recommended that this be done whenever possible. A free standing device may not be activated or may be deactivated because the alarm is annoying and not be reactivated again. Simply educating staff not to turn off an alarm does not eliminate the problem because even knowledgeable, conscientious, and experienced personnel occasionally forget to turn an alarm to the on position (98).

Alarm signals should be both audible and visible. It may be difficult to pinpoint the source of an alarm if more than one alarm device is used unless a visible indicator is present. The signal should persist only for the duration of the adverse pressure condition.

Most pressure alarms have a delay (reset, mute, silencing) switch which can be activated by the user and which will delay the audible signal. This feature may be crucial for user acceptance. Alarms that cannot be temporarily silenced may be so annoying that they are shut off permanently and forgotten. However, it should not be possible to silence an alarm permanently.

If battery power is used there should be a means to determine if there is sufficient power (99). A backup battery is desirable.

Alarms can be tailored to detect more than one dangerous pressure condition. By including several variables in one alarm a greater number of potential hazards can be detected.

LOW PRESSURE (VENTILATION FAILURE ALARM, PRESSURE FAILURE ALARM, DISCONNECT ALARM)

These are designed to alert the user to failure to achieve a certain predetermined or user-selected pressure within a predetermined or user-selected time span (100, 101). Alarms that allow the user to select the pressure may have distinct values (Fig. 5.13) or allow continuous variation. The time span should be long enough that the peak pressure must fall below the alarm point for several successive breaths before the alarm will sound. This will avoid false alarms due to short-term disturbances in the ventilatory pattern (101).

Conditions that can be detected by a low pressure alarm include a disconnection or major leak in the breathing system, a leaking tracheal tube cuff, failure of the ventilator to cycle, an unconnected ventilator, too low a setting on the ventilator, and failure of the gas supply to the ventilator or from the machine. Disconnects are the most frequent complications leading to mortality and morbidity (102), so use of low-pressure alarms should be mandatory when artificial ventilation is used.

The low pressure alarm should be set just

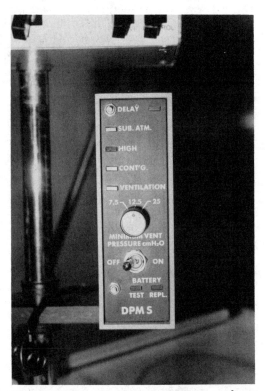

Figure 5.13. Free-standing pressure alarm. In addition to the low-pressure alarm (which is adjustable to 7.5, 12.5, or 25 cm H_2O), this unit features subatmospheric pressure, high-pressure and continuing pressure alarms. In addition, there is a delay (silencing) feature.

below the peak pressure reached during inspiration. If the pressure is set too low, the alarm may be fooled (103, 104). When a choice of low pressures is available the highest pressure that is below peak inspiratory pressure should be set.

Placement of the sensor is of great importance. Two general locations have been employed: in the ventilator and in the breathing system with a tubing connecting to the alarm mechanism. Locating the sensor in the ventilator is unsatisfactory for several reasons. Under certain circumstances, a combination of a high inspiratory flow rate and breathing system resistance can create sufficient back pressure to generate a false positive signal at the bellows sensor (105). These alarms can also be fooled by obstruction in the inspiratory limb, failure of the ventilator to cycle (106) and application of negative pressure to the outside of the bellows by scavenging system malfunction (107). Some manufacturers who have made ventilators with sensors built into the ventilator now offer conversion kits to allow placement of the sensor in the breathing system.

The preferred location for the sensor is in the breathing system as close as possible to the patient port. The closer the sensor is to the patient, the closer the pressure monitored is to that of the patient's airway and not that of the ventilator. Many manufacturers supply a 15-mm T for the sensor. This should be placed at the tracheal tube connector—not at the fresh gas inlet on the absorber (108).

The next best site is on the exhalation side of the circle system on the patient side of the unidirectional valve. Placement on the inspiratory side is less desirable, but the user should read and follow the directions for each alarm because some manufacturers suggest placement in the inspiratory limb upstream of any humidifier to avoid subjecting the probe to excessive condensed water vapor. From the standpoint of pressure monitoring, this site is not optimal. Components such as humidifiers may create sufficient back pressure to allow the peak of the pressure wave to reach the alarm point even though a disconnection has taken place.

Problems with disconnect alarms have been reported. Water in the line between the breathing system and alarm can prevent it from activating during a low pressure situation (109) or may cause a false alarm (110). A disconnect alarm can be fooled by use of a PEEP valve if the end-expiratory pressure falls above the selected low pressure. Even when the sensor is located at the tracheal tube connector, the alarm may be inhibited if there is a disconnection and the breathing system connector lodges against some object like a pillow or if there is a kinked or obstructed tracheal tube. Those operating on batteries will not alarm if the batteries fail (111). Failure of these alarms to detect low-pressure situations have been reported (112–114). It is essential that the alarm be checked before use.

SUSTAINED ELEVATED PRESSURE

Sustained elevated (continuing) pressure occurs when there is an elevated pressure, but the pressure increase is limited by a bag or ventilator bellows. It may arise from several mechanisms (115): accidental activation of the oxygen flush valve; system defects which limit or prevent exhalation; an improperly adjusted relief valve; occlusion of the scavenging system; ventilator failure during inspiration; malfunction of a ventilator relief valve and incorrect connection of the patient to a ventilator.

The device compares the airway pressure waveform with a preset level to ensure that part of the waveform falls below that level (101). If it does not, an alarm sounds. Some alarms incorporate a valve that opens after 10 sec of sustained pressure. This allows the pressure in the system to drop (116).

HIGH PRESSURE

A high-pressure alarm senses pressures that generally occur only when the pressure is not buffered by a bag or ventilator bellows. Situations where this might occur are airway obstruction, a kinked or occluded endotracheal tube, a punctured ventilator bellows, occlusion or obstruction of the expiratory limb of the breathing system, or a patient coughing or straining against the endotracheal tube.

SUBAMBIENT PRESSURE

Pressures less than atmospheric in the system can be generated by a patient who is trying to inhale against an empty reservoir bag, a blocked inspiratory limb or during a ventilator's expiratory phase. Other causes of subatmospheric pressure include malfunction of an active scavenging system, a nasogastric tube placed in the trachea (117), or a ventilator attempting to refill its descending bellows after a significant gas loss from the system.

PEEP PRESSURE

Although positive end expiratory pressure is not often utilized during anesthesia, alarms are available which are activated if the PEEP level falls below a preset level.

RESPIRATORY RATE

Pressure alarms which measure respiratory rate and have alarms for high and low frequencies are also available.

Anesthetic Agent Monitoring

Anesthetic agent monitors are useful for several reasons.

1. They allow the user to check the accuracy of calibration of vaporizers to detect malfunctions and determine when maintenance is needed. For this purpose, the sensor should be placed in the fresh gas line of the machine.

2. They are useful when a concentration of agent below the lowest calibration on a vaporizer is dialed or when the vaporizer is used with gas flows outside those for which it is calibrated.

3. They can detect when a vaporizer is inadvertently on or when a vaporizer turned off is allowing a leak of vapor into the fresh gas line.

4. They provide information on the anesthetic agent uptake. The difference between inspired and expired concentrations provides a measure of patient saturation. Anesthetic uptake or elimination by the patient and breathing system can be calculated by taking the difference between the mean concentration delivered into the system (measured in the fresh gas line) and the mean concentration leaving the breathing system (measured in mixed gases from the outlet of the relief valve) and multiplying by the fresh gas flow.

5. They are useful in demonstrating the relationship between concentrations in the fresh gas line and those in the breathing system. This makes them useful in teaching situations, especially for teaching use of low flow or closed system anesthesia.

6. They provide information on anesthetic depth, allowing one to evaluate and control the progress of the anesthetic. Anesthetic depth is directly related to alveolar gas concentrations. If an anesthetic agent monitor is placed in the expiratory limb, the concentration registered will be a guide to alveolar concentration, especially as patient uptake and the ratio of fresh

gas flow to alveolar ventilation decrease. (*Note:* End-tidal gases are a better reflection of alveolar gases than mixed expired gases, but measurement of end-tidal concentrations require a very fast response time and placement of the sensor very near the patient in the breathing system.) Anesthetic agent monitors should not be regarded as a replacement for other means of measuring depth, but as an additional source of information.

There are a number of different methods of determining anesthetic agent concentrations in addition to the mass spectrometer, which will be discussed separately.

SILICONE RUBBER RELAXATION (NARKOTEST, NORTH AMERICAN DRAGER)

This method depends on the variation in the elasticity of silicone rubber strips when exposed to anesthetic agents. The strips are connected by a lever to a pointer on a scale which is calibrated in volumes percent. Response to inhaled anesthetics is linear (118).

This instrument was designed for measurement of halothane. Several authors have calibrated this instrument for other agents and have determined conversion factors for those agents (118–120). These are shown in Table 5.2.

The reading on the scale should be multiplied by the conversion factor to obtain the concentration in volumes percent. Use of more than one agent will result in an additive effect. Elastance is affected by nitrous oxide so the instrument needs to be set to 0 with the nitrous oxide–oxygen mixture to be used.

The conversion factors are proportional to anesthetic rubber/gas and oil/gas solubility and inversely proportional to silicone rubber retention time. Since anesthetic potency is correlated with oil/gas solubility it has been suggested that this instrument approximates a "MAC meter" (122). Readings at 1 MAC are shown in Table 5.2.

The instrument can be used as a breathethrough device on either the inspiratory or expiratory side or it can be mounted on a flat surface. There is minimal resistance to the passage of gases (120, 123). Compensation for humidity is built into the meter. Saturated water at room temperature will not affect the readings, but at 37°C, saturated water vapor will register 0.45% after equilibration (120). Temperature compensation is incorporated into the meter and

Table 5.2.
Conversion Factors for Narkotest

Agent	Conversion Factor	Reading at 1 MAC*	Response Time†
			sec
Enflurane	1.46–1.64	1.2–1.0	100
Halothane	1.0	0.8	108
Methoxyflurane	0.16–0.20	1.0–0.8	843
Isoflurane	1.8	0.7	119

* MAC, minimum anesthetic concentration.
† Time to reach 95% of maximum response (121).

is effective within the range of ambient temperatures. It tends to read high at low temperatures and low at high temperatures (120).

The accuracy is ±0.10–0.15% halothane (120, 122) and it is accurate over a wide range of gas flows (120). The speed of response is shown in Table 5.2.

The apparatus is simple, portable, inexpensive, reliable, and requires no electrical input. It does not have an alarm, which limits its usefulness as a vigilance aid.

CRYSTAL OSCILLATION METHOD (ENGSTROM MULTIGAS MONITOR FOR ANAESTHESIA; EMMA)

Another method of anesthetic agent monitoring uses a quartz crystal coated with a layer of silicone oil that can adsorb or release halogenated anesthetic molecules (124, 125). Such a crystal placed in a resonance circuit will oscillate with a frequency determined partly by the crystal's mass (125). When a gas containing halogenated hydrocarbons is passed through a cell containing such a crystal, molecules of the agent are quickly adsorbed onto the crystal, causing a change in its mass which in turn changes the frequency of oscillation. By use of an electronic system consisting of two oscillating circuits, one of which has an uncoated (reference) crystal and the other a coated (detector) crystal, an electric signal which is proportional to the vapor concentration can be obtained.

The coated and reference crystals are housed in a measuring head that incorporates a heating element to avoid water condensation. The measuring head is inserted into the breathing system or fresh gas line. It is connected by a cable to the display unit where the concentration is shown on a meter. Upper and lower alarms (with visible and audible signals) can be set on the meter. A recording device may be connected to the unit to keep a record of concentrations.

The device can be used to measure halothane, isoflurane, trichlorethylene, enflurane, and methoxyflurane and will record from 0–5% for each agent.

The measuring head can be mounted anywhere in the gas circuit, including between the Y-piece and the patient. It cannot differentiate among the various detectable agents, so the vapor to be measured must be identified in advance and the gas selection knob set.

A 15-min warm-up time is recommended before use, but 30 min may be preferable to avoid zero drift (125). The instrument can be calibrated using special test gases or with a special calibration transducer.

Oxygen and nitrogen have no measurable effect and the effect of carbon dioxide is insignificant in clinical situations; 80% nitrous oxide produces a deflection of approximately 0.1%. Certain organic gases such as acetone and alcohol will cause interference.

The instrument is sensitive to water vapor and this can produce a sizable deflection at elevated temperatures and 100% relative humidity (122, 123). The interference is greater with isoflurane than with halothane or enflurane (122). The effect can be lessened by inserting a heat and moisture exchanger between the measuring head and the patient and can be compensated for if the gas temperature and relative humidity remain constant (126). Water vapor will not be a problem if dry gases are measured in the fresh gas line (122).

The response time is short enough to allow breath-by-breath analysis. It varies with the agent (being shortest for isoflurane and longest for methoxyflurane) (124), gas flows (being faster at higher flows) (125, 126), and agent concentration (being faster with higher concentrations). Lag time is minimal.

Accuracy is claimed by the manufacturers to be 0.1% or 5% of the reading, whichever is larger. The sensitivity is 0.02% and the stability is good (127).

This device has many advantages. It is compact, rugged, and easy to use and transport. The measuring head has low resistance and minimal dead space (13 ml). It can monitor five gases, making it more versatile than most other devices. Its cost is reasonable. Hayes and co-workers (126) felt that the unit was satisfactory for

measuring concentrations delivered by vaporizers and average inspired or expired concentrations, but that accurate end-tidal concentrations could not be obtained. Linstromberg and colleagues (122) felt that it could be used to measure the output of vaporizers, but that in-circle measurements were not accurate because of the humidity effects. Problems with this instrument have been reported (128, 129).

INFRARED ANALYSIS (130)

All of the anesthetic gases have one or more absorption bands in the infrared spectral region. In an infrared analyzer, an infrared light beam of the proper wavelength is passed through two chambers, one of which contains a standard gas and the other the gas to be analyzed. Since the anesthetic gas absorbs some infrared light, less light will be detected by the photocell in the test chamber than in the control chamber. The differences can be computed in terms of gas concentration.

This instrument is easy to use and has a fast response time. All of the anesthetic agents, including nitrous oxide, can be monitored, but only one gas at a time can be measured (125). The response curve using the halothane head can be applied to measurement of enflurane without modification (131).

ULTRAVIOLET ANALYSIS

Halothane absorbs ultraviolet light at certain wavelengths. By measuring the loss of light in a chamber of fixed size through which the anesthetic mixture is passed, an equivalent of halothane concentration can be obtained.

Ultraviolet measurement of halothane has been performed for many years (132). Recently improvements in these devices have made them more useful (133, 134).

The device is relatively inexpensive and easily portable. It has a rapid response and can be used for breath-by-breath analysis. End-tidal concentrations can be obtained (133). It is not affected by nitrous oxide. Only one gas can be monitored at a time.

Ultraviolet measurement is controversial because of the finding that exposure of mice to halothane that had been irradiated by ultraviolet light resulted in toxicity (135, 136). A valve to prevent returning of gas exposed to ultraviolet light to the breathing system should be used (133).

Capnometry and Capnography

Capnometry is the measurement of the concentration of carbon dioxide during the respiratory cycle. Capnography is the display of this concentration on either a screen or a paper graph. Analysis of carbon dioxide in respiratory gases has been available for many years. Only recently, however, has the technology been advanced to the point where its routine use in the operating room is practical.

PRINCIPLES OF OPERATION

The most commonly used monitors are based on the ability of some gases to absorb infrared light. Infrared light filtered at a certain wavelength is passed through a reference chamber containing carbon dioxide-free gas and also through a sample chamber containing gas whose carbon dioxide concentration is to be measured. Infrared light is absorbed by carbon dioxide in the sample gas. Both beams fall on collectors and the difference in intensity between them is measured. This difference is related to the concentration of carbon dioxide in the sample chamber.

Of the commonly used anesthetic agents, only nitrous oxide has a significant spectral overlap. Most carbon dioxide monitors designed for use in anesthesia provide a means to eliminate this interference. Some require calibration with the nitrous oxide-containing mixture to be used.

The concentration of carbon dioxide may be displayed continuously or as peak (normally end-tidal) values. Minimum inspired concentration may also be shown. Other parameters such as respiratory rate, minute volume, carbon dioxide production, and tidal volume may also be displayed.

TYPES OF INSTRUMENTS

There are two basic types of instruments available. One utilizes direct measurement at the sampling site and the other withdrawal of the sample to the instrument.

Flow-Through Devices

In these the sensor, which is connected to the analyzer by a cable, is placed directly in the breathing system using a special adaptor. The sensor is heated to avoid water condensation. There is no limitation on the length of the cable, so the monitor need not be near the patient.

These monitors do not require a standard gas for calibration.

It is essential that the adaptor be placed in the breathing system as close to the patient as possible to avoid contamination with gases from the breathing system and so that the end-tidal concentration will approximate the alveolar concentration as closely as possible.

Disadvantages of this type of monitor include the fact that the sensor is heavy and cumbersome and can exert enough drag on the endotracheal tube to cause extubation. It is also very fragile and expensive. The adaptor for the sensor may have considerable dead space, making it unacceptable for use with pediatric patients. Special low dead space adaptors may reduce this problem (137).

One of these analyzers, the Siemens Sirecust 300, resets itself to 0 automatically during each inspiratory phase, assuming this sample contains no carbon dioxide. This eliminates the need for periodic calibration, but if there is carbon dioxide in the inspired mixture, the analyzer measures only the increase over that concentration, and will underestimate the true level (138–140).

One complication of these analyzers has been reported (141). Thermal skin burns, apparently produced by radiant energy, occurred with use of a flow-through analyzer, despite use of multiple layers of gauze which kept the sensor from direct contact with the skin. To prevent this, it may be necessary to interpose a piece of aluminum foil between two pieces of soft material. The aluminum will reflect the radiant energy.

Aspiration Devices

Aspiration (withdrawal) analyzers continuously draw a small volume of gas from the point of sensing through a thin plastic tube into the monitor where it is analyzed. If the patient is intubated, the end of the sampling tube can be placed in the breathing system. A special adapter can be used or a hole which will accept a small tubing can be drilled into a component such as the Y-piece or corrugated tubing. The small tubing should extend down into the tracheal tube. If the patient is not intubated the end of the tube can be placed just in front of or inside the patient's nostril. If the patient is a mouth breather, it can be placed through an oxygen mask.

On most monitors the flow rate can be varied.

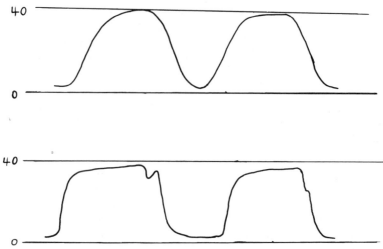

Figure 5.14.   Effects of incorrect flow rates with aspiration devices. *Upper curve:* The flow rate is too low. It is raised above the baseline and the plateau is absent. If the flow is reduced still further, the curve becomes sinusoidal. *Lower curve:* If the flow rate is too high, a dip in the plateau is sometimes seen, caused by the admixture of other gases.

It should be adjusted according to the size of the patient and his respiratory rate (142). A low flow rate should be used for patients with low tidal volumes (143). If the flow rate is too low the curve on the capnogram will be raised above the baseline and the plateau will be absent (Fig. 5.14). If the flow rate is too high, a dip in the plateau may be seen (Fig. 5.14), caused by the admixture of other gases, and a falsely low value may be obtained (144).

These analyzers are calibrated using a gas of known concentration. Excessive moisture getting into the analyzer can be a problem. There is usually either a filter (which must be changed periodically) or a water trap (which must be emptied periodically).

Advantages of this type of analyzer include the ability to sample gas from patients who are not intubated and are breathing spontaneously. Disadvantages include the need for a short length of sample tubing. If it is too long the response time will be slow. The monitor must be scavenged or the gases returned to the system, necessitating another tube. Water, blood or moisture may clog the tubing, making the measured value incorrect.

INTERPRETATION OF CAPNOMETRY

Carbon dioxide is formed in the body cells as a product of metabolism, transported by the blood, and excreted by the lungs. If the patient is connected to a breathing system, it has to travel through this before it is eliminated. Changes in exhaled carbon dioxide may reflect changes in metabolism, circulation, respiration, or apparatus. Tables 5-3 to 5-6 list some causes of changes in exhaled carbon dioxide.

Metabolism

Every cell in the body produces carbon dioxide. During an anesthetic, carbon dioxide production varies. Table 5.3 lists some causes of increased or decreased carbon dioxide production. It falls with decreased temperature, increased muscle relaxation and increased depth of anesthesia. It is increased by intense muscle activity, as seen with seizures. End-tidal carbon dioxide will rise when carbon dioxide is absorbed from the peritoneal cavity during laparoscopy and following injection of sodium bicarbonate.

Of particular interest to the anesthesiologist is early diagnosis of the syndrome known as malignant hyperpyrexia. This syndrome is characterized by a hypermetabolic state with a massive increase in carbon dioxide production. The increase occurs early, before the rise in temperature. Carbon dioxide monitoring is more sensitive than temperature measurement for early detection of this syndrome.

Circulation

Carbon dioxide is transported from the cells to the lungs by the circulatory system. Anything which interferes with this will cause a decrease

Table 5.3.
Capnography and Capnometry with Altered Carbon Dioxide Production

	Waveform on Capnograph	End-Tidal CO_2	Inspiratory CO_2	End-Tidal to Arterial Gradient
Absorption of carbon dioxide from peritoneal cavity	Normal	↑	0	Normal
Injection of sodium bicarbonate	Normal	↑	0	Normal
Pain, anxiety, shivering	Normal	↑	0	Normal
Increased muscle tone (as from muscle relaxant reversal)	Normal	↑	0	Normal
Convulsions	Normal	↑	0	Normal
Hyperthermia	Normal	↑	0	Normal
Hypothermia	Normal	↓	0	Normal
Increased depth of anesthesia (in relation to surgical stimulus)	Normal	↓	0	Normal
Use of muscle relaxants	May see curare cleft	↓	0	Normal

Normal end-tidal carbon dioxide is 38 torr (5%). Inspired carbon dioxide is normally 0. The arterial to end-tidal gradient is normally less than 5 torr.

Table 5.4.
Capnographic and Capnometric Alterations as a Result of Circulatory Changes

	Waveform on Capnograph	End-Tidal CO_2	Inspired CO_2	End-Tidal to Arterial Gradient
Decreased transport of carbon dioxide to the lungs (impaired peripheral circulation)	Normal	↓	0	Normal
Decreased transport of carbon dioxide through the lungs (pulmonary embolus, either air or thrombus; surgical manipulations)	Normal	↓	0	Elevated
Right to left shunt	Normal	↑	0	Elevated
Increased patient dead space	Normal	↓	0	Elevated
Increased transport of carbon dioxide to the lungs (restoration of peripheral circulation after it has been impaired, e.g., after release of a tourniquet)	Normal	↑	0	Normal

in exhaled carbon dioxide. Capnometry is of great value as an indication of the quality of circulation. As long as the production of carbon dioxide is constant and the tissues are in equilibrium with the blood, the elimination of carbon dioxide by the lungs should also be constant.

If the end-tidal carbon dioxide suddenly falls, carbon dioxide delivery, and hence blood flow, to the lungs, may be decreased. This could be caused by a drop in cardiac output, cardiac depression, decreased venous return to the heart secondary to hypovolemia, or by an obstruction of the pulmonary artery or its branches resulting from pulmonary embolism, surgical manipulations during thoracic surgery, or air embolism. Table 5.4 lists some circulatory causes of changes in end-tidal carbon dioxide.

Capnometry has been used to measure the adequacy of circulation during controlled hypotension (145). It is of proven usefulness for detecting air embolism (146, 147). Although not as sensitive as the Doppler, it is not affected by electrocautery and can be used in major ENT cases where the Doppler method is not applicable.

The capnogram is a far better guide to the absence of circulation than the pulse or blood pressure (144). Cardiac arrest in the face of electrocardiographic activity can be detected by the absence of carbon dioxide in the exhaled gases and the effectiveness of cardiac resuscitation can be gauged by capnometry.

Respiration

Elimination of carbon dioxide depends upon

Table 5.5.
Capnometry and Capnography with Respiratory Problems

	Waveform on Capnograph	End-Tidal CO_2	Inspiratory CO_2	End-Tidal to Alveolar Gradient
Disconnection	Absent		0	
Apneic patient, stopped ventilator	Absent		0	
Endobronchial intubation	May show sloping ascending limb	↑	0	Elevated
Hyperventilation	Normal	↓	0	Normal
Hypoventilation, mild to moderate	Normal	↑	0	Normal
Hypoventilation, extreme	Abnormal	↓	0	Elevated
Upper airway obstruction	Abnormal	↑	0	Elevated
Rebreathing (under drapes, for example	Baseline elevated	↑	↑	Normal
Esophageal intubation	Absent		0	

Table 5.6.
Capnographic and Capnometric Alterations Seen with Equipment Problems

	Waveform on Capnograph	End-Tidal CO_2	Inspired CO_2	Arterial to End-Tidal Gradient
Increased apparatus dead space	Baseline Elevated	↑	↑	Normal
Circle system: Faulty unidirectional valve, faulty or exhausted absorbent, bypassed absorber	Baseline Elevated	↑	↑	Normal
Inadequate fresh gas flow to a Mapleson system	Baseline Elevated	↑	↑	Normal
Problems with the inner tube of a Bain system	Baseline Elevated	↑	↑	Normal
Malfunctioning non-rebreathing valve with rebreathing	Baseline Elevated	↑	↑	Normal
Obstruction to expiration in the breathing system	Abnormal	↑	0	Elevated
Leakage in breathing system	Abnormal	↓	0	Elevated
Water in sampling cell	Abnormal	↑	↑	Elevated
Water blocking sampling line	Absent			
Leakage in sampling line	Abnormal	↓	0	Elevated
Too low a flow rate with aspiration devices	Abnormal	↓	↑	Elevated
Too high a flow rate with aspiration devices	Abnormal	↓	0	↑
Inadequate seal around endotracheal tube	Abnormal	↓	0	↑

the state of the lungs and airways and functioning of the whole respiratory mechanism. Alveolar hyperventilation and hypoventilation can be detected by capnometry, allowing more precise control of arterial carbon dioxide. This is especially important in neurosurgical cases. A capnometer with appropriate alarms can serve as a disconnection or apnea monitor. Table 5.5 lists some respiratory causes of increased and decreased end-tidal carbon dioxide.

Capnometry is of great value in monitoring the respiration of sedated patients who are not intubated and who are breathing spontaneously. In cases where a plastic drape is placed over the head, and ventilation of the breathing space is inadequate, rebreathing will occur. This can be detected by monitoring the inspired carbon dioxide concentration. If this rises, rebreathing is occurring and ventilation of the air space needs to be increased.

A dependable means to determine when an endotracheal tube has been positioned correctly in the tracheobronchial tree is obviously of great value. In one study of misadventures in anesthesia, placement of the tracheal tube in the esophagus was the leading cause of death or cerebral damage (148). Movement of the reservoir bag and chest can occur with the tube in the esophagus. Auscultation of breath sounds can be misleading. After pre-oxygenation, it may be a long time before the patient's color changes. If exhaled carbon dioxide is measured, there can be no question about the tube's position.

Breathing System Function

If there is a problem with the breathing system which causes an increase in inspired carbon dioxide concentration, exhaled carbon dioxide will rise. Examples of such problems are listed in Table 5.6 and include absent or incompetent unidirectional valves, faulty or exhausted absorbent, or a bypassed absorber in the circle system; increased dead space; inadequate fresh gas flow to a Mapleson system; defects in the inner tube of a Bain system; and malfunctioning non-rebreathing valves.

CORRELATION BETWEEN ARTERIAL AND END-TIDAL CONCENTRATIONS

Measurement of end-tidal carbon dioxide concentrations is important because there is a significant correlation between end-tidal and arterial concentrations. In one study of adult patients under anesthesia, the arterial carbon dioxide concentration exceeded the end-tidal concentration by an average of only 1.7 torr (152). In a study in children breathing spontaneously with halothane anesthesia, a median arterial to end-tidal carbon dioxide tension difference of 5 torr was found (149). The difference was greater as the level of carbon dioxide rose. However, alveolar plateaus were not always seen, so true end-tidal values were not always obtained.

There are situations where the correlation between these two values will not be good. Tables 5.4 to 5.6 show some conditions with increased arterial to alveolar gradients. The most common problem is failure to obtain an alveolar sample. Common causes are shallow breathing and incorrect placement or kinking of the sample catheter. This can be recognized by monitoring the waveforms on a capnograph. If a nearly horizontal plateau (Fig. 5.15) is not seen, the numerical value obtained may not be equivalent to the end-tidal concentration. Therefore capnography should always be used in conjunction with capnometry. In infants, even appearance

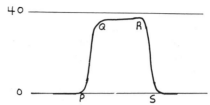

Figure 5.15. Normal capnogram. R, S, P is the inspiratory phase. At P, as expiration begins, dead space containing no carbon dioxide is the first gas exhaled. As alveolar gas appears, the curve slopes upward quickly and levels out into a horizontal plateau which represents outflowing of alveolar carbon dioxide. When the slope between Q and R is nearly horizontal, the numerical value obtained from the capnometer will be equivalent to the alveolar concentration. R is the peak expired concentration. After this, inhalation begins and the value quickly drops to 0, where it stays for the remainder of inspiration.

of a plateau may not be a sufficient condition to ensure reliability of end-tidal sampling (143, 150).

Another instance when arterial and end-tidal concentrations may not correlate well is when there is a ventilation perfusion (V/Q) mismatch with an increase in dead space. In the lung, the ideal unit has a normally ventilated alveolus adjacent to a normally perfused pulmonary capillary. This results in an arterial-to-alveolar gradient of less than 5 torr (151). In an inadequately perfused alveolus (low V/Q), there is decreased transfer of carbon dioxide between blood and lung with a resultant increase in the alveolar-to-arterial gradient. A venous admixture (high V/Q) or right-to-left shunt will also cause an increased gradient, but the effect is less than that caused by an increase in alveolar dead space (151).

The difference between end-tidal and arterial carbon dioxide concentrations will be increased in patients with lung disease, but the difference tends to be relatively stable (151, 152). When pulmonary impairment is present, arterial blood gases can be determined to establish the difference between arterial and end-tidal carbon dioxide. Once the difference is established, end tidal values provide a reliable estimate of arterial carbon dioxide. Presence of lung disease can frequently be diagnosed by examination of the carbon dioxide waveform.

Measurement of end-tidal carbon dioxide should allow better control of ventilation with fewer blood gas determinations and a cost saving. End-tidal analysis has the advantages of being noninvasive and available on a breath-by-breath basis. Hyperventilation induced by drawing of arterial blood samples resulting in erroneously low arterial carbon dioxide concentrations is not a problem with end-tidal analysis.

CAPNOGRAPHY

The ability to see and interpret exhaled carbon dioxide waveforms greatly enhances the usefulness of carbon dioxide analysis. Waveforms can be displayed on an oscilloscope or can be printed on graph paper. If a paper is used, trends can be followed by running the paper at a slow speed (Fig. 5.16). Faster speeds are used for examination of individual wave forms.

The waveform should be examined for height, frequency, rhythm, baseline, and shape. Height depends on the concentration of carbon dioxide. Frequency depends on respiratory rate. Rhythm depends on the state of the respiratory center or ventilator function. The baseline should be zero (unless carbon dioxide is deliberately added to the inspired gases).

A complete analysis of wave forms is beyond

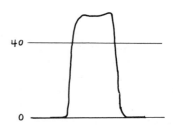

Figure 5.18. Hypoventilation (or increased production of carbon dioxide with constant ventilation). The alveolar plateau is seen, so the end-tidal concentration represents alveolar gas. Note increased height of the curve.

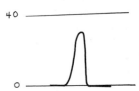

Figure 5.19. Extremely low tidal volume. Since an alveolar plateau is not seen, the end-tidal concentration on the capnometer will not represent alveolar concentration of carbon dioxide.

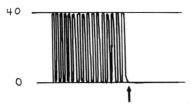

Figure 5.16. Normal capnograph at slow paper speed with sudden cessation of respiration (*arrow*). Note that on the normal capnograph the curves are long, thin and close together and the heights are even. Sudden stoppage is most commonly due to a disconnection or a stopped ventilator.

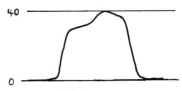

Figure 5.20. Camel curve. Seen with patients in the lateral position. Changes in the V-Q ratios of the two lungs leads to differences in their expired carbon dioxide concentrations. The gas exhaled from one lung reaches the capnograph before that from the other. The result is varying height in the two halves of the curve. Hyperventilation favors mixing of expired gases and diminishes this effect. Hypotension aggravates perfusion differences between the lungs and accentuates the effect (144).

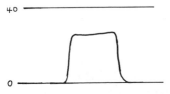

Figure 5.17. Hyperventilation (or decreased production of carbon dioxide with constant ventilation). The shape of the curve is normal, but the end-tidal concentration is lower than normal.

the scope of this book. The reader is referred to the excellent atlas of capnography by Smallhout (144). Some common waveforms are shown in Figures 5.14 through 5.27. There is only one normal waveform in adults (Fig. 5.15). Capnograms recorded from normal infants and small children show several characteristics different from those of adults (144).

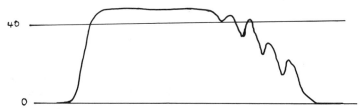

Figure 5.21. Bradypnea with cardiogenic oscillations. Cardiogenic oscillations are usually seen under the following circumstances (144): negative intrathoracic pressure; pulse/respiratory rate of at least 5.4 in adults and at least 4 in children; low vital capacity/size of heart; low inspiratory/expiratory ratio; prolongation of the expiratory phase; apnea; very low tidal volume; muscular relaxation.

Figure 5.22. Rebreathing. With the onset of rebreathing, the inspired carbon dioxide concentration fails to return to 0. When rebreathing is eliminated, the inspired carbon dioxide returns to 0 and the peak concentration returns to normal.

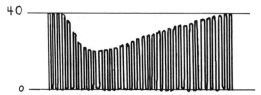

Figure 5.24. Sudden fall in exhaled carbon dioxide. This is most commonly due to a sudden circulatory event, such as air embolism, but could be caused by sudden kinking of an endotracheal tube.

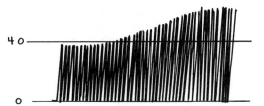

Figure 5.23. Hypoventilation following normal ventilation.

Mass Spectrometry (153–159)

Used primarily in the past as a research tool and later in the respiratory intensive care, the mass spectrometer is now used frequently in the operating room to monitor oxygen, nitrogen, carbon dioxide, nitrous oxide, and volatile anesthetic agents.

THEORY OF OPERATION

The operation of the mass spectrometer is based on the ability to separate and identify substances according to their molecular mass. A small volume of gas is drawn from the sampling area by a pump and passed into an ionization chamber where the gas molecules are bombarded with an electron beam. The beam causes loss of electrons, converting molecules into positively charged ions which are then accelerated, focused by means of an electrical field, and drawn into an analysis chamber. Within the analysis chamber is a magnetic field at right angles to the direction of travel of the ions. The ions are deflected into circular trajectories whose radii are determined by the masses or more specifically, by the mass-to-charge ratios. By suitable positioning of electrometers that measure the intensity of the bombardment, the quantity of ions of any particular mass can be determined.

DESCRIPTION AND USE

The mass spectrometer serves as the brains of a system which collects and samples gases from many locations. One centrally located mass spectrometer can service up to 16 operating rooms. Gases are collected from a catheter attached to the elbow connector between the mask or endotracheal tube and the breathing system (158). It may be desirable to extend the catheter down into the endotracheal tube. The gases are then drawn through small tubings to the mass spectrometer. There a switching mechanism causes gases from all active stations to be ana-

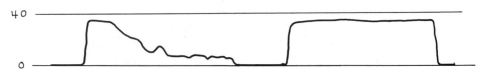

Figure 5.25. Effect of a leak. The downward slope of the plateau blends with the descending limb. Peak value will usually be below the alveolar concentration. The second wave, which is normal, follows correction of one leak.

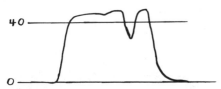

Figure 5.26. Curare cleft or notch. Seen during spontaneous ventilation. This is most commonly due to inadequate muscle relaxant reversal. It is also seen in patients with cervical transverse lesions. It is caused by a lack of synchronous action between the intercostal muscles and the diaphragm. The cleft is in the third part of the plateau. The depth of the cleft is proportional to the degree of muscle paralysis. The level of carbon dioxide varies. A cleft can also be seen with a flail chest, hiccup, pneumothorax and when a patient tries to breathe while on a respirator (144).

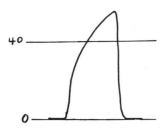

Figure 5.27. Airway or equipment problem limiting exhalation (bronchospasm, bronchitis, asthma, emphysema, herniated endotracheal tube cuff, foreign body). The ascending limb slopes toward the right and the alveolar plateau slopes upward. The angle (Q) between the ascending limb and the plateau is wider than normal and in extreme cases cannot be identified. The carbon dioxide level may be normal or elevated, but the actual alveolar concentration is usually higher than the capnograph suggests.

lyzed on a rotating (time-shared) basis. Samples from any individual station will be analyzed as often as every 20 sec or up to every several minutes, depending on the system and the number of locations on line at any one time. The information on each analysis is then relayed to the display units in each operating room. Units may emit a "beep" when a new analysis is displayed (158). Alarms can be set in each operating room for concentrations outside appropriate limits. Wave forms of exhaled carbon dioxide can be displayed.

A computer is usually part of the system. This will allow trends to be made and displayed on the video monitor. Printouts of data collected can also be obtained.

ADVANTAGES

The mass spectrometer has many advantages. It is accurate, versatile and easy to calibrate and operate. It has good stability and a fast response time (154). Inspired and end-tidal measurements can be made.

There is only one instrument to monitor many parameters. The display units in the operating rooms take up less space than would be taken up by individual monitors.

It has the ability to monitor nitrogen. This can be of value in detecting and quantifying pulmonary air embolism (158, 160, 161) and in detecting inward leakage of air into the breathing system around a poorly fitting mask or through a malfunctioning relief valve or ventilator (158).

The long-term trending and printout capabilities are very useful, especially for teaching or research.

DISADVANTAGES

There are several disadvantages to the use of a mass spectrometer. The primary disadvantage is that if problems occur which result in inoperability, the entire operating room suite may be without proper monitoring. The system is quite expensive. Central units require a separate room which may need independent air conditioning (154). Special ductwork to each operating room must be installed.

While the response time is rapid, the delay

while other locations are being sampled may be unacceptable for detection of sudden changes or verifying placement of a tracheal tube. Use of more than one mass spectrometer may be necessary in larger institutions.

Problems have been encountered in pediatric patients because of the routine use of uncuffed tracheal tubes (155). Gas loss around the tube can invalidate end-tidal readings unless the probe is inserted well into the tracheal tube, where it is more likely to become blocked by secretions.

There is a need to have one or more staff physicians who are interested in it and can guide its design, installation, and use. Without this level of physician interest the system's capabilities are unlikely to be realized.

MASS SPECTROMETER VERSUS INDIVIDUAL MONITORS

The decision whether to purchase a mass spectrometer or individual vigilance aids is difficult. Cost is of great significance. Use of a mass spectrometer probably has little merit in a small hospital since other devices can perform most of the same functions. In larger hospitals, the mass spectrometer may be more cost effective.

Teaching institutions may value the mass spectrometer for its instructional capabilities, but trainees should learn the use of other vigilance aids, since most of the hospitals where they will practice anesthesia after leaving training will not have mass spectrometers.

The question of backup equipment needs to be addressed. What will be done if the system is down? At the very least, individual oxygen monitors must be available. Carbon dioxide analyzers should be available for at least selected cases. However, if their use is the standard of care for that particular institution or community, backup units must be available. A recent report from a major university indicates an inoperative time of less than 2% (158).

HUMIDIFICATION METHODS

Moistening Breathing Tubes and Bag

Chase and co-workers (162) showed that moistening the inside of the breathing tubes and bag with water prior to use increased the humidity in the circle system significantly. However, the humidity level declined with passage of time as evaporation produced cooling.

This has the advantage of simplicity, but there is a limit to the increase in humidity. Sterile water should be used to avoid transmission of bacteria.

Addition of Water to an In-System Vaporizer

Another simple way to add humidity is to put water in an in-system vaporizer and turn it to the ON position. This has the same limits as moistening the tubes and bag. In addition, these vaporizers are usually very difficult to sterilize, so transmission of bacteria could be a significant problem. Confusion may also arise and liquids other than water may be placed in the vaporizer.

Heat and Moisture Exchanger (163–175) (Condenser Humidifier, Swedish Nose, Artificial Nose, Passive Humidifier, Regenerative Humidifier)

DESCRIPTION

A heat and moisture exchanger (HME), shown in Figure 5.28, comes with standard male and female 15-mm connections for placement between the endotracheal tube and the breathing system. Inside the HME is an exchange medium which has a large surface area and thermal capacity. A variety of materials in various configurations have been used for the exchange medium. A newer development is the hygroscopic condenser humidifier (163). This consists of an HME plus a hygroscopic unit, which actively binds the water molecules in expired gases. The relative humidity of expired gas passing through a conventional humidifier is approximately 100%. The relative humidity of

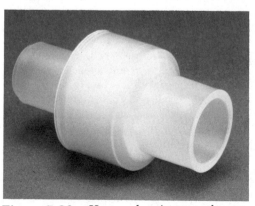

Figure 5.28. Heat and moisture exchanger. (Courtesy of Portex, Inc.)

expired gas passing through a combined HME and hygroscopic unit is much less (115).

Older model HMEs were not disposable, but could be cleaned and sterilized. Newer models have either permanent housing and the medium is replaced or the whole HME is disposable. Pediatric HMEs which offer less dead space and resistance than adult models are available.

ACTION

The HME works in a similar fashion to the upper respiratory tract, condensing water and capturing heat during exhalation and humidifying and warming inspired gases. During exhalation, warm moist gas from the patient passes through the relatively cool element; the gas is cooled and the element is warmed. Water condenses onto the element. During inspiration, cooler and drier gases enter the device and in passing through the relatively warm, wet element become warmed and humidified.

The inspired humidity that is achieved using an HME will depend on the humidity of gases reaching it during inspiration and to some extent on ventilatory rate and tidal volume (164, 174). Even the best HME can do no more than return to the patient all of the water exhaled. Heat and moisture exchangers vary in their ability to provide adequate inspired moisture (174, 175). Some can be wetted to increase efficiency, but others cannot. The directions with each device should be read carefully. Some cannot be used with humidifiers or nebulizers in the breathing system.

ADVANTAGES

These devices have been used for humidification of inspired gases for patients with tracheostomies for over 20 years (163). They closely reproduce the normal fluctuating temperature and humidity in the respiratory tract. They are inexpensive, easy to use, small, lightweight, reliable, of simple design, and silent in operation. They can be used with any breathing system or ventilator. They do not require a source of water or electric power and are not associated with overhydration or overheating. Water condensation in the expiratory circuit is greatly reduced. Bacterial contamination is not a significant problem (177). They are free of the dangers of overhydration and overheating.

DISADVANTAGES

In the past, cross-infection has been a problem but this has been eliminated by the introduction of disposable HMEs. Most precautions pertain to dead space and resistance (30). Resistance of HMEs is comparable to normal airway resistance, although the presence of viscous secretions will increase the resistance greatly, necessitating changing of the HME (178). Added dead space is of particular significance in small children and spontaneously breathing patients. Dead space varies considerably among the HMEs available (174, 175). Smaller units are available for use on patients with low tidal volumes. Use of an HME provides another possible site for a disconnection. Airway obstruction is a possible hazard.

The main disadvantage is that there is a limit to the inspired humidity these devices can deliver. Loss of water from the trachea may still occur. Therefore less efficient HMEs may be unacceptable, particularly for lengthy cases with high flows of non-humidified gases (174, 175).

Heated Humidifiers (Vaporizers)

A humidifier is an instrument that emits water vapor by passing a stream of gas over or through a water reservoir, across wicks dipped into water or a rain of water droplets (120). Heated humidifiers are the most popular way of supplying humidity during prolonged mechanical ventilation in intensive care units. However, most of those constructed for intensive care use are not suitable for use in anesthesia because their high internal resistance makes them unacceptable for spontaneously breathing patients (26, 32).

Heated humidifiers designed for use in anesthesia are now available from a number of manufacturers. There is a standard on humidifiers available from the American National Standards Institute (179), and a humidifier should not be considered for purchase unless it meets this standard. With some humidifiers the water reservoir is disposable. Others require refilling. In those with separate humidifying chambers and reservoirs, either or both components may be disposable (180).

METHOD OF OPERATION

The moisture output of an unheated humidifier diminishes with time because vaporization cools the water, thereby reducing the vapor pressure. Addition of heat will maintain constant humidification. Most heated humidifiers utilize electricity to supply heat. Humidifiers utilizing the heat of reaction in the absorber have also been devised (181–184).

Keeping the temperature just above ambient will prevent water condensation in the delivery tube. However, when gases saturated at room temperature are inhaled, water will still be lost from the tracheobronchial tree, since the relative humidity drops as the gases are warmed during inspiration. To prevent this water loss, the inspired gases must be saturated and at near body temperature. This can be accomplished in two ways: (a) the water reservoir can be heated above body temperature or (b) the conducting tube can be modified to conserve the heat content of the gas.

Superheating

Some devices superheat the water reservoir in order to maintain adequate heat content on the patient's end of the delivery tube. With a heated humidifier and no hose heating, normal ambient temperatures cool the gases in the delivery tubing. As a result, water will rain out. Condensation will be less with higher flows (180, 185). This is because with a high gas flow the rate of passage of the warmed gases through the breathing or delivery tube is rapid and there is less time to cool towards ambient temperature. Clear tubing should be used so the accumulated water can be seen and this water must be drained periodically.

Modifying the Delivery Tube

Less cooling and condensation in the delivery tube and lower water bath temperature can be achieved by shortening, insulating, or heating the delivery tube. This will prevent condensation. The tube should be warmed right up to the tracheal tube (or as close as possible).

Various methods of heating the delivery tube have been devised including a heating wire (186–188), external heating tape (189), incorporation of an air or water jacket around the tube (34, 190), and placing the inspiratory limb inside the expiratory limb (31, 184, 191, 192). The heated wire has the advantage of still allowing clear visualization of the delivery tube.

Humidifiers can be used with both circle and non-rebreathing systems. With Mapleson systems and systems employing non-rebreathing valves the humidifier is included in the fresh gas line (185). If possible, it should be placed near the end of the fresh gas flow to decrease conden-

sation in the tube. However, this may present problems in mounting.

In the circle system it can be interposed in the inspiratory line, downstream of the unidirectional valve, but if a bacterial filter is used, the humidifier must be placed downstream to prevent the filter from becoming clogged. Humidifiers should always be placed lower than the patient to prevent aspiration of large volumes of water if the apparatus is accidentally tipped.

It is mandatory that a heated humidifier have controls to prevent hyperthermia. It should be used only in conjunction with a thermometer near the patient's airway. The temperature must be monitored at the patient end of the circuit and kept near normal body temperature by manual or servo-control of the humidifier heater. The monitor should include an alarm. A cut-out system to prevent excessive heating is highly desirable (193).

ADVANTAGES

Heated humidifiers are highly efficient and capable of producing saturated gas at body temperature even at high flowrates. Monitoring and adjustment of airway temperature of the patient allows production of any desired temperature and humidity in the inspired gases. Many reviewers have concluded that this is the most physiological method of supplementing inspired humidity (194).

DISADVANTAGES

Humidifiers are bulky and may be difficult to mount. They are somewhat complex and some effort is required to operate them satisfactorily. Monitoring of the temperature of inspired gases at the patient end is necessary. Periodic draining of condensed water may be necessary. They are costly and may be difficult to clean and sterilize. Sepsis can be a problem, although infectious problems are less than with nebulizers (195, 196). There is one case reported where a leak in a humidifier in the fresh gas line caused a decreased fresh gas flow to the breathing system with significant rebreathing (51). Adding a humidifier changes the breathing system volume and compliance significantly (197).

The high humidity may cause problems with sticking of non-rebreathing, unidirectional, or relief valves. Bacterial filters may become clogged. If the delivery hose or inspiratory line is not heated, water will condense, resulting in noisy bubbling. There is always danger of the water draining into the endotracheal tube. If the humidifier is placed in the fresh gas line condensed water could obstruct it and an obstruction downstream could result in a splash back into the anesthesia machine or vaporizer (26).

The need for supplying heat creates many problems. Control of the temperature may be unsatisfactory and failure could result in hyperthermia and damage to the respiratory tract (53). Breakdown products of undetermined nature and toxicity have been found when a heated humidifer was used with halothane (54). Flammable anesthetic agents cannot be used and fires and electrocutions are hazards.

Nebulizers (Aerosol Generators, Atomizers)

A nebulizer is an instrument that emits water in the form of droplets (aerosol) (198). They are of two types: jet (high-pressure, compressed gas) and ultrasonic. Both can be heated.

MECHANISM OF ACTION

With the high-pressure nebulizer, a jet of high pressure gas encounters the liquid, inducing shearing forces and producing its dissociation into a mist. Since a high flow must be used, this type of nebulizer should be placed in the fresh gas line (199).

With an ultrasonic nebulizer, the liquid is subjected to intense ultrasonic vibration and a stable mist is produced. There is no need for a driving gas to cause nebulization. It can be used in the fresh gas line or in the inspiratory limb (45).

ADVANTAGES

Nebulizers can deliver gases saturated with water without heat, and if desired, can produce gases carrying more water.

DISADVANTAGES

Nebulizers are somewhat costly and difficult to operate. Jet nebulizers require high gas flows. Ultrasonic nebulizers require a source of electricity, so electroshock and fires are possible hazards and flammable anesthetic agents cannot be used. Back pressure created by some nebulizers can cause inaccuracy of flowmeters or vaporizers (199).

Transmission of infections is a particular problem with nebulizers since bacteria can be suspended in the water droplets (200–203).

Nebulizers may produce a positive water balance and result in fluid overload, particularly in infants and small children. Nebulization may have deleterious effects on the lungs if used for prolonged periods (49). There may be considerable water deposition in the tubings, requiring frequent draining and posing the dangers of water draining into the patient or blockage of the fresh gas line.

CLASSIFICATION OF BREATHING SYSTEMS

A favorite pastime among anesthesiologists has been the classification of breathing systems. The result has been a hopelessly confused terminology. Probably the most widely used nomenclature is that using the terms open, semi-open, semi-closed and closed. Unfortunately, various authors have defined these terms differently. As can be seen from Table 5.10, the T-piece has been variously described as open, semi-open and semi-closed. The nomenclature of the other systems is no less varied.

In an attempt to provide some relief from this confusion, a description of various authors' classifications will be presented. Subsequently, a nomenclature will be described which the authors feel is superior.

Existing Classifications

1. Dripps RD, Echenhoff JE, Vandam LD: *Introduction to Anesthesia*, ed 3. Philadelphia, W. B. Saunders, 1968.

This classification is summarized in Table 5.7. They classify their techniques of inhalation anesthesia into five categories according to the presence or absence of: (a) a reservoir bag in the breathing circuit, (b) rebreathing of exhaled gases, (c) an absorber to remove expired carbon dioxide and (d) directional valves in the breathing circuit. The five techniques are insufflation, open, semi-open, semi-closed and closed.

The insufflation system is one in which anesthetic gases and oxygen are delivered directly into the mouth or trachea. There are no valves, reservoir bag or carbon dioxide absorption.

In the open system, the patient inhales only the anesthetic mixture delivered by the anesthesia machine. Valves direct each exhaled breath into the atmosphere. A reservoir bag may or may not be present. Rebreathing is minimal and there is no carbon dioxide absorption. This includes systems used with intermittent flow machines and systems which use nonrebreathing valves.

Table 5.7.
Classification of Breathing Systems*

	Reservoir Bag	Rebreathing of Exhaled Gases	Carbon Dioxide Absorption	Directional Valves
Insufflation	No	Least	No	No
Open (non-rebreathing)				
1. Demand	No	Minimal	No	Two
2. Non-rebreathing valves	Yes	Minimal	No	Two
Semi-open				
1. Open drop	No	Partial	No	None
2. T-piece	No	Partial	No	None
3. Magill	Yes	Partial	Yes	Two
Semi-closed	Yes	Partial	Yes	Two
Closed				
1. To and fro	Yes	Complete	Yes	None
2. Circle	Yes	Complete	Yes	Two

*From Dripps RD, Echenhoff JE, Vandam LD: *Introduction to Anesthesia*, ed 3. Philadelphia, W. B. Saunders, 1968.

In the semi-open system, exhaled gases flow into the surrounding atmosphere and also to the inspiratory line of the apparatus to be rebreathed. There is no chemical absorption of exhaled carbon dioxide. Rebreathing depends on the fresh gas flow. A reservoir bag and a directional valve are optional.

In the semi-closed system, part of the exhaled gases passes into atmosphere whereas part mixes with fresh gases and is rebreathed. Chemical absorption of carbon dioxide is used. Directional valves are employed and a reservoir bag is present.

In the closed system there is complete rebreathing of expired gas. Carbon dioxide absorption, a reservoir bag and directional valves are present.

2. Moyers J: A nomenclature for methods of inhalation anesthesia. *Anesthesiology* 14:609–611, 1953.

Moyers (204) based his classification (shown in Table 5.8) of open, semi-open, semi-closed and closed on the presence or absence of a reservoir bag and rebreathing. An open system has no reservoir or rebreathing. The semi-open system has a reservoir but no rebreathing. The semi-closed system has a reservoir and partial rebreathing, whereas the closed has a reservoir and complete rebreathing. This system does not provide for classification of insufflation with flows low enough to allow rebreathing.

3. Collins VJ: *Principles of Anesthesiology*, ed 1. Philadelphia, Lea & Febiger, 1966.

Collins' classification is shown in Table 5.9. He defined an open system as one in which an anesthetic agent is brought to the patient's respiratory tract with atmospheric air as the diluent agent. The respiratory tract has access to the atmosphere during both inspiration and expiration. There is no reservoir or rebreathing.

A semi-open system is one in which the patient's respiratory system is open to atmosphere both during inspiration and expiration. There is a reservoir that is open to atmosphere, rebreathing is technically absent and atmospheric air either carries or dilutes the anesthetic agent.

The semi-closed system is defined as one in which the patient's respiratory system is completely closed to atmosphere on inspiration but open on expiration. A reservoir closed to atmosphere is present.

The closed system is one which allows no escape of anesthetic mixtures. There is no access to atmosphere either on inspiration or expiration. Rebreathing is complete and a reservoir is required.

4. Adriani J: *The Chemistry and Physics of*

Table 5.8.
Classification of Breathing Systems*

	Reservoir	Rebreathing
Open	No	No
Semi-open	Yes	No
Semi-closed	Yes	Yes, partial
Closed	Yes	Yes, complete

*From Moyers J: A nomenclature for methods of inhalation anesthesia. *Anesthesiology* 14:609–611, 1953.

Table 5.9.
Classification of Breathing Systems*

	Reservoir	Rebreathing	Access to Atmosphere Inspiration	Access to Atmosphere Expiration
Open	No	No	Yes	Yes
Semi-open	Yes	No	Yes	Yes
Semi-closed	Yes	No Partial	No	Yes
Closed	Yes	Yes, complete	No	No

*From Collins VJ: *Principles of Anesthesiology*, ed 1. Philadelphia, Lea & Febiger, 1966.

Anesthesia. Springfield, Ill., Charles C Thomas, 1962.

Adriani's systems (Table 5.10) are divided into open vaporization, insufflation, semi-closed and closed (rebreathing). An open system is one employing the open-drop mask. With the insufflation technique a continuous stream of gas flows to the patient's nasopharynx, oropharynx or trachea. He defines the semi-closed system as one in which there is complete enclosure of the inspired atmosphere and no air dilution. The closed system permits complete rebreathing.

5. Conway CM: *Anaesthetic Circuits, Foundations of Anaesthesia*, ed 1. Edited by C Scurr and S Feldman. Philadelphia, F. A. Davis, 1970.

Conway (4) (Table 5.11) also used the terms open, semi-open, semi-closed and closed. An open system is one with infinite boundaries and no restriction to fresh gas flow. The semi-open system is one partially bounded, with some restriction to fresh gas flow. The closed circuit is defined as having no provision for gas overflow.

Table 5.10.
Classification of Breathing Systems*

Open vaporization
Insufflation
Semi-closed
1. Rebreathing permitted
2. No rebreathing
Closed

*From Adriani J: *The Chemistry and Physics of Anesthesia*. Springfield, Ill., Charles C Thomas, 1962.

Table 5.11.
Classification of Breathing Systems*

Open	A circuit with infinite boundaries and no restriction upon the entry of fresh gas
Semi-Open	A partially bounded circuit with some restriction of fresh gas entry
Closed	A fully bounded circuit with no provision for gas overflow
Semi-closed	A fully bounded circuit with provision for venting of excess gas

1. Semi-closed rebreathing circuits
2. Semi-closed absorption circuits
3. Non-rebreathing circuits

*From Conway CM: Anaesthetic circuits. In Scurr C, Feldman S (eds): *Scientific Foundations of Anaesthesia*. Philadelphia, F. A. Davis, 1970.

The semi-closed system is one allowing for overflow of excess gas. It is divided into semi-closed rebreathing, semi-closed absorption and semi-closed non-rebreathing circuits.

6. Hall J: *Wright's Veterinary Anaesthesia*, ed 6. London, Bailliere, Tindall & Cox, 1966.

This book describes a British nomenclature using the terms open, semi-open, semi-closed and closed (Table 5.12). In this classification, the open system has no reservoir bag or re-

Table 5.12.
Classification of Breathing Systems*

	Reservoir Bag	Rebreathing
Open	No	No
Semi-open	No	Partial
Semi-closed		
1. Without absorption	Yes	Partial
2. With absorption	Yes	Partial
Closed	Yes	Complete

*From Hall J: *Wright's Veterinary Anaesthesia*, ed 6. London, Baillière Tindall & Cox, 1966.

Table 5.13.
Classification of Breathing Systems*

Open	No rebreathing
Semi-closed	Partial rebreathing
Closed	Total rebreathing

*From McMahon J: Rebreathing as a basis for classification of inhalation technics. *J Am Assoc Nurse Anesthetists* 19:133–158, 1951.

Table 5.14.
Classification of Breathing Systems*

Carbon dioxide wash-out circuits
   1. Open (no reservoir bag)
      Open mask (drop)
      Insufflation
      T-piece
   2. Semi-open (with reservoir bag)
      Magill circuit
      Rees system
Carbon dioxide absorption circuits
   1. Closed (fresh gas flow equals uptake by patient)
   2. Semi-closed (fresh gas flow greater than uptake)

*From Baraka A: Functional classification of anaesthesia circuits. *Anaesth Intensive Care* 5:172, 1977.

Table 5.15.
Classification of Breathing Systems

	Insufflation	Non-rebreathing Valves	T-Piece	Magill and Mapleson B, C and D Systems	Open Drop	Circle System	To and Fro
Dripps	Insufflation	Open	Semi-open	Semi-open	Semi-open	Semi-closed / Closed	Semi-closed / Closed
Collins	Open	Semi-closed non-rebreathing	Open (no exp. arm) / Semi-open (with exp. arm)	Semi-closed / Partial rebreathing / No rebreathing	Open / Semi-open (if towels added)	Semi-closed partial rebreathing / Closed	Semi-closed partial rebreathing / Closed
Adriani	Insufflation	Semi-closed non-rebreathing	Semi-closed (if no air dilution)	Semi-closed	Open	Semi-closed / Closed	Semi-closed / Closed
Conway	Open	Semi-closed non-rebreathing	Semi-closed rebreathing / Semi-open (low gas flow and short exp. limb)	Semi-closed / Rebreathing / Non-rebreathing	Semi-open with occlusive packing	Semi-closed absorption / Closed	Semi-closed absorption / Closed
Moyers	Open	Semi-open	Open (no exp. limb) / Semi-open (with exp. limb and high fresh gas flow) / Semi-closed (with exp. limb and low fresh gas flow)	Semi-open (high fresh gas flow) / Semi-closed (low fresh gas flow)	Open / Semi-closed with towels or thick mask	Semi-closed / Closed	Semi-closed / Closed
Wright's	Open		Semi-closed without absorption / Semi-open (if exp. limb occluded during inspiration)	Semi-closed without absorption	Open / Semi-open with occlusive packing	Semi-closed with absorption / Closed	Semi-closed with absorption / Closed
McMahon	Open	Open	Open / Semi-closed	Open / Semi-closed	Open / Semi-closed	Semi-closed / Closed	Semi-closed / Closed
Baraka	Open	Open (no bag) / Semi-open (with bag)	Open (no bag) / Semi-open (with bag)	Semi-open	Open	Semi-closed / Closed	Semi-closed / Closed

breathing. The semi-open system also has no reservoir bag but has partial rebreathing. Semi-closed systems have a reservoir bag and partial rebreathing. They are divided into those with and those without carbon dioxide absorption. The closed system has complete rebreathing and a reservoir.

7. McMahon J: Rebreathing as a basis for classification of inhalation technics. *J Am Assoc Nurse Anesth* 19:133–158, 1951.

McMahon (18) (Table 5.13) used rebreathing as the basis for classification of systems into open, semi-closed and closed. An open technique is one in which no rebreathing is employed. This includes techniques in which gases are administered at a total flowrate equal to or greater than the respiratory minute volume. Techniques with flows less than the respiratory minute volume would also be considered as open if there were no increase in dead space. The semi-closed system would employ some rebreathing. The closed system employs total rebreathing.

8. Baraka (205) classified breathing systems according to their mechanisms of carbon dioxide elimination. His system is shown in Table 5.14. Carbon dioxide is eliminated from the circuit either by wash-out or by absorption. Open systems are those that eliminate carbon dioxide by washout and have no reservoir bag. Semi-open systems also wash out carbon dioxide, but have a reservoir bag. Semi-closed systems utilize carbon dioxide absorption and have a fresh gas flow that exceeds patient uptake. Closed systems also utilize carbon dioxide absorption and have a fresh gas flow that equals patient uptake.

9. The International Standards Organization has devised a classification of breathing systems based on the amount of rebreathing that occurs. Systems are classified as non-rebreathing systems, partial rebreathing systems and complete rebreathing.

Proposed Classification

Hamilton (206) recognized the shortcomings of the nomenclature described above and advanced a nomenclature which we feel gives the maximum information. He proposed that the terms open, semi-open, etc. be dropped in favor of a description of the equipment and the total fresh gas flow to the system. The description of the equipment will be familiar to the reader after having read the next three chapters. The flow will determine the amount of rebreathing, if any, that takes place. When this is given, the reader will have precise, meaningful information. Table 5.15 shows the various systems according to the equipment and the various authors' classifications.

References

1. Macintosh R, Mushin WW, Epstein HG: *Physics for the Anaesthetist.* Oxford, Blackwell Scientific Publications, 1963.
2. Gaensler EA, Maloney JV, Bjork VO: Bronchospirometry. II. Experimental observations and theoretical considerations of resistance breathing. *J Lab Clin Med* 39:935–953, 1952.
3. Brown ES, Hustead RF: Resistance of pediatric breathing systems. *Anesth Analg* 48:842–849, 1969.
4. Conway CM: Anaesthetic circuits. In Scurr C, Feldman S (eds): *Scientific Foundations of Anaesthesia.* Philadelphia, F. A. Davis, 1970, pp 399–405.
5. Cain CC, Otis AB: Some physiological effects resulting from added resistance to respiration. *J Aviation Med* 20:149–160, 1949.
6. Davies JM, Hogg MIJ, Rosen M: Upper limits of resistance of apparatus for inhalation analgesia during labour. *Br J Anaesth* 46:136–144, 1974.
7. Fujita M: Resistance to breathing through various anesthesia apparatus: safety limit of external resistance during general anesthesia. *Far East J Anesthesia* 3:8–16, 1960.
8. Graff TD, Sewall K, Lim HS, Kanatt O, Morris RE, Benson DW: The ventilatory response of infants to airway resistance. *Anesthesiology* 27:168–175, 1966.
9. Nunn JF, Ezi-Ashi TI: The respiratory effects of resistance to breathing in anesthetized man. *Anesthesiology* 22:174–185, 1961.
10. Cheney FW, Hornbein TF, Crawford EW: The effect of expiratory resistance on the blood gas tensions of anesthetized patients. *Anesthesiology* 28:670–676, 1967.
11. Proctor DF: Studies of respiratory air flow. IV. Resistance to air flow through anesthesia apparatus. *Bull Johns Hopkins Hosp* 96:49–58, 1955.
12. Silverman L, Lee G, Plotkin T, Sawyers LA, Yancey AR: Air flow measurements on human subjects with and without respiratory resistance at several work rates. *Arch Indust Hyg* 3:461–478, 1951.
13. Smith WDA: The effects of external resistance to respiration. Part I. General review. *Br J Anaesth* 33:549–554, 1961.
14. Whitelaw WA, Derenne JP, Coutre J, Milic-Emili J: Adaptation of anesthetized men to breathing through an inspiratory resistor. *J Appl Physiol* 41:285–291, 1976.
15. Bentley RA, Griffin OG, Love RG, Muir DCF, Sweetland KF: Acceptable levels for breathing resistance of respiratory apparatus. *Arch Environ Health* 27:273–280, 1973.
16. Hogg MIJ, Davies JM, Mapleson WW, Rosen M: Proposed upper limit of respiratory resistance for inhalation apparatus used in labour. *Br J Anaesth* 46:149–152, 1974.
17. Rosen M: Recent advances in pain relief in chil-

dren. I. Inhalation and systemic analgesia. *Br J Anaesth* 43:837–848, 1971.

18. McMahon J: Rebreathing as a basis for classification of inhalation technics. *J Am Assoc Nurse Anesthetists* 19:133–158, 1951.

19. Sykes MK: Nonrebreathing valves. *Br J Anaesth* 31:450–455.

20. Sykes MK: Rebreathing circuits. *Br J Anaesth* 40:666–674, 1968.

21. Spoerel WE, Aitken RR, Bain JA: Spontaneous respiration with the Bain breathing circuit. *Can Anaesth Soc J* 25:30–35, 1978.

22. Dykes MHM, Chir MB, Laasberg LH: Clinical implications of halothane contamination of the anesthetic circle. *Anesthesiology* 35:648–649, 1971.

23. Samulksa HM, Ramaiah S, Noble WH: Unintended exposure to halothane in surgical patients: halothane washout studies. *Can Anaesth Soc J* 19:35–41, 1972.

24. Murray WJ, Fleming P: Patient exposure to residual fluorinated anesthetic agents in anesthesia machine circuits. *Anesth Analg.* 52:23–26, 1973.

25. Dery R, Pelletier J, Jacques A, Clavet M, Houde JJ: Humidity in anesthesiology. Heat and moisture patterns in the respiratory tract during anaesthesia with the semi-closed system. *Can Anaesth Soc J* 14:287–298, 1967.

26. Amirdivani M, Siegel D, Chalon J, Ramanathan S, Turndorf H: A heated water humidifier with a rotating wick. *Anesth Analg* 58:244–246, 1979.

27. Chase HF, Kilmore MA, Trotta R: Respiratory water loss via anesthesia systems: mask breathing. *Anesthesiology* 22:205–209, 1961.

28. Forbes AR: Humidification and mucus flow in the intubated trachea. *Br J Anaesth* 45:874–878, 1973.

29. Weeks DB, Broman KE: A method of quantitating humidity in the anesthesia circuit by temperature control: semiclosed circle. *Anesth Analg* 49:292–296, 1970.

30. Boys JE, Howells TH: Humidification in anaesthesia. *Br J Anaesth* 44:879–886, 1972.

31. Chalon J, Patel C, Ramanathan S, Turndorf H: Humidification of the circle absorber system. *Anesthesiology* 48:142–146, 1978.

32. Tausk HC, Miller R, Roberts RB: Maintenance of body temperature by heated humidification. *Anesth Analg* 55:719–723, 1976.

33. Stone DR, Downs JB, Paul WL, Perkins HM: Adult body temperature and heated humidification of anesthetic gases during general anesthesia. *Anesth Analg* 60:736–741, 1981.

34. Racz GB: Humidification in a semiopen system for infant anesthesia. *Anesth Analg* 50:995–1002, 1971.

35. Rashad KF, Benson DW: Role of humidity in prevention of hypothermia in infants and children. *Anesth Analg* 46:712–718, 1967.

36. Fonkalsrud EW, Calmes S, Barcliff LT, Barrett CT: Reduction of operative heat loss and pulmonary secretions in neonates by use of heated and humidified anesthetic gases. *J Thorac Cardiovasc Surg* 80:718–723, 1980.

37. Chalon J, Ali M, Turndorf H, Fischgrund GK: *Humidification of Anesthetic Gases.* Springfield, Ill., Charles C Thomas, 1981.

38. Rashad K, Wilson K, Hurt HH Jr, Graff TD, Banson DW: Effect of humidification of anesthetic gases on static compliance. *Anesth Analg* 46:127–133, 1967.

39. Chalon J, Loew DAY, Malebranche J: Effects of dry anesthetic gases on tracheobronchial ciliated epithelium. *Anesthesiology* 37:338–343, 1972.

40. Mackuanying N, Chalon J: Humidification of anesthetic gases for children. *Anesth Analg* 53:387–391, 1974.

41. Tayyab MA, Ambiavagar M, Chalon J: Water nebulization in a non-rebreathing system during anaesthesia. *Can Anaesth Soc J* 20:728–735, 1973.

42. Burton JDK: Effects of dry anesthetic gases on the respiratory mucous membrane. *Lancet* 1:235–238, 1962.

43. Chalon J, Patel C, Ali M, Ramanathan S, Capan L, Tang C, Turndorf H: Humidity and the anesthetized patient. *Anesthesiology* 50:195–198, 1979.

44. Gawley TH, Dundee JW: Attempts to reduce respiratory complications following upper abdominal operations. *Br J Anaesth* 53:1073–1078, 1981.

45. Stevens HL, Kennedy RL: The ultrasonic approach to humidification of anesthesia gases. *J Asthma Res* 5:325–333, 1968.

46. Knudsen J, Lomholt N, Wisborg K: Postoperative pulmonary complications using dry and humidified anaesthetic gases. *Br J Anaesth* 45:363–368, 1973.

47. Noguchi H, Takumi Y, Aochi O: A study of humidification in tracheostomized dogs. *Br J Anaesth* 45:844–848, 1973.

48. Hayes B: Humidification in anaesthesia. *Br J Anaesth* 51:389–390, 1979.

49. Modell JH, Giammona ST, Davis JH: Effect of chronic exposure to ultrasonic aerosols on the lung. *Anesthesiology* 28:680–688, 1967.

50. Garg GP: Correspondence. *Anesth Analg* 54:618–620, 1975.

51. Nimocks JA, Modell JH, Perry PA: Carbon dioxide retention using a humidified "nonrebreathing" system. *Anesth Analg* 54:271–273, 1975.

52. Kirch TJ, DeKornfeld TJ: An unexpected complication (hyperthemia) while using the Emerson postoperative ventilator. *Anesthesiology* 28:1106–1107, 1967.

53. Klein EF, Graves SA: "Hot pot" tracheitis. *Chest* 65:225–226, 1974.

54. Karis JH, O'Neal F, Weitzner SW: Alteration of halothane in heated humidifiers. *Anesth Analg* 59:518, 1980.

55. *Standard for 22 mm Anesthesia Breathing Circuit Connectors.* Pamphlet M-1, Compressed Gas Association, Inc., 500 Fifth Ave., New York, N.Y. 10036, 1972.

56. Wyant GM: Rebreathing bag. *Br Med J* 1:112, 1970.

57. Parmley JB, Tahir AH, Dascomb HE, Adriani J: Disposable versus reusable rebreathing circuits: advantages, disadvantages, hazards, and bacteriologic studies. *Anesth Analg* 51:888–894, 1972.

58. Johnstone RE, Smith TC: Rebreathing bags as pressure-limiting devices. *Anesthesiology* 38:192–194, 1973.

59. Stone DR, Graves SA: Compliance of pediatric rebreathing bags. *Anesthesiology* 53:434–435, 1980.

60. *Anesthesia Reservoir Bags.* Z-79, 4-1974, American National Standards Institute, 1430 Broadway, New York, N.Y. 10018.

61. Parmley JB, Tahir AH, Dascomb HE, Adriani J: Disposable versus reusable rebreathing circuits. *Items Topics*, pp 1–4, 1974.

62. Parmley JB, Tahir AH, Adriani J: Disposable plastic breathing bags and tubes. *JAMA* 217:1842–1844, 1971.

63. *Breathing Tubes.* A-79.6-1974, American National Standards Institute, 1430 Broadway, New York, N.Y. 10018.

64. Smith WDA: The effects of external resistance to respiration. Part II. Resistance to respiration due to anaesthetic apparatus. *Br J Anaesth* 33:610–627, 1961.

65. Kirby RA: Mechanical ventilation in acute ventilatory failure: facts, fiction, and fallacies. *Curr Probl Anesth Crit Care Med* 1:1, 1977.

66. Mushin WW, Rendell-Baker L, Thompson P, Mapleson WW: *Automatic Ventilation of the Lungs*, ed 3. Oxford, Blackwell Scientific Publications, 1980.

67. Cottrell JE, Bernhard W, Turndorf H: Hazards of disposable rebreathing circuits. *Anesth Analg* 55:743–744, 1976.

68. Cottrell JE, Chalon J, Turndorf H: Faulty anesthesia circuits: a source of environmental pollution in the operating room. *Anesth Analg* 56:359–362, 1977.

69. Carden E, Chir B: A tube-supporting "fork." *Canad Anaesth Soc J* 15:505, 1968.

70. Ciola LF: Universal breathing tube support. *Anesthesiology* 22:844–846, 1961.

71. Harris JA, Aldrete JA: An anesthetic tubing support. *Anesthesiology* 33:462, 1970.

72. Mushin WW, Mapleson WW: Pressure-flowrate characteristics of expiratory valves. *Br J Anaesth* 26:3–10, 1954.

73. Mehta S, Behr G, Chari J, Kenyon D: A passive method of disposal of expired anesthetic gases. *Br J Anaesth* 49:589–593, 1977.

74. Morgan BA, Nott MR: Wear in plastic exhaust valves. *Anaesthesia* 35:717–718, 1980.

75. Nott MR, Norman J: Resistance of Heidbrink-type expiratory valves. *Br J Anaesth* 50:477–480, 1978.

76. Sykes MK: Three nonrebreathing valves for use in anaesthesia. *Br J Anaesth* 31:446–449, 1959.

77. Egbert LD, Laver MB: Accuracy of manual ventilation: comparison of closed and semiclosed breathing systems. *Anesthesiology* 25:93–94, 1964.

78. Egbert LD, Bisno D: The educated hand of the anesthesiologist: a study of professional skill. *Anesth Analg* 46:195–200, 1967.

79. Conway CM, Schoonbee C: Factors affecting the performance of circle systems used without carbon dioxide absorption. *Br J Anaesth* 53:115P, 1981.

80. Frumin MJ, Lee ASJ, Papper EM: New valve for nonrebreathing systems. *Anesthesiology* 20:383–385, 1959.

81. Mushin WW, Rendell-Baker L, Thompson PW, Mapleson WW: *Automatic Ventilation of the Lungs*. Oxford, Blackwell Scientific Publications, 1980, pp 823–847.

82. Eger EI: Anesthetic systems: construction and function. In *Anesthetic Uptake and Action*. Baltimore, Williams & Wilkins, 1975.

83. Smith RJ, Volpitto PP: Volume ventilation valve. *Anesthesiology* 20:885–886, 1959.

84. Steen SN, Lee ASJ: Prevention of inadvertent excess pressure in closed systems. *Anesth Analg* 39:264–266, 1960.

85. Hough VJ: Prevention of ventilator accident. *Anesthesiology* 49:226–227, 1978.

86. Love JB: Misassembly of a Campbell ventilator causing leakage of the driving gas to a patient. *Anaesth Intensive Care* 8:376–377, 1980.

87. Longmuir J, Craig DB: Inadvertent increase in inspired oxygen concentration due to defect in ventilator bellows. *Can Anaesth Soc J* 23:327–329, 1976.

88. Marsland AR, Solomos J: Ventilator malfunction detected by O_2 analyzer. *Anaesth Intensive Care* 9:395, 1981.

89. Cooper JB: Prevention of anesthetic mishaps. Conference on Technology and Equipment in Anesthesiology, Cleveland, Ohio, May 18–20, 1979.

90. Figallo EM, Smith RB, Pautler S, Reilly KR: Continuous oxygen analyzers in clinical anesthesia. *Anesth Rev* 5:25–31, 1978.

91. *Requirements for Oxygen Analyzers for Monitoring Patient Breathing Mixtures.* Z-79,10-1979, American National Standards Institute, 1430 Broadway, New York, N.Y. 10018.

92. Steward DJ, Pelton DA: Audio vs visual oxygen alarm. *Anesthesiology* 52:192, 1980.

93. Hewitt K, Marshall RD: The IL 404 oxygen alarm monitor. *Anaesthesia* 31:1291–1292, 1976.

94. Cooper JB: Selecting an oxygen monitor. Workshop on Anesthesia Safety, American Society of Anesthesiologists, New Orleans, La., 1977.

95. Westenskow DR, Jordan WS, Jordan R, Sillman ST: Evaluation of oxygen monitors for use during anesthesia. *Anesth Analg* 60:53–56, 1981.

96. Anonymous: Portable oxygen analyzers. *Health Devices* 1:203–215, 1972.

97. Mazza N, Wald A: Failure of battery-operated alarms. *Anesthesiology* 53:246–248, 1980.

98. Altman P, Pumphrey D, Bailey WC: Modification to prevent deactivation of Bennett spirometer alarm system during mechanical ventilation. *Resp Care* 18:294–295, 1973.

99. Fodor I, Bloomfield D, Fisher A, Kerr JH: A control-free ventilator alarm. *Anaesthesia* 32:1026–1029, 1977.

100. Cooper JB: Prevention of anesthetic mishaps. In Technology and Equipment in Anesthesiology, Case Western Reserve University, Cleveland, Ohio, May 18–20, 1979.

101. Ventilation alarms. *Health Devices* 10:204–220, 1981.

102. Cooper JB, Newbower RS, Long CD, McPeek B: Preventable anesthesia mishaps: a study of human factors. *Anesthesiology* 49:399–406, 1978.

103. McEwen JA, Small CF, Saunders BA, Jenkins

LC: Hazards associated with the use of disconnect monitors. *Anesthesiology* 53:S391, 1980.

104. Reynolds AC: Disconnect alarm failure. *Anesthesiology* 58:488, 1983.

105. Medical device alert, Ohio Medical Products, December 8, 1976.

106. Sarnquist FH, Demas K: The silent ventilator. *Anesth Analg* 61:713–714, 1982.

107. Heard SO, Munson ES: Ventilator alarm nonfunction associated with a scavenging system for waste gases. *Anesth Analg* 62:230–232, 1983.

108. Anesthesia ventilator distal sensing tee. *Items Topics* 31:23, 1982.

109. Anonymous: Airway pressure monitor. *Biomed Safety Standards* 12:123, 1982.

110. Hommelgaard P, Nissen T: A water-insensitive ventilator alarm. *Anaesthesia* 34:1048–1051, 1979.

111. Mazza N, Wald A: Failure of battery-operated alarms. *Anesthesiology* 53:246–248, 1980.

112. Hazard: Bunn Model 65 ventilation alarm. *Technol Anesth* 2:1, 1981.

113. Anonymous: Canadian government issues alert on Monaghan/Hospal 703 ventilator alarm. *Biomed Safety Standards* 10:135, 1980.

114. Ventilation monitor/ventilator incompatibility. *Health Devices* 11:328–329, 1982.

115. Rendell-Baker L, Meyer JA: Accidental disconnection and pulmonary barotrauma. *Anesthesiology* 58:286, 1983.

116. Seed RF: Alarms for lung ventilators. *Br J Clin Equip* 4:114–121, 1978.

117. Spielman FJ, Sprague DH: Another benefit of the subatmospheric alarm. *Anesthesiology* 54:526–527, 1981.

118. Lowe HJ, Hagler K: Clinical and laboratory evaluation of an expired anesthetic gas monitor (Narko-Test). *Anesthesiology* 34:378–382, 1971.

119. Velasquez JL, Feingold A: Calibration of the Narkotest gas monitor for isoflurane. *Anesth Analg* 55:441–442, 1976.

120. White DC, Wardley-Smith B: The "Narkotest" anesthetic gas meter. *Br J Anaesth* 44:1100–1104, 1972.

121. Velazquez JL, Feingold A, Walther P: Response time of the Narkotest anesthetic gas monitor. *Anesth Analg* 56:395–397, 1977.

122. Linstromberg JW, Muir JJ: Non-uniform interference by water vapor in the Engstrom EMMA. *Anesthesiology* 57:A163, 1982.

123. Bennetts FE: Closed circuit halothane anaesthesia. Use of the Narkotest as an in-line monitor in a nonpolluting technique. *Anaesthesia* 31:644–650, 1976.

124. Luff NP, White DC: Evaluation of the EMMA anaesthetic gas monitor. *Br J Anaesth* 53:1102, 1981.

125. Kay B, Cohen AT, Wheeler MF: A laboratory investigation of a multigas monitor for anaesthesia (EMMA). *Anaesthesia* 37:446–450, 1982.

126. Hayes JK, Westenskow DR, Jordan WS: Continuous monitoring of inspiratory and end-tidal anesthetic vapor using a piezoelectric detector. *Anesthesiology* 57:A180, 1982.

127. Geoeon A, Hamilton K, Kindlund A, Lundstrom I, Mebius C, Haggmark S, Reiz S: A new sensitive method for breath-by-breath monitoring of anaesthetic gases. Reprinted from International Congress Series No. 538, *Anaesthesiology*, Proceedings of the Seventh World Congress of Anaesthesiologists, Hamburg, Germany, Sept. 14–21, 1980, Zindler M, Rugheimer E (eds). Amsterdam, Excerpta Medica, 1980, pp 656–659.

128. Kay B, Calpin M, Beatty P, et al: Another source of inaccuracy of the EMMA. *Anaesthesia* 37:608, 1982.

129. White DC, Luff DD: Are vaporizers and gas analysers accurate? A source of error. *Anaesthesia* 37:607, 1982.

130. Paredes R, Zapata A, Palacios N, Tejada V: The calibration of anesthesia vaporizers by infrared spectroscopy. *Anesthesiology* 36:107–110, 1963.

131. Goldman E, Sherrill D, de Campo T, Aldrete JA: Calibration curves of enflurane using the Beckman LB2 gas analyzer with the halothane head. *Anesthesiology* 53:79–81, 1980.

132. Robinson A, Denson JS, Summers FW: Halothane analyzer. *Anesthesiology* 23:391–394, 1962.

133. Tatnall ML, West PG, Morris P: A rapid-response UV halothane meter. *Br J Anaesth* 50:617–621, 1978.

134. Diprose KV, Epstein HG, Redman LR: An improved ultra-violet halothane meter. *Br J Anaesth* 52:1155–1160, 1980.

135. Bosterling B, Trevor A, Trudell JR: Binding of halothane-free radicals to fatty acids following UV irradiation. *Anesthesiology* 56:380–384, 1982.

136. Karin JH, O'Neal FO, Menzel DB: Toxicity of ultraviolet (UV) irradiated halothane in mice. *Anesthesiology* 53:S245, 1980.

137. Fisher DM, Swedlow DB: Estimating PaCO$_2$ by end-tidal gas sampling in children. *Crit Care Med* 9:287, 1981.

138. Dunn GL, Morison DH, Ahston JC: Siemens PCO$_2$ gas analyzer. *Can Anaesth Soc J* 30:318, 1983.

139. Fletcher R, Werner O, Nordstrom L, Jonson B: Sources of error and their correction in the measurement of carbon dioxide elimination using the Siemens-Elema CO$_2$ analyzer. *Br J Anaesth* 55:177–185, 1983.

140. Olsson SG, Fletcher R, Jonson B, Nordstrom L, Prakash O: Clinical studies of gas exchange during ventilatory support—a method using the Siemens-Elema CO$_2$ analyzer. *Br J Anaesth* 52:491–499, 1980.

141. Reder RF, Brown EG, DeAsla RA, Jurado RA: Thermal skin burns from a carbon dioxide analyzer in children. *Ann Thorac Surg* 35:329–330, 1983.

142. Nuzzo PF: Capnography in infants and children. *Perinatol Neonatol* May/June, 1978.

143. Reznik AM, Epstein MAF, Epstein RA: End tidal sampling of CO$_2$ in infants. *Anesthesiology* 51:S387, 1979.

144. Smalhout B, Kalenda Z: *An Atlas of Capnography*, ed 2, vol 1, Utrecht-Zeist, The Netherlands, 1982.

145. Greenway RE, Heeneman H, Keeri-Szanto M: Circulatory monitoring using a carbon dioxide analyzer during planned hypotension: a clinical note. *Can Anaesth Soc J* 24:282–285, 1977.

146. Brechner TM, Brechner VL: An audible aarm for monitoring air embolism during neurosurgery. *J Neurosurg* 47:201–204, 1977.

147. Bethune RWM, Brechner VL: Detection of venous air embolism by carbon dioxide monitoring. *Anesthesiology* 29:178, 1968.

148. Utting JE, Gray TC, Shelley FC: Human misadventure in anaesthesia. *Can Anaesth Soc J* 26:472–478, 1979.

149. Valentin N, Lomholt B, Thorup M: Arterial to end-tidal carbon dioxide tension difference in children under halothane anaesthesia. *Can Anaesth Soc J* 29:12–15, 1982.

150. Jordan WS, Westenskow DR, Hayes J, Roberts LS: Should capnometry replace capnography in pediatric anesthesia? *Anesthesiology* 57:A421, 1982.

151. Watts CE: Carbon dioxide elimination and capnography. *Resp Ther* 25:107–113, 1980.

152. Whitesell R, Asiddao C, Gollman D, Jablonski J: Relationship between arterial and peak expired carbon dioxide pressure during anesthesia and factors influencing the difference. *Anesth Analg* 60:508–512, 1981.

153. American Society for Hospital Engineering of the American Hospital Association: *Mass Spectrometer Respiratory Monitoring Systems.* AHA catalog no. 1167, American Hospital Association, 840 N. Lakeshore Dr., Chicago, Ill. 60611, 1980.

154. Gillbe CE, Heneghan CPH, Branthwaite MA: Respiratory mass spectrometry during general anaesthesia. *Br J Anaesth* 53:103–109, 1981.

155. Gothard JWW, Busst CM, Branthwaite MA, Davies NJH, Denison DM: Applications of respiratory mass spectrometry to intensive care. *Anaesthesia* 35:890–895, 1980.

156. Hill DW: Production of accurate gas and vapour mixtures. *Br J Appl Physics* 12:410–413, 1961.

157. Mapleson WW, Willis BA, Williams B: Blood-gas tension measurement in anaesthesia by bubble equilibration and mass spectrometry. *Br J Anaesth* 52:1061–1070, 1980.

158. Ozanne GM, Young WG, Mazze WJ, Severinghouse JW: Multipatient anesthetic mass spectrometry: rapid analysis of data stored in long catheters. *Anesthesiology* 55:62–70 1981.

159. Severinghouse JW, Ozanne G: Multioperating room monitoring with one mass spectrometer. *Acta Anaesthesiol Scand (Suppl)* 70:186–187, 1978.

160. Losee JM, Sherrill D, Virtue RW, Lechner AJ: Quantitative detection of venous air embolism in the dog by mass spectrometry measurement of end tidal nitrogen. *Anesthesiology* 57:A146, 1982.

161. Air embolism detected by mass spectrometry. *Anesthesiology News 8,* 9:1–11, 1982.

162. Chase HF, Trotta R, Kilmore MA: Simple methods for humidifying nonrebreathing anesthesia gas systems. *Anesth Analg* 41:249–256, 1962.

163. Gedeon A, Mebius C: The hygroscopic condenser humidifier. A new device for general use in anaesthesia and intensive care. *Anaesthesia* 34:1043–1047, 1979.

164. Steward DJ: A disposable condenser humidifier for use during anaesthesia. *Can Anaesth Soc J* 23:191–195, 1976.

165. Mapleson WW, Morgan JG, Hillard EK: Assessment of condenser-humidifiers with special reference to multiple-gauze model. *Br Med J* 1:300–305, 1963.

166. Shanks CA: Clinical anesthesia and multiple-gauze condenser humidifier. *Br J Anaesth* 46:773–777, 1974.

167. Weeks DB: Evaluation of a disposable humidifier for use during anesthesia. *Anesthesiology* 54:337–340, 1981.

168. Weeks DB: Humidification of anesthetic gases with an inexpensive condenser-humidifier in the semiclosed circle. *Anesthesiology* 41:601–604, 1974.

169. Weeks DB, Chalon J: Humidification of gas mixtures delivered by miniature ventilators. *Anaesthesia* 29:191–193, 1974.

170. Walker AKY, Bethune DW: A comparative study of condenser-humidifiers. *Anaesthesia* 31:1086–1093, 1976.

171. Toremalm NG: A heat and moisture exchanger for post-tracheotomy care. *Acta Otolaryngol* 52:461–472, 1960.

172. Shanks CA, Sara CA: A reappraisal of the multiple gauze heat and moisture exchanger. *Anaesth Intensive Care* 1:428–432, 1973.

173. Revenas B, Lindholm CE: The foam nose—a new disposable heat and moisture exchanger. A comparison with other similar devices. *Acta Anaesth Scand* 23:34–39, 1979.

174. Weeks DB, Ramsey FM: Laboratory investigation of six artificial noses for use during endotracheal anesthesia. *Anesth Analg* 62:758–763, 1983.

175. Heat and moisture exchangers. *Health Devices* 12:155–167, 1983.

176. Hay R, Miller WC: Efficacy of a new hygroscopic condenser humidifier. *Crit Care Med* 10:49–51, 1982.

177. Pennington JH, Lumley J, O'Grady F: The growth of pseudomonas pyocyanea in Garthur condenser humidifiers. *Anaesthesia* 21:211–215, 1966.

178. Reynolds FB: Humidification and humidifiers. Problems in the performance of anesthetic and respiratory equipment. *Int Anesthesiol Clin* 12/3:79–91, 1974.

179. *Humidifiers and Nebulizers.* Z-79.9-1979, American National Standards Institute, 1430 Broadway, New York, N.Y. 10018.

180. Heated humidifiers. *Health Devices* 9:167–180, 1980.

181. Chalon J, Ramanathan S: Water vaporizer heated by the reaction of neutralization by carbon dioxide. *Anesthesiology* 41:400–404, 1974.

182. Chalon J, Goldman C, Amirdivani M, Rothblatt A, Ramanathan S, Turndorf H: Humidification in a modified circle system. *Anesth Analg* 58:216–220, 1979.

183. Chalon J, Simon R, Patel C, Ramanathan S, Sessler S, Turndorf H: An infant circuit with a water vaporizer warmed by carbon dioxide neutralization. *Anesth Analg* 57:307–312, 1978.

184. Paspa P, Tang CK, Dwarkakanath R, Ramanathan S, Chalon J, Fischgrund GK, Turndorf H: A percolator vaporizer heated by reaction of neutralization of lime by carbon dioxide. *Anesth*

Analg 60:146–149, 1981.

185. Garg GP: Humidification of the Rees-Ayre T-piece system for neonates. *Anesth Analg* 52:207–209, 1973.

186. Spence M, Melville AW: A new humidifier. *Anesthesiology* 36:89–93, 1972.

187. Shanks CA, Gibbs JM: A comparison of two heated water-bath humidifiers. *Anaesth Intensive Care* 3:41–47, 1975.

188. Baker JD, Wallace CT, Brown CS: Maintenance of body temperature in infants during surgery. *Anesthesiol Rev* 4:21–25, 1977.

189. Berry FA, Hughes-Davies DI, Difazio CA: A system for minimizing respiratory heat loss in infants during operation. *Anesth Analg* 52:170–175, 1973.

190. Epstein RA: Humidification during positive pressure ventilation of infants. *Anesthesiology* 35:532–536, 1971.

191. Chalon J, Simon R, Ramanathan S, Patel C, Klein G, Rand P, Turndorf H: A high-humidity circle system for infants and children. *Anesthesiology* 49:205–207, 1978.

192. Ramanathan S, Chalon J, Turndorf H: A compact, well-humidified breathing circuit for the circle system. *Anesthesiology* 44:238–242, 1976.

193. Whitehurst P, St Andrew D: Temperature alarm and cut-out system for use with heated water humidifiers. *Br J Anaesth* 52:557–558, 1980.

194. Weeks DB: Evaluation of a disposable humidifier. *Anesthesiology* 40:511–515, 1974.

195. Schulze T, Edmondson EB, Pierce AK, Sanford JP: Studies of a new humidifying device as a potential source of bacterial aerosols. *Am Rev Resp Dis* 96:517–519, 1967.

196. Vesley D, Anderson J, Halbert MM, Wyman L: Bacterial output from three respiratory therapy humidifying devices. *Resp Care* 24:228–234, 1979.

197. Cote CJ, Ryan JF, Wood JB, Robinson MA, Vacanti FX, Welch JP: Wasted ventilation with eight anesthetic circuits used on children. *Anesthesiology* 55:A334, 1981.

198. Chalon J: Humidity control in anesthetic circuitry and ventilators. *ASA Refresher Courses in Anesthesiology* 2:27–38, 1974.

199. Fortin G, Blanc VF: Miniature ventilators with interrupted non-rebreathing circle systems and other anaesthetic circuits. *Can Anaesth Soc J* 17:613–623, 1970.

200. Edmondson EM, Reinzrz JA, Pierce AK, Sanford JP: Nebulization equipment. A potential source of infection in gram-negative pneumonias. *Am J Dis Child* 111:357–360, 1966.

201. Rhoades ER, Ringrose R, Mohr JA, Brooks L, McKown BA, Felton F: Contamination of ultrasonic nebulization equipment with gram negative bacteria. *Arch Intern Med* 127:228–232, 1971.

202. Spaepen MS, Bodman HA, Kundsin RB, Berryman JR, Fenel V: Microorganisms in heated nebulizers. *Health Lab Sci* 12:316–320, 1975.

203. Spaepen MS, Berryman JR, Bodman HA, Kundsin RB, Fenel V: Prevalence and survival of microbe contaminants in heated nebulizers. *Anesth Analg* 57:191–196, 1978.

204. Moyers J: A nomenclature for methods of inhalation anesthesia. *Anesthesiology* 14:609–611, 1953.

205. Baraka A: Functional classification of anaesthesia circuits. *Anaesth Intensive Care* 5:172–178, 1977.

206. Hamilton WK: Nomenclature of inhalation anesthetic systems. *Anesthesiology* 25:3–5, 1964.

CHAPTER 6

The Breathing System. II. The Mapleson Systems

There is a group of breathing systems characterized by the absence of directional valves to direct gases to or from the patient. Since there is no clear separation of inspired and expired gases the composition of the inspired mixture is highly dependent on the fresh gas flows used.

These systems were classified by Mapleson into five basic types: A through E. A sixth, the Mapleson F system, was later added to the classification (1).

This classification is shown diagrammatically in Figure 6.1. The components include a reservoir bag, corrugated tubing, port for the fresh gas inflow, relief valve, and patient connection (for mask or tracheal tube connector). A humidifier may be added to any of these systems by placing it in the fresh gas line. Some of the components are absent from certain systems. Arrangement of the components differs among the various systems and this greatly influences their performance. Within these six systems there are some commonly used variations and these will be discussed under the individual systems.

MAPLESON A SYSTEM (MAGILL SYSTEM, MAGILL ATTACHMENT)

Description of Equipment

CLASSIC FORM

The Magill system is shown diagrammatically in Figure 6.1A. It consists of the following parts: fresh gas inlet near the reservoir bag; a reservoir bag located between the fresh gas inlet and the corrugated tubing; corrugated tubing; relief valve of the high-pressure type located at the patient end of the corrugated tubing; and patient connection.

An oxygen analyzer should always be used, preferably placed between the relief valve and the corrugated tubing. In adults, it may be placed between the relief valve and the patient, but in children this could result in excessive dead space. It could also be placed at the neck of the bag, between the bag and the corrugated tubing, or in the fresh gas line, but in these locations the concentration of oxygen shown on the monitor may differ substantially from the inspired concentration, especially during controlled ventilation.

MODIFICATIONS

Several modifications have been described which allow the Magill system to be changed easily into another type of system (2–5). It has also been modified to make it more suitable for use with controlled ventilation (6, 7).

In the Lack modification (8, 9), the relief valve is at the bag end of the corrugated tubing. This makes it easier for the anesthesiologist to adjust the valve and facilitates scavenging of excess gases. An inner "expiratory" limb allows gas to pass from the patient to the relief valve.

Techniques of Use

For spontaneous ventilation the relief valve is opened fully. Excess gas is discharged through the relief valve during late exhalation.

For controlled or assisted ventilation, intermittent positive pressure is applied to the bag. The relief valve is tightened so that when the bag is squeezed sufficient pressure can be built up to inflate the lungs. Under these conditions, the relief valve opens during inspiration.

Functional Analysis

SPONTANEOUS RESPIRATION (10, 11)

The sequence of events during the respiratory cycle using the Magill system with spontaneous ventilation is shown in Figure 6.2. As the patient

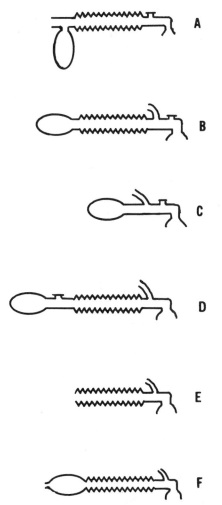

Figure 6.1. The Mapleson classification. Components include a reservoir bag, corrugated tubing, relief valve, fresh gas inlet, and patient connection. The patient connection is at the right and has an internal diameter of 15 mm and an outside diameter of 22 mm for attachment to a mask or endotracheal tube connector. (Redrawn from Mapleson WW: The elimination of rebreathing in various semiclosed anesthetic systems. *Br J Anaesth* 26:323–332, 1954.)

exhales (*C*), the exhaled gases, first the dead space gas and then alveolar gas, pass into the corrugated tubing toward the bag. At the same time, fresh gas flows into the bag. When the bag is full, the pressure in the system rises until the relief valve opens. The first gas discharged will be alveolar gas. The remainder of exhalation—containing only alveolar gas—exhausts through the open valve. In addition, the continuing inflow of fresh gas reverses the flow of exhaled gases in the corrugated tubing. Alveolar gas which had passed the relief valve now returns and exits.

If the fresh gas flow is high (*A*), it will force the dead space gas out also; if the fresh gas is intermediate (*D*), some of the dead space gas may be rebreathed. If the fresh gas flow is low (*E*), alveolar gas will be left in the corrugated tubing.

At the start of inspiration, the first gas inhaled will be from dead space between the patient and the relief valve. The next gas will be either alveolar gas (if the fresh gas flow is very low), exhaled dead space gas (if the fresh gas flow is adequate) or fresh gas (if the fresh gas flow is high). By adjustment of the fresh gas flow, a situation can be obtained in which all or most of the patient's dead space gas is inhaled with each inspiration. Since this is dead space gas, it will have a composition similar to fresh gas.

Should the fresh gas flow be so low that alveolar gas is inhaled, the tidal volume or respiratory rate may increase, but this will not compensate because the increased volume of gas drawn in will contain a larger volume of alveolar gas. Unlike some of the other Mapleson systems, the respiratory waveform does not affect the required fresh gas flow (10).

Various investigators have determined both theoretically and experimentally the fresh gas flow needed to prevent rebreathing of alveolar gas. Mapleson predicted that rebreathing of gases which had been in contact with the alveoli would be prevented if the fresh gas flow was at least equal to the patient's minute ventilation (12). Laboratory work (13–15) and clinical measurements (2, 16, 17) have substantiated this.

Several investigators have shown that rebreathing does not occur until the fresh gas flow is approximately equal to alveolar ventilation (70–71% of minute volume) (11, 18–20). However, Conway (18) points out that when this critical level is approached, normal variations in tidal volume and alveolar ventilation may cause a transient disparity between ventilatory requirements and the fresh gas flow. Should carbon dioxide accumulation occur, the patient will respond by increasing minute volume. This may set up a vicious circle, since increased ventilation will require an increased fresh gas flow to prevent rebreathing. A progressive state could develop in which increasing ventilation increases the disparity between the fresh gas flow and the alveolar ventilation. For this reason, it

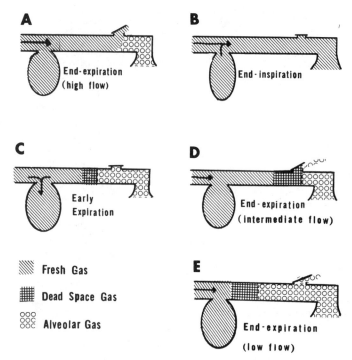

Figure 6.2. Magill system with spontaneous ventilation. See text for details. (Redrawn from Kain ML, Nunn JF: Fresh gas economies of the Magill circuit. *Anesthesiology* 29:964–974, 1968.)

is suggested that the fresh gas flow be at least equal to minute volume.

Experimentally in adults, investigators have found no appreciable concentration of carbon dioxide occurred if the fresh gas flow was at least 7 to 8 liters/min (13, 15, 16, 17, 21). Ungerer (22) found no rebreathing until the fresh gas flow was reduced below 80 ml/kg/min.

For the system to function correctly, the corrugated tubing must be large enough to contain exhaled alveolar gas. With earlier versions of the Lack modification, the capacity of the inspiratory (outer) limb was too small so that alveolar gas reached the bag with relatively high fresh gas flows (23). High resistance in the expiratory limb contributed to this. When this occurred, the system acted as a mixing device and a much higher fresh gas flow was needed to prevent rebreathing. In later versions of the Lack modification the inspiratory (outer) limb is enlarged and the resistance of the expiratory limb is less (24).

The relatively low fresh gas flows needed to operate the Magill system with spontaneous respiration will result in a relatively high humidity in the inspired gases.

CONTROLLED OR ASSISTED VENTILATION

During controlled or assisted ventilation (Fig. 6.3), the pattern of flow of gases in the circuit changes. During exhalation (Fig. 6.3A), the pressure in the system will remain low and no gas will escape through the relief valve, if the bag does not become taut. All exhaled gases, both dead space and alveolar, will remain in the corrugated tubing, with the alveolar gas nearest the patient. If the tidal volume is large, some alveolar gas may spill into the bag.

At the start of inspiration, the exhaled gases flow into the patient. Since alveolar gases occupy the space nearest the patient, some will be forced into the lungs (Fig. 6.3B). As the pressure in the system rises, the relief valve opens so that gas both escapes from the relief valve and continues to enter the patient. When all the exhaled gas has been driven from the tube, fresh gas reaches the relief valve and the patient (Fig. 6.3C). Some enters the patient but some is lost through the valve. Thus during controlled ventilation some rebreathing of alveolar gases occurs and some fresh gas is wasted. Most inves-

A

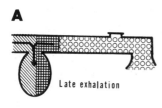

Late exhalation

B

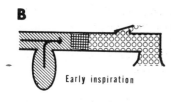

Early inspiration

C

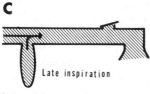

Late inspiration

Figure 6.3. Magill system with controlled ventilation. See text for details.

tigators feel that this is an illogical system to use for controlled respiration. Rebreathing of alveolar gas may be decreased by increasing the tidal volume or the fresh gas flow. It can also be decreased by using a low-pressure relief valve such as the Steen or Georgia valve (10). This prevents the loss of gas during inspiration and causes the relief valve to open during the latter part of expiration.

Various investigators have found differing fresh gas flows necessary when the Magill system is used with controlled ventilation, with values as low as 5 liters/min and as high as 20 liters/min recommended in adults (14, 21, 25, 26). This wide disparity can be explained by differences in tidal volumes and minute ventilation.

Hazards

If a pressure-limiting reservoir bag is used with the Magill system, gases may preferentially flow back toward the reservoir bag and a dangerous amount of rebreathing can occur (27).

A mechanical ventilator which relieves excess gases cannot be used with this system, since the entire breathing system would then become dead space.

Earlier models of the Lack system had high resistance in the inner expiratory limb and too small an inspiratory limb (23). These problems have been corrected with later models (24).

A case has been reported in which a Lack circuit was incorrectly manufactured so that the inner expiratory tube which should have been connected to the relief valve was connected to the reservoir bag (28). This arrangement converted the entire tubing to dead space.

MAPLESON B SYSTEM

Description of Equipment

The Mapleson B system is shown in Figure 6.1B. It is composed of the following parts: fresh gas inlet located near the patient end of the system; a relief valve also located near the patient connection; corrugated tubing between the bag and the fresh gas flow; and a bag located at the end of the corrugated tubing.

The oxygen analyzer is best placed between the corrugated tubing and the fresh gas inlet. It may also be placed in the fresh gas line, or, for adults, between the fresh gas inlet and the relief valve.

Techniques of Use

SPONTANEOUS RESPIRATION

To use the Mapleson B system with spontaneous respirations, the relief valve is opened completely. Excess gas is discharged through the valve during exhalation.

ASSISTED OR CONTROLLED RESPIRATION

This is accomplished by tightening the relief valve sufficiently to allow the lungs to be inflated. Excess gas overflows during inspiration.

Functional Analysis

SPONTANEOUS RESPIRATION

As the patient exhales, the bag fills to its full capacity. The bag then contains gas from the anatomical and equipment dead space as well as some fresh gas and alveolar gas. The corrugated tubing will contain alveolar gas and some fresh gas, which is pushed back into the tubing. After the bag has reached its full capacity, the relief valve opens. Because of the closed limb and the proximity of the relief valve to the fresh gas inlet, the gas lost from the system is mainly fresh gas (12). As the patient begins to inspire, the relief valve closes and he will draw in fresh gas and gas from the corrugated tubing. No gas should be drawn from the bag as long as the volume in the corrugated tubing exceeds the tidal volume.

The amount of rebreathing will depend on the fresh gas flow. The lower the flow, the greater the part of the tidal volume that will come from the corrugated tube. With low fresh gas flows, there will be less mixing of exhaled gas with fresh gas and the amount of gas rebreathed will be higher. To completely avoid rebreathing, the fresh gas flow must be equal to peak inspiratory flow rate (normally 20–25 liters/min) (29, 30). A fresh gas flow more than double minute volume will, in most clinical circumstances, reduce rebreathing to acceptable levels (12, 30).

CONTROLLED OR ASSISTED VENTILATION

The behavior of the Mapleson B system during controlled or assisted ventilation is similar to that during spontaneous ventilation. Rebreathing is slightly less because fresh gas accumulates at the patient end of the tubing during the expiratory pause (30). During inspiration, fresh gas is pushed into the lungs while mixed expired gas is vented through the relief valve (30). A fresh gas flow of 2 to 2.5 times minute volume is recommended to prevent excessive rebreathing (30, 31).

MAPLESON C SYSTEM

Description of Equipment

The Mapleson C system, shown in Figure 6.1C, is identical to the Mapleson B system except that the corrugated tubing is omitted. The bag attaches directly to the fresh gas inflow tube.

Techniques of Use

The Mapleson C system allows respirations to be spontaneous, assisted, or controlled. Use of this system is similar to that described for the Mapleson B system.

Functional Analysis

The Mapleson C system behaves similarly to the Mapleson B system. However, the re-

breathed gas contains more alveolar gas than the B system. "Acceptable" levels of rebreathing during spontaneous ventilation are achieved when the fresh gas flow is twice the minute volume. During controlled ventilation fresh gas flow must be 2 to 2.5 times minute volume (12, 21, 29, 30, 32).

MAPLESON D SYSTEM

While used primarily for anesthesia, this system has also been employed in long-term ventilation of infants and children (33, 34). It is also used to ventilate patients during transport and resuscitation.

Description

CLASSIC FORM

The Mapleson D system is shown diagrammatically in Figure 6.1D and in Figure 6.4. It consists of the following parts: a fresh gas inlet at the patient end; a length of corrugated tubing connecting the fresh gas inlet to the relief valve; a relief valve of the high-pressure type; and a reservoir bag adjacent to the relief valve. The length of the tubing has no functional importance as long as the volume of the tube and reservoir bag exceed the patient's tidal volume (35), but does determine the distance the user can be from the patient.

The oxygen analyzer may be placed between the bag and the mounting, or in the fresh gas line or between the corrugated tubing and the fresh gas inlet. In adults, it may be placed between the fresh gas inlet and the patient connection.

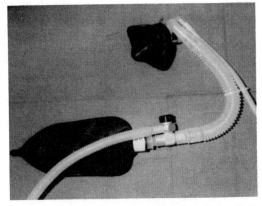

Figure 6.4. Mapleson D system. A tube leading to the scavenging interface is attached to the relief valve.

Devices for administration of continuous positive airway pressure applicable to the Mapleson D system are available (36–38).

BAIN MODIFICATION

In the Bain coaxial modification (39) the fresh gas tubing is incorporated inside the exhalation limb. This decreases the bulk of the system and the additional drag of a second tube.

The Bain coaxial modification is available with a metal head with channels drilled into it (Fig. 6.5). This provides a fixed position for the reservoir bag and makes it accessible for ventilating the patient. It includes mounting brackets for attachment to the anesthesia machine or an IV pole, a relief valve, and attachments for the bag and exhalation tubing. Some heads also have a pressure monitor. The fresh gas port may be part of the permanent attachment (40) or may be on the tubing. The tubing is available in a disposable form (40).

Techniques of Use

The Mapleson D system offers the anesthesiologist the ability to manually assist or control respirations, control ventilation using a ventilator (34, 39, 41, 42) or it may be used with spontaneous ventilation.

Manually controlled ventilation is instituted by partially closing the relief valve and squeezing the bag. Artificial controlled ventilation is achieved by connecting the hose of a mechanical ventilator in place of the reservoir bag and closing the relief valve. Any ventilator can be used provided that the anesthetic gases are not needed to power the ventilator itself. For spontaneous respirations, the relief valve is left completely open.

Functional Analysis (12, 21, 43)

SPONTANEOUS BREATHING

It has been shown that the Mapleson D system is identical to the Mapleson F in terms of function during spontaneous respiration. Thus studies on rebreathing with the Mapleson F system may be applied to the Mapleson D system as well.

During exhalation exhaled gases mix with fresh gases and move through the corrugated tube away from the patient and toward the bag.

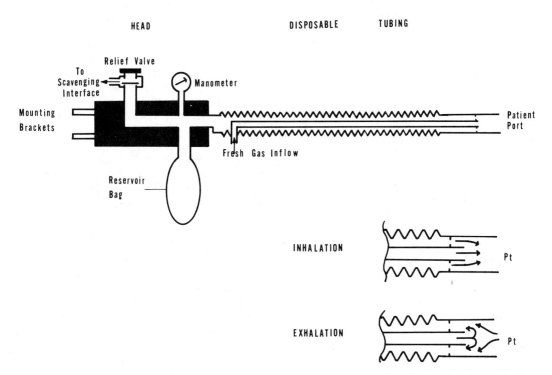

Figure 6.5. Bain modification of the Mapleson D system. The fresh gas inflow line is inside the corrugated tubing.

After the bag has filled, the mixture exits via the relief valve. During the expiratory pause, fresh gases pass along the corrugated tubing, moving the other gases down the tube.

During inspiration the patient will inhale gas from the fresh gas inlet and the large corrugated tube. The gas drawn from the corrugated tube may be entirely fresh gas or a mixture of fresh and exhaled gas. If rebreathing of carbon dioxide-contaminated gas occurs, it will be during the latter part of inspiration. Three factors will determine the amount of rebreathing that occurs: the tidal volume, the respiratory waveform and the fresh gas flow.

Respiratory Waveform (44)

The respiratory waveform may affect rebreathing. Factors that tend to decrease rebreathing include a high inspiratory/expiratory time ratio, a slow rise in inspiratory flow rate, a low flow rate during the last part of expiration, and a long expiratory pause (30). All these factors provide time for the fresh gas flow to flush the expiratory limb and minimize the quantity of alveolar gas which is re-inhaled. Byrick and co-workers (45) and Spoerel (46) showed that a higher fresh gas flow was required to prevent rebreathing in patients breathing halothane than in patients breathing enflurane. This was attributed to the different respiratory waveforms with the different agents.

The Fresh Gas Flow

When the Mapleson D circuit is used with spontaneous respiration, a crucial decision about fresh gas flow requirements must be made. If the fresh gas flow is high, it will flush the corrugated tube, pushing the alveolar gas into the bag or through the relief valve. Then it will be the minute ventilation of the patient that determines the $PaCO_2$. If the fresh gas flow is not high enough, there will be rebreathing of expired CO_2.

There have been a large number of studies on the fresh gas flow needed to prevent rebreathing, or to maintain normal arterial carbon dioxide, and there is no general agreement. Byrick and co-workers (47) found that the fresh gas flow required to eliminate rebreathing varied widely from patient to patient. Recommendations have been made in terms of minute volume, patient weight, and patient surface area.

Minute Volume. Most studies have recom-mended that the fresh gas flow be two to three times the predicted minute volume to prevent significant rebreathing (1, 2, 10, 12, 15, 16, 29–31, 44, 48–56). A few have recommended lower values (57, 58).

Body Weight. A flow of 100 ml/kg has been suggested for adults (46, 59, 60) and this is the recommended flow in package inserts, but others have suggested that this figure is too low (22, 47, 61, 62). Other recommendations include greater than 150 ml/kg (22), 200–300 ml/kg (62), 200 ml/kg (30), and 250 ml/kg (47). Byrick and colleagues (45) recommended 100 ml/kg/min for patients breathing halothane but 70 ml/kg/min for patients breathing enflurane.

Body Surface Area. In terms of body surface area, Rayburn recommended a fresh gas flow of 4000 ml/m²/min in larger children and adults to maintain normal arterial carbon dioxide (63).

Higher flows should be used (or ventilation controlled) in patients with an increase in carbon dioxide production (fever, hyperalimentation, small children), those with an increased dead space (use of mask, lung disease, advancing age), and patients with decreased minute ventilation (51, 63).

Several authors have suggested using another system for spontaneous ventilation (61, 64, 65).

CONTROLLED VENTILATION

During expiration, exhaled gases flow from the patient down the corrugated tubing. At the same time, a steady flow of fresh gas flows into the tubing. During the expiratory pause the fresh gas flow continues and flushes the exhaled gases down the tubing.

During inspiration, when the bag is squeezed, fresh gas and gas from the corrugated tubing go into the patient. Thus practically all the fresh gas is pushed into the patient.

CONTROLLED OR ASSISTED VENTILATION

If the fresh gas flow is low, some expired gases mixed with fresh gases may be forced back through the corrugated tubing. Thus the patient may receive some mixed expired gases along with fresh gases from the fresh gas port.

A great deal has been written about the correct fresh gas flow needed for controlled ventilation with the Mapleson D system, and there are many different opinions.

Theoretical analyses have been performed and formulas devised relating fresh gas flow to carbon dioxide tension or to the prevention of rebreathing. Recommendations have been based on body weight (29, 35, 42, 44, 51, 57, 66–75), minute volume (1, 12, 15, 29, 44, 48, 49, 51, 52, 54), and body surface area (76).

It has been pointed out (66) that in most of the reported work, emphasis has been placed upon the prevention of rebreathing rather than carbon dioxide retention by the patient. With controlled ventilation, this goal may be achieved despite the occurrence of considerable rebreathing. Later recommendations are lower than some of the original recommendations, probably due to the realization that with partial rebreathing end-tidal carbon dioxide may exceed normal limits while the patient remains normocarbic (63). Other studies have used end-tidal rather than mixed expired carbon dioxide and this has caused excessive fresh gas flows to be recommended (63).

In analyzing the performance of these systems when ventilation is controlled, two relationships become evident (51). (a) When the fresh gas flow is very high, the $PaCO_2$ becomes ventilation-limited (51, 67). The higher the minute volume, the lower the $PaCO_2$. (b) When the minute volume exceeds the fresh gas flow substantially, the fresh gas flow is the controlling factor for carbon dioxide elimination (provided at least predicted alveolar ventilation is met). The higher the fresh gas flow, the lower the $PaCO_2$. How high a minute volume is necessary is still a matter of debate, with suggestions ranging from 1.5 to 3 times fresh gas flow (51, 75–77).

Combining these influences, a graph can be constructed, as shown in Figure 6.6. An infinite number of combinations of fresh gas flow and minute volume can be chosen to produce a given $PaCO_2$. One can use high fresh gas flows and low minute volumes or high minute volumes and low fresh gas flows or combinations in between.

Shown in Figure 6.6, *left*, with a high fresh gas flow, the circuit is a non-rebreathing one. The high flows are uneconomical and associated with low humidity, heat loss, and increased operating room pollution. Also the predictability of the $PaCO_2$ level becomes dependent on the accuracy of the minute volume. Accurate adjustment can be difficult, especially for small children (51).

On the *right* is the region of deliberately controlled rebreathing. Carbon dioxide levels can then be regulated by adjusting the fresh gas flow (62). Lower flows (and increased rebreathing)

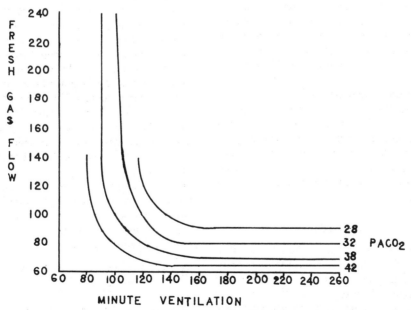

Figure 6.6. Mapleson D system used with controlled ventilation. Each isopleth represents a constant level of $PaCO_2$. Note that essentially the same $PaCO_2$ is achieved for fresh gas flows from 100 to 240 ml/kg/min. (Redrawn from Froese AB: Anesthesia circuits for children. ASA Refresher Courses, 1978.)

are associated with higher humidity, less heat loss and greater economy of fresh gases. Large tidal volumes can be used without inducing hypocarbia.

Individual differences in dead space/tidal volume are minimized at high levels of minute volume (51, 63). For these reasons it would appear, in most cases, advantageous to aim for the right side of the graph. Exceptions might be made for patients with stiff lungs, poor cardiac performance and/or hypovolemia.

HUMIDITY OF THE BAIN SYSTEM

The design of the Bain circuit is conducive to humidification of inspired gases. With other circuits, fresh gas, once warmed and humidified, must traverse the distance from the humidifier to the airway through noninsulated tubing. This results in a progressive decrease in temperature and humidity with rainout in the inspiratory limb. In the Bain circuit, the inspiratory line is insulated by the warm exhaled gas in the outer expiratory tubing. Consequently the temperature and humidity drop in the inspired gas is minimized.

Ramanathan and colleagues (43) found that the Bain system initially delivered 14 mg H_2O/liter, and this rose to 21 mg H_2O/liter after 70 min of use at a flow rate of 5 liters/min. Using high minute volumes, Rayburn achieved an initial humidity of 21 mg H_2O/liter, which increased over the first 30 min and then remained stable between 24 and 25 mg H_2O/liter (78). However, Chalon and co-workers (79) were unable to obtain a moisture output above 21 mg H_2O/liter under the same conditions.

Holtzman used the Bain system for long-term mechanical ventilation of children (33). They found there was less cooling of the inspired gases over the length of the inspiratory tubing than when conventional ventilator circuits were used. Thus a lower humidifier temperature could be used.

Hazards

Any situation which causes the fresh gas flow to be lowered presents a hazard, since dangerous rebreathing may occur. This has been reported with emptying of a nitrous oxide tank (80), loss of gas through a loose vaporizer filler cap (81) and a leak in a humidification device (82).

Special hazards are associated with the Bain system. The system should not be used with an intermittent-flow machine (83) unless the machine is set to give continuous flow (84).

If the inner tube of the Bain system becomes detached from its connections at the machine end (85, 86), or the fresh gas tube becomes kinked or twisted (87–89), the entire exhalation limb becomes dead space (85, 86). The outer tube should always be transparent to allow inspection of the connections. It has been suggested that the inner tube be fixed at the patient end to avoid twisting (88). If a Bain circuit is washed it should not be stretched as this may cause the inner tube to detach from its connection at the machine end. Some new coaxial circuits have been developed that eliminate many of these problems.

In another case the Bain system was incorrectly assembled so that the fresh gas line was mistakenly connected to the nipple for the pressure manometer while the manometer was connected to the inflow orifice (90). The entire volume of the outer tube became dead space.

The connection of the inner tube can be confirmed by turning on a flowmeter and occluding the inner tube with a finger while observing the flowmeter indicator. If the inner tube is intact and correctly connected, the indicator will fall (91).

The integrity of the inner tube can be confirmed by using a test described by Pethick (92) in which the bag is filled while holding a hand over the patient port. After removing the hand from the patient end, the oxygen flush is activated. A Venturi effect created by the oxygen flow at the end of the tube will cause a negative pressure in the exhalation tubing, and this will cause the bag to deflate. If the inner tube is not intact, this maneuver will cause the bag to inflate slightly. However, this test would not expose a faulty Bain system in which the inner tube were omitted (93), or did not extend to the patient port.

In departments that use both a Bain circuit and other circuits such as the Mapleson A, a conventional wide-bore tubing may be attached to the system instead of the Bain (94). This will result in total rebreathing.

MAPLESON E (THE T-PIECE SYSTEM)

The T-piece, first described by Ayre in 1937 (95), was developed in response to the need for apparatus with low resistance and minimal dead space for pediatric anesthesia.

Description of Equipment

The T-piece itself is a simple piece of metal with three limbs and a port at the end of each limb. One port is for the fresh gas and is attached to the delivery hose from the anesthesia machine. The second port attaches to the endotracheal tube or mask connector. The third limb is the expiratory limb. A length of tubing may be attached to form a reservoir for the gases. If too small a diameter tube is used for the expiratory limb, a significant rise in airway pressure may occur during expiration. For children the exhalation connection should be at least 1 cm in diameter (96, 97). A 1-cm diameter tube attached to this end would therefore contain 2 cc of volume per inch of tubing (103). For adults a slightly larger tubing connection, about 1.25 cm is recommended. Tubing attached to this connection would contain 3 cc of volume per inch.

The oxygen analyzer may be placed in the fresh gas line or between the expiratory port of the T-piece and the expiratory tubing. In larger patients it may be placed between the T-piece and the patient, but this should be avoided in small patients because it adds to the dead space.

Scavenging may be performed by enclosing the expiratory port in a plastic chamber from which excess gases are suctioned.

Modifications

Innumerable modifications of the original T-piece have been made (96, 98). Several modifications have the fresh gas inlet extending inside the body of the T-piece toward the patient connection to minimize dead space.

A pressure-limiting device may be added to the system (99–102).

In the Bain modification of the T-piece, the fresh gas tube is incorporated into the expiratory limb.

Harrison (48) reviewed the modifications of the expiratory limb and classified them into three categories. Type I had no expiratory limb, type II had an expiratory limb volume greater than the patient's tidal volume. In type III, the expiratory limb volume was less than the tidal volume. He concluded the most useful was type II.

Techniques of Use

The T-piece system may be used with either spontaneous or controlled ventilation. Manually controlled ventilation is possible by intermittently occluding the exhalation limb with the finger and letting the fresh gas flow inflate the lungs. This makes it difficult to gauge the depth of respiration. Addition of a bag or mechanical ventilator to the expiratory limb converts it into a Mapleson F system which will be discussed in the next section. Without a reservoir bag to transmit respiratory information and to squeeze at the optimal time, satisfactory assisted respiration is hard to achieve.

Functional Analysis

The sequence of events during the respiratory cycle is shown in Figure 6.7. When the patient exhales, exhaled gases pass down the expiratory limb and mix with fresh gases entering via the fresh gas inlet. During the expiratory pause, the fresh gas flow continues to sweep the exhaled gases away from the T-piece and down the expiratory limb.

During inspiration, the gases initially inhaled come from the fresh gas reserve plus the fresh gas which inflows constantly. The latter part of inspiration may contain some diluted alveolar gas.

The fresh gas flow requirements are extremely complex. The presence or absence and the amount of rebreathing or air dilution in a clinical situation will depend on the fresh gas flow, the patient's minute volume, the volume of the exhalation limb, the type of ventilation (spontaneous or controlled) and the respiratory pattern (44).

REBREATHING

Rebreathing occurs when the patient inspires gases from the expiratory limb which were previously exhaled. If there is no exhalation limb, no rebreathing can occur. If there is an expiratory limb, the fresh gas flow needed to prevent rebreathing will be the same as for the Mapleson D system (see previous section).

During controlled ventilation there can be no rebreathing since if the finger occludes the exhalation limb, only fresh gas will be used to inflate the lungs.

AIR DILUTION

Air dilution occurs when the patient inspires, from the expiratory limb, air drawn in from the atmosphere. If the exhalation tubing has a volume greater than the tidal volume, air dilution cannot occur.

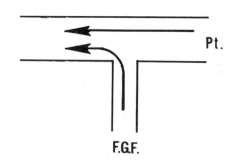

Figure 6.7. Functional analysis of the T-piece system. See text for details.

If there is no expiratory limb, or if the volume of the expiratory limb is less than the patient's tidal volume, air dilution can occur. It can be prevented by providing a fresh gas flow which exceeds the peak inspiratory flow rate, normally 3 to 5 times the minute volume during spontaneous breathing (48, 97, 103). No air dilution can occur during controlled ventilation since the finger occludes the exhalation port.

Hazards of the T-Piece System

EXCESSIVE PRESSURE

When respiration is controlled by intermittently occluding the expiratory limb with the finger, there is a steady, rapid rise in pressure. Prolonged occlusion may lead to overinflation and barotrauma. Overinflation is a great danger with this system because the anesthesiologist does not have the "feel" of inflation which he has with a bag system. Also the pressure-buffering effect of the bag is absent.

The T-piece system is positioned close to the patient. When surgery around the head is performed, the system may be obscured from view by drapes and the expiratory limb may become occluded by pressure from drapes or instruments (100). The outlet tube should be visible whenever possible, and care should be exercised to prevent its occlusion.

To overcome this potential hazard, it has been recommended that a pressure-limiting device be placed in the system (99–102).

OTHER

A case has been reported where the right angle connection between the straight endotracheal tube connector and the T-piece caused obstruction to inflow (104).

MAPLESON F SYSTEM JACKSON-REES SYSTEM, REES SYSTEM

This is the most commonly used form of the T-piece system.

Description of Equipment

The Jackson-Rees modification of the T-piece system (105) consists of the addition of a bag with an opening in it to the exhalation limb of the T-piece (Figs. 6.1*F* and 6.8). The hole in the bag most commonly is in the tail. It may be fitted with a device to prevent the bag from collapsing but at the same time allowing excess gases to escape. Alternately, the hole may be in the side of the bag so the user can place his finger over it.

Scavenging can be performed by enclosing the bag in a plastic chamber from which waste gases are suctioned (51) or by attaching various devices to the relief mechanism in the bag.

Techniques of Use

The system can be used with spontaneous, controlled, or assisted respirations. For spontaneous respiration the valve or relief mechanism is left fully open. For assisted or controlled respirations the relief mechanism is sufficiently occluded to allow the bag to remain distended. Respirations can then be managed by squeezing the bag. Alternately, the hole in the bag can be occluded by the user's finger during inspiration.

If it is desired to use a mechanical ventilator, the bag is replaced by the hose from the ventilator.

FUNCTIONAL ANALYSIS

The system functions very much like a Mapleson E system. The addition of a bag to the expiratory limb will not affect the function of the system provided the bag is separated from the patient by a tube with an internal volume which exceeds the patient's tidal volume. If the tube volume is too small, re-inhalation of mixed expired gas from the bag may occur. The system

then approximates to a Mapleson C circuit (30, 95).

SPONTANEOUS RESPIRATION

The flows required to prevent rebreathing during spontaneous respiration are the same as those required with the Mapleson D system (see previous section).

CONTROLLED RESPIRATION

During controlled ventilation, the system functions like a Mapleson D system and the flow requirements are similar. However, two authors have found higher carbon dioxide levels with hand (as compared with mechanical) controlled ventilation (69, 73). They suggested this may be due to the difficulty in maintaining an adequate bag volume for ventilation in small children. They suggest increasing the fresh gas flowrate or converting to a Mapleson D system when ventilation is controlled manually.

Positive end-expiratory pressure does not affect end-tidal carbon dioxide during controlled respiration, but causes an increase during spontaneous breathing when fresh gas flows are less than 3 times minute volume (106).

Hazards

These are the same as those described for the Mapleson E system. However, excessive pressure is less likely to develop, since there is a bag in the system.

EVALUATION OF SYSTEMS
Advantages

1. The simplicity of design makes these systems easy to assemble and use.

2. All parts of the system can be disassembled and disinfected or sterilized in a variety of ways.

3. These systems are quite light and are not likely to cause excessive drag on the mask or endotracheal tube, facial distortion, or accidental extubation.

4. With the exception of the relief valve, there are no moving parts so the equipment is not prone to malfunction.

5. The equipment is inexpensive.

6. Resistance to respiration is low.

7. These systems can be conveniently positioned.

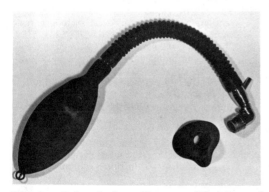

Figure 6.8. Jackson-Rees modification of Ayre's T-piece. Hole is in center of bag. See text for details.

Disadvantages

1. These systems require relatively high gas flows. This results in poor economy and loss of heat and humidity (except with partial rebreathing and the Bain and Magill systems). Assessment of ventilation may be hampered by the high inflow rates required. When comparing the systems during spontaneous ventilation, the relative order of merit is A, D, F, E (with an expiratory limb), C, and B. During controlled ventilation the order becomes D, F, E (with an expiratory limb), B, C, and A.

2. The correct gas flow may be difficult to determine. With some systems it is necessary to change the gas flow when going from spontaneous to controlled.

3. With all of these systems should the fresh gas flow be too low for any reason, dangerous rebreathing may occur.

4. A disadvantage of the Mapleson A, B, and C systems is that they have a relatively heavy relief valve located close to the patient's face, where it may be inaccessible to the anesthesiologist. Also scavenging becomes rather awkward. These disadvantages can be overcome by using the Lack modification of the Mapleson A.

5. The Mapleson E and F systems are difficult to scavenge and air dilution is a problem with the Mapleson E system.

References

1. Willis BA, Pender JWM, Mapleson WW: Rebreathing in a T-piece: Volunteer and theoretical studies of the Jackson-Rees modification of Ayre's T-piece during spontaneous respiration. *Br J Anaesth* 47:1239–1246, 1975.
2. Baraka A, Brandstater B, Muallem M, Seraphim C: Rebreathing in a double T-piece system. *Br J Anaesth* 41:47–53, 1969.
3. Esplen JR: Three-in-one anaesthetic assembly. *Br J Anaesth* 24:312–314, 1952.
4. Manicom AW, Schoonbee CG: The Johannesburg A-D circuit switch, a valve device for converting a co-axial Mapleson D into a co-axial Mapleson A system. *Br J Anaesth* 51:1185–1187, 1979.
5. Waters DJ: A composite semiclosed anaesthetic system suitable for controlled or spontaneous respiration. *Br J Anaesth* 33:417–418, 1961.
6. Carden E, Nelson D: A new and highly efficient circuit for paediatric anaesthesia. *Can Anaesth Soc J* 19:572–582, 1972.
7. Carden E: Efficient positive pressure ventilation with a modified Magill circuit in adults. *Can Anaesth Soc J* 21:242–250, 1974.
8. Lack JA: Pollution control by co-axial circuits. *Anaesthesia* 31:561–562, 1976.
9. Lack JA: Theatre pollution control. *Anaesthesia* 31:259–262, 1976.
10. Eger EI: Anesthetic systems: construction and function. In *Anesthetic Uptake and Action.* Baltimore, Williams & Wilkins, 1975.
11. Kain ML, Nunn JF: Fresh gas economies of the Magill circuit. *Anesthesiology* 29:964–974, 1968.
12. Mapleson WW: The elimination of rebreathing in various semiclosed anaesthetic systems. *Br J Anaesth* 26:323–332, 1954.
13. Bracken A, Sanderson DM: Carbon dioxide concentrations found in various anaesthetic circuits. *Br J Anaesth* 27:428–435, 1955.
14. Sykes MK: Rebreathing during controlled respiration with the Magill attachment. *Br J Anaesth* 31:247–257, 1959.
15. Woolmer R, Lind B: Rebreathing with a semiclosed system. *Br J Anaesth* 26:316–322, 1954.
16. Davies RM, Verner IR: Carbon dioxide elimination from semiclosed systems. *Br J Anaesth* 28:196–200, 1956.
17. Lowe SG deC: Carbon dioxide in anaesthesia. *Proc R Soc Med* 49:220–223, 1956.
18. Conway CM, Davis FM, Knight HJ, Leigh JM, Preston TD, Tennant R: An experimental study of gaseous homeostasis and the Magill circuit using low fresh gas flows. *Br J Anaesth* 48:447–455, 1976.
19. Kain ML: Fresh gas flow and rebreathing in the Magill circuit with spontaneous respiration. *Proc R Soc Med* 60:749–750, 1962.
20. Norman J, Adams AP, Sykes MK: Rebreathing with the Magill attachment. *Anaesthesia* 23:75–81, 1968.
21. Waters DJ, Mapleson WW: Rebreathing during controlled respiration with various semiclosed anaesthetic systems. *Br J Anaesth* 33:374–381, 1961.
22. Ungerer MJ: A comparison between the Bain and Magill anaesthetic systems during spontaneous breathing. *Can Anaesth Soc J* 25:122–124, 1978.
23. Barnes PK, Seeley HF, Gothard JWW, Conway CM: The Lack anaesthetic system. *Anaesthesia* 31:1248–1253, 1976.
24. Norman JF, Nott M, Walters F: Performance of the Lack circuit. *Anaesthesia* 32:673, 1977.
25. Marshall M, Henderson GA: Positive pressure ventilation using a semiclosed system: a reassessment. *Br J Anaesth* 40:265–269, 1958.
26. Obiaya MO, Dakaraju P: Magill circuit and controlled ventilation. *Can Anaesth Soc J* 23:135–142, 1976.
27. Waters DJ: Use and misuse of a pressure-limiting bag. *Anaesthesia* 22:322–325, 1967.
28. Muir J, Davidson-Lamb R: Apparatus failure—cause for concern. *Br J Anaesth* 52:705–706, 1980.
29. Greene NM: Flow rates into anaesthetic circuits. Ninth Annual Anesthesiology Symposium, Naval Regional Medical Center, Portsmouth, Va; Aug. 31–Sept. 2, 1978.
30. Sykes MK: Rebreathing circuits. *Br J Anaesth* 40:666–674, 1968.
31. Christensen KN, Thomsen A, Hansen OL, Jorgensen S: Flow requirements in the Hafnia mod-

ification of the Mapleson circuits during spontaneous respiration. *Acta Anaesth Scand* 22:27–32, 1978.

32. Christensen KN: The flow requirement in a nonpolluting Mapleson C circuit. *Acta Anaesth Scand* 20:307–312, 1976.

33. Holzman BH, Trapana Y, Mora J, MacIntyre S: Modified Mapleson D system for long-term mechanical ventilation of infants and children. *Crit Care Med* 9:481–486, 1981.

34. Bain JA, Reid D: A simple way to ventilate babies utilizing a Mark VII Bird ventilator and a modified Mapleson D breathing circuit. *Can Anaesth Soc J* 22:202–207, 1975.

35. Bain JA, Spoerel WE: Low flow anesthesia utilizing a single limb circuit. In Aldrete JA, Lowe JH, Virtue RW (eds): *Low Flow and Closed System Anesthesia*. New York, Grune & Stratton, 1979, pp 151–164.

36. Bagger M: A simple and inexpensive device for administration of continuous positive airway pressure breathing. *Br J Anaesth* 52:627–628, 1980.

37. Erceg GW: PEEP for the Bain breathing circuit. *Anesthesiology* 50:542–543, 1979.

38. Hagerdal M, Lecky JH: Anesthetic death of an experimental animal related to a scavenging system malfunction. *Anesthesiology* 47:522–523, 1977.

39. Bain JA, Spoerel WE: A streamlined anaesthetic system. *Can Anaesth Soc J* 19:426–435, 1972.

40. Henville JD, Adams AP: A co-axial breathing circuit and scavenging valve. *Anaesthesia* 31:257–258, 1976.

41. Adams AP: The Bain circuit. Prevention of anaesthetic mixture dilution when using mechanical ventilators delivering nonanaesthetic gases. *Anaesthesia* 32:46–49, 1977.

42. Henville JD, Adams AP: The Bain anaesthetic system: an assessment during controlled ventilation. *Anaesthesia* 31:247–256, 1976.

43. Ramanathan S, Chalon J, Capan L, Patel C, Turndorf H: Rebreathing characteristics of the Bain anesthesia circuit. *Anesth Analg* 56:822–825, 1977.

44. Harrison GA: The effect of the respiratory flow pattern on rebreathing in a T-piece system. *Br J Anaesth* 36:206–211, 1964.

45. Byrick RJ, Janssen EG: Respiratory waveform and rebreathing in T-piece circuits: a comparison of enflurane and halothane waveforms. *Anesthesiology* 53:371–378, 1980.

46. Spoerel WE: Aitkieh RR, Bain JA: Spontaneous respiration with the Bain breathing circuit. *Can Anaesth Soc J* 25:30–35, 1978.

47. Byrick RJ: Respiratory compensation during spontaneous ventilation with the Bain circuit. *Can Anaesth Soc J* 27:96–105, 1980.

48. Harrison GA: Ayre's T-piece: a review of its modifications. *Br J Anaesth* 36:115–120, 1964.

49. Mapleson WW: Theoretical considerations of the effects of rebreathing in two semi-closed anaesthetic systems. *Br Med Bull* 14:64–68, 1958.

50. Willis BA, Pender JW, Mapleson WW: Estimation of rebreathing in the Jackson-Rees modification of Ayre's T-piece system. *Br J Anaesth* 47:638, 1975.

51. Froese AB: Anesthesia circuits for children. ASA Refresher Courses, 1978.

52. Onchi Y, Hayashi T, Ueyama H: Studies on the Ayre T-piece technique. *Far East J Anesth* 1:30–40, 1957.

53. Gibb DB, Prior G, Pollard B: Methods of conserving carbon dioxide in artificially ventilated patients. *Anaesth Intensive Care* 5:122–127, 1977.

54. Inkster JS: The T-piece technique in anaesthesia. An investigation into the inspired gas concentrations. *Br J Anaesth* 28:512–519, 1956.

55. Conway CM, Seeley HF, Barnes PK: Spontaneous ventilation with the Bain anaesthetic system. *Br J Anaesth* 49:1245–1249, 1977.

56. Seeley HF, Barnes PK, Conway CM: Fresh gas requirements during spontaneous ventilation with the Bain anaesthetic system. *Br J Anaesth* 50:78, 1978.

57. Soliman MG, Laberge R: The use of the Bain circuit in spontaneously breathing paediatric patients. *Can Anaesth Soc J* 25:276–281, 1978.

58. Meakin G, Coates AL: Effect of anaesthesia on rebreathing in the Bain circuit. *Anesthesiology* 53:S327, 1980.

59. Bain JA, Spoerel WE: Spontaneous breathing with the Bain circuit. *Can Anaesth Soc J* 25:336–337, 1978.

60. Bain JA, Spoerel WE: Bain circuit. *Can Anaesth Soc J* 26:65–66, 1979.

61. Goodwin K: Letters to the editor. *Can Anaesth Soc J* 23:675, 1976.

62. Rose DK, Byrick RJ, Froese AB: Carbon dioxide elimination during spontaneous ventilation with a modified Mapleson D system: studies in a lung model. *Can Anaesth Soc J* 25:353–365, 1978.

63. Rayburn RL: Pediatric anaesthesia circuits. ASA Refresher Courses, 1981.

64. Mansell WH: Spontaneous breathing with the Bain circuit at low flow rates: a case report. *Can Anaesth Soc J* 23:432–434, 1976.

65. Nott MR, Norman J: The Bain and Lack breathing systems. *Anaesthesia* 36:635–636, 1981.

66. Nightengale DA, Richards CC, Glass A: An evaluation of rebreathing in a modified T-piece system during controlled ventilation of anaesthetized children. *Br J Anaesth* 37:762–771, 1965.

67. Bain JA, Spoerel WE: Flow requirements for a modified Mapleson D system during controlled ventilation. *Can Anaesth Soc J* 20:629–636, 1973.

68. Bain JA, Spoerel WE: Carbon dioxide output and elimination in children under anaesthesia. *Can Anaesth Soc J* 24:533–539, 1977.

69. Akkineni S, Patel KP, Bennett EJ, Grundy EM, Ignacio AD: Fresh gas flow to limit $PaCO_2$ in T and circle systems without CO_2 absorption. *Anesthesiol Rev* 4:33–37, 1977.

70. Chu YK, Rah KH, Boyan CP: Is the Bain breathing circuit the future anaesthesia system? An evaluation. *Anesth Analg* 56:84–87, 1977.

71. Froese AB: The experts opine. *Surv Anesthesiol* 23:396–397, 1979.

72. Patel KP, Bennett EJ, Ignacio AD, Grundy EM: CO_2 control in infants and children with Mapleson D and F systems. Abstracts of Scientific

Papers, ASA Meeting, 1976, pp 11–12.

73. Kuwabara S, McCaughey TJ: Artificial ventilation in infants and young children using a new ventilator with the T-piece. *Can Anaesth Soc J* 13:576–584, 1966.

74. Goodloe SL, Wolfson B, Siker ES: The effect of minute volume on PCO_2 using the Bain circuit. *Anesthesiology* 51:S379, 1979.

75. Rose DK, Froese AB: The regulation of $PaCO_2$ during controlled ventilation of children with a T-piece. *Can Anaesth Soc J* 26:104–113, 1979.

76. Rayburn RL, Graves SA: A new concept in controlled ventilation of children with the Bain anesthetic circuit. *Anesthesiology* 48:250–253, 1978.

77. Keenan RL, Boyan CP: How rebreathing anaesthetic systems control $PaCO_2$ studies with a mechanical and a mathematical model. *Can Anaesth Soc J* 25:117–121, 1978.

78. Rayburn RL, Watson RL: Humidity in children and adults using the controlled partial rebreathing anaesthesia method. *Anesthesiology* 52:291–295, 1980.

79. Chalon J, Ali M, Turndorf H, Fischgrund GK: *Humidification of Anesthetic Gases.* Springfield, Ill., Charles C Thomas, 1981.

80. Dunn AJ: Empty tanks and Bain circuits. *Can Anaesth Soc J* 25:337, 1978.

81. Mullin RA: Letter to the editor. *Can Anaesth Soc J* 25:248–249, 1978.

82. Nimocks JA, Modell JH, Perry PA: Carbon dioxide retention using a humidified "nonrebreathing" system. *Anesth Analg* 54:271–273, 1975.

83. Sugg GR: Misuse of coaxial circuits. *Anaesthesia* 32:293–294, 1977.

84. Padfield A, Perks ER: Misuse of coaxial circuits. *Anaesthesia* 33:77–78, 1978.

85. Hannallah R, Rosales JK: A hazard connected with reuse of the Bain's circuit: a case report. *Can Anaesth Soc J* 21:511–513, 1974.

86. Breen M: Letters to the editor. *Can Anaesth Soc J* 22:247, 1975.

87. Inglis MS: Torsion of the inner tube. *Br J Anaesth* 52:705, 1980.

88. Nagvi NH: Torsion of inner tube. *Br J Anaesth* 53:193, 1981.

89. Mansell WH: Bain circuit: The hazard of the hidden tube. *Can Anaesth Soc J* 23:227, 1976.

90. Paterson JG, Vanhooydonk V: A hazard associated with improper connection of the Bain breathing circuit. *Can Anaesth Soc J* 22:373–377, 1975.

91. Foex P, Crampton-Smith A: A test for coaxial circuits. *Anaesthesia* 32:294, 1977.

92. Pethick SL: Correspondence. *Can Anaesth Soc J* 22:115, 1975.

93. Peterson WC: Bain circuit. *Can Anaesth Soc J* 25:532, 1978.

94. Boyd CH: Another hazard of coaxial circuits. *Anaesthesia* 32:675, 1977.

95. Ayre P: Anaesthesia for intracranial operation. *Lancet* 1:561–563, 1937.

96. Brooks W, Stuart P, Gabel PV: The T-piece technique in anaesthesia: an examination of its fundamental principle. *Anesth Analg* 37:191–196, 1958.

97. Lewis A, Spoerel WE: A modification of Ayre's technique. *Can Anaesth Soc J* 8:501–511, 1961.

98. Hallen B, Reiners N: A mask attachment for the T-piece technique. *Anaesthesia* 24:110–112, 1969.

99. Freifeld S: Modification of the Ayre T-piece system. *Anesth Analg* 42:575–577, 1963.

100. Taylor C, Stoelting VK: Modified Ayre's T-tube technic—anesthesia for cleft lip and palate surgery. *Anesth Analg* 42:55–62, 1963.

101. Keuskamp DHG: Automatic ventilation in paediatric anaesthesia using a modified Ayre's T-piece with negative pressure during expiratory phase. *Anaesthesia* 18:46–56, 1963.

102. Ramanathan S, Chalon J, Turndorf H: A safety valve for the pediatric Rees system. *Anesth Analg* 53:741–743, 1976.

103. Ayre P: The T-piece technique. *Br J Anaesth* 28:520–523, 1956.

104. Haley FC: Letters to the Editor. *Can Anaesth Soc J* 22:628–629, 1975.

105. Rees GJ: Anaesthesia in the newborn. *Br Med J* 2:1419–1422, 1950.

106. Dobbinson TL, Fawcett ER, Bolton DPG: The effects of positive and expiratory pressure on rebreathing and gas dilution in the Ayre's T-piece system—laboratory study. *Anaesth Intensive Care* 6:19–25, 1978.

CHAPTER 7

The Breathing System. III. Systems Employing Non-Rebreathing Valves

Systems employing non-rebreathing valves are used in the operating room primarily for pediatric anesthesia. The high fresh gas flows required have made them less popular for adults. Another important use for non-rebreathing valves is in portable resuscitation apparatus.

DESCRIPTION OF EQUIPMENT

The two commonly used systems employing non-rebreathing valves are shown in Figure 7.1. They consist of the following components: a non-rebreathing valve, fresh gas inlet, bag, tubing, relief valve and oxygen analyzer.

Non-Rebreathing Valve (Inflating Valve)

A non-rebreathing valve directs fresh gas to the patient and releases exhaled gas to atmosphere or a scavenging system.

VALVE TERMINOLOGY (1)

The Valve Body Assembly

The valve body assembly is a housing with associated internal parts, including one or more movable parts which opens, shuts, or partially obstructs one or more parts.

The Valve Body

The valve body constitutes the housing for the valve body assembly.

The Valve Seat

The valve seat or seating is the surface, usually but not always annular, with an opening which may be partially or completely obstructed by a movable part to direct or obstruct the flow.

Inlet of the Valve

The inlet is the part through which fresh gas enters the valve. It usually has a 22-mm male connection.

The Patient Port

The patient port is the part of the valve attached to the mask or endotracheal tube connector. It usually has a 15-mm female with a concentric 22-mm male connector.

The Exhalation Port

The exhalation port is the channel through which exhaled gases escape to atmosphere or scavenging system after having passed through the valve.

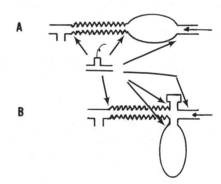

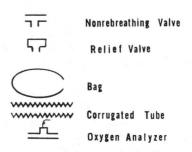

Figure 7.1. Systems employing non-rebreathing valves. See text for details.

Positional Valve

A positional valve is one which must remain horizontal as it requires gravity to close it completely.

Nonpositional Valve

A nonpositional valve is closed by elastic tension of rubber or by a spring and may be used in any position.

Flap Valve

A flap valve is one in which the movable part is made of a flexible material and is secured at its center or its edge.

Fishmouth Valve

A fishmouth valve is a special type of flap valve in which two flaps approximate at a midpoint. The flow of gas in one direction causes the flaps to open like a fishmouth. Reversal of the flow causes the flaps to meet and prevents the retrograde flow of gas.

Disc Valve

A disc valve is one in which the movable part consists of a flat disc made of plastic or metal. It is held onto its seat by gravity or a spring.

Mushroom Valve

A mushroom valve is a hollow balloon-like device which when inflated occludes an opening.

CLASSIFICATION OF VALVES

A number of classifications of non-rebreathing valves have been devised (1–3). Most are based on mechanical characteristics of the valve, such as the presence or absence of springs, rubber flaps, knife edge, etc. While structural differences are important, the writers feel it is essential that the practitioner have a knowledge of their function. The following classification, proposed by Sykes (4), is a functional one based on whether the valve was mainly intended for use with spontaneous or controlled ventilation or both.

From a functional standpoint, the main difference between spontaneous and controlled ventilation is the pressure inside the valve during inspiration. With spontaneous ventilation, the patient exerts a negative pressure which is transmitted to the inside of the valve. When respiration is controlled, a positive pressure exists inside the valve during inspiration.

Valves Designed for Spontaneous Respiration

These valves are designed to be used only with the spontaneously breathing patient. During inspiration, the negative pressure exerted by the patient closes the exhalation port. During exhalation the pressure in the valve increases and gas escapes through the exhalation port.

If this type of valve is used with controlled or assisted respirations, it is necessary to close the exhalation port with a finger during inspiration. This has the serious limitation of requiring use of both hands so that the anesthesiologist can do little else except manage ventilations (5).

Valves Designed for Controlled Respiration

In this type of valve, a pressure increase opens the inlet and closes the exhalation port. If the patient is allowed to breathe spontaneously, he will inspire room air through the exhalation port.

When it is desired to shift from controlled or assisted to spontaneous ventilation, additional equipment must be available to administer the desired gas mixture. Valves solely for controlled ventilation are usually intended for use with respirators or resuscitation apparatus and are not generally used for anesthesia (6).

Valves Designed for Both Spontaneous and Controlled Ventilation

In this type of valve, the exhalation port is closed and the inlet opens during inspiration with either controlled or spontaneous respirations. During expiration, the exhalation port is unblocked to permit free exhalation and the inspiratory port is blocked to prevent rebreathing. Valves designed for controlled ventilation and valves designed for both spontaneous and controlled ventilation are known as automatic non-rebreathing valves (7).

SPECIFIC VALVES

Ambu Valve

Classification. Controlled respiration.

Construction. A diagram of the Ambu valve is shown in Figure 7.2. The valve body may be of clear plastic or metal. It contains two seats, A and B. The movable part consists of a yellow

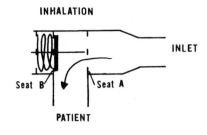

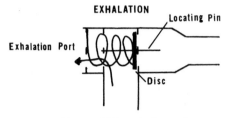

Figure 7.2. Ambu valve.

plastic disc which is held onto seat A by a spring. A locating pin centers the disc on the seat.

Function. When the bag is squeezed, the force of the gas pushes the disc against seat B, closing the exhalation port and allowing the patient's lungs to be inflated. During exhalation, the pressure on the inlet side of the disc falls and the spring pushes the disc onto seat A. Exhaled gases then pass from the patient out through the exhalation port.

If the patient is breathing spontaneously, the disc will not move and the patient will inhale room air.

The valve is most often used with the Ambu resuscitation bag.

Care and Cleaning. The valve can be disassembled for cleaning. When reassembling the valve, it is essential to insert the guide pin through the appropriate channels. The valve should be checked for competence after it has been reassembled.

The Ambu E, Ambu Hesse and Ambu E2 Valves

Classification. Spontaneous or controlled respiration.

Construction. The Ambu E valve is shown in Figure 7.3. It is made of transparent plastic, with the inlet connection colored blue. It contains two molded shutters, one for inhalation and one for exhalation. An outlet cover is available. The Ambu Hesse valve is similar to the Ambu E valve but is slightly larger. The Ambu

E2 valve is shown in Fig. 7.4. It differs from the Ambu E in that it has no exhalation shutter at the end of the exhalation channel.

Function. In the use of the Ambu E and Ambu Hesse valves the negative pressure created by the patient during spontaneous inspiration closes the exhalation shutter and gas is drawn in through the inhalation shutter. When ventilation is assisted or controlled, the positive pressure from bag squeezing opens the inspiratory shutter so that the end of the shutter occludes the exhalation channel. During exhalation, the inspiratory shutter collapses. The exhalation channel is opened and gas passes to atmosphere through the exhalation shutter. When there is excess gas in the system, both shutters open just enough to vent the excess gas.

In the use of the Ambu E2 valve the negative pressure created by the patient during spontaneous inspiration opens the inhalation shutter. It also draws in air from the exhalation channel.

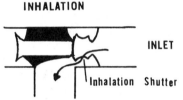

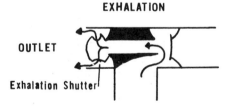

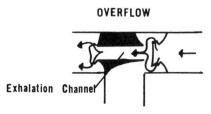

Figure 7.3. Ambu E valve.

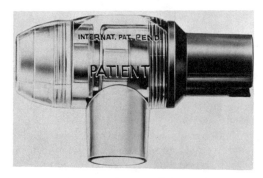

Figure 7.4. Ambu E2 valve. (Courtesy of Ambu International.)

The result is that a mixture of fresh gas and air is inhaled. During controlled or assisted respiration, the positive pressure from bag squeezing causes the inspiratory shutter to occlude the exhalation channel, so that fresh gases pass to the patient. During exhalation, the inhalation shutter closes and the exhaled gases pass through the exhalation channel to atmosphere.

Evaluation. Resistance of the Ambu E on inspiration ranges from 0.6–2.1 cm H_2O at flows from 5–40 liters/min. Resistance on exhalation at the same flows ranges from 0.6–2.5 cm H_2O. The dead space is 10 ml. Back leak is 9.0% of tidal volume with a retarded bag release and 1.8% with a rapid release (8).

Resistances of the Ambu Hesse valve on inspiration range from 0.2–0.7 cm H_2O at flows from 5–40 liters/min. Resistances on exhalation range from 0.2–0.9 cm H_2O at the same flows. The dead space is 14 ml. Back leak is 7.3% of tidal volume with a retarded bag release and 0.9% with a rapid release (8).

Resistances of the Ambu E2 are not available. The dead space is 10 ml. The back leak is 9.0% of tidal volume with a retarded bag release and 1.8% with a rapid release (8).

Care and Cleaning. The valves can be disassembled for cleaning. The parts can be cleaned with soapy water or other cleaning or sterilizing solutions. Agents harmful to polycarbonate cannot be used, however. The parts may be boiled, autoclaved or gas sterilized.

When reassembled, care must be taken to place the shutters in the correct positions. Three cases have been reported where a leaflet was placed over the inlet to the exhalation channel in the Ambu E valve (9–11). The patient could inspire normally, but the exhalation channel was blocked. This resulted in complete rebreathing.

The Fink Valve

Classification. Spontaneous or controlled respiration.

Construction. The Fink valve is shown in Figures 7.5 and 7.6. The valve body is metal. A flexible diaphragm is positioned above the exhalation port. A pressure tube leads from the inlet side of the inspiratory flap valve to the space over the diaphragm. This space can communicate with the atmosphere through a vent at the top. At the top of the valve is an adjustable knob which is connected to a rotating disc. If the knob is turned to its maximum counterclockwise position, the pressure tube communicates with the space above the diaphragm and the vent to atmosphere is closed. When the knob is turned to its maximum clockwise position, the rotating disc occludes both the pressure tube and the vent at the top. At an intermediate position both the pressure tube and the vent are partially open.

The valve is supplied in two forms: the straight valve as diagrammed and a right-angle valve in which the gas inlet is perpendicular to the patient opening and vent. The latter type is for attachment to a mask.

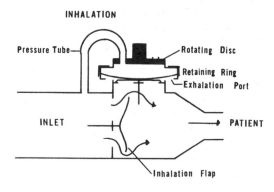

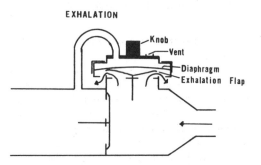

Figure 7.5. Fink valve.

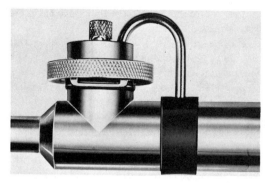

Figure 7.6. The Fink valve. (Courtesy of Ohio Medical Products, a division of Airco, Inc.)

Function. For *spontaneous respiration*, the knob is turned clockwise. During inspiration, the negative pressure exerted by the patient opens the inhalation flap and closes the exhalation flap. Gas flows past the inhalation flap to the patient. Upon exhalation, the inspiratory valve is closed by the exhaled gases which flow past the expiratory flap valve and through the exhalation port.

For *controlled respiration*, the knob is turned to its maximum counterclockwise position. When the bag is squeezed, the pressure in the inlet increases. This pressure is transmitted to the space above the diaphragm. The diaphragm is pushed downward onto the exhalation flap, preventing it from opening. Gases flow past the inhalation flap to the patient.

During exhalation, the pressure at the inlet decreases, the inhalation flap closes, the diaphragm moves upward, the exhalation flap opens and the exhaled gases pass to atmosphere (12).

With the knob in an intermediate position, gas passes through the pressure tube to the space above the diaphragm and vents to atmosphere. The amount of leak can be adjusted by turning the knob.

Evaluation. The dead space of the valve is 11.5 cc.

Loehning and co-workers (13) found no back leak with this valve, even with a retarded bag release.

Orkin and colleagues (14) studied the resistance of the Fink valve. They found that with the straight valve the pressure on exhalation increased from 0.5 to 8 cm H_2O as the flow increased from 10 to 90 liters/min. In the right-angled valve the pressure increased from 1 to 4 cm H_2O at the same flows. Pressures during inspiration at the same flows ranged from 1–2.75 cm H_2O for the straight valve and 1–3 cm H_2O for the right-angled valve.

Sykes (4) also studied the resistance of the Fink valve. His results are shown in Table 7.1.

Care and Cleaning. The valve can be disassembled for cleaning by unscrewing the retaining ring. The parts can then be washed with soap and water and the entire valve can be gas-sterilized.

The Frumin Non-Rebreathing Valve (15)

Classification. Spontaneous or controlled ventilation.

Construction. The Frumin non-rebreathing valve is diagrammed in Figure 7.7. Two configurations are available. The 90-degree model is diagrammed in Figure 7.7. In the other model the inlet and patient ports are 180 degrees from each other.

The valve consists of a clear plastic body containing a rubber or silicone inspiratory flap valve and an inflating rubber mushroom valve which covers the exhalation port (15). A pressure channel connects the inlet with the cavity of the mushroom valve.

Function. In *controlled ventilation* the pressure on the mushroom and in the common chamber is the same during inspiration. However, the surface area of the mushroom is larger

Table 7.1.
Resistances of Some Non-Rebreathing Valves*

Valve	Inspiration Flow (liters/min)						Expiration Flow (liters/min)					
	15	20	30	40	50	60	15	20	30	40	50	60
	in cm water						*in cm water*					
Fink	0.9	1.3	1.9	2.5	3.1	4.0	0.4	0.5	0.8	1.3	1.8	2.1
Ruben	0.7	0.8	1.1	1.4	1.8	2.0	0.4	0.5	0.8	1.5	2.4	3.5
Stephen-Slater	0.9	1.1	1.7	2.1	2.5	2.8	0.6	0.8	1.3	2.0	2.6	3.5

* From Sykes MK: Non-rebreathing valves. *Br J Anaesth* 31:450–455, 1959.

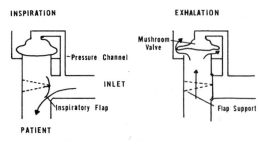

Figure 7.7. Frumin valve.

than that of the expiratory valve seat. Therefore, the downward force (pressure × area) is greater than the upward force. The mushroom is inflated and this prevents gas from passing out the expiratory port.

At the start of exhalation, the pressure at the inlet drops and the mushroom deflates. The pressure from the patient's exhalation closes the inspiratory flap valve and gases pass around the mushroom valve to atmosphere.

In *spontaneous respiration*, on inspiration, the inspiratory flap valve is pulled open and fresh gas is drawn toward the patient. The normal resting position of the mushroom seals off the exhalation port.

If, during spontaneous breathing, there is inadequate fresh gas flow, negative pressure generated by the patient will be transmited to the inhalation port and, therefore, also into the mushroom. Atmospheric pressure will collapse the mushroom, raise it off the exhalation port and allow room air to be drawn in. A negative pressure of less than 1 mm Hg will produce this effect.

Evaluation. The valve has a resistance of 1.5 cm H_2O at a flow of 60 liters/min during either inspiration or expiration (15).

Loehning and co-workers (13) found no back leak with this valve, even with a retarded bag release.

Care and Cleaning. The valve can be disassembled and the parts washed. The entire valve can be gas sterilized.

Laerdal Anesthesia Valve

Classification. Spontaneous or controlled ventilation.

Construction. The Laerdal anesthesia valve is shown diagrammatically in Figure 7.8. A disassembled valve is shown in Figure 7.9. It has a clear plastic body and contains a yellow rubber inspiratory fishmouth valve with a circular

flange. A circular exhalation flap valve occludes the exhalation ports.

Function. In *spontaneous respiration* the fishmouth valve opens and allows gas to pass to the patient during inspiration. The exhalation flap prevents room air from being inhaled through the exhalation ports. During exhalation, the fishmouth valve closes. The gas then passes through the exhalation ports to atmosphere.

In *controlled ventilation* the pressure at the inlet opens the fishmouth valve and pushes the flange against the exhalation ports during inspiration. This allows fresh gas to pass to the patient and prevents its loss through the exhalation ports. During exhalation, the valve functions the same as with spontaneous respirations.

Evaluation. Resistances are given in Table 7.2.

Care and Cleaning. The valve can be disassembled to clean or repair broken parts. It can be cleaned with chemical solutions, boiling or autoclaving. When reassembling, it is important not to leave out the fishmouth valve.

A case has been reported in which an additional expiratory leaflet was inserted at the inlet side of the exhalation port. This second leaflet blocked exhalation (16).

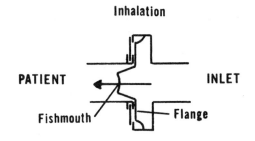

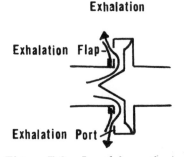

Figure 7.8. Laerdal anesthesia valve.

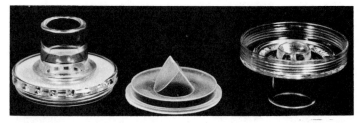

Figure 7.9.   Laerdal anesthesia valve. The disassembled valve is shown. At *left* is the portion of the valve closest to the patient. The exhalation flap encircles the valve housing. In the *center* is the rubber fishmouth portion. The *right* part is the part of the housing closest to the bag.

Table 7.2.
Resistances of the Laerdal Anesthesia Valve*

	Inspiratory			Expiratory		
Flow in liters/min	4.7	20.7	44.6	5.0	27.0	54.4
Resistance in cm H$_2$O	0.32	0.84	1.82	0.16	1.31	2.83

* Courtesy of Laerdal Medical Corporation.

Lewis-Leigh Inflation Valve (17)

Classification. Spontaneous or controlled respiration.

Construction. The Lewis-Leigh inflation valve is shown in Figures 7.10 and 7.11. It consists of a clear plastic body with a chimney which may be rotated 90 degrees. This changes the position of the exhalation valve seat at the bottom of the chimney. A disc-type valve is located at the top of the exhalation chimney.

In the upper two drawings, the chimney is rotated clockwise for controlled ventilation. The rubber flap valve can seat either on a ridge of the body or on the lower end of the chimney. During inspiration, the rubber flap valve blocks the exhalation chimney and gas passes to the patient. During exhalation, the flap valve seats on the ridge and gas passes up the chimney, lifting the disc valve. When the chimney is rotated counterclockwise the flap valve is prevented from seating on the chimney but not on the ridge. This is the position for spontaneous respiration. During inspiration gas passes the flap valve and travels to the patient. The disc valve in the chimney prevents room air from being drawn into the valve. During exhalation, the flap valve seats on the ridge and exhaled gases pass into the chimney. Should the fresh gas flow exceed the patient's minute ventilation, excess gases can pass up the chimney, as shown in the lower drawing.

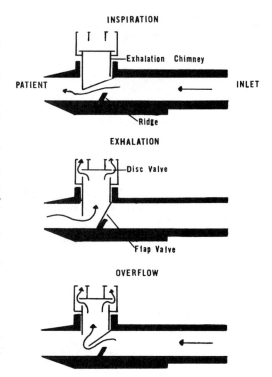

Figure 7.10.   Lewis-Leigh valve.

The Lewis-Leigh valve is a modification of the Digby Leigh valve. The Digby Leigh valve had a simple disc-type exhalation valve instead of the chimney. It was necessary to close the exhalation valve with the finger when controlled or assisted ventilation was used.

Function. During inspiration, the flap valve moves away from its seat on the body and closes over the base of the chimney. The disc valve in the chimney prevents air from being drawn into the valve during spontaneous ventilation. Gas then flows toward the patient.

At the end of inspiration, when the pressure in the system returns to atmospheric, the flap valve returns to its resting position over the fresh gas inlet. As the patient exhales, the increased pressure lifts the disc valve so that gas escapes to atmosphere. When the chimney is rotated 90 degrees counterclockwise, gas can then leak through the valve to atmosphere. This

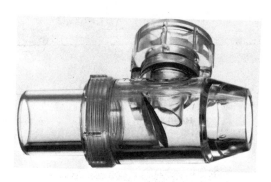

Figure 7.11. Lewis-Leigh valve. (Courtesy of Harris-Lake, Inc.)

provides a safety factor by preventing pressure increases in the system (17).

Evaluation. Loehning and co-workers (13) investigated back leak with two Lewis-Leigh valves and found that when the bag was released rapidly back leak was 8–11% of tidal volume. If the bag release was retarded, however, the back leak was 10–29% of tidal volume.

Brown and Hustead (18) found a resistance of 0.1 cm H_2O with flows of 3 and 5 liters/min.

The Lewis-Leigh valve is sometimes used in conjunction with a breathing bag as a resuscitation unit called the Pulmonator.

Care and Cleaning. The valve can be gas sterilized or cold chemical sterilization techniques can be used.

The Ruben Valve (19)

Classification. Spontaneous or controlled ventilation.

Construction. A diagram of the Ruben valve is shown in Figure 7.12. It consists of a clear plastic body with metal fittings. The fittings are colored as follows: blue inlet, red patient connection, and gold outlet. Inside the body is a spool-shaped piston which is held onto seat A by a spring. A disc-type valve is near the exhalation port. An attachment is available to prevent obstruction of the outlet valve (20).

Function. During inspiration, the piston is pushed to the right by the force of the incoming

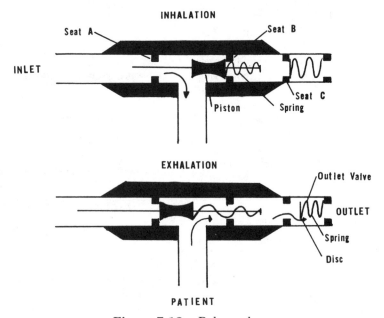

Figure 7.12. Ruben valve.

gas. At its maximum right position it seals against seat B. Gas is prevented from passing to the outlet and passes on toward the patient. The outlet valve prevents the inrush of air during spontaneous breathing. When the pressure at the inlet drops, the force of the spring pushes the piston against seat A. During exhalation, the pressure of the exhaled gases causes the disc valve to open. Gas then passes to atmosphere.

When the valve is to be used with resuscitation equipment, the exhalation valve is not present (21). This allows the patient to inspire from atmosphere.

Evaluation. Sykes (4) investigated the resistance of the Ruben valve. His results are shown in Table 7.1. Ruben (19) found resistance on inspiration to be 0.8 cm H_2O and on expiration 1.0 cm H_2O with a flow of 25 liters/min. If the outlet valve is absent, the expiratory resistance is 0.

Cilliers (22) found gas leakage on inspiration to be less than 5%.

Loehning and colleagues (13) tested the Ruben valve for back leak. They found that with a rapid and complete bag release the back leak was 10–12% of tidal volume. If the bag release was retarded, the back leak was 32–44% of tidal volume. If the patient had increased resistance or decreased compliance, the back leak could be as high as 76% of tidal volume.

Dead space of the valve is 9 ml (19).

The valve in use causes a clicking noise which may be disturbing (4). Askrog and co-workers (23), found that the valve tended to stick in the inspiratory position. Wisborg and colleagues (11) described several serious malfunctions with the Ruben valve. Most common were sticking of the bobbin and the exhalation valve so that neither inspiration nor exhalation could occur. If only the expiratory port was blocked, dangerously high pressures could result. Either the bobbin or the spring or both may be incorrectly assembled. This may result in increased resistance to inspiration and exhalation and partial or total rebreathing.

Waters and co-workers (24) found that when the Ruben valve was used with controlled ventilation, a considerable amount of fresh gas was lost when the bag was squeezed through the expiratory port before the bobbin completed its excursion to the inflation position. The patient's total ventilation was therefore less than the fresh gas flow.

Care and Cleaning. The valve can be cleaned by flushing the channels with soap and

water. It tolerates most chemical solutions but deteriorates if exposed to heat (19). The valve can be gas sterilized.

The Stephen-Slater Valve (25–28)

Classification. Spontaneous respiration.

Construction. The Stephen-Slater valve is shown in Figures 7.13 and 7.14. The valve body is made of metal. The valve has two rubber flap valves, each secured by a shaft at its center. A right-angled form of the valve is available with the inlet and patient ends at right angles.

Function. During inspiration, the negative pressure exerted by the patient opens the inhalation flap valve, allowing gas to flow toward the patient. The negative pressure helps to keep the expiratory flap valve closed. During exhalation, the pressure in the valve rises. The inspiratory flap closes and the expiratory flap opens. Gas then flows to atmosphere.

During the expiratory pause, fresh gas flow can keep both flap valves open if the fresh gas flow is greater than 3 liters/min. This feature

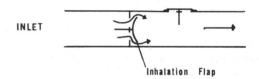

INHALATION

INLET   Inhalation Flap

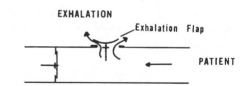

EXHALATION   Exhalation Flap

PATIENT

Figure 7.13. Stephen-Slater valve.

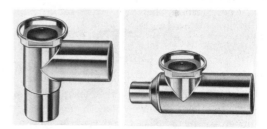

Figure 7.14. Stephen-Slater non-rebreathing valve. (Courtesy of Ohio Medical Products.)

allows some additional wash-out of the valve body and lowers the resistance (11).

If controlled respiration is desired, the expiratory flap valve must be held closed as the bag is squeezed (25). Then no gas can escape in spite of the increased pressure in the valve.

Evaluation. Stephen (29) found a resistance of 1.75 cm of water on inspiration and 1.0 cm H_2O on exhalation using a flow of 15 liters/min. Orkin and colleagues (14) found resistance to be lower. At flows between 10 and 90 liters/min, the inspiratory resistance varied between 1 and 2 cm H_2O. The expiratory resistance was slightly lower at the same flows. Brown and Hustead (18) found a resistance of 0.2 cm H_2O with a flow of 5 liters/min and 0.1 cm H_2O with a flow of 3 liters/min. Sykes (4) investigated the resistances of the valve. His results are shown in Table 7.1.

Slater and Stephen (26) found a dead space of 10 cc. Another study found the dead space to be 7.2 cc with no flow and 0.3 cc with a flow of 3 liters/min or more (30).

Foregger (1) found a back leak of 30 cc with a tidal volume of 500 ml.

With prolonged or repeated use, the exhalation leaflet may curl, allowing air dilution (5).

Care and Cleaning. The valve can be washed. The rubber flap valves can be removed for cleaning. They should not be boiled or autoclaved but may be cleaned with a sponge dampened with ether (31). The entire unit can be gas sterilized.

Fresh Gas Inlet

This may be through an opening in the tail of the bag (Fig. 7.1*A*) or near the neck of the bag (Fig. 7.1*B*).

The Reservoir Bag

The bag acts as a reservoir to collect fresh gas during exhalation and the expiratory pause. Usually it is a thin-walled rubber bag similar to that described in Chapter 5. A self-refilling bag is commonly used with resuscitation equipment.

Tubing

This component is optional. In some systems the bag connects directly to the non-rebreathing valve. In others, however, a length of corrugated rubber tubing is placed between the non-rebreathing valve and the bag. This will enable the anesthesiologist to sit at a distance from the patient's head and still maintain control and vigilance over the bag.

Relief Valve

This is also optional, but is highly recommended. If the fresh gas flow is too high, the pressure in the inspiratory line will increase and may cause the non-rebreathing valve to jam in an inspiratory position, preventing exhalation. To prevent this, some non-rebreathing valves are designed to vent the excess gas to atmosphere. Alternately, a relief valve, either high or low pressure, may be included in the system (Fig. 7.1).

Oxygen Analyzer

An oxygen analyzer may be placed in the fresh gas line between the bag and the inspiratory tubing or between the inspiratory tubing and the non-rebreathing valve (Fig. 7.1).

Humidifier

A humidifier may be placed in the fresh gas line or the inspiratory line. However, many of the non-rebreathing valves tend to stick when wet.

USE OF THE SYSTEM

Before use each valve should be tested for proper function during both inspiration and expiration (11, 16, 32). This can be easily done using a reservoir bag as a test lung.

Spontaneous Ventilation

For spontaneous ventilation, the total flow from the anesthesia machine is adjusted so that the reservoir bag is ¾ full at the beginning of inspiration (22). If a relief valve is used, the fresh gas flow can be set above the minute volume and excess gases will overflow during exhalation.

Controlled Ventilation

The total fresh gas flow is set approximately equal to the desired minute volume. The anesthesiologist squeezes the bag briskly at the start of inspiration and quickly relaxes his grip when inspiration is complete. If the squeeze is not brisk, fresh gas may pass out the exhalation port. This reduces the tidal volume delivered to the patient. If bag relaxation is retarded, there may be back leak with certain valves (13).

If a relief valve is present in the system, the fresh gas flow may be set above the desired minute volume. Excessive gases will be vented during inspiration.

Some valves may emit a single click but should not chatter.

With certain valves, the valve may be kept "floating" by a high flow of gas (30). This will provide wash-out of the valve body and reduce dead space.

If, for some reason the bag must be left unattended when the patient is apneic, the fresh gas flow can be turned off, or the relief valve opened fully.

FUNCTIONAL ANALYSIS

If the non-rebreathing valve is competent, there should be no mixing of inhaled and exhaled gases beyond the mask or endotracheal connector. The dead space of the entire breathing system is equal to the dead space of the valve. The patient inhales fresh gas from the reservoir bag and exhaled gas is blown free into the atmosphere. Air dilution may occur with some valves.

The patient's minute volume during controlled respiration should equal the fresh gas flow provided (a) there are no leaks; (b) there is no pressure applied to the reservoir bag during exhalation and (c) the reservoir bag is grasped briskly at the start of inspiration to move the moving parts quickly with minimum leakage of gas (22).

In a number of valves exhaled gas can leak past the inspiratory valve into the inspiratory limb. Fortunately, it is usually only the dead space portion of exhaled gas that is reinhaled (33).

HAZARDS (7, 34–37)

All automatic non-rebreathing valves carry the danger of a sudden occlusion of the exhalation port (4). This may be caused by:

1. External occlusion. This may be from drapes, assistant's hands, etc. With continued inflow of fresh gas into the valve and accumulation of exhaled gas, a sudden release of the outlet obstruction may cause the valve to stick in the inspiratory position (20). Some valves have arrangements to protect the exit port (20).

2. Internal occlusion. This could result from a squeeze or bump on the bag, excessive fresh gas flow, operation of the oxygen flush valve or the patient coughing. A dangerous time is when changing abruptly from controlled to spontaneous ventilation, when apnea or hypoventilation may persist for several minutes. The fresh gas flow quickly distends the bag and the pressure inside the valve rises rapidly, holding the expiratory port closed. Unless the pressure is decreased to release the locked valve, inflow will cause a continuous and possibly dangerous rise in pressure (38).

To lessen this danger, a high-pressure relief valve may be incorporated into the inspiratory limb (39). A low-pressure relief valve may also be used, but it has the disadvantage that a sudden increase in pressure will close it.

A high-pressure alarm may also be helpful in warning the user that such a problem exists.

ADVANTAGES (4, 12, 22, 25, 40–42)

1. Hazards of carbon dioxide absorption (heat retention, inhalation of irritant dust, exhausted soda lime) are eliminated. Trichloroethylene may be used.

2. The equipment is compact, lightweight and mobile.

3. The equipment is inexpensive.

4. The equipment is simple with a minimum number of parts.

5. The system can be used to estimate minute volume.

6. Dead space and rebreathing are minimal if the valve functions properly. Resistance is generally low.

7. The composition of the inspired mixture is close to that delivered by the machine (4, 41). The concentrations of gases in the inhaled mixture can be changed rapidly so that denitrogenation, oxygenation and saturation with nitrous oxide can be achieved rapidly.

8. The only two distensible parts of the system are the patient's lungs and the reservoir bag. Therefore, the "feel" of the bag may be a better indicator of changes in compliance than in systems employing relief valves.

9. The patient's minute volume can be estimated by adjusting the fresh gas flow until the reservoir bag is kept ¾ inflated at the end of expiration. The sum of gas flows recorded on the flowmeters equals minute volume (4, 22).

DISADVANTAGES

1. For adult patients a relatively large total gas flow is required. This results in increased cost, operating room contamination and an explosive hazard when a flammable agent is used. However, it should be noted that the recommended fresh gas flow is less than that needed for most of the Mapleson type systems (22, 43).

2. Some of the valves are noisy and stick, particularly when wet.

3. There may be considerable loss of heat and humidity from the patient.

4. The feel of the bag is different from that in other systems. The anesthesiologist's hand must be re-educated.

5. With some valves it is necessary to use both hands to assist or control respirations.

6. Cleaning and sterilization are somewhat difficult.

7. The valve must be located at the patient's head. Its bulk may be troublesome with certain operations or may cause the endotracheal tube to kink (44).

8. When used on adult patients, the higher gas flows required may cause an undesirable amount of resistance (14).

9. With some valves there may be considerable rebreathing, especially if the bag release is retarded.

10. Some of the valves are difficult to use with a scavenging system.

11. Sticking of the expiratory valve during spontaneous ventilation can lead to inhalation of air.

12. During controlled ventilation some gas often slips past the expiratory valve in the initial part of inspiration, reducing the tidal volume delivered (22, 45). This is known as forward leak.

13. There is a lack of standardization among the valves, so that with some valves the anesthesiologist must rotate the control mechanism clockwise to set it for controlled ventilation and counterclockwise on other valves (6).

14. The dead space of some valves is relatively large for pediatric patients (6).

15. Fresh gas inflow must be matched to minute volume and this may require frequent adjustments. Too low an inflow produces obstruction with most non-rebreathing valves and in the remainder causes dilution of the inspired gas with ambient air (46).

References

1. Foregger R: The classification and performance of respiratory valves. *Anesthesiology* 20:296–308, 1959.
2. Kay G: The respiratory valve. *Med J Aust* 2:234–239, 1949.
3. Mushin WW, Rendell-Baker L, Thompson PW, Mapleson WW: Valves for use in controlled ventilation. In *Automatic Ventilation of the Lungs*, ed 2. Philadelphia, F. A. Davis, 1969, pp 771–806.
4. Sykes MK: Nonrebreathing valves. *Br J Anaesth* 31:450–455, 1959.
5. Anonymous: A piston-type nonrebreathing valve. *Anesthesiology* 16:1037, 1955.
6. Rayburn RL: Pediatric anesthesia circuits. ASA Refresher Course, 1981.
7. Steen SN, Chen JL: Automatic non-rebreathing valve circuits: some principles and modifications. *Br J Anaesth* 35:379–382, 1963.
8. Personal communication: R.O. Jonsson, Ambu International.
9. Kelly MP: Ventilation equipment. *Br Med J* 2:176, 1968.
10. Grogono AW, Porterfield J: Ambu valve: danger of wrong assembly. *Br J Anaesth* 42:978, 1970.
11. Wisborg K, Jacobsen E: Functional disorders of Ruben and Ambu-E valves after dismantling and cleaning. *Anesthesiology* 42:633–634, 1975.
12. Fink BR: A nonrebreathing valve of new design. *Anesthesiology* 15:471–474, 1954.
13. Loehning RW, Davis G, Safar P: Rebreathing with "nonrebreathing" valves. *Anesthesiology* 25:854–856, 1964.
14. Orkin LR, Siegal M, Rovenstine EA: Resistance to breathing by apparatus used in anesthesia II valves and machines. *Anesth Analg* 36:19–27, 1957.
15. Frumin MJ, Lee ASJ, Papper EM: New valve for nonrebreathing systems. *Anesthesiology* 20:383–385, 1959.
16. Dolan PF, Shapiro S, Steinbach RB: Valve misassembly—manually operated resuscitation bag. *Anesth Analg* 60:66–67, 1981.
17. Lewis G: Nonrebreathing valve. *Anesthesiology* 17:618–619, 1956.
18. Brown ES, Hustead RF: Resistance of pediatric breathing systems. *Anesth Analg* 48:842–849, 1969.
19. Ruben H: A new nonrebreathing valve. *Anesthesiology* 16:643–645, 1955.
20. Hoskins CH: Attachment for the Ruben valve. *Anaesthesia* 16:366–367, 1961.
21. Ruben H, Hesse H, Eng D: Adjustable respiratory valves offering low resistance to flow of gas. *Anesthesiology* 17:782–786, 1956.
22. Cilliers AJ: The use of the Ruben non-rebreathing valve in anaesthesia for thoracic surgery. *Anaesthesia* 17:444–454, 1962.
23. Askrog V, Soren E: Experiments with non-rebreathing anesthesia systems during controlled ventilation. *Anesth Analg* 45:348–351, 1966.
24. Waters DJ, Mapleson WW: Rebreathing during controlled respiration with various semiclosed anaesthetic systems. *Br J Anaesth* 33:374–381, 1961.
25. Stephen CR, Slater HM: A nonresisting nonrebreathing valve. *Anesthesiology* 9:550–552, 1948.
26. Slater HM, Stephen CR: Anesthesia for infants and children. *Arch Surg* 62:251–289, 1951.
27. Stephen CR, Slater HM: Agents and techniques employed in pediatric anesthesia. *Anesth Analg* 29:254–262, 1950.
28. Shuman RC: Modified nonrebreathing valve.

Anesthesiology 17:749–750, 1956.

29. Stephen CR: Techniques in pediatric anesthesia. The nonrebreathing valve. *Anesthesiology* 13:77–85, 1952.
30. Brown ES, Hustead RF: Dead space in pediatric equipment. *Items Topics* 13:1–3, 1967.
31. Campbell MB: Nonrebreathing technics. *J Am Assoc Nurse Anesthetists* 22:97–105, 1954.
32. Pauca AL, Jenkins TE: Airway obstruction by breakdown of a non-rebreathing valve: How foolproof is foolproof? *Anesth Analg* 60:529–531, 1981.
33. Sykes MK: Rebreathing circuits. *Br J Anaesth* 40:666–674, 1968.
34. Lee S: A universal valve for anaesthetic circuits. *Br J Anaesth* 36:318–321, 1964.
35. Davenport HT, Kleenleyside HB: Interstitial emphysema and pneumothorax associated with the use of a modified non-rebreathing valve. *Can Anaesth Soc J* 4:126–130, 1957.
36. Potter GL: Some clinical aspects of the nonrebreathing valve. *Anesth Analg* 38:114–117, 1959.
37. Lee S: Exhalation tunnel for nonrebreathing techniques. *Anesthesiology* 25:716–717, 1964.
38. Eger EI, Epstein RM: Hazards of anesthetic equipment. *Anesthesiology* 25:490–504, 1964.
39. Holland R: Special committee investigating deaths under anaesthesia: memorandum on the dangers of nonrebreathing valves. *Med J Aust* 2:46–47, 1970.
40. Campbell MB: Choice of equipment for pediatric anesthesia. *J Am Assoc Nurse Anesthetists* 35:193–205, 1967.
41. Mapleson WW: The concentration of anaesthetics in closed circuits, with special reference to halothane I. Theoretical study. *Br J Anaesth* 32:298–309, 1960.
42. Smith RM: General anesthesia systems in pediatrics. *JAMA* 205:808–809, 1968.
43. Sykes MK: Rebreathing during controlled respiration with the Magill attachment. *Br J Anaesth* 31:247–257, 1959.
44. Holm HH: A new valve for paediatric anaesthesia. *Acta Anaesthesiol Scand* 12:75–79, 1968.
45. Scurr C, Feldman S: *Scientific Foundations of Anaesthesia.* Philadelphia, F.A. Davis, 1970.
46. Eger EI: Anesthetic systems; construction and function. In *Anesthetic Uptake and Action.* Baltimore, Williams & Wilkins, 1975.

CHAPTER 8

The Breathing System. IV. The Circle System

The most frequently used system for adult anesthesia in the United States today is the circle system. It is so named because the assembled components form the configuration of a circle. Certain components, such as the absorber and unidirectional valves, are standard equipment on most anesthesia machines.

COMPONENTS

The circle system which is diagrammed in Figure 8.1 consists of the following components: (*a*) absorber, (*b*) absorbent, (*c*) fresh gas inlet, (*d*) unidirectional valves, (*e*) relief valve, (*f*) pressure gauge, (*g*) breathing tubes, (*h*) reservoir bag, (*i*) Y-piece, (*j*) oxygen sensor, and (*k*) optional pieces of equipment such as a circulator, bacterial filter, in-system vaporizer, pressure sensor, and selector valve.

Absorber

The absorber for adult breathing systems is a heavy, bulky component which is usually attached to the anesthesia machine, but may be a separate unit. Completely disposable absorbers are available.

CANISTER
Contents

The canister contains the absorbent and makes up the main part of the absorber. The sidewalls may be of metal, plastic, or glass. Prepacked plastic disposable canisters are available. Plastic and glass allow observation of the absorbent for indicator change. Some canisters have metal cases outside to conduct static electricity.

An absorber may contain one or two canisters. Most modern canisters utilize two interchangeable canisters placed in apposition (Fig. 8.2). Another type of absorber contains one canister which is divided in the middle into two chambers. This is also called a reversible chamber absorber. An older type absorber utilized a canister with a single chamber and is called a single chamber absorber.

With fresh absorbent in both chambers, the carbon dioxide is absorbed mostly in the upstream chamber. As the absorbent becomes exhausted, the carbon dioxide will enter the downstream chamber where absorption will continue. After the absorbent in the upstream canister is exhausted, the chamber is removed and the exhausted absorbent discarded and replaced with fresh absorbent. The downstream canister containing partially used absorbent is then placed in the upstream position. With the reversible chamber absorber the exhausted absorbent is discarded and the canister turned 180 degrees so the chamber which was downstream becomes the upstream chamber. Fresh absorbent is in the downstream chamber.

Size

Each canister should provide an air space equal to or greater than the maximum tidal volume (1). Then the downstream canister should trap all carbon dioxide passing through the absorber even when the upstream canister is no longer active. The volume of air in a filled canister is approximately 50% of that in the empty canister.

Canisters of considerably varying capacity have been employed. Modern canisters are of much larger size than older ones. Advantages of larger canisters include better utilization of absorbent, more complete removal of carbon dioxide and longer intervals between absorbent changes. Canisters with large cross-sections allow a lower flow velocity and less turbulence, so that resistance and the hazard of absorbent dust migration are reduced (2). Disadvantages of large canisters include bulkiness and increased

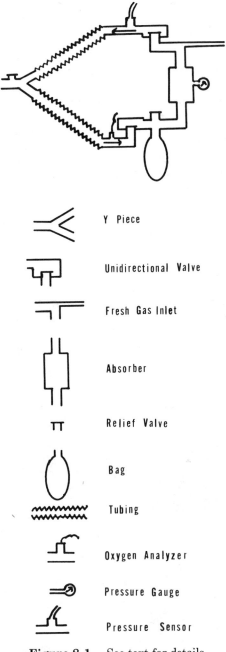

Y Piece

Unidirectional Valve

Fresh Gas Inlet

Absorber

Relief Valve

Bag

Tubing

Oxygen Analyzer

Pressure Gauge

Pressure Sensor

Figure 8.1. See text for details.

chance of cross-infection because more patients exhale into a given charge.

Pattern and Direction of Flow

Flow through the canister is pulsatile. During exhalation, newly exhaled gases push the gases in the absorber further through. If the reservoir bag is on the upstream side of the absorber, fresh gas flow may cause a reversed flow through the absorber during the expiratory pause.

Absorbent is not consumed in a simple advancing pattern. The pattern of absorption within a correctly packed canister is shown in Figure 8.3. It makes no difference whether the gases enter at the top or bottom of the absorber. The first absorption occurs at the inlet and along the sides (3). The tendency of gas to travel along the inside periphery of the canister is known as the "wall effect." Granules on the outer layer are in contact with the smooth wall and the open space between these granules and the wall is greater than elsewhere because no protuberances from other granules are available to fill the hollows. Hence the flow resistance is less and gas finds its way along this path. The wall effect can be minimized by baffles in the canister.

HEAD AND BASE

The head and base of the absorber fit tightly against the interposed canisters. They are

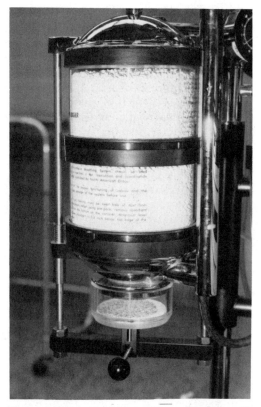

Figure 8.2. Double canister absorber with dust/moisture trap at bottom and external tube to the right.

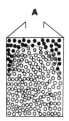
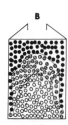
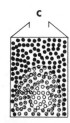

Figure 8.3. Pattern of carbon dioxide absorption in a canister. Darkened circles represent exhausted absorbent. *A*, canister after limited use. Absorption of carbon dioxide occurs primarily at the inlet and to a lesser extent along the sides. The granules at the inlet are becoming exhausted. A zone of partial exhaustion occurs along the sides. *B*, canister after extensive use. The absorbent granules at the inlet and along the sides are exhausted. Granules near the center of the inlet end of the canister form a zone of partial exhaustion. *C*, at exhaustion a "blind spot" in the distal third of the canister remains where the granules are still capable of absorbing carbon dioxide. (Redrawn from Adriani J, Rovenstein EA: Experimental studies on carbon dioxide absorbers for anesthesia. *Anesthesiology* 2:10, 1941.)

tightened together to effect a seal and loosened to allow the absorbent to be changed.

There are spaces at the top and bottom for incoming gases to disperse before passing through the absorbent or for outgoing gases to collect before passing on through the circle. This promotes even distribution of flow through the absorber (1). In the base this space also allows dust and condensed water to accumulate. This prevents caking of the absorbent due to excessive water in the dependent layers of absorbent. Some bases have drain cocks to allow removal of accumulated water. Other bases have a special dust and moisture trap (Fig. 8.2).

SCREENS AND BAFFLES

Baffles, annular rings which serve to direct the path of gas travel toward the central area of the canister, are frequently placed at the top, bottom, and middle of the absorber. They increase the path of travel by gases at the periphery and thus compensate for the reduced resistance to flow along the walls of the canister (1, 4, 5). Screens are usually present at the bottom of each canister and frequently at the top of the absorber. They hold the absorbent firmly in place. The screen and baffle may be one unit, separate, or may attach to each other.

SIDE OR CENTER TUBE

When gas both enters and leaves the absorber at the top, a means must be incorporated to return the gases to the top of the absorber after the gases have passed through the absorbent or to carry them to the bottom of the absorber before they pass upwards through the absorbent. This is accomplished by an internal tube in the center of the canister (Fig. 8.4) or by an external side tube (Fig. 8.2). A center tube tends to increase channeling (3, 6) because the sidewalls are smooth and offer a pathway of low resistance. It also makes filling the canisters more difficult. If the center tube does not fit into the head tightly, gas may escape through the leak and bypass the absorbent (7).

BYPASS (CUT-OUT CONTROL)

A bypass mechanism is optional on some absorbers. There are two types of bypasses: complete and partial. A complete bypass is capable of diverting all of the gases entering the absorber to the outlet without passing through the absorbent. A partial bypass allows only a portion of the incoming gas to bypass the absorbent when fully open.

A bypass allows an increase in $PaCO_2$ without

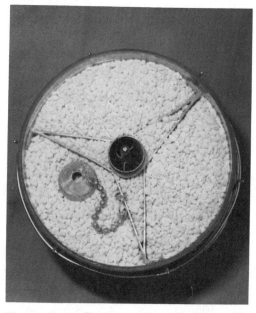

Figure 8.4. Canister with an internal tube. The cap on the chain should be placed over the tube when the canister is filled to prevent granules from falling into the base of the absorber.

hypoventilation. A complete bypass allows the absorbent to be changed without interrupting ventilation. Also if there is a leak in the absorber, the bypass can be turned on to stop loss of gases from the system.

Some anesthesiologists turn the bypass on at the conclusion of an anesthetic. It may still be in that position at the beginning of the next case. Dangerous hypercapnia can result, especially if the bypass is complete. The degree of hypercapnia will depend on the fresh gas flow (8). With high gas flows the danger is less, but even if high flows are used, the bypass should always be checked before starting a case. On one common absorber the bypass is located on the side of the absorber opposite from where the operator normally stands or sits and is not easily seen (Fig. 8.5). Since it is easily overlooked, checking this should be standard procedure.

Carbon Dioxide Absorption

ADVANTAGES

Carbon dioxide absorption is used to allow rebreathing of exhaled gases, which has the following advantages (9):

1. The cost of anesthesia is reduced because lower fresh gas flows can be used.

2. Operating room pollution is reduced.

3. Inflammable mixtures are enclosed, reducing the hazard of explosion.

4. Heat and moisture are conserved.

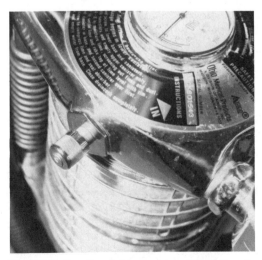

Figure 8.5. Partial bypass at side of the absorber. This is located on the side of the absorber opposite from where the user normally stands and is easily overlooked.

5. The inhaled mixture will be of a more nearly constant composition. The level of anesthesia may be easier to maintain.

ABSORBENTS

Carbon dioxide absorption employs the general principle of a base neutralizing an acid (3). The acid is carbonic acid formed by the reaction of carbon dioxide with water. The base is the hydroxide of an alkali or alkaline earth metal. The end products of the reaction are water and a carbonate (10).

There are two absorbents in common use today, soda lime and barium hydroxide lime.

Soda Lime

Composition (11). The composition of soda lime has varied over the years. The soda lime most used today is the so-called "wet" or "high-moisture" variety. By weight it is 4% sodium hydroxide, 1% potassium hydroxide, 14–19% water and enough calcium hydroxide to make 100%. In addition, small amounts of silica and kieselguhr (for hardening) and indicators are present.

The water is present as a thin film of absorbent sodium hydroxide and calcium hydroxide solution on the granule surface (3). The moisture content is essential because the reactions take place between ions which exist only in the presence of water (12). Absorbents with low moisture show rapid exhaustion owing to dehydration. On the other hand, those with higher moisture have a slower rate of absorption, stickiness, and increased resistance (4, 13). The humidity of the gas does not affect the capacity of soda lime to absorb carbon dioxide (6, 14). Absorption is as effective when the gases are dry as when they are humidified, provided the soda lime has a high moisture content.

Increasing the sodium hydroxide content increases the activity because it is a more active base than calcium hydroxide. However, the sodium base is hygroscopic and readily absorbs water from atmospheres of high humidity. This causes clogging of the pores of the granules, "caking" during use and excessive heating (3, 15).

Chemistry. To initiate the chemical reaction, carbon dioxide must first react with the water on the surface of the granule to form carbonic acid:

$$CO_2 + H_2O \rightleftharpoons H_2CO_3$$

This is a weak acid and is incompletely dissociated into its ions:

$$H_2CO_3 \rightleftharpoons H^+ + HCO_3^-$$
$$\downarrow$$
$$H^+ + CO_3^{-2}$$

The sodium hydroxide and calcium hydroxide are likewise dissociated into their ions:

$$NaOH \rightleftharpoons OH^- + Na^+$$

$$Ca(OH)_2 \rightleftharpoons 2OH^- + Ca^{2+}$$

The sodium and calcium ions combine with the carbonate ions, forming as end products sodium carbonate and calcium carbonate:

$$2NaOH + 2H_2CO_3 + Ca(OH)_2 \rightleftharpoons$$
$$CaCO_3 + Na_2CO_3 + 4H_2O$$

Water is also formed from the hydrogen and hydroxyl ions. Heat is liberated at the rate of 13,700 calories per mole of water produced (or CO_2 absorbed). This heat does not affect absorption efficiency (15, 16), but may be significant with regard to the patient.

A phenomenon known as "peaking" or "regeneration" was seen with soda lime. The absorption efficiency of the soda lime would fall off after several hours of use. When the charge was set aside and allowed to remain idle and then used again, absorption would proceed nearly as efficiently as before but for a shorter period of time. In other words, the soda lime appeared to be reactivated with rest. The amount of regeneration depended on the length of the period of rest (17). After a number of such periods of efficient absorption with intervening periods of rest, terminal exhaustion occurred. The explanation for regeneration was advanced by Adriani (3, 18).

He pointed out that sodium hydroxide is more soluble and active than calcium hydroxide and combines preferentially with carbon dioxide to form sodium carbonate. Sodium carbonate, because it is soluble, would dissolve in the moisture on the granules. It could then penetrate into the granule and react with the less active and less soluble calcium hydroxide to form calcium carbonate, which is insoluble, and sodium hydroxide. The regenerated sodium hydroxide would then impart renewed activity to the absorbent.

There is general agreement that with modern "wet" soda lime the absorption capacity regenerated with rest is slight (19) and affords no appreciable improvement of the over-all life of the absorbent (20).

Regeneration does have some importance when indicators are used, however. Soda lime which shows an exhausted color, if allowed to rest, will often show a reversal of color. The absorptive capacity, however, of that soda lime will be low and the exhausted color will reappear after only a brief exposure to carbon dioxide.

Shape and Size of Granules. Soda lime is supplied in granular form. The granules have irregular surfaces to provide a maximum of surface area for absorption.

The size of the granules is important. Small granules provide greater surface area on which the reaction can take place and decrease channeling (21, 22). They cause more resistance (21, 22, 23) and "caking" (10, 21), however. Larger granules cause a lower resistance to air flow but offer less surface area for absorption. Experimental and clinical studies have shown that a blend of larger and smaller granules has the effect of minimizing resistance with little sacrifice in absorptive efficiency (24).

Soda lime granules are graded in size by mesh number. A 4-mesh strainer has four openings per inch whereas one of 8-mesh has eight openings per inch. Soda lime granules graded 4 mesh will pass through the 4-mesh strainer but not through a strainer with smaller holes. In other words, the higher the mesh number, the smaller the particles. Soda lime in use in anesthesia today consists of granules 4–8 mesh (3). Smaller sizes are available for special needs.

Hardness. Soda lime granules tend to fragment easily, producing alkaline dust ("fines"). Excessive powder produces channeling resistance to flow, caking and may be blown through the system to the patient. To prevent this, small amounts of silica are added to soda lime to increase hardness (3). Silica tends, however, to clog the pores of the soda lime and reduce its efficiency, a drawback overcome by the addition of kieseguhr (12).

Hardness is tested by placing a weighed amount of absorbent in a pan with steel ball bearings and agitating it. The soda lime is then sifted onto an 8-mesh screen. The percentage of the original sample remaining on the screen is the hardness number. The hardness number should be greater than 75 (3). There may be some variations in the dust content of different brands of absorbent (25). Some manufacturers coat the outside of the granules with an antidusting film to which dust particles adhere (4).

Barium Hydroxide Lime

Composition. Barium hydroxide lime is a mixture of approximately 20% barium hydroxide and 80% calcium hydroxide. It may also contain some potassium hydroxide and an indicator (12). Barium hydroxide is the more active component of the mixture, acting much as sodium hydroxide in soda lime.

Moisture in barium hydroxide lime is incorporated into the structure of the barium hydroxide as an octahydrate, $(Ba(OH)_2 \cdot 8H_2O)$. Some moisture is also present on the surface, as with soda lime. Compared with soda lime, the water content is less variable and less likely to be lost by evaporation. Water will be lost, however, if the barium hydroxide lime is heated over 100°C.

Chemistry. The reactions between barium hydroxide lime and carbon dioxide are as follows:

$$Ba(OH)_2 8H_2O + CO_2 \rightarrow BaCO_3 + 9H_2O$$

$$9H_2O + 9CO_2 \rightarrow 9H_2CO_3$$

$$9H_2CO_3 + 9Ca(OH)_2 \rightarrow 9CaCO_3 + 18H_2O$$

$$2KOH + H_2CO_3 \rightarrow K_2CO_3 + 2H_2O$$

$$Ca(OH)_2 + K_2CO_3 \rightarrow CaCO_3 + 2KOH$$

Heat and water formation vary little from soda lime under identical conditions (26). There is some regeneration with barium hydroxide lime (27, 20).

Size and Shape. Barium hydroxide lime is presently supplied in granular form (4–8 mesh) similar to soda lime. It was formerly supplied in the form of pellets which had a much shorter life than the granular form.

Hardness. It is not necessary to add a hardening agent to barium hydroxide lime because the water of crystallization present imparts sufficient hardness to prevent dust formation (10, 28).

Compatibility of Absorbents and Anesthetic Agents

Ideally, the removal of carbon dioxide should be the sole effect of an absorbent on the gases passing through the canister. The majority of inhalation anesthetics are stable in the presence of absorbents. Trichloroethylene is a notable exception, producing toxic breakdown products and should never be used with the circle system.

One study (29) found that halothane reacts with soda lime, producing a metabolite that is toxic to mice. However, even with a system closed for 4 hr, the concentration of this metabolite remained quite low.

Absorbents will absorb considerable amounts of anesthetics (30–32). Dry absorbent material absorbs more anesthetic agent than wet.

INDICATORS

Indicators are acids or bases whose color depends on hydrogen ion concentration. They are added to the absorbent to indicate when exhaustion has occurred. The indicator does not affect absorption. Some of the commonly used indicators and their colors are shown in Table 8.1. Indicators may produce confusion because one indicator when fresh is white while another brand when expired is white (33). It is important for the user to be aware of which particular indicator is in the absorbent being used.

CONTENTS (20, 34)

The volume of the canister is divided into two segments: the granular space and the air space.

Granular Space

The granular space is occupied by solid absorbent. This is measured by bulk density, which is defined as the weight of absorbent in a given volume. It is affected by the size of the absorbent granules and how well the canister is packed. The smaller the granules and the closer the packing, the greater will be the bulk density. Well packed soda lime has a bulk density of 0.9 g/cc. For barium hydroxide lime, it is 1 g/cc.

Air Space

The air space occupies from 48–55% of the volume of the canister (20). It is divided into two parts: the void space and the pore space.

Void Space. The void space (intergranular or interstitial space) is between the granules. It

Table 8.1.
Indicators for Absorbents

Indicator	Color when Fresh	Color when Exhausted
Phenolphthalein	White	Pink
Ethyl violet	White	Purple
Clayton yellow	Red	Yellow
Ethyl orange	Orange	Yellow
Mimosa Z	Red	White

varies with the size of the granules and how tightly they are packed. The smaller the granules and the closer they fit together, the smaller the void space. The void space of soda lime is 40–47% of its volume (20). For barium hydroxide lime, the figure is 45% (27).

Pore Space. The pore space (intragranular space) is that found within the pores of the granules. It is here that the reaction between the base and the carbonic acid takes place. The pore volume for fresh absorbent is 8% of the total volume. The pore space varies inversely with the moisture content of the absorbent (3, 34). As absorption proceeds, the pore space decreases, because carbonate occupies the spaces (3).

STORAGE, HANDLING, AND USE OF ABSORBENTS

Absorbents are supplied in several types of containers: resealable packages, disposable prefilled canisters, pails, cans, and cartons. Packages and pails, once opened, should be resealed as soon as possible to prevent reaction of the absorbent with carbon dioxide in the air. Opened packages of absorbent, especially soda lime, are also subject to moisture loss, particularly at elevated temperatures. This moisture loss can result in a decrease in absorptive activity (21). High temperatures in the storage area will have no effect on absorbents if the containers are sealed, but any temperature below freezing is harmful (35). The moisture content, when frozen, will expand and cause fragmentation of the granules.

All personnel concerned with the handling of absorbent should be periodically warned that it is caustic. Absorbent dust is strongly irritant to the eyes and respiratory tract. Skin is also subject to attack, particularly when damp. Absorbents should always be handled gently to avoid fragmentation and dust formation.

When a canister is emptied, it should be washed out with soap and water, using a brush. Care should be taken to remove dust particles along the rubber surfaces. These particles will cause the seals to warp, making it difficult to achieve a tight fit. Screens should be cleared of dust particles and granules. If they are allowed to become clogged, resistance to respiration will be increased.

Used absorbent should be placed at least temporarily in a trash container where it is exposed to room air so that the anesthetic vapors are permitted to dissipate.

Proper filling of the canister is indispensable to good absorptive activity and should always be performed with care. The canister should be held over a suitable trash container when being filled, to avoid getting dust particles on the floor. Absorbent should be slowly poured into the canister while it is rotated, stopping occasionally to tap the sides to settle the granules (5). The canister should be filled completely but not overfilled. The upper layer of the absorbent should be level. Screens should not be forced over absorbent because this will cause granules to be crushed. Resulting dust (fines) may cause damage to the respiratory tract (36) or facial burns (37). A small space should remain at the top to provide a distribution area and more even flow for gases passing through the canister.

With prefilled canisters, it is important to remove the top and bottom labels, if present, before insertion (38). If this is not done, gas will not flow through the canister.

CHANGING THE ABSORBENT

The interval between absorbent changes cannot be determined with complete confidence for every situation. Some general guidelines can be set forth. Measuring the carbon dioxide contentration in the inspiratory gas stream is the only reliable method to assure complete carbon dioxide removal. The anesthesiologist should always be alert for signs of carbon dioxide accumulation and err toward too frequent changes rather than too few.

Indicator Color Change

The color change showing through the transparent walls of a canister requires experience for correct interpretation. It is not always a dependable indication of the absorption capacity; nevertheless, if understanding is exercised, it can be a practical guide.

When the color change shows strongly, the absorbent is at or near the point of clinical exhaustion. When little or no color change shows, active absorbent is present, but the amount is indeterminate and may be quite small.

Guidelines. *Double Canister Absorber.* The absorbent in a double canister absorber should be changed when the color change reaches the second canister (18).

Single Canister Absorber. When a single canister absorber is used, it is difficult to determine when the absorbent should be changed. Jorgensen and co-workers (39) using a single canister that held 600 g of soda lime found that the absorbent should be replaced when the color shift had progressed to ⅔ of the charge.

Modifying Factors. The following must be borne in mind when using a color indicator and interpreting its significance.

Change in Color with Rest. When a canister is rested, the color may revert back to its pre-exhaustion level. The change may occur even when the absorbent is sufficiently exhausted to be of no further value clinically. Upon reuse, the color will rapidly return to its exhausted state. The rested canister, therefore, can give a false impression of its usefulness.

Channeling. Channeling refers to the passage of gas preferentially along low-resistance pathways, bypassing the bulk of the absorbent. It is caused by loose packing of the absorbent and/or faulty canister design. Channeling frequently occurs at the contacting part of the absorber on-off valve and the internal tube.

When channeling occurs, the color change will proceed quite rapidly along the channels while occurring more slowly in the rest of the absorbent. The absorbent along the channels will soon become exhausted and carbon dioxide will filter through the canister.

Reaction with Antistatic Spray. The indicator may react with materials used in antistatic sprays with premature discoloration of the absorbent along the canister sides (40). This could lead to the discarding of fresh absorbent in the mistaken belief it is spent.

Absence of Indicator. Cases of use of absorbent without indicators have been reported (41, 42). Most absorbents can be ordered without indicator. These absorbents could be substituted by mistake.

Heat in the Canister

The chemical reaction involving the absorption of carbon dioxide is exothermic. Heat generation occurs in proportion to the amount of carbon dioxide absorbed. Noting the temperature of a canister periodically is useful. Some heat production should be apparent unless very high flows are used. Interpretation of heat in a canister must be done with caution. While a rising temperature within a canister indicates that absorption is proceeding, there is no correlation with the amount of absorbent capacity remaining because it may reflect heat production in one part of the canister while another part is allowing exhaled gases to pass through

without removal of carbon dioxide. Some of the variables affecting heat generation in a canister are the rate of carbon dioxide production by the patient, his temperature, ambient room temperature, and the fresh gas flow.

A hot canister may indicate efficient absorption of carbon dioxide, a very high carbon dioxide production rate, or residual heat in a canister that is no longer functioning efficiently. A canister will remain warm to the touch even long after the absorbent has become exhausted. A cool canister may indicate a very low rate of carbon dioxide production, a canister not in the breathing system, exhausted absorbent, or an absorbent just starting to react with carbon dioxide.

INDICES OF PERFORMANCE

Theoretical Maximum Absorption Capacity

Absorber. For absorbents, theoretical absorption capacity refers to the total volume of carbon dioxide that can be absorbed by a given weight of absorbent if the absorbent were fully utilized. The absorbent capacity of barium hydroxide lime is 27.1 liters of carbon dioxide per 100 g of absorbent. For soda lime it is 25.1 liters per 100 g (43).

Canister. For a given canister, the theoretical absorption capacity is the total volume of carbon dioxide that can be absorbed by the absorbent contained in the canister if it is fully utilized. This will depend on the size of the canister.

Efficiency of Utilization of Absorbent

When exhaustion occurs, the entire charge in the absorber will not be exhausted. The efficiency of utilization of absorbent is the percentage of the maximum absorption capacity used when exhaustion occurs. This will vary with the type of canister and the point at which exhaustion is said to occur. The larger the canister, the higher the efficiency (6, 44, 45).

Absorption Capacity

This is the theoretical maximum absorbent capacity times the efficiency of utilization of absorbent. It may be expressed either as carbon dioxide absorbed per 100 g of absorbent or total carbon dioxide absorbed by a given canister filled with absorbent.

Carbon Dioxide Absorption Efficiency (20, 22, 46) (Carbon Dioxide Absorption Ratio)

Carbon dioxide absorption efficiency is the amount of carbon dioxide absorbed as a percentage of the amount entering a canister. An efficiency of 90% means that 90% of the carbon dioxide entering the canister is absorbed, whereas 10% goes through. As a canister is used, the efficiency will fall. The absorption rate depends on the effectiveness of the absorbent, absence of channeling and the duration of contact. The longer the contact time, the better the absorption efficiency. With higher flow rates through the absorber less carbon dioxide is absorbed (20, 47). Tidal volume has minimal effect on absorption efficiency (20, 46).

Exhaustion Time

Exhaustion time refers to the total length of time a canister may be used before it fails to keep the carbon dioxide concentration at an acceptable level. It is influenced by many factors, including the following:

1. The acceptable inspired carbon dioxide level. The level judged unacceptable varies from 0.1 to 1% with different authors (3, 6, 13, 22, 39, 44, 45, 48–51).

2. Channeling. Channeling due to improper packing or canister design will reduce the exhaustion time.

3. Size of the absorber. The larger the absorber, the longer the exhaustion time.

4. Rate of carbon dioxide production by the patient. The higher the rate of carbon dioxide production, the shorter the exhaustion time.

5. Pattern of ventilation. A high flow rate through the canister will reduce the absorption efficiency and shorten the exhaustion time.

6. Position of the absorber in relation to other components in the system. This will be discussed fully later in this chapter.

7. Fresh gas flow. The higher the fresh gas flow, the longer the exhaustion time.

Because of these many variables it is not possible to predict the exhaustion time of a particular canister.

Fresh Gas Inlet

The fresh gas inlet is the point at which gas from the anesthesia machine enters the system. It is usually connected by a flexible rubber tubing (delivery hose) to the common gas outlet on the machine. It may be located in several positions, but in most cases it is attached to the absorber.

Unidirectional Valves (Flutter Valves, One-Way Valves, Directional Valves, Dome Valves, Flap Valves, Non-Return Valves, Inspiratory and Expiratory Valves)

Two unidirectional valves are used in each circle system. They direct the flow of gas toward the patient in one tubing and away from the patient in the other. The valves in use today are placed in either of two locations: attached to the absorber or in the Y-piece.

A typical absorber-mounted unidirectional valve is shown diagrammatically in Figure 5.1F. It consists of a disc covered with a clear plastic dome which allows visual inspection of the valve. The disc seats horizontally on an annular seat. A guide to prevent the disc from becoming dislodged laterally and/or vertically may be present. Gas enters at the bottom and flows through the center of the valve, raising the disc from its seat. The gas then passes under the plastic dome and on through the breathing system. Reversing the gas flow will cause the disc to contact the seat, stopping further retrograde flow. Absorber-mounted unidirectional valves are positional and must be vertical for the disc to seat properly.

Unidirectional valves incorporated into a Y-piece consist of discs or rubber flaps similar to those found in most non-rebreathing valves.

As can be seen in Figure 5.1F, turbulence results from gas flow through a unidirectional valve. While this was a significant problem with older valves (52, 53), present valves have light discs and present only slight resistance.

The most common problem with unidirectional valves is incompetency. The mushroom type may become "fluted" (54). The disc of the absorber-mounted type may adhere to the dome unless a guard is present (2). Wetting may cause the disc to stick. Electrostatic charges may cause the disc to remain attracted to the dome (55). The sealing gasket may be missing (56). The threads on a guide pin may catch the disc and hold it open (55). Foreign material such as absorbent granules may hold a valve open (2). Since an open valve provides less resistance to flow than a closed valve which must open, the flow of gas will be primarily through the incompetent side, with rebreathing (50, 54).

Valves may fail to open properly or completely (57). Wetting of a valve may cause it to stick unless it is constructed of a nonwettable material (2). This is more likely to be a problem with the exhalation unidirectional valve.

Another hazard of the unidirectional valve was reported by Dean (58). During cleaning, the disc was lost and not recovered. Several months later it was found out of sight below the seat. At that time it had moved into such a position that it covered the opening to the bag mount and functioned as a one-way valve. Gas could pass from a ventilator into the system, but not back again. It is important that all components of this valve be accounted for.

The valved Y-piece presents special problems, especially if used in a department which also has machines with unidirectional valves mounted on the absorber. If a valved Y-piece is inadvertently placed in a circle system containing unidirectional valves near the absorber, there is a 50% chance that the valves will be opposed. In this case, the reservoir bag may or may not fill but the patient cannot be ventilated or breathe spontaneously. Near fatal accidents have resulted (59–61). Some non-valved Y-pieces look the same as their valved counterparts externally, so the mistake is relatively easy to make. The other possible situation is that a circle system will be assembled with no unidirectional valves in it (62). Since some of the valves in Y-pieces are not easily visualized, it may be assumed that they are present when, in fact, they are not. In this event the patient would be able to breathe or be ventilated, and, to all external appearances, the circuit would function normally, but in fact there would be comparatively little absorption of carbon dioxide, which would accumulate.

The ASA Committee on Mechanical Equipment has discouraged use of the valved Y-piece. Certainly they should not be present in a department that also has valves on the absorber. If it is the determination of an individual anesthesia department that valved Y-pieces are preferred, all the anesthesia machines in the hospital should conform to this. Otherwise the potential hazards described will always be present.

Relief Valves

Relief valves were discussed in Chapter 5. The most commonly used are the high-pressure relief valves. During spontaneous breathing the relief valve opens at the end of the expiratory pause. The valve should be adjusted to a low opening pressure. When manually assisted or controlled ventilation is used, the relief valve must be adjusted to the maximum required inspiratory ventilation pressure. The relief valve then opens at the end of the inspiratory phase. Various types of collection devices are attached to these valves for scavenging as discussed in Chapter 9.

Pressure Gauge (Manometer)

Circle systems have a pressure gauge attached to the absorber (Fig. 8.6). These gauges usually are calibrated in both centimeters of water and millimeters of mercury with positive and negative scales.

The gauge is usually of the diaphragm type shown in Figure 8.6. Changes in pressure in the system are transmitted to the space beneath the diaphragm, causing it to move to the left or right. Movements of the diaphragm are transmitted to the pointer which moves over a calibrated scale.

Breathing Tubes

Breathing tubes were discussed in Chapter 5. The length of the tubes does not influence the

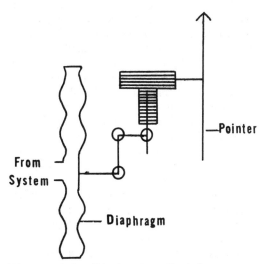

Figure 8.6. Diaphragm-activated pressure gauge. A double pair of thin metal diaphragms possessing a certain degree of elasticity are sealed together, trapping some atmospheric air between them. The pressure of the gases trapped by the diaphragms varies as the pressure of the atmosphere on the outer surface of the enclosure changes. The diaphragms bulge outward or are compressed inward. A series of levers is activated, moving the pointer, which records the pressure.

amount of dead space or rebreathing in the circle system.

Most breathing tubes in use today are disposable plastic. Unfortunately they are sometimes defective. Problems include kinking, indentations, leaks, and separation of components (63, 64).

Reservoir Bags

Bags were discussed in Chapter 5. Bag size should be suited to the size of the patient and the anesthesiologist's hand. Usually bags of 3–5 liters capacity are used for adults. A large bag increases the response time between an alteration in the concentration of the fresh gas and the effect on the inspiratory concentration (55).

The bag is attached to the bag mount (bag extension). When a ventilator is used, the bag is removed and the ventilator connecting hose attached to the bag mount, unless there is a ventilator selector switch. A case has been reported where the reservoir bag mount broke off (65), preventing use of the system.

The Y-Piece (Y-Connector)

The Y-piece is used to join the inspiratory and expiratory tubes to the mask or endotracheal tube. In most disposable systems, the Y-piece and the tubings are permanantly attached. All Y-pieces have two 22-mm male connectors to connect to the breathing tubes. The patient connection port has a 15-mm female connector. This will receive the 15-mm male tracheal tube connector or the mask adaptor which was discussed in Chapter 5. In most cases the patient connection port will have a 22-mm male fitting coaxial with the 15-mm female one. This will allow direct connection between the Y-piece and the mask (Fig. 8.7). The Y-piece may be designed so that the coaxial patient port swivels. A relief valve of the high pressure type may be on top of the Y-piece. A septum extending to the patient connection port may be present to decrease dead space. Some Y-pieces contain unidirectional valves (see section on unidirectional valves).

Swivel Y-pieces found on some disposable systems may be prone to leak (63). Some Y-pieces which are part of a disposable tubing may become detached from the breathing tubes (64).

The Ohio No. 100 inhaler valve which has a shut-off plunger valve mounted on the front part of the Y-piece is shown in Figure 8.8. Figures 8.9 shows a diagram of the inhaler valve. As the knob is turned counterclockwise (A), the stem moves outward. The Y-piece then functions similarly to other Y-pieces. When the knob is turned clockwise (B), the stem moves inward. The gas from the system is prevented from passing to the patient and an opening occurs between patient and atmosphere. The patient can then inhale room air, if breathing spontaneously. This position can be used to check the system for leaks and to prevent loss of gas during intubation, insertion of airways, etc.

The special features of the No. 100 inhaler valve pose a potential hazard. Since this is not a widely used piece of equipment, a user unfa-

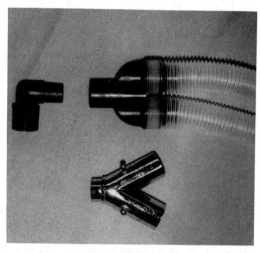

Figure 8.7. Y-pieces. Both Y-pieces shown have a 15-mm female connector and will accept the mask/endotracheal tube adaptor at left. The top Y-piece, which is part of a disposable system, has a coaxial 22-mm male fitting so that it can be attached directly to a mask.

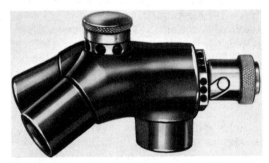

Figure 8.8. No. 100 inhaler valve. (Courtesy of Ohio Medical Products, a division of Airco, Inc.)

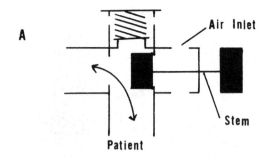

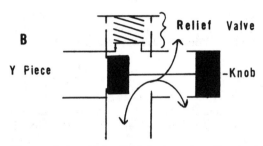

Figure 8.9. Ohio 100 inhaler valve. See text for details.

miliar with it may not be aware that the patient can be excluded from the breathing system. If the valve is in the B position it may be impossible to ventilate the patient.

When a metal Y-piece is used, it is important that care be taken that is does not exert undue pressure on the supraorbital nerve.

Sensor for the Oxygen Monitor

The sensor for the oxygen monitor is usually fitted into the right angle portion of a T-shaped adapter fitted into the breathing system. An alternate adapter is in a specially designed plastic dome over a unidirectional valve. The sensor should be placed so that the tip points downward. This will prevent water from accumulating on the membrane.

Plastic T-shaped adapters may pose special problems. The rocking motion associated with placing the breathing tube on the adapter can cause the adapter to crack. Unless it becomes totally broken, it is difficult to detect. The crack is usually in a ridge and if the plastic is black, it is difficult to see.

Optional Equipment

CIRCULATORS

A circulator is used in the circle system to minimize dead space under the face mask, re-

duce resistance to breathing (especially inspiratory resistance), increase the heat and humidity (66), and reduce the work of breathing (67, 68). The smaller the patient, the more important these considerations become. With a circulator, gases and vapors are mixed more rapidly within the system, eliminating abrupt changes in inspiratory concentrations. The time for changes in fresh gas composition to produce changes in the inspired concentration is also reduced.

The circulator consists of a method of moving gases rapidly around the circle. A Y-piece containing a septum is used to clear exhaled gases from under the mask, reducing the dead space. The same effect can be achieved by using concentric pipes for the mask connection.

The Revell Circulator (67, 70, 71) (Fig. 8.10) employs a turbine-driven fan powered by oxygen, compressed air, or suction. The Neff circulator (72, 73) utilizes the fresh gas flow to run a Venturi device. This eliminates the need for an auxiliary source of power. A magnetic drive circulator powered by compressed air has been developed (68).

To use a circulator, the rate of circulation should be set just high enough to float the discs in the unidirectional valves. The discs will be seen to move slightly with inspiration and expiration. If either unidirectional valve seats momentarily at the patient's peak respiratory flow during either inhalation or exhalation, the effectiveness of the circulator is not impaired as long as the valves are open during the pause before inspiration because it is during this interval that exhaled gases are swept toward the absorber (69). Increasing the rate of circulation beyond

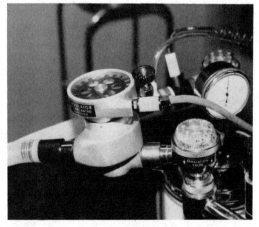

Figure 8.10. Revell circulator. The small black knob is used to regulate the flow.

the point of float by the disc may increase resistance due to turbulence. With increased flow beyond this point, the pressure in the system will rise, accentuating leaks. This rate of circulation needed to float the valve disc will be accompanied by minimal changes in pressure at the patient port. Proper use of a circulator will result in a pressure of up to 1 cm H_2O at the patient connection (55). This is approximately equal to the opening pressure of most relief valves. Resistance to respiration will be less than without the circulator since the unidirectional valves are held open.

Use of a circulator does not affect the fluctuations of the bag with respiration or the anesthesiologist's assisting or controlling respirations by bag squeezing.

Use of a circulator has certain disadvantages. With some types there must be an accessible source of power. The increased pressure may magnify leaks in the system (72). If the circulator is used in a circle containing an in-system vaporizer, vaporization may be accelerated to a hazardous level by the additional flow provided by the circulator (74). It may be necessary to turn off an in-circle vaporizer at least intermittently when a circulator is in use.

With the Neff circulator resistance to the flow of fresh gas will result in a pressure transmitted back to the anesthesia machine (73). This pressure may exaggerate leaks in the machine, change the output of vaporizers and make flowmeter readings erroneous.

BACTERIA FILTERS

One of the disadvantages of the circle system is that it is difficult to clean and/or sterilize certain components, particularly the absorber, ventilator, and unidirectional valves. To help solve this problem, filters have been developed. They have three purposes: (a) protection of the patient from contaminated inspired gases; (b) protection of anesthesia equipment and the hospital environment from exhaled contaminants; and (c) trappings of airborne particulate matter such as dirt, absorbent dust, metallic flakes, etc.

Several different kinds of filters are available for use in anesthesia. Most are disposable, but a few can be sterilized and reused. Most are bidirectional, but a few are unidirectional. They are supplied in three forms: (a) attached to the breathing tube of a disposable circle system; (b) attached to a ventilator hose; and (c) as a separate component (Fig. 8.11).

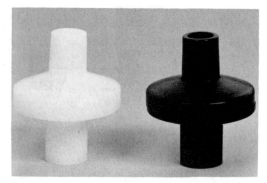

Figure 8.11. Bacterial filter, both conductive and non-conductive versions. (Courtesy of Ohio Medical Products, a division of Airco, Inc.)

Filtration may be accomplished either by a sieve action (porosity or membrane filter) or by employing electrostatic principles to attract and hold microorganisms (depth filter). Porosity filters have small pores. The assumption is that screening out particles of a given size will also screen out pathogenic organisms of a corresponding size. Most pathogenic bacteria are larger than 0.5 μm (75). Filters effective in trapping bacteria down to 0.2–1 μm in size have been produced. Their effectiveness is rated by particulate filtration efficiency, which measures the percentage of a given number of particles of a given size retained by the filter.

Filters employing electrostatic principles rely on the natural electrostatic charge carried by living bacteria and viruses. The filter acts as a magnet. These filters are rated in effectiveness by biological filtration efficiency, which is the percentage of a given number of biologically active organisms in an aerosol retained by the filter.

A variety of materials including fiberglass, foam, and paper have been used for the filter media (76). Most are now treated to reduce wetting.

There are a number of problems with filters. With most resistance increases, sometimes to a hazardous level, with humidity (76, 77). Obstruction of filters due to exhaled blood (78), edema fluid (79), manufacturing defects (80, 81), washing or sterilizing a filter not designed to be washed or sterilized (75, 82), and using a unidirectional filter backwards have all been reported. Some filters absorb significant amounts of anesthetics (75). Soda lime has been noted to penetrate a filter because of inadequate seal of the media edges (76).

The use of bacteria filters is highly controversial and many have questioned whether their inclusion in a breathing system is really necessary. Recent authors have indicated that cross-contamination by breathing systems is not significant (83, 84) and that routine use of filters does not reduce contamination of the equipment or patient or reduce postoperative pulmonary infections (85–89). The use of filters may be indicated in patients requiring respiratory isolation at the time of surgery or to protect patients at increased risk for developing an infection.

In-Circle Vaporizers

In-circle vaporizers were discussed in Chapter 4. They are not used frequently. The vapor output is less predictable than that of out-of-system vaporizers and with today's potent agents this is a great disadvantage.

SELECTOR VALVES (SWITCH VALVES, MODE SELECTOR VALVES, BAG-VENTILATOR SWITCH VALVES, SWITCHING VALVES)

Selector valves provide a rapid and convenient method of changing between manual and automatic ventilation. They may be mounted either on the absorber or the ventilator.

Absorber-Mounted Selector Valve

An absorber-mounted selector valve is shown in Figure 8.12. It has connections for the reservoir bag and for the hose to a ventilator. This device is diagrammed in Figure 8.13A and B. By turning the valve, either the bag or ventilator hose will be included in the system. Another absorber-mounted selector valve is shown in Figure 8.13C. The relief valve on the circle system is included on the bag mount side of the valve so that when the valve is switched to the ventilator mode the relief valve is excluded from the breathing system. This eliminates the necessity of closing the relief valve when switching to the ventilator mode. Selector valves eliminate the need to move the bag and connect the ventilator hose when switching from manual to automatic ventilation and vice versa. They also prevent loss of anesthetic gases and vapors into the room when switching between these modes. The ventilator hose is kept off the floor. Since the bag stays mounted, there is no danger of its becoming lost when the ventilator is in use.

Confusion can result from use of these devices if the user is not familiar with them. If the

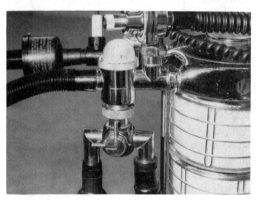

Figure 8.12. Absorber-mounted selector valve.

Breathing System

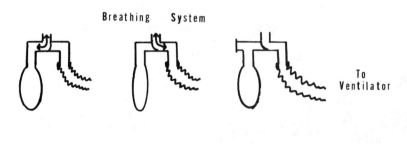

A B C

To Ventilator

Figure 8.13. Absorber-mounted selector valves. *A* shows the bag mode, *B* the ventilator mode. Switching from the bag to ventilator mode is accomplished by turning the valve. This eliminates the need to remove the bag and connect the ventilator hose. *C* shows a newer type of selector valve. The relief valve is on the bag mount side of the valve. When the ventilator mode is selected, the relief valve is excluded from the system. This eliminates the need to close the relief valve when switching to the ventilator mode.

selector valve is in the ventilator mode, but it is intended that the bag be used, confusion may result when increasing the fresh gas flow or using the oxygen flush fails to fill the bag. Pressure buildup in the system will be limited by the pressure-limiting device on the ventilator, however. If the selector valve is in the bag mode when it is intended that the ventilator be used, the patient will not the ventilated, even though the ventilator will continue to cycle. Pressure buildup will be limited by the reservoir bag (see Chapter 5).

A hazard with one of these valves has been reported. A missing retainer ring allowed the valve handle to be positioned so that when the bag was squeezed, gas escaped toward the ventilator. This resulted in a leak in the breathing system (90).

Ventilator-Mounted Selector Valves

This device is shown in Figure 8.14 and diagrammed in Figure 8.15. These devices have been manufactured both as integral parts of ventilators and as accessories. They have three ports. The right-hand port may be part of the ventilator, or provide a port for attachment of a hose leading to the ventilator. The port leading downward is for a bag. The port pointing to the left is for a hose leading to the breathing system.

Hazards exists with these devices. If the hose leading to the breathing system is accidentally connected to the bag port (Figure 8.15C) when the device is in the ventilator mode, the ventilator will continue to cycle, but the patient will

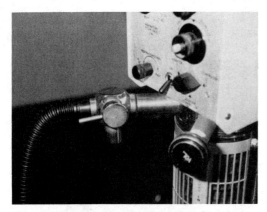

Figure 8.14. Ventilator-mounted selector valve. The port pointing downward is for a bag. Because of hazards associated with this device, it is recommended that these be removed and destroyed.

not be ventilated. Also, since there is no bag in the breathing system to buffer pressure increases (and the relief valve will usually be closed when switching to the ventilator mode) a very rapid pressure buildup will occur (91–93). If the hose is connected to the bag port with the selector valve positioned so that the bag outlet is in circuit (Fig. 8.15D), gas will escape to atmosphere.

One manufacturer altered the selector valve so that the hose from the breathing system would not fit the bag mount (93). Other manufacturers and authors have recommended that ventilator selector valves be removed and destroyed (94, 95).

ARRANGEMENT OF COMPONENTS

Objectives

The following are general objectives in the placement of components.

1. Selective inspiration of fresh gas and ventings of alveolar gas. Fresh and dead space gas should be preferentially included in the inspired gases so that the inspired concentrations approach those in the fresh gas. For this to occur, the system must be able to store fresh gas unmixed with expired gas (96). This increased control over the composition of the inspired mixture will result in faster inductions and awakenings.

The lower the fresh gas flow, the more important this objective becomes, since the lower the fresh gas flow, the longer it takes for changes in fresh gas flow concentrations to be reflected by changes in inspired concentrations.

Faster inductions and emergence will also be aided by selective venting of alveolar gases. During induction when the concentration of anesthetic agent in the fresh gas is higher than in inspired mixtures, it is advantageous that alveolar gases containing low concentrations of anesthetic agents, rather than fresh or dead space gases containing higher concentrations, be eliminated through the relief valve. During emergence, the opposite is true.

2. Minimal consumption of absorbent (97). For efficient absorbent use, the gas vented through the relief valve should have the highest possible concentration of carbon dioxide. This will occur when (a) the exhaled gas does not pass through the absorber before being vented; (b) the exhaled gas is diluted as little as possible either by fresh gas or by previously exhaled gas

Breathing System

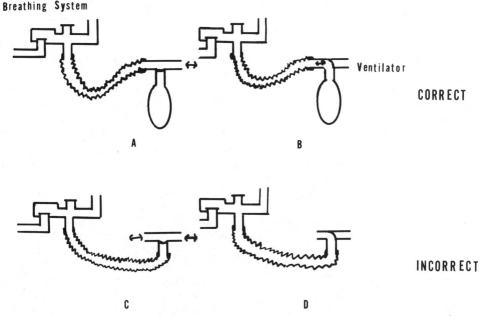

Figure 8.15. Ventilator-mounted selector valve. Switching from the bag mode (B) to the ventilator mode (A) is accomplished by turning the valve. In C and D the hose leading to the breathing system is incorrectly placed on the bag port. With the valve turned to the ventilator mode (C), a dangerous pressure rise will occur in the breathing system, since fresh gas flow into the system will continue and there is no mechanism for buffering or releasing the pressure. The ventilator will continue to cycle and may give no indication that there is a problem. If the ventilator has a disconnection alarm with the sensor in the breathing system, the alarm will not sound. If the sensor is in the ventilator, the alarm will sound. In D the valve is turned to the bag mode, and the hose is open to atmosphere. This will result in a gross leak and it will be impossible to generate enough pressure in the breathing system to ventilate the patient.

that has passed through the absorber; and (c) the vented gas is that exhaled late in exhalation because the first gas exhaled is that from the dead space and contains a very low concentration of carbon dioxide.

As fresh gas flow is reduced, more and more inspired gas must pass through the absorbent, so this objective becomes less important. When using a totally closed system, the arrangement of components should have no effect on the utilization of absorbent, since all the gases will pass through the absorber.

3. Accurate readings from a respirometer placed in the system (98–101). If the fresh gas inlet is positioned so that the fresh gas continuously flows through the respirometer, the respirometer will not measure ventilatory volume accurately.

4. Maximal humidification of inspired gases.

5. Minimal dead space.

6. Low resistance to respiration.

7. Avoidance of hazards. The benefit-to-risk ratio of each arrangement should be considered.

8. Convenience.

Components should be so arranged that they do not create difficulties during use. Tubings and wires should not become tangled. Components should not exert pull on the endotracheal tube or mask. Components should fit securely together and not leak.

Unfortunately, there is no one arrangement of components of the circle system which will meet all of the above objectives. Certain clinical situations may demand that particular objectives be given priority. For example, in pediatric anesthesia, dead space, resistance, and humidification are more significant than in adult anesthesia. In some cases the placing of components may result in a conflict of objectives. For example, venting carbon dioxide upstream of the absorber will conserve absorbent but will tend to reduce inspired humidity, because the amount of heat and humidity produced are directly proportional to the volume of carbon dioxide entering the canister.

Consideration of Individual Components

FRESH GAS INLET

Figure 8.16 shows possible locations of the fresh gas inlet. It is most commonly placed upstream of the inspiratory unidirectional valve and downstream of the absorber (position *A*). In this position fresh gas will collect in the absorber and components between the expiratory unidirectional valve and the absorber during exhalation. The gas between the fresh gas inlet and the bag is pushed backwards during the expiratory phase. At low fresh gas flows, gas vented through the relief valve will be gas that has not yet passed through the absorber. With higher flows, some gas that has been in the absorber may be vented. At very high flows, some fresh gas may be vented.

Placing the fresh gas inflow upstream of the absorber (position *B*) would cause the fresh gas to be diluted before reaching the patient. During induction, anesthetic agent in the fresh gas would be retained in the absorber, resulting in lower concentrations of anesthetic in the inspired mixture and a slower induction (30). Another problem with placing the fresh gas inlet in position *B* is that dust from the absorbent may be blown into the inspiratory limb when a high flow is used, as for example, when the oxygen flush is activated.

Placing the fresh gas inlet in position *B* will prevent gas that has passed into the absorber from being vented through the relief valve. But location of the fresh gas inlet near the relief valve increases the likelihood that fresh gas will be vented.

Position *B* does have an advantage in that it will improve humidification (102–105). This will result in more drying of the absorbent, especially if high gas flows are used. Since dry absorbent absorbs more anesthetic agent than humidified absorbent, more agent will be retained in the absorbent, slowing induction. Also subsequent patients will be subjected to more volatile agent as it is released by the absorbent.

Placing the fresh gas flow upstream of the bag and relief valve (position *E*) would have all the disadvantages of position *B* and would result in considerable venting of fresh gas.

Placing the fresh gas inflow upstream of the expiratory unidirectional valve (position *D*) has all the disadvantages of positions *B* and *E*. In addition, during inspiration the fresh gas flow would force exhaled gases back toward the patient, causing dangerous rebreathing.

Position *C* was originally advocated to reduce the dead space by sweeping exhaled gases out of the Y-piece during exhalation (97). If the unidirectional valves are competent, there should be only slight retrograde flow at the Y-piece. With incompetent valves, even a high inflow cannot prevent the rebreathing of exhaled gases (97). If the Y-piece has a septum, placement of the fresh gas inlet in this position will wash out dead space under a mask.

With the inflow in position *C*, during exhalation, fresh gas would join the exhaled gases and escape though the relief valve without reaching the patient. This would result in poor economy of fresh gas (106) and inefficient use of absorbent (97) because fresh gas would dilute the concentration of carbon dioxide in the gas vented through the relief valve.

Another disadvantage of placing the fresh gas inlet downstream of the inspiratory unidirectional valve is that a respirometer placed on the exhalation side of the circuit will not record tidal or minute volumes accurately (55, 98–101). The reason for this is that during exhalation both exhaled and fresh gases will be passing through the respirometer. The respirometer will continue to register flow even if the patient is apneic. Accurate respirometer readings can still be obtained by turning off the fresh gas flow temporarily (100), or by placing the respirometer

Fresh Gas Inlet Placement

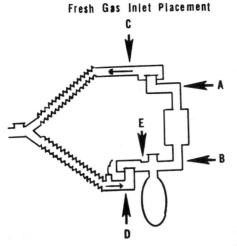

Figure 8.16. Possible locations for the fresh gas inlet. See text for details.

between the Y-piece and the mask or tracheal tube connector (101).

A final disadvantage of position C is that if the oxygen flush were used and if there were an obstruction in the exhalation limb of the breathing system, the patient would be exposed to a sudden rapid increase in pressure (107). With the fresh gas inlet in other positions the increase in pressure would be slower because it would be dissipated through the relief valve and buffered with the bag.

Position C was found to be advantageous compared to position A in an experimental model using controlled ventilation without carbon dioxide absorption (108). The authors attributed the greater efficiency to variations in the degree of mixing of fresh and exhaled gas in the system.

THE RESERVOIR BAG

Figure 8.17 shows possible locations for the reservoir bag. The most common location is between the exhalation unidirectional valve and the absorber (position A).

During spontaneous ventilation, absorbent use is equally efficient if the bag is on the inspiratory (position D) or the expiratory side of the absorber (position A) (97). During controlled or assisted ventilation, more efficient use occurs with the bag on the exhalation side (position A) (97). If the bag is on the inspiratory side exhaled gases would pass through the absorber to the bag during exhalation. Squeezing the bag during inhalation would cause the gases to reverse flow and pass retrograde through the

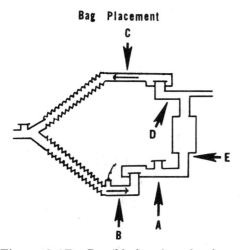

Bag Placement

Figure 8.17. Possible locations for the reservoir bag. See text for details.

absorber, to be vented through the relief valve. This would result in inefficient absorbent use, since gases cleared of carbon dioxide would be vented.

Bag position is also important because when a mechanical ventilator is used, the relief valve in the system is closed and excess gases are vented through the ventilator. The position of the bag will determine the position of the relief valve when a ventilator is used. If the bag is placed in position D, fresh gas will be lost through the relief valve and exhaled gases must pass through the absorber before being vented.

Placing the bag on the exhalation side will result in decreased resistance to exhalation because the patient does not exhale through the absorber (109). During spontaneous ventilation, this advantage may be offset by the increase in inspiratory resistance but during controlled or assisted ventilation, only expiratory resistance need be considered because the inspiratory effort will be supplied by the anesthesiologist's hand or the ventilator.

A disadvantage of placing the bag on the exhalation side is that the sudden increase in pressure from squeezing the bag may force dust from the absorber into the inspiratory tubing (110).

Another possible position for the bag is position E, at the bottom of an absorber on the downstream side. An advantage may be better humidification. Chalon and co-workers (111, 112) pointed out that condensation of water occurs in the space below the absorbent. Location of the bag at the bottom of the absorber would provide maximum passage of gas over this water. A disadvantage to position E is that dust from the absorbent may collect in this area. A hard squeeze of the bag could force a cloud of this dust into the inspiratory limb of the breathing system (37).

If the bag is placed between the patient and either of the unidirectional valves (positions B or C), it would form a reservoir for exhaled gases which would then be rebreathed.

UNIDIRECTIONAL VALVES

Two locations have been used for the unidirectional valves (Fig. 8.18): in the Y-piece (position B) or attached to the absorber (position A).

Placing the valves in the Y-piece offers the advantage of eliminating backflow of exhaled gases into the inspiratory tubing if there is a

Unidirectional Valve Placement

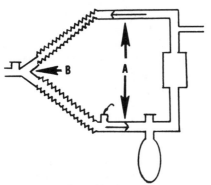

Figure 8.18. Possible locations for the unidirectional valves. See text for details.

leak between the absorber and the patient. This is not a frequent problem. In normal circumstances backflow into this tubing is insignificant.

During spontaneous ventilation, the location of the unidirectional valves does not affect the life of the absorbent. With controlled ventilation, placing the valves in the Y-piece results in more efficient use (97). This is because, with controlled ventilation, a higher pressure is present during inspiration. This causes the breathing tubings to expand so that the volume of gas in them is increased. During exhalation the pressure in the system falls and if the unidirectional valves are at the absorber, this additional gas mixes with the expired gases. This lowers the carbon dioxide concentration of the gas flowing through the relief valve. Locating the valves in the Y-piece prevents the mixing of fresh gases with exhaled gases during exhalation. There is also greater economy of fresh gas with the unidirectional valves in the Y-piece during controlled ventilation.

Disadvantages of placing the valves in the Y-piece include the fact that they are bulky (especially with scavenging apparatus attached), difficult to see, and have a higher resistance than large unidirectional valves placed on the absorber (113). Also, flushing with oxygen will not clear the inspiratory limb.

Of great significance are the serious accidents that have occurred when a valved Y-piece was placed by error into a system with an absorber which also had valves (59–61). If the valves are not in phase with each other, the patient cannot be ventilated or breathe spontaneously (see discussion of the Y-piece.)

HIGH-PRESSURE RELIEF VALVE

Figure 8.19 indicates the possible locations for the relief valve in the system.

Spontaneous Respiration

During spontaneous respiration, the most efficient use of absorbent occurs with the relief valve on the Y-piece (position *A*) (97, 113). This is because during spontaneous respiration overflow occurs in the latter part of exhalation. Gas exhaled during the first part of exhalation is dead space gas with a low concentration of carbon dioxide. Because the relief valve is not open, this gas passes by the relief valve. When the bag is filled, the pressure in the system rises and the relief valve opens. Since this opening occurs during the latter part of exhalation, the gases coming from the patient (and being expelled through the relief valve) consist mainly of alveolar gas (with a high carbon dioxide content). No such discrimination is possible when the relief valve is distant from the patient (113).

Problems may occur with the relief valve at the Y piece. The added weight (especially when scavenging apparatus is added) may increase the incidence of disconnections. Transfer tubing from this position to the scavenging interface may become entangled with other things. In addition, the valve will be difficult to adjust in head and neck cases.

Absorbent use is quite inefficient if the relief valve is at *C* or *D*, since any gas vented would have passed through the absorber. If the relief valve is placed between the patient and the

Relief Valve Placement

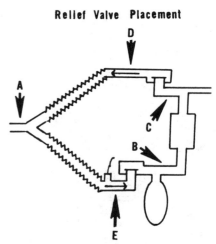

Figure 8.19. Possible locations for the relief valve. See text for details.

absorber (positions *E* or *B*) only gas that has not passed through the absorber will be vented.

If the relief valve is placed at *C*, much of the fresh gas will be vented. Fresh gas may be vented if the relief valve is at *B*, but only if the fresh gas flow is quite high.

If the relief valve is in position *D*, exhaled gases will move retrograde into the inspiratory tubing on expiration, causing an increase in dead space.

Controlled or Assisted Ventilation

During controlled or assisted ventilation, overflow occurs during inspiration. If the relief valve is at the Y-piece (position *A*), fresh gas and gas that has previously passed through the absorbent are vented to atmosphere. This results in inefficient use of absorbent (97, 113). The same holds true if the relief valve is located at *C* or *D*. Locating the relief valve between the patient and the absorber (positions *E* or *B*) should result in more efficient use of absorbent, although some fresh gas may dilute the carbon dioxide being vented at *E* and at *B* there may be venting of gas that has contacted absorbent.

Considerable venting of fresh gas will occur with the relief valve at *C*, *D*, or *A*. There will be some venting if it is located at *E*. Fresh gas will be vented at *B* only if the fresh gas flow is quite high.

An exception to using position *A* with controlled or assisted respiration is if the unidirectional valves are in the Y-piece (113). Then the most economical arrangement is with the relief valve on the downstream side of the exhalation unidirectional valve near the patient (106, 113).

THE LOW-PRESSURE RELIEF VALVE

With both spontaneous and controlled ventilation, the low-pressure relief valve vents gas at the end of the expiratory pause. The most efficient position for the low-pressure relief valve for both spontaneous and controlled respiration is position *A* (Fig. 8.19) at the Y-piece near the patient. This results in good economy of fresh gas and efficient absorbent use (113–115). A disadvantage of this location is that the force of the patient's exhalations will be greatest at this position and may close the valve.

Positions *E* and *B* do not allow as much discrimination between alveolar and dead space as position *A*, because of their distance from the patient, but may be used if there are difficulties with the valve in position *A*.

Placing a low-pressure relief valve in positions *C* or *D* will result in overflow of fresh gas. Placing it in position *D* will also allow retrograde flow in the inspiratory tubing during exhalation.

BACTERIA FILTERS

As shown in Figure 8.20, four positions have been recommended for placement of bacteria filters. Another possible location is in the ventilator hose.

Position *A* is between the inhalation tubing and the Y-piece. A filter here will protect the patient from contamination and absorbent dust, but does not protect the absorber or the operating room environment. This puts the filter near the patient, which may be a problem if the filter is heavy or bulky. Bacteria filters should not be located at position *A* if a humidifier is located upstream.

Position *B* is between the Y-piece and the exhalation tubing. In this position the absorber and exhalation tubing will be protected. If the filter is upstream of the relief valve, the operating room environment will be protected. Water, mucus, or edema fluid can collect in the filter in this position, causing an increase in resistance or obstruction (79). The weight of the filter may make it unsuitable to this location. Most disposable systems do not allow the interposition of a filter at positions *A* or *B*.

Position *C* is between the inspiratory tubing and the inspiratory unidirectional valve. A filter in this position will protect the patient from contamination from the absorber and its attached parts but not the inhalation tubing. It

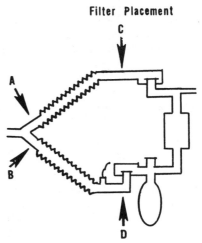

Filter Placement

Figure 8.20. Possible locations for bacterial filter. See text for details.

will catch absorbent dust. It does not protect the absorber or the operating room air from contamination by the patient. The size or weight of the filter is not a problem in this position. If a humidifier is used, it should be downstream of the filter.

Position D is between the exhalation unidirectional valve and the exhalation tubing. In this position the filter will protect the internal parts of the absorber and other components from contamination, but the exhalation tubing will become contaminated. If the filter is upstream from the relief valve, the operating room environment is protected. Since the filter is on the expiratory side, obstruction with fluid may occur (79).

IN-SYSTEM VAPORIZER

Two positions are commonly used for in-system vaporizers. One is on the inspiratory side downstream of the fresh gas inlet and the alternate on the exhalation side upstream of the relief valve and unidirectional valve. Either of these locations allow secure anchoring to the absorber so the vaporizer will not be tipped.

Placing an in-circle vaporizer on the inspiratory side results in faster inductions since the fresh gas must pass through the vaporizer before delivery to the patient. An additional advantage is since the fresh gas is dry, the problem of water condensation in the vaporizer is less.

Placing the vaporizer on the expiratory side has the following disadvantages:

1. Moisture from exhaled gases may condense in the vaporizer, decreasing its output.

2. Induction will be slower than with the vaporizer on the inhalation side for several reasons: (a) Before reaching the patient, the vaporizer output will be diluted by gas in the tubings and in the absorber by fresh gas entering the system. (b) During the passage around the circle, some vapor will be absorbed by the tubings and the absorbent. (c) Some vapor will be lost through the relief valve.

SENSOR FOR OXYGEN MONITOR

Figure 8.21 shows possible locations for the oxygen monitor sensor. In positions H and I the sensor is inserted into the dome of a unidirectional valve.

Positions B, F, A, and H are on the inspiratory side. Position B, between the Y-piece and the tracheal tube or mask, has several disadvantages. Placing the sensor at this point will increase dead space, which may be significant in small patients. Placing the sensor at this location may cause the cable to the analyzer box to stretch and cause a pull on the Y-piece and increases the likelihood that it will become entangled with other tubings and wires.

Position F has the disadvantage that most disposable systems do not allow interposition at this point. In addition, pull from the cable may be a problem. With positions A and H the cable usually will not be stretched.

Positions G, E, I, and C are on the exhalation side of the system. If low fresh gas flows are used, the reading may be considerably lower than on the inspiratory side. Even with a closed system the inspired-expired difference is only about 4–6%. Placing the sensor on the expiratory side will usually expose it to more humidity, but with most sensors this is not a problem. Most disposable systems will not permit the sensor to be placed at G.

It has been advocated that the sensor be placed in a position near the Y-piece (positions G, F or B), so that the oxygen analyzer will act as a disconnect alarm in the event of disconnection at the tracheal tube. While it is true that this is the most common site for disconnections, they may occur in other locations. With a high fresh gas flow, the oxygen concentration may not fall sufficiently for the alarm to sound. An oxygen analyzer should *not* be regarded as a disconnect alarm.

Position D is on the hose which delivers anesthetic gas to the breathing system. If the sensor is placed in this position, the monitor will indicate only the concentration of oxygen delivered to the breathing system, and not the concentration the patient is breathing.

CIRCULATOR

A circulator may be placed either on the exhalation or inhalation side of the absorber. Its weight and positional requirements make other locations impractical.

The mean under-mask pressure that occurs when a circulator is used depends on where in the circle the circulator is placed (70). If placed on the inspiratory side there will be an increase in pressure under the mask, which increases with circulation. If the circulator is placed on the expiratory side, the under-mask pressure will be negative.

SPIROMETER

A spirometer may be placed in several locations in the circle system. Some have special adaptors for attaching them securely at particular locations.

They are usually placed on the expiratory side. During spontaneous respiration they will read accurately. During controlled respiration, they will overread, due to expansion of the tubings (100, 101).

A spirometer placed between the tracheal tube connector or mask and the Y-piece will record accurately with both spontaneous and controlled ventilation. Some are too bulky to place in this position and the increase in dead space may be significant in pediatric patients. Also when used in this position they are frequently dropped on the floor.

They may be placed on the inspiratory side, but if there is a leak between the spirometer and the patient, the volume recorded will be higher than that received by the patient. During controlled ventilation, they will overread, due to expansion of the tubings.

PRESSURE SENSOR

Pressure sensors can be placed anywhere in the breathing system that the oxygen sensor can be placed (Fig. 8.21). Most disposable systems do not allow placement at positions F or G. Position B has the same disadvantages as placing the oxygen sensor at that point. In order to

place the pressure sensor in the fresh gas line (position D) a special adaptor would be needed. In addition the small diameter of the tubing and high flow of gas might give false readings.

Positions A, C, I, E, and H provide a stable place to locate the sensor. In order to use positions I or H special modifications would need to be made to the domes over the unidirectional valves. T-piece adaptors could be used in positions A, E, and C. Positions C and E on the expiratory side would have an advantage over position A because the flow of gas from the oxygen flush would have less effect of that location. Also the sensor is less likely to be "fooled" by an obstruction to flow in the inspiratory limb if placed on the exhalation side.

RESISTANCE OF THE CIRCLE SYSTEM

The most important components in the circle influencing resistance are the relief valve, the unidirectional valves (23, 116) and the canister (23, 117–119). Use of a circulator will reduce the resistance imposed by unidirectional valves.

Figures for the total resistance of a circle system are difficult to obtain. It will depend on, among other things, the fresh gas flow (which influences the flow through the relief valve) and the pattern of ventilation (which influences the flowrate through the canister and valves).

Figures for the total resistance of a circle system containing a modern absorber and with the relief valve closed are shown in Table 8.2. The influence of the pattern of ventilation on resistance is seen in this table. The pressure swings increase with increases in respiratory rate and tidal volume.

One of the main objections to the use of an adult circle system for small children has been

O₂ Analyzer Placement

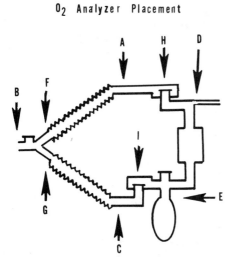

Figure 8.21. Possible locations for sensor for oxygen monitor. See text for details.

Table 8.2.
Resistance to Ventilation of Circle System*

Frequency	Tidal Volume	Pressure Swing
min	*cc*	*cm H₂O*
12	500	$-1 + \frac{1}{2}$
12	1000	$-1 + 1$
12	1600	$-2 + 1\frac{1}{2}$
24	500	$-1 + 1$
24	1000	$-3 + 1\frac{1}{2}$
44	500	$-4 + 3$

* From Young TM: Carbon dioxide absorber. *Anaesthesia* 26:78, 1971.

that it causes a high resistance. However, since resistance depends on flowrate and flowrates for children are small, an adult circle system may be used with spontaneously breathing infants (120–122). Other problems, such as dead space, should be considered before this is attempted, however.

DEAD SPACE IN THE CIRCLE SYSTEM

In the circle system dead space extends into the Y-piece as far as the partition. Using a Y-piece with a septum will decrease dead space. The dead space does not extend the entire length of the breathing tubes to the unidirectional valves on the machine. Immediately before closure of the unidirectional valves, the columns of gases in the breathing tubes move in the opposite direction from their usual flow until stopped abruptly by closure of the valves. This regurgitation of gases is referred to as "backlash" and causes a slight increase in dead space. If the valves are competent, however, backlash will be clinically insignificant.

HEAT AND HUMIDITY

Several investigators (123–125) have found that gases in the inspiratory limb of a modern circle system are near room temperature. Shanks and co-workers (126) found that with low fresh gas flows (1 liter/min) the inspired gases were approximately 2° C above room temperature.

Chalon and associates (123) studied the humidity of the circle system. Their results for a "standard adult" system, using a fresh gas flow of 5 liters/min are shown in Figure 8.22. The inspired humidity initially was 30%. This rose to 61% in 100–120 min, stabilizing at this level. These values may be altered by:

1. Changing the fresh gas flow. Decreasing the fresh gas flow from 5 liters/min to 500 ml/min resulted in an initial humidity of 47.5% which increased to 93% where it stabilized.

2. Changes in carbon dioxide output by the patient. Chalon and co-workers (123) found that reduction of the patient's carbon dioxide output decreased the initial and final humidity slightly.

3. Changes in minute ventilation. Increasing ventilation, by mobilizing water from the absorber, will increase the humidity (123).

4. Prior use of the system. Chalon (123) found that prior use of the system resulted in an initially higher humidity that stabilized in the same period of time at the same final humidity.

5. Position of components of the system. Several investigators (103, 105, 127, 128) found that a significant increase in humidity of inspired gas is attained by directing the fresh gas through the absorber before it goes to the inspiratory limb.

6. Wetting the inspiratory tubing (129, 130).

7. Heating the canister (127).

8. Use of a circulator (66, 131). The addition of a circulator provides a dramatic increase in humidity as well as an increase in temperature.

9. Unusual modifications to the circle system. Modifications to the circle system to increase inspired humidity include coaxial inspiratory and expiratory tubings (111, 112, 132–134), utilizing the heat of reaction to vaporize water (132, 133, 135) and directing the fresh gas flow through the absorber (111, 122).

In the circle system moisture is available from three sources (125): (a) exhaled gases; (b) the water content of the absorbent granules, both in

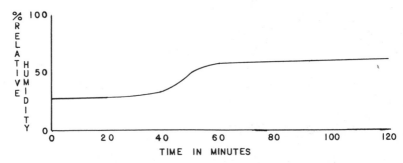

Figure 8.22. Humidity changes in the circle system with use. Fresh gas flow 5000 ml/min; CO_2 inflow 200 ml/min; respiratory rate 12/min and tidal volume 500 ml. (From Chalon J, Kao ZL, Dolorico VN, Atkin DH: Humidity output of the circle absorber system. *Anesthesiology* 38:462, 1973.)

the granular and perigranular spaces; and (c) water liberated from the neutralization of carbon dioxide. Dery and colleagues (125) showed that most of the inspired humidity in the circle system was supplied by the water content of the granules with exhaled gases making a small contribution. The amount of water derived from the reaction of carbon dioxide was negligible.

The temperature rise in an upstream canister is due to the heat of reaction of neutralization. The temperature in the downstream canister, until the absorbent in the upstream canister is exhausted, is influenced by warm gases from the upstream canister flowing through it. Water evaporated by the heat of neutralization moves downstream and condenses. The upstream absorbent gets drier and the downstream becomes wetter.

Inside a modern absorber Lumley found that the temperature rarely exceeds 40°C (136), although Chalon and co-workers (123) recorded temperatures as high as 43°C. The temperature at the center of an absorber is consistently higher than that at the periphery.

RELATIONSHIP BETWEEN INSPIRED AND DELIVERED CONCENTRATIONS

In a system with no rebreathing, the concentrations of gases and vapors in the inspired mixture will be close to those in fresh gas. With rebreathing, however, the concentrations in the inspired mixture may differ considerably from those in the fresh gas.

The four principal components of the inspired mixture will be considered: nitrogen, carbon dioxide, oxygen, and anesthetic agents.

Nitrogen

The importance of nitrogen lies in the fact that when it is a large component of the inspired mixture it hinders the establishment of high tensions of anesthetic agents (primarily nitrous oxide) and may cause low inspired oxygen tensions.

Before any fresh gas is delivered to the breathing system, nitrogen is present in approximately 80% concentration. It enters the system from exhaled gases and leaves through the relief valve and leaks.

The rate of elimination of nitrogen from the breathing system during the early part of an anesthetic is influenced primarily by the amount of rebreathing. Using high gas flows for a few minutes to eliminate most of the nitrogen in the system and the patient's functional residual capacity and well perfused body tissues is called "denitrogenation." The rate of denitrogenation in a circle system was studied by Hamilton and associates (137). Figure 8.23 shows denitrogenation curves with fresh gas flows of 5 and 10 liters/min. Using flows in excess of 5 liters/min decreased the time of denitrogenation only slightly. Most authorities recommend that when nitrous oxide is used with a circle system that high flows of fresh gas be used initially to achieve denitrogenation.

After an initial period of high rate, nitrogen elimination by the patient will proceed at a slower rate. In a closed system, the nitrogen concentration will gradually rise. Provided denitrogenation has been carried out, even if all the body's nitrogen is exhaled, the concentration of nitrogen cannot increase to more than 10% (138).

Carbon Dioxide

Carbon dioxide enters the circle only from the patient. Unlike nitrogen, the rate of carbon dioxide elimination from the patient does not usually change substantially with time.

WITH ABSORBENT

The inspired carbon dioxide concentration should be near 0. Accumulation of carbon dioxide may arise from failure of one or both unidirectional valves (54, 139), exhausted absorbent, or the absorber bypass mechanism being turned on. Fresh gas flow should have no effect on carbon dioxide concentration in the inspired gases. Arterial carbon dioxide concentration should depend only on ventilation.

WITHOUT ABSORBENT

A number of investigations using the circle system without absorbent have been published (140–151), with various recommendations for fresh gas flow and ventilation. The arterial carbon dioxide level achieved will depend on the fresh gas flow, the arrangement of circle system components, and ventilation. Suggested advantages of not using absorbent include the following: (a) ability to achieve the desired level of carbon dioxide with hyperventilation; (b) elimination of possible inhalation of absorbent dust; (c) no dependence on absorbent to eliminate CO_2; and (d) low resistance. Disadvantages in-

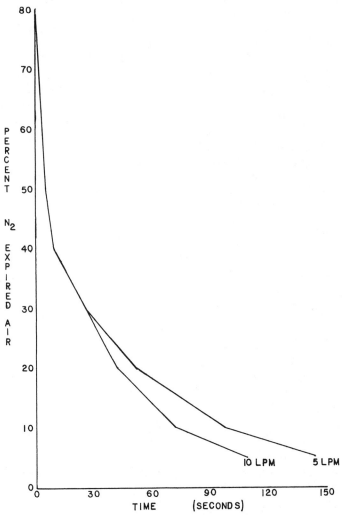

Figure 8.23. Denitrogenation curves of circle system. Flows in excess of 5 liters/min decrease denitrogenation time only slightly. (From Hamilton WK, Eastwood DW: A study of denitrogenation with some inhalation anesthetic systems. *Anesthesiology* 16:861–867, 1955.)

clude the need for uneconomical high flows and difficulty in predicting arterial carbon dioxide.

Oxygen

Oxygen enters the system by way of the fresh gas flow. It leaves through patient uptake, the relief valve and leaks in the system. The gas mixture inspired by the patient will be composed of a combination of fresh gas flow and gas previously exhaled that has traversed the circle. Except during induction using high concentrations of nitrous oxide and when the concentration of oxygen in the fresh gas flow is lowered,

the concentration of oxygen in exhaled gas will be lower than that in the fresh gas.

The following influence the concentration of oxygen in the inspired mixture: (a) uptake and elimination of other gases by the patient; (b) arrangement of the components of the circle; (c) oxygen uptake by the patient; (d) ventilation; (e) fresh gas flow and (f) the concentration of oxygen in the fresh gas.

UPTAKE AND ELIMINATION OF OTHER GASES BY THE PATIENT

Of the common anesthetic gases, only nitrous oxide is administered in sufficiently high concentrations for this to have an appreciable effect. The higher the uptake of nitrous oxide, the higher the inspired oxygen concentration. The highest uptake of nitrous oxide occurs during the first few minutes of administration. Uptake then falls, the rate of fall depending on ventilation and the fresh gas flow. Even after anesthesia has been in progress for a considerable period of time great variations in uptake will be present.

ARRANGEMENT OF COMPONENTS OF THE CIRCLE

Arranging the components of the circle system so as to achieve selective inspiration of fresh gas (see section on arrangement of components) will increase the inspired oxygen concentration.

UPTAKE OF OXYGEN BY THE PATIENT

The greater the patient's oxygen uptake, the lower the oxygen concentration in expired gases and therefore in the inspired gas mixture. Oxygen uptake is affected by many factors, shows great variation among patients, and may vary during the course of anesthesia (152).

VENTILATION

If the fresh gas flow remains the same while alveolar ventilation is increased, the percentage of oxygen in the inspired mixture will decrease because more of the inspired gas must be derived from previously exhaled gas. This has a limiting value because as ventilation increases the concentration of oxygen in the exhaled gases will increase.

FRESH GAS FLOW

The higher the fresh gas flow, the higher the inspired oxygen concentration will be. The difference between delivered and inspired oxygen is increased by decreasing the fresh gas flow.

CONCENTRATION OF OXYGEN IN THE FRESH GAS FLOW

The higher the concentration of oxygen in the fresh gas flow, the higher its concentration will be in the inspired mixture.

Thus inspired oxygen concentration is affected by a number of factors that vary greatly. Only three—ventilation, fresh gas flow, and con-

centration of oxygen in the fresh gas—can usually be varied by the anesthesiologist. Ventilation cannot be varied much without risking arterial hypoxemia and hypercapnia. Both fresh gas flow and concentration of oxygen in the fresh gas flow can be varied over a wide range. It is a common practice to use high fresh gas flows to keep the difference between the inspired and fresh gas concentrations small. Use of high flows is uneconomical and has other disadvantages and use of lower flows is becoming more popular.

Irrespective of what flows or agents are used, the authors of this book feel that the use of a reliable, calibrated oxygen analyzer is mandatory for safe anesthesia. In these days of technological development and sophisticated equipment, there should be no room for guesswork when such an important matter as inspired oxygen concentration is concerned.

Anesthetic Agent

The concentration of an anesthetic agent in the inspired mixture in the circle system is a complex subject. For discussion purposes, it can be divided into two situations: with the vaporizer inside the circle and the vaporizer outside the circle. Anesthetic gases such as nitrous oxide and cyclopropane which are supplied from outside the circle behave the same as anesthetic vapors from out-of-circle vaporizers. Only induction will be considered.

VAPORIZER OUTSIDE THE CIRCLE

With the vaporizer outside the circle vaporization is effected by fresh gas flow only. During induction the highest concentration of anesthetic agent will be in the fresh gas line. The following factors will influence the concentration of agent in the inspired mixture: (a) uptake by the patient; (b) uptake by components of the system; (c) arrangement of system components; (d) uptake and elimination of other gases by the patient; (e) volume of the system; (f) concentration in the fresh gas flow and (g) fresh gas flow.

Uptake of Anesthetic Agent by the Patient

Uptake of anesthetic agent by the patient will lower the concentration in the exhaled, and hence in the inspired, mixture. The rate of uptake will depend on the concentration in the inspired mixture, ventilation, factors relating to the patient such as dead space, pulmonary shunting, and time. Rate of uptake is usually high initially then falls—fairly rapidly at first, then more and more slowly.

Uptake by Components of the Circle

Anesthetic agents will be taken up by rubber, plastic, metal, and absorbent (30–32, 153–156). This will delay the rise of concentration in the inspired mixture.

Arrangement of Components of the Circle

Achievement of high inspired concentrations of anesthetic agent will be enhanced by an arrangement of circle system components that favors selective inspiration of fresh gases (see discussion on arrangement of components).

Uptake and Elimination of Other Gases

Uptake of other gases, including oxygen, by the patient will cause the concentration of anesthetic agent in the exhaled gas to rise. This in turn will raise the concentration in the inspired mixture. Elimination of nitrogen will dilute concentrations and slow induction. Carbon dioxide elimination should have little effect because it will be absorbed.

Volume of the System

The greater the volume of the system, the more dilution of exhaled gases will occur. This will lower the exhaled concentration of anesthetic agent and so slow the rise of inspired agent concentration. Pediatric circle systems with low volume allow more control over the inspired concentration at low fresh gas flows than do larger systems.

Concentration of the Fresh Gas Flow

The higher the concentration of anesthetic agent in the fresh gas the higher the inspired concentration.

Fresh Gas Flow

The higher the fresh gas flow the faster the inspired concentration will approach that of the fresh gas. As fresh gas flow increases the effect of other factors such as uptake by the patient and components of the circle system decreases.

Because of these many factors, it is never possible to predict the concentration of gases within the circle accurately unless a high fresh gas flow is used. The greatest variation occurs during induction, when anesthetic uptake is high and nitrogen excretion by the patient dilutes the gases in the circuit. For this reason, most authors recommend that anesthesia be begun with high fresh gas flows (96, 158). Several devices are now available to measure the concentration of anesthetic agent in the inspired or expired gas mixture.

VAPORIZER INSIDE THE CIRCLE

With the vaporizer inside the circle, vaporization is brought about by mixed fresh and exhaled gases passing through the vaporizer. The concentration of anesthetic agent will be highest in the gas leaving the vaporizer and 0 in the fresh gas flow. The vaporizer concentration will not be equal to the vaporizer output except at the start of an anesthetic. As time passes and anesthetic agent recirculates, the vaporizer output will tend to rise. This will be offset by two factors. First, most in-circle vaporizers have minimal temperature compensation, so that the vaporizer output will fall with time if the setting remains the same. Secondly, with time water from the absorbent or patient will condense in the vaporizer. The specific gravity of most anesthetic agents is greater than water, so the water will tend to remain on the surface, decreasing vaporization.

With an in-circle vaporizer, vaporization depends on ventilation. The greater the ventilation, the greater the amount of agent vaporized. Increased ventilation also results in increased uptake by the patient, which may lower the concentration. This provides the in-circle vaporizer with a safety factor during spontaneous ventilation. Most anesthetic agents depress respirations, reducing the gas flow through the vaporizer so that the concentration in the circle rises less rapidly. With controlled ventilation this safety factor is lost. Controlled ventilation with an in-circle vaporizer is dangerous because the higher minute volume will result in increased vaporization.

Prediction of inspired anesthetic concentrations with the vaporizer inside the circle is so complex that it is impossible for all practical purposes. For this reason and the dangers of using controlled ventilation, most anesthesiologists prefer to have the vaporizer outside the circle.

PEDIATRIC CIRCLE SYSTEMS

Several pediatric circle systems have been described. All employ the same basic components as the adult systems. Smaller tubings, bags, and absorbers are used. The Y-piece usually has a septum to reduce dead space.

Bloomquist Pediatric Circle System (159)

Figure 8.24 shows a diagram of two possible arrangements of the Bloomquist pediatric circle system. The system is mounted on a flat metal base in which two horizontal parallel channels have been drilled. A relief valve and pressure gauge connect to one channel. At one end of each channel are located a unidirectional valve and connection for a breathing tube. The other end of either channel can be connected to either the fresh gas inlet or the reservoir bag. A third arrangement is to connect both the fresh gas inlet and the bag to the same hole and plug the unused hole, as originally described by Bloomquist. By interchanging positions of the tubes, plug and bag, the direction of flow through the canister can be varied. Arrangement *B* (Figure 8.24), with the fresh gas flow on the upstream side of the canister, results in increased humidity (160).

Two vertical holes are drilled into the surface of the block, each connecting with one of the two horizontal channels. The first vertical hole contains a circular mounting into which a small

transparent canister will seat. The second vertical hole accommodates a tube connecting to the upper end of the absorber.

The Bloomquist system is shown in Figure 8.25. The base contains a central mounting hose to receive the post of the support boom supplied with the unit. Components have 15-mm male and female fittings with a sequence of female to male in the direction of gas flow. The system is available with a valved Y-piece and a high-pressure relief valve attached to the Y-piece, as shown in Figure 8.25. A disadvantage of the Bloomquist is that the absence of a drain in the bottom of the absorber may cause water to accumulate in the channels with resultant corrosion (160).

Ohio Infant Circle Absorber System

The Ohio infant circle absorber system is shown in Figure 8.26. The fresh gas inlet is downstream of the inspiratory unidirectional valve and the Y-piece contains a septum. This combination provides a steady flow of gas to wash out the dead space under the face mask (161).

The relief valve is on the inspiratory side of the absorber. This causes increased resistance to exhalation because the patient must exhale through the absorber. Absorbent use is ineffi-

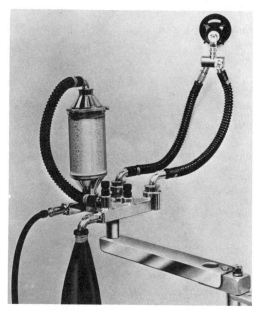

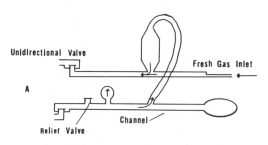

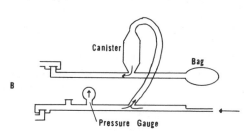

Figure 8.24. Bloomquist pediatric circle system. (From Bloomquist ER: Pediatric circle absorber. *Anesthesiology* 28:787–789, 1957.)

Figure 8.25. Bloomquist pediatric circle system. (Courtesy of Foregger, Division of Puritan-Bennett Corporation.)

cient because all exhaled gases must pass through the absorber before being vented through the relief valve.

Two bag connections (*A* and *B*) are present, one on each side of the absorber (Fig. 8.27), so that the bag may be positioned on either the exhalation or inhalation side of the absorber. Placing the bag on the exhalation side (position *B*) causes less expiratory resistance. A plastic cap is provided for the unused opening.

If the fresh gas inflow is at the alternate (*B*) bag port which allows the fresh gas to first pass through the absorber, the inspired humidity will be increased (105, 162).

The canister is divided vertically by a septum. The gases rise through one side and descend through the other. When the canister is rotated counterclockwise, the absorber is cut out of the

breathing circuit so that the absorbent can be changed while anesthesia is being administered. Two sizes of canisters are available.

The Ohio infant circle absorber system is shown in Figure 8.27. It is easily mounted on an operating table. The top of the absorber is made of clear plastic so that the color change of the absorbent can be observed.

Columbia Pediatric Valve Circle System (163)

The Columbia circle valve (163) is a modified Y-piece plus mask adaptor. The unidirectional valves are incorporated into it and the inspiratory and expiratory pathways are divided so that the dead space is low. Usually a high-pressure relief valve is placed just distal to the expiratory unidirectional valve.

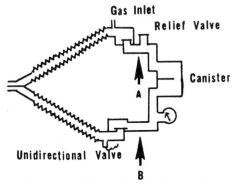

Figure 8.26. Ohio infant circle absorber system.

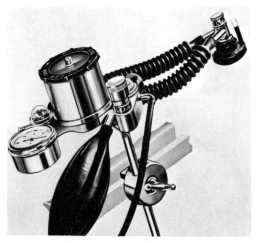

Figure 8.27. Ohio infant circle absorber system. (Courtesy of Ohio Medical Products, a division of Airco, Inc.)

USE OF THE CIRCLE SYSTEM WITH LOW FLOWS

Closed system anesthesia was used in the 1940s and 1950s to conserve expensive anesthetic agents and to reduce the explosive hazard with flammable anesthetics. Following the introduction of halothane and other potent inhalation anesthetics frequently used with nitrous oxide, the technique was largely abandoned. In recent years, considerable interest has been shown in the use of low-flow techniques.

Definitions (164)

Low-flow anesthesia has been variously defined as any inhalation technique in which a circle system with absorbent is used with a fresh gas inflow (*a*) less than the patient's alveolar minute volume, (*b*) 1 liter/min or less (164) or (*c*) 3 liters/min or less (165). Closed system anesthesia is a form of low-flow anesthesia in which the fresh gas inflow equals uptake of anesthetic gases and oxygen by the patient and system. No excess gas is vented through the relief valve.

Anyone wishing to employ low-flow or closed circuit anesthesia should first become familiar with the literature on this topic. The following is a summary of some of the most important principles of this technique.

Equipment

Administration of low flow or closed circuit anesthesia requires no extraordinary equipment.

ANESTHESIA MACHINE

A standard anesthesia machine can be used, but it is necessary that it have an oxygen flowmeter that will accurately register flows as low as 100 cc/min. For pediatric work, even lower flows may be required. The flowmeter to an empty kettle vaporizer may be used for such a purpose if the diluent flowmeters do not accurately meter such low flows.

CIRCLE SYSTEM

A standard circle system with the absorber filled with active absorbent is used. It is suggested that if the absorber has a bypass mechanism that this be removed or the absorber replaced with one that does not have a bypass. Should the bypass be inadvertently left in the ON position during closed or low-flow anesthesia, extreme hypercarbia would result.

The system must be free from leakage. This includes the appropriate patient interface. Endotracheal intubation with a cuffed tube or a gas-tight fit between the mask and the face is required. In pediatric anesthesia, it is often customary to use a loose fitting cuffless tracheal tube. Since this leak must be compensated for by high fresh gas flows, low flow anesthesia cannot be used.

OXYGEN ANALYZER

With low flows there is no reliable relationship between the oxygen concentration in the inspired and fresh gases, so use of a reliable, calibrated oxygen analyzer is mandatory (166).

VAPORIZER

Vapor can be added to the circle in three ways: (a) syringe injections into the expiratory limb (138, 167–175). If this method is used, great care must be taken that only small amounts are injected at a time and that the syringe containing the liquid agent is not confused with those containing agents for intravenous injection. (b) In-circle vaporizer (168, 169, 175–184). These were discussed in Chapter 4. (c) Out-of-system vaporizers (138, 182, 185). For this a vaporizer capable of producing high output concentrations is needed. Unfortunately some vaporizers cannot deliver high concentrations and some do not function well at low flows (186).

Downing and co-workers (182) found that having the vaporizer out of the circle provided more satisfactory anesthesia than having it in the circle.

VENTILATOR

It has been suggested (187) that a ventilator whose bellows rises during exhalation be used because this will result in easier detection of leaks. With these ventilators anesthetic gases can only leak out, resulting in collapse of the bellows. If a ventilator whose bellows descends during exhalation is used, leaks may lead to entrainment of driving gas during exhalation or air may be entrained into the circuit.

ANESTHETIC AGENT MONITOR

The concentrations of anesthetic agents can be monitored using a variety of devices, but an absolute knowledge of inspired concentrations is not necessary for safe anesthesia (188).

CARBON DIOXIDE MONITOR

Monitoring carbon dioxide is highly desirable when using low-flow techniques. Hypercarbia can occur as a result of inactive absorbent, incompetent unidirectional valves, or an absorber bypass in the ON position. The consequences of these problems are greater than when high flows are used.

Techniques

INDUCTION

Induction with low-flow anesthesia is difficult for several reasons but may be accomplished with an in-circuit vaporizer or by injection of measured amounts of liquid anesthetic directly into the expiratory limb of the circuit. If a low fresh gas flow is used for the start of administration, excretion of nitrogen into the system will severely dilute all other gases present. This will not usually present problems if nitrous oxide is not being used. If nitrous oxide is being used, the nitrogen will prevent establishment of high concentrations without hypoxia. Patient awareness may result.

More commonly induction is accomplished by high flow to allow denitrogenation, establishment of anesthetic concentrations, and provision of oxygen well in excess of consumption during the unsteady states associated with induction. Closed or low-flow anesthesia is established after gas exchange has stabilized.

MAINTENANCE

During maintenance it is necessary to monitor three factors: oxygen concentration (using an oxygen monitor), depth of anesthesia (done the same way as when higher flows are used), and circuit volume. Nitrous oxide and oxygen inflows should be adjusted to maintain a satisfactory oxygen concentration and constant circuit volume and agent inflow to obtain the desired level of anesthesia.

Constant circle volume can be achieved by one of several means (173):

Constant Bag Size

A constant bag position at end-tidal volume indicates constant volume.

Ventilator with Upright Bellows

This type of ventilator exhausts excess gas when the bellows expands to the top of its cage. Constant volume can be achieved by adjusting the fresh gas flow so that the bellows height is maintained 100 to 200 ml below the top at the end of exhalation.

Ventilator with Inverted (Hanging) Bellows

In these ventilators the weight of the bellows results in a negative airway pressure during exhalation (descent). In a totally closed system the return to atmospheric pressure is slowed so that the pressure gauge registers 0 just prior to the next inspiration. If it does not reach 0, fresh gas flow should be increased. If the negative pressure reaches 0 prior to the beginning of the next respiratory cycle, an excess of fresh gas over that needed for a closed circuit is being delivered.

If rapid changes in any component are required, it is necessary to increase the fresh gas flow. Examples of such circumstances include too light or too deep anesthesia, malignant hyperthermia (where it is desirable to rapidly eliminate anesthetic agent from the system), and any circumstance where it is desirable to increase the oxygen concentration. Whenever the integrity of the circle is broken, high flows with the desired anesthetic and nitrous oxide concentrations should be administered for several minutes before returning to low flows.

If closed system anesthesia is used, it is recommended that high flows be used for 1 to 2 min at least once an hour to eliminate gases such as nitrogen, carbon monoxide, etc. that accumulate in the system.

EMERGENCE

Recovery from anesthesia is extremely slow when low flows are used. Anesthesiologists familiar with the technique frequently will shut off or reduce delivered anesthetic concentrations in anticipation of surgery completion "coasting" (138, 164, 189, 190). High flows are frequently needed at least briefly to clear nitrous oxide.

Advantages

REDUCTION OF OPERATING ROOM AND ENVIRONMENTAL POLLUTION

With lower flows, there will be less anesthetic agent put into the operating room if an efficient scavenging system is not in use. However, use of low-flow techniques does not eliminate the need for a scavenging system, since high flows are still necessary at times. Since the amount of excess gases and vapors that must be removed from the operating room is reduced, there will be a savings in energy if an active scavenging system is used.

Stratospheric pollution is also important. Fluorocarbons are known to attack the earth's protective ozone layer (191). With the use of low flows, the ecological dangers from fluorocarbons are minimized.

ESTIMATION OF ANESTHETIC AGENT UPTAKE AND OXYGEN CONSUMPTION

Low flow technique gives the user information pertaining to trends and magnitude of uptake of oxygen and anesthetic agents. At equilibrium, the patient-circuit volume is constant as fresh gas inflow is matched by the patient's uptake of oxygen and anesthetic agents. Changes in volume may be attributed to changes in uptake of oxygen or nitrous oxide since the volume contributed by the vapors of the potent inhalational agents is not significant.

INCREASED HEAT AND HUMIDITY

Low-flow anesthesia unquestionably results in higher humidity than higher flows. The magnitude of the humidity achieved is not great and is less than that achieved with some other systems unless a circulator is used. Use of low flows may not eliminate the need to provide other sources of humidity for certain patients and procedures.

GRADUAL CHANGES OF ANESTHETIC DEPTH

Low flows allow the circle system to exert a "buffering" effect so that changes in concentrations of components in the inspired mixture occur more gradually. This is partly because the fresh gas flow is low in relation to system volume. Also with low flows uptake of anesthetic agent by the patient can significantly decrease the concentration in the system and this decrease will limit uptake.

ECONOMY (192, 193)

This is unquestionably a major advantage of low flow anesthesia. Significant savings can be achieved with lower flows of nitrous oxide and oxygen, but the greatest savings occurs with the potent volatile agents. Savings are somewhat offset by increased absorbent usage, but this is small in relation to other expenses.

Disadvantages

MORE ATTENTION REQUIRED

More attention is required because gas flow into the system must be kept in balance with uptake and inspired concentration will not be equal to those in the fresh gas flow. Constant adjustment of flowmeters is required and this could lead to insufficient attention to other aspects of a patient's care.

INABILITY TO QUICKLY ALTER INSPIRED CONCENTRATIONS

This is a significant disadvantage only if the user insists on using low flows at all times. The user of low flows must realize that there are times when high flows should be used.

DANGER OF HYPERCARBIA

The degree of hypercarbia from inactive absorbent, incompetent unidirectional valves or the bypass on the absorber being left in the ON position will be greater when low flows are used.

GREATER KNOWLEDGE REQUIRED

Use of low flow anesthesia does require more knowledge of uptake and distribution than use of high flows. However, it is arguable whether the need to acquire this knowledge is a disadvantage.

ACCUMULATION OF UNDESIRED GASES AND VAPORS IN THE SYSTEM

This is probably only a problem with closed circuit anesthesia, since low flows provide a continuous flush of the system. Also periodic "flushing" with high flows will decrease the accumulation.

Carbon Monoxide

Middleton and co-workers (194) reported that carbon monoxide from the breakdown of hemoglobin accumulated in the closed circle system. However, the levels reported were not likely to cause clinically significant effects. Another study (138) found that carboxyhemoglobin concentrations actually decreased during closed circuit anesthesia.

Acetone, Methane, and Hydrogen

Morita and associates (195) reported that methane and acetone accumulated in the circle system and suggested that during prolonged cases methane and hydrogen could possibly increase to flammable or explosive concentrations.

Ethanol

Ethanol is commonly eliminated partly through the lungs. Use of low flows would slow elimination.

Toxic Metabolites of Anesthetic Agents

Chloroform and trichlorethylene both react with absorbent to produce toxic products but are not commonly used at this time. Sharp and colleagues (29) demonstrated that low concentrations of two volatile metabolites of halothane and a metabolic decomposition product (which has been shown to be mutagenic in one study (196) but not in another (197), could be found in exhaled gases of patients anesthetized with halothane using a circle system, but not a system without absorbent. The levels of these products were higher with lower flows. Eger (198) pointed out that the levels found were well below those found to be toxic in laboratory animals.

ADVANTAGES OF THE CIRCLE SYSTEM

1. The advantages of rebreathing (low fresh gas flows resulting in less operating room pollution and containment of inflammable mixtures, conservation of heat and moisture and absence of abrupt fluctuations in anesthetic depth) are present.

2. The lengths of the tubings can be varied so that the canister may be placed away from the patient to allow optimal surgical exposure in head and neck surgery.

3. $PaCO_2$ depends only on ventilation, not fresh gas flow.

DISADVANTAGES OF THE CIRCLE SYSTEM

1. It is composed of many parts which can be disarranged or may malfunction (9). One example of this is when opposing unidirectional valves are placed in the same system.

2. Resistance is greater than with most other systems. It lacks the ability to give the anesthesiologist a good "feel" of the patient's lungs because of the compliance inherent in the circuit itself (199).

3. Some of the components are difficult to clean so that cross-infection between patients may be a problem.

4. The system is bulky and not easily portable.

5. Inspired concentrations cannot be accurately predicted at low fresh gas flows.

6. Ventilatory minute volume must be restricted to prevent hypercarbia.

7. The large gas volume in the system means a relatively large volume change in the bag is needed to deliver a small amount of gas (due to compression of gases and the compliance of the tubes). With small patients the volume delivered is such a small fraction of the total that it is difficult for the user to consistently deliver the same volume.

References

1. Elam JO: The design of circle absorbers. *Anesthesiology* 19:99–100, 1958.
2. Eger EI, Epstein RM: Hazards of anesthetic equipment. *Anesthesiology* 25:490–504, 1964.
3. Adriani J: Disposal of carbon dioxide from devices used for inhalational anesthesia. *Anesthesiology* 21:742–758, 1960.
4. *The Sodasorb Manual of Carbon Dioxide Adsorption in Inhalation Anesthetic Apparatus.* Dewey and Almy Chemical Division of W. R. Grace & Company, 1962.
5. Elam JO: Channeling and overpacking in carbon dioxide absorbers. *Anesthesiology* 19:403–404, 1958.
6. Miles G, Adriani J: Carbon dioxide absorption. *Anesth Analg* 38:293–300, 1959.
7. Whitten MP, Wise CC: Design faults in commonly used carbon dioxide absorbers. *Br J Anaesth* 44:535–537, 1972.
8. Bergman JJ, Eisele JH: The efficiency of partial soda-lime bypass circuits. *Anesthesiology* 36:94–95, 1972.
9. Adriani J: *Techniques and Procedures.* Springfield, Ill., Charles C Thomas, 1964.
10. Adriani J, Batten DH: The efficiency of mixtures of barium and calcium hydroxides in the absorption of carbon dioxide in rebreathing appliances. *Anesthesiology* 3:1–10, 1942.
11. Grant WJ: *Medical Gases. Their Properties and Uses.* Chicago, Year Book Medical Publishers, pp 133–134, 1978.
12. Hale DE: The rise and fall of soda lime. *Anesth Analg* 46:648–655, 1967.
13. Brown ES, Bakamjian V, Seniff AM: Performance of absorbents: effect of moisture. *Anesthesiology* 20:613–617, 1959.
14. Bracken A: Carbon dioxide absorption. *Anaesthesia* 13:207, 1958.
15. Adriani J, Rovenstine EA: Experimental studies on carbon dioxide absorbers for anesthesia. *Anesthesiology* 2:1–19, 1941.
16. Adriani J, Byrd ML: A study of carbon dioxide absorption appliances for anesthesia: the canister. *Anesthesiology* 2:450–455, 1941.
17. Foregger R: The regeneration of soda lime following absorption of carbon dioxide. *Anesthesiology* 9:15–20, 1948.
18. Adriani J: Elimination of carbon dioxide from devices used for inhalation anesthesia. *Int Anesth Clin* 12:3:47–78, 1974.
19. Jorgensen B, Jorgensen S: The 600 gram CO_2 absorption canister: an experimental study. *Acta Anaesth Scand* 21:437–444, 1977.
20. Sato T: New aspects of carbon dioxide absorption in anesthetic circuits. *Med J Osaka Univ* 22:173–206, 1971.
21. Bracken A, Sanderson DM: Some observations on anaesthetic soda lime. *Br J Anaesth* 27:422–427, 1955.
22. Lund I, Lund O, Erikson H: Model experiments on absorption efficiency of soda lime. *Br J Anaesth* 29:17–20, 1957.
23. Hunt HK: Resistance in respiratory valves and canisters. *Anesthesiology* 16:190–205, 1955.
24. Adriani J: The removal of carbon dioxide from rebreathing appliances. *J Aviation Med* 12:304–309, 1941.
25. Maycock E: Soda lime dust. *Anaesth Intensive Care* 8:217, 1980.
26. Adriani J: Rebreathing in anesthesia. *South Med J* 35:798–804, 1942.
27. Nuhn LJ: Personal communication.
28. Batten DH: The absorption of carbon dioxide from anesthesia apparatus. *N Y State J Med* 43:539–544, 1943.
29. Sharp JH, Trudell JR, Cohen EN: Volatile metabolites and decomposition products of halothane in man. *Anesthesiology* 50:2–8, 1979.

30. Grodin WK, Epstein RA: Halothane adsorption by soda lime. *Anesthesiology* 51:S317, 1979.

31. Grodin WK, Epstein MAF, Epstein RA: Enflurane and isoflurane adsorption by soda lime. *Anesthesiology* 55:A124, 1981.

32. Grodin WK, Epstein RA: Halothane adsorption complicating the use of soda-lime to humidify anaesthetic gases. *Br J Anaesth* 54:555–559, 1982.

33. Davis R: Soda lime dust. *Anaesth Intensive Care* 7:390, 1979.

34. Brown ES: Voids, pores and total air space of carbon dioxide absorbents. *Anesthesiology* 19:1–6, 1958.

35. *The Sodasorb Manual of Carbon Dioxide Adsorption in Inhalation Anesthetic Apparatus.* Dewey and Almy Chemical Division, W. R. Grace & Company, 1974.

36. Geikler H, Kunze D, Ziegan J: Acute inflammation of the respiratory mucous membrane following soda lime instillation. *Surv Anesthesiol* 14:462, 1970.

37. Lauria JI: Soda-lime dust contamination of breathing circuits. *Anesthesiology* 42:628–629, 1975.

38. Feingold A: Carbon dioxide absorber packaging hazard. *Anesthesiology* 45:260, 1976.

39. Jorgensen B, Jorgensen S: Carbon dioxide elimination from circle systems. *Acta Anaesth Scand(Suppl)* 53:86–93, 1973.

40. Houghton IT, Farrelly PJ: The use of antistatic sprays with soda-lime containing an indicator. *Br J Anaesth* 43:206, 1971.

41. Barasch ST, Booth S, Modell J: Hypercapnia during cyclopropane anesthesia: a case report. *Anesth Analg* 55:439–441, 1976.

42. Detmer MD, Chandra P, Cohen PJ: Occurrence of hypercarbia due to an unusual failure of anesthetic equipment. *Anesthesiology* 52:278–279, 1980.

43. Spain JA: Cost of delivery of anesthetic gases reexamined. III. *Anesthesiology* 55:711–712, 1981.

44. Bracken A, Cox LA: Apparatus for carbon dioxide absorption. *Br J Anaesth* 40:660–665, 1968.

45. Muneyuki M: Absorption effeciency of carbon dioxide in various models of canisters—an experimental study by the use of a lung model. *Far East J Anesth* 4:10–30, 1963.

46. Lund I, Andersen KL, Erikson H: Efficiency of carbon dioxide absorption by soda lime in a closed system. *Br J Anaesth* 28:13–19, 1956.

47. Brown ES: Performance of absorbents: continuous flow. *Anesthesiology* 20:41–44, 1959.

48. Woolmer R, Lind B: Rebreathing with a semiclosed system. *Br J Anaesth* 26:316–322, 1954.

49. Brown ES: Factors affecting the performance of absorbents. *Anesthesiology* 20:198–203, 1959.

50. Brown ES, Elam JO: Practical aspects of carbon dioxide absorption. *N Y State J Med* 23:3436–3442, 1955.

51. Mousel LH, Weiss WA, Gilliom LA: A clinical study of carbon dioxide absorption during anesthesia. *Anesthesiology* 7:375–398, 1946.

52. Proctor DF: Studies of respiratory air flow. IV. Resistance to air flow through anesthesia apparatus. *Bull Johns Hopkins Hosp* 96:49–58, 1955.

53. Orkin LR, Siegcl M, Rovenstine EA: Resistance to breathing by apparatus used in anesthesia. II. Valves and machines. *Anesth Analg* 36:19–27, 1957.

54. Kerr JH, Evers JL: Carbon dioxide accumulation: valve leaks and inadequate absorption. *Can Anaesth Soc J* 5:154–160, 1958.

55. Schreiber P: *Anaesthesia Equipment. Performance, Classification, and Safety.* New York, Springer-Verlag, 1974.

56. Schweitgzer SA, Babarczy AJ: An unexpected hazard of the Boyles machine. *Anaesth Intensive Care* 4:72–73, 1976.

57. Fogdall RP: Exacerbation of iatrogenic hypercarbia by PEEP. *Anesthesiology* 51:173–175, 1979.

58. Dean HN, Parsons DE, Raphaely RC: Case report: bilateral tension pneumothorax from mechanical failure of anesthesia machine due to misplaced expiratory valve. *Anesth Analg* 50:195–198, 1971.

59. Dogu TS, Davis HS: Hazards of inadvertently opposed valves. *Anesthesiology* 33:122–123, 1970.

60. Rendell-Baker L: Another close call with crossed valves. *Anesthesiology* 31:194–195, 1969.

61. White CW: Hazards of the valved Y-piece. *Anesthesiology* 32:567, 1970.

62. Smith RH, Volpitto PP: Volume ventilation valve. *Anesthesiology* 20:885–886, 1959.

63. Cottrell JE, Chalon J, Turndorf H: Faulty anesthesia circuits: a source of environmental pollution in the operating room. *Anesth Analg* 56:359–362, 1977.

64. Cottrell JE, Bernhard W, Turndorf H: Hazards of disposable rebreathing circuits. *Anesth Analg* 55:743–744, 1976.

65. Stevenson PH, McLeskey CH: Breakage of a reservoir bag mount, an unusual anesthesia machine failure. *Anesthesiology* 53:270–271, 1980.

66. Jordan M, Flynn P, Askill S, Morris LE: Maximum inspired humidity produced by forced circulation. *Anesthesiology* 55:A365, 1981.

67. Morris LE: The circulator concept. *Int Anesthesiol Clin* 12,3:181–197, 1974.

68. Neff WB, Sullivan MT, Poulter TC: A magnetic drive circulator designed for completely closed carbon dioxide absorption systems. *Anesthesiology* 51:169–170, 1979.

69. Revell DG: An improved circulator for closed circle anaesthesia. *Can Anaesth Soc J* 6:104–107, 1959.

70. Roffey PJ, Revell DG, Morris LE: An assessment of the Revell circulator. *Anesthesiology* 22:583–590, 1961.

71. Revell DG: A circulator to eliminate mechanical dead space in circle absorption systems. *Can Anaesth Soc J* 6:98–103, 1959.

72. Jones PL, Prosser J: An assessment of the Neff circulator. *Can Anaesth Soc J* 20:659–674, 1973.

73. Neff WB, Burke SF, Thompson R: A venturi circulator for anesthetic systems. *Anesthesiology* 29:838–841, 1968.

74. Morris LE: Revell circulator and vapor concentration measurements. In Aldrete JA, Lowe HJ, Virtue RW (eds): *Low Flow and Closed System Anesthesia.* New York, Grune & Stratton, 1979, pp 273–276.

75. Bryan-Brown CW: Bacterial filters. *Int Anesthe-*

siol Clin 10:147–156, 1972.

76. Dryden GE, Dryden SR, Brown DG, Schatzle KC, Godzeski C: Performance of bacteria filters. *Resp Care* 25:1127–1135, 1980.

77. Loeser EA: Water-induced resistance in disposable respiratory-circuit bacterial filters. *Anesth Analg* 57:269–271, 1978.

78. Mason J, Tackley R: An acute rise in expiratory resistance due to a blocked ventilator filter. *Anaesthesia* 36:335, 1981.

79. Kopman AF, Glaser L: Obstruction of bacterial filters by edema fluid. *Anesthesiology* 44:169–170, 1976.

80. *Ventilator Breathing Circuits.* Health Devices Alerts, Vol. 5, 1981.

81. Escobar A, Aldrete JA: Bacteria filters for anesthesia apparatus. *Anesthesiol Rev* 4:25A–25B, 1977.

82. Grundy EM, Bennett EJ, Brennan T: Obstructed anesthetic circuits. *Anesthesiol Rev* 31:35–36, 1976.

83. DuMoulin GC, Saubermann AJ: The anesthesia machine and circle system are not likely to be sources of bacterial contamination. *Anesthesiology* 47:353–358, 1977.

84. Ping FC, Oulton JL, Smith JA, Skidmore AG, Jenkins LC: Bacterial filters—are they necessary on anaesthetic machines? *Can Anaesth Soc J* 26:415–419, 1979.

85. Pace NL, Webster C, Epstein B, Matsumiya S, Coleman M, Britt MR, Garibaldi RA: Failure of anesthesia circuit bacterial gas filters to reduce postoperative pulmonary infections. *Anesthesiology* 51:S362, 1979.

86. Rigor BM, Astrello JM, Landry M, Haynes G: Prevention of contamination in anesthesia circuits. Abstracts of the 52nd Congress of International Anesthesia Research Society, 1978, p 86.

87. Feeley TW, Hamilton WK, Xavier B, Moyers J, Eger EI: Sterile anesthesia breathing circuits do not prevent postoperative pulmonary infection. *Anesthesiology* 54:369–372, 1981.

88. Garibaldi RA, Britt MR, Webster C, Pace NL: Failure of bacterial filters to reduce the incidence of pneumonia after inhalation anesthesia. *Anesthesiology* 54:364–368, 1981.

89. Mazze RI: Bacterial air filters. *Anesthesiology* 54:359–360, 1981.

90. Warren PR, Gintautas J: Problems with Dupaco ventilator valve assembly. *Anesthesiology* 53: 524–525, 1980.

91. Sears BE, Bocar ND: Pneumothorax resulting from a closed anesthesia ventilator port. *Anesthesiology* 47:311–313, 1977.

92. Norry HT: A pressure limiting valve for anaesthetic and respirator circuits. *Can Anaesth Soc J* 19:583–588, 1972.

93. Morrow DH, Dixon WM, Townley NT, Herbert CL: A safety modification of the Air-Shields ventimeter ventilator. *Anesthesiology* 26:361–362, 1965.

94. *Medical Device Alert,* Ohio Medical Products, December 8, 1981.

95. Cooper JB: Prevention of ventilator hazards. *Anesthesiology* 48:299–300, 1978.

96. Conway CM: Alveolar gas relationships during use of the circle system with carbon dioxide absorption. *Br J Anaesth* 53:1135–1146, 1981.

97. Brown ES, Seniff AM, Elam JO: Carbon dioxide elimination in semiclosed systems. *Anesthesiology* 25:31–36, 1964.

98. Briere C, Patoine JG, Audet R: Inaccurate ventimetry by fresh gas inlet position. *Can Anaesth Soc J* 21:117–119, 1974.

99. Campbell DI: Change of gas inflow siting on Boyle MK3 absorbers. *Anaesthesia* 26:104, 1971.

100. Campbell DI: Volumeter attachment on Boyle circle absorber, *Br J Anaesth* 43:206–207, 1971.

101. Purnell RJ: The position of the Wright anemometer in the circle absorber system. *Br J Anaesth* 40:917–918, 1968.

102. Bain JA, Spoerel WE: A streamlined anaesthetic system. *Can Anaesth Soc J* 19:426–435, 1972.

103. Weeks DB: Higher humidity, an additional benefit of a disposable anesthesia circle. *Anesthesiology* 43:375–377, 1975.

104. Shanks CA, Sara CA: Estimation of inspiratory-limb humidity in the circle system. *Anesthesiology* 40:99–100, 1974.

105. Berry FA, Hughes-Davies DI: Methods of increasing the humidity and temperature of the inspired gases in the infant circle system. *Anesthesiology* 37:456–462, 1972.

106. Harper M, Eger EI: A comparison of the efficiency of three anesthesia circle systems. *Anesth Analg* 55:724–729, 1976.

107. Russell WJ, Drew SE: A potential hazard with an inspiratory valve of a circle system. *Anaesth Intensive Care* 5:269–271, 1977.

108. Schoonbee CG, Conway CM: Factors affecting carbon dioxide homeostasis during controlled ventilation with circle systems. *Br J Anaesth* 53:471–477, 1981.

109. Fujita M: Resistance to breathing through various anesthesia apparatus: safety limit of external resistance during general anesthesia. *Far East J Anesth* 3:8–16, 1960.

110. Amaranath L, Boutros AR: Circle absorber and soda lime contamination. *Anesth Analg* 59:711–712, 1980.

111. Chalon J, Patel C, Ramanathan S, Turndorf H: Humidification of the circle absorber system. *Anesthesiology* 48:142–146, 1978.

112. Chalon J, Simon R, Ramanathan S, Patel C, Klein G, Rand P, Turndorf H: A high humidity circle system for infants and children. *Anesthesiology* 49:205–207, 1978.

113. Eger EI, Ethans CT: The effects of inflow, overflow and valve placement on economy of the circle system. *Anesthesiology* 29:93–100, 1968.

114. Eger EI: Anesthetic systems: construction and function. In Eger EI (ed): *Anesthetic Uptake and Action.* Baltimore, Williams & Wilkins, 1975.

115. Rendell-Baker L: On the promise of economy denied. *Anesthesiology* 29:5–6, 1968.

116. Brown ES, Hustead RF: Resistance of pediatric breathing systems. *Anesth Analg* 48:842–849, 1969.

117. Adriani J: Rebreathing in anesthesia. *Bull Am Assoc Nurse Anesthetists* 9:189–196, 1941.

118. Young TM: Carbon dioxide absorber. *Anaesthesia* 26:78–79, 1971.

119. Young TM: Performance of two carbon dioxide absorbers. The MIE Jumbo and BOC Mk III. *Anaesthesia* 24:417–427, 1969.

120. Graff TD, Holzman RS, Benson DW: Acid-base balance in infants during halothane anesthesia with the use of an adult circle absorption system. *Anesth Analg* 43:583–589, 1964.

121. Jasinska MT, Goudsouzian NG, Ryan JF: Evaluation of carbon dioxide retention in children using three anesthetic circuits. *Anesth Rev* 1:17–19, 1974.

122. Lewis GB Jr: The experts opine. *Surv Anesthesiol* 23:397–398, 1979.

123. Chalon J, Kao ZL, Dolorico VN, Atkin DH: Humidity output of the circle absorber system. *Anesthesiology* 38:458–465, 1973.

124. Dery R, Pelletier J, Jacques A, Clavet M, Houde JJ: Humidity in anaesthesiology. Heat and moisture patterns in the respiratory tract during anaesthesia with the semi-closed system. *Can Anaesth Soc J* 14:287–298, 1967.

125. Dery R, Pelletier J, Jacques A, Clavet M, Houde JJ: Humidity in anaesthesiology II. Evolution of heat and moisture in the large carbon dioxide absorbers. *Can Anaesth Soc J* 14:205–219, 1967.

126. Shanks CA, Sara CA: Airway heat and humidity during endotracheal intubation. III. Rebreathing from the circle absorber at low fresh gas flows. *Anaesth Intensive Care* 1:415–417, 1973.

127. Berry FA, Ball CG, Blankenbaker WL: Humidification of anesthetic systems for prolonged procedures. *Anesth Analg* 54:50–54, 1975.

128. Weeks DB, Broman KE: A method of quantitating humidity in the anesthesia circuit by temperature control: semiclosed circle. *Anesth Analg* 49:292–296, 1970.

129. Chase HF, Kilmore MA, Trotta R: Respiratory water loss via anesthesia systems: mask breathing. *Anesthesiology* 22:205–209, 1961.

130. Shanks CA, Sara CA: Airway heat and humidity during endotracheal intubation. 4. Connotations of delivered water vapour content. *Anaesth Intensive Care* 2:212–220, 1974.

131. Flynn PJ, Morris LE: Humidity in anaesthetic systems. *Br J Anaesth* 53:1096, 1981.

132. Chalon J, Goldman C, Amirdivani M, Rothblatt A, Ramanathan S, Turndorf H: Humidification in a modified circle system. *Anesth Analg* 58:216–220, 1979.

133. Paspa P, Tang CK, Dwarkmanath R, Ramanathan S, Chalon J, Fischgrund GK, Turndorf H: A percolator vaporizer heated by reaction of neutralization of lime by carbon dioxide. *Anesth Analg* 60:146–149, 1981.

134. Ramanathan S, Chalon J, Turndorf H: Compact well-humidified breathing circuit for the circle system. *Anesthesiology* 44:238–242, 1976.

135. Chalon J, Ramanathan S: Water vaporizer heated by the reaction of neutralization of carbon dioxide. *Anesthesiology* 41:400–404, 1974.

136. Lumley J, Morgan M: The temperature inside carbon dioxide absorbers. *Anaesthesia* 31:63–68, 1976.

137. Hamilton WK, Eastwood DW: A study of denitrogenation with some inhalation anesthetic systems. *Anesthesiology* 16:861–867, 1955.

138. Lowe HJ, Ernst EA: *The Quantitative Practice of Anesthesia. Use of Closed Circuit.* Baltimore, Williams & Wilkins, 1981.

139. Schultz EA, Buckley JJ, Oswald AJ, Van Bergen FH: Profound acidosis in an anesthetized human: report of a case. *Anesthesiology* 21:285–291, 1960.

140. Akkineni S, Patel KP, Bennett EJ, Grunty EM, Ignacio AD: Fresh gas flow to limit PaCO$_2$ in T and circle systems without CO$_2$ absorption. *Anesthesiol Rev* 4:33–37, 1977.

141. Conway CM, Schoonbee C: Factors affecting the performance of circle systems used without carbon dioxide absorption. *Br J Anaesth* 53:115P, 1981.

142. deSilva AJC: Normocapnic ventilation using the circle system. *Can Anaesth Soc J* 23:657–666, 1976.

143. Benson DW, Graff TD, Hurt HH, Lim HS: The circle semi-closed system control of PaCO$_2$ by inflow rates of anesthetic gases and hyperventilation. *Anesthesiology* 29:174, 1968.

144. Gibb DB, Prior G, Pollard B: Methods of conserving carbon dioxide in artificially ventilated patients. A clinical investigation. *Anaesth Intensive Care* 5:122–127, 1977.

145. Harris PHP, Kerr JH, Edmonds-Seal J: Artificial ventilation using a circle circuit without an absorber. *Anaesthesia* 30:269–270, 1975.

146. Keenan RL, Boyan CP: How rebreathing anaesthetic systems control PaCO$_2$ studies with a mechanical and mathematical model. *Can Anaesth Soc J* 25:117–121, 1978.

147. Ladegaard-Pedersen HJ: A circle system without carbon dioxide absorption. *Acta Anaesth Scand* 22:281–286, 1978.

148. Suwa K, Yamamura H: The effect of gas inflow on the regulation of CO$_2$ levels with hyperventilation during anesthesia. *Anesthesiology* 33:440–445, 1970.

149. Scholfield EJ, Williams NE: Prediction of arterial carbon dioxide tension using a circle system without carbon dioxide absorption. *Br J Anaesth* 46:442–445, 1974.

150. Snowdon SL, Powell DL, Fadl ET, Utting JE: The circle system without absorber. *Anaesthesia* 30:323–332, 1975.

151. Patel K, Bennett EJ, Grundy EM, Ignacio A: Relation of PaCO$_2$ to fresh gas flow in a circle system. *Anesth Analg* 55:706–708, 1976.

152. Lawler PG, White DC: The measurement of oxygen uptake during anesthesia. *Br J Anaesth* 49:511–512, 1977.

153. Lowe HJ, Titel JH, Hagler KJ: Absorption of anesthetics by conductive rubber in breathing circuits. *Anesthesiology* 34:283–289, 1971.

154. Dykes MHM, Chir B, Laasberg LH: Clinical implications of halothane contamination of the anesthetic circle. *Anesthesiology* 35:648–649, 1971.

155. Eger EI, Larson CP, Severinghaus JW: The solubility of halothane in rubber, soda lime and various plastics. *Anesthesiology* 23:356–359, 1964.

156. Eger EI, Brandstater B: Solubility of methoxyflurane in rubber. *Anesthesiology* 24:679–683, 1963.

157. Grodin WK, Epstein MAF, Epstein RA: Mechanisms of halothane adsorption by dry soda-lime. *Br J Anaesth* 54:561–565, 1982.

158. Eger EI: Factors affecting the rapidity of alteration of nitrous oxide concentration in a circle system. *Anesthesiology* 21:348–355, 1960.

159. Cullen SC: Pediatric circle absorber. *Anesthe-*

siology 28:787–789, 1957.

160. Ramanathan S, Chalon J, Turndorf H: Humidity output of the Bloomquist infant circle. *Anesthesiology* 43:679–682, 1975.

161. Brown ES, Hustead RF: Rebreathing in pediatric anesthesia systems. *Anesthesiology* 288:241–242, 1967.

162. Berry FA, Hughes-Davies DI, DiFazio CA: A system for minimizing respiratory heat loss in infants during operation. *Anesth Analg* 52:170–175, 1973.

163. Rackow H, Salanitre E: A new pediatric circle valve. *Anesthesiology* 29:833–834, 1968.

164. Stone SB, Greene NM: Low-flow anesthesia. *Curr Rev Clin Anesth* 1:114, 1981.

165. Spence AA, Alison RH, Wishart HY: Low flow and "closed" systems for the administration of inhalation anaesthesia. *Br J Anaesth* 53:69S–73S, 1981.

166. Smith TC: Nitrous oxide and low inflow circle systems. *Anesthesiology* 27:266–271, 1966.

167. Wolfson B: Closed circuit anaesthesia by intermittent injections of halothane. *Br J Anaesth* 34:733–737, 1962.

168. Gusterson FR, Clark JM: The use of the Goldman halothane vaporizer in the closed circuit. *Br J Anaesth* 32:388–393, 1960.

169. Jones PIE, Robertson G, Ware RJ, Strunin L: Enflurane in a closed circle-absorber system: vaporizer inside the circle. *Br J Anaesth* 51:994P, 1979.

170. Ramagnoli A, Cohen M, Diamond MJ: A safe and economical method of administering fluothane in closed circuit anaesthesia. *Can Anaesth Soc J* 7:186–190, 1960.

171. Weingarten M, Lowe HJ: A new circuit injection technic for syringe measured administration of methoxyflurane: a new dimension in anesthesia. *Anesth Analg* 52:634–642, 1973.

172. Spain JA, Ernst EA, Lowe HJ: Computer assisted closed circuit anesthesia. *Anesthesiology* 53:S366, 1980.

173. Lowe HJ: The anesthetic continuum. In Aldrete JA, Lowe HJ, Virtue RW (eds): *Low Flow and Closed System Anesthesia.* New York, Grune & Stratton, 1979, pp 11–37.

174. Hawes DW, Ross JA, White DC, Wloch RT: Servo-control of closed circuit anaesthesia. *Br J Anaesth* 54:229P–230P, 1982.

175. Garlington L, Neff WB: A simple in-circuit vaporizer for closed-circuit anaesthesia. *Anesthesiology* 54:434–435, 1981.

176. Older P: In-circle halothane anaesthesia. In *Proceedings of the Third Asian and Australian Congress of Anesthesiology.* London, Butterworth, 1970, pp 207–210.

177. Titel JH, Lowe HJ, Elam JO, Grosholz JR: Quantitative closed-circuit halothane anesthesia. A clinical study employing a new pressurized temperature-compensated vaporizer. *Anesth Analg* 47:560–569, 1968.

178. Mapleson WW: The concentration of anaesthetics in closed circuits, with special reference to halothane. I. Theoretical study. *Br J Anaesth* 32:298–309, 1960.

179. Mushin WW, Galloon S: The concentration of anaesthetics in closed circuits with special reference to halothane. III. Clinical aspects. *Br J Anaesth* 32:324–333, 1960.

180. Galloon S: The concentration of anaesthetics in closed circuits with special reference to halothane. II. Laboratory and theatre investigations. *Br J Anaesth* 32:310–323, 1960.

181. Salamonsen RF: A vaporizing system for programmed anaesthesia. *Br J Anaesth* 50:425–433, 1978.

182. Downing JW, Brock-utne JG: "Closed" circuit (rebreathing) enflurane anaesthesia. *S Afr Med J* 52:514–517, 1977.

183. Jordan MJ, Bushman JA: Closed-circuit enflurane using an in-circle Goldman vaporizer. *Br J Anaesth* 53:185P, 1981.

184. Jordan MJ, Bushman JA: Closed-circuit halothane and enflurane using an in-circle Goldman vaporizer. *Br J Anaesth* 53:1285–1290, 1981.

185. Nunn JF: Control of vapor concentrations. In Aldrete JA, Lowe HJ, Virtue RW (eds): *Low Flow and Closed System Anesthesia.* New York, Grune & Stratton, 1979, pp 213–224.

186. Lin C: Assessment of vaporizer performance in low-flow and closed-circuit anesthesia. *Anesth Analg* 59:359–366, 1980.

187. Lin CY, Mostert JW, Benson DW: Closed circle systems. A new direction in the practice of anesthesia. *Acta Anaesth Scand* 24:354–361, 1980.

188. Hamilton WK: Low-flow systems without calculus (or even algebra). *ASA Refresher Courses in Anesthesiology* 8:79–86, 1980.

189. Feingold A: Controlled emergence from anesthesia using the closed-circle system. *Anesth Analg* 53:869–875, 1974.

190. Weingarten M: Low flow and closed circuit anesthesia. In Aldrete JA, Lowe HG, Virtue RW (eds); *Low Flow and Closed System Anesthesia.* New York, Grune & Stratton, 1979, pp 67–70.

191. Virtue RW: Anesthetic gas flows, costs, and pollution. *Anesthesiol Rev* 5:14–16, 1978.

192. Herscher E, Yeakel AE: Nitrous oxide-oxygen based anesthesia: the waste and its cost. *Anesthesiol Rev* 4:29–31, 1977.

193. Nunn JF: Potential economics of using closed circuit anesthesia. In Aldrete JA, Lowe HJ, Virtue RW (eds): *Low Flow and Closed System Anesthesia.* New York, Grune & Stratton, 1979, pp 109–112.

194. Middleton V, Poznak AV, Artusio JF, Smith SM: Carbon monoxide accumulation in closed circle anesthesia systems. *Anesthesiology* 26:715–719, 1965.

195. Morita S, Latta W, Hambro K, Snider MT: Accumulation of methane, acetone, and nitrogen in the inspired gas during closed circuit anesthesia. *Anesth Analg* 60:267–268, 1981.

196. Garro AJ, Phillips RA: Mutagenicity of the halogenated olefin, 2-bromo-2-chloro-1,1-difluoroethylene, a presumed metabolite of the inhalation anesthetic, halothane. *Environ Health Persp* 21:65–69, 1977.

197. Waskell L: Lack of mutagenicity of two possible metabolites of halothane. *Anesthesiology* 50:9–12, 1979.

198. Eger EI: Dragons and other scientific hazards (editorial). *Anesthesiology* 50:1, 1979.

199. Carden E, Nelson D: A new and highly efficient circuit for paediatric anaesthesia. *Can Anaesth Soc J* 19:572–582, 1972.

CHAPTER 9

Controlling Trace Gas Levels

It has been well documented that administration of anesthesia may be toxic to a patient, but only in recent years has it been appreciated that a risk may also apply to those who work in the area where anesthesia is administered.

In the past the usual practice was to exhaust excess anesthetic gases and vapors directly into room air; as a consequence operating room personnel were exposed to trace concentrations of these drugs. Such chronic exposure results in sustained blood levels of anesthetics, induction of drug-metabolizing enzymes, and increased biodegradation of the anesthetics.

For many decades anesthesiologists worked in this environment without serious regard for any detrimental effects that might accrue from such chronic exposure. In recent years, however, questions have been raised about hazards, real or imagined, to operating room personnel from exposure to trace amounts of anesthetic gases and vapors.* Unfortunately, attempts to understand the situation have been hampered by the existence of tenuous, confusing and often conflicting evidence. The situation is far from clear cut and much more work needs to be done before it can be stated with any conviction that a problem even exists.

METHODS OF STUDY

A trace level of an anesthetic gas is a level far below that needed for clinical anesthesia. Trace gas levels are usually expressed in parts per million (ppm), which is volume/volume (100% of a gas is 1,000,000 ppm; 1% is 10,000 ppm).

Reported trace gas concentrations found in the absence of control measures vary greatly, depending on the fresh gas flows in use, the ventilation system, the length of time that anesthesia has been administered, where the concentration is measured, and other variables.

Halothane: Levels in operating rooms average 1–10 ppm, with many higher and lower values being reported (1–34). In recovery rooms levels from 0–8.2 ppm have been found (24, 27, 28, 35).

Nitrous oxide: In unscavenged rooms levels from 400–3000 ppm have been found (1, 2, 4, 6–8, 11, 12, 20, 22, 24, 27–29, 31, 36–44). In recovery rooms levels varying from 15–1660 ppm have been found (24, 27, 28, 39, 45).

Enflurane: Levels in operating rroms from 5–46 ppm have been reported (8).

Methoxyflurane: Levels from 1–10 ppm have been reported (4, 7, 8, 27, 37).

To better interpret the data it is first necessary to understand how it was gathered. There have been four basic methods of study (46). All have major limitations and disadvantages.

Animal Investigations

In these studies laboratory animals are exposed to varying levels of gases for varying amounts of time and studied to determine effects. These studies must be interpreted warily. It has been shown in animals that diets affect tumor susceptibility; stress affects reproductive abilities; hypoxia can cause congenital malformations; and low anesthetic levels cause behavior patterns to change (47). Toxicity usually depends on both exposure time and concentration, making it difficult to correlate exposure time in animals with that in humans, since the lifespans are so different. Finally, variations in drug effects among species increases the uncertainty about the relevance of these findings to man.

Human Volunteer Studies

Human volunteers have been used to study possible effects of trace gases on skilled performance, immune responses, and patterns of drug metabolism.

---

* Through the remainder of this chapter anesthetic gases and vapors will be referred to as gases, since most vapors behave as gases.

Epidemiological Studies of Exposed Personnel

There have been a number of epidemiological studies of exposed personnel. All have serious flaws. Most have been retrospective and involve unsupported questionnaires, usually obtained by mail. They suffer from low response rates, inappropriate control groups, misrecollections and biases on the part of the respondents, poor wording, failure to include significant points in the questionnaires, and misinterpretations due to differences in education and experience on the part of the respondents. Interpretation of the data is hampered by a lack of agreement as to what level of significance to accept (48). Finally, they have not been designed to test the cause-effect relationship between trace gas levels and problems in exposed personnel. Some studies predict increased risk for specific groups but do not make such predictions for other equally exposed groups (47). Other studies have shown problems in groups with and without exposure to the operating room environment, suggesting that the result may not be related to trace gas exposure.

Mortality Studies

Studies on the causes of death and the age at which death occurred among anesthesiologists have provided some very interesting and valuable data, despite some questions about the appropriateness of the control group and rather small numbers.

PROBLEMS

Spontaneous Abortions

EPIDEMIOLOGICAL STUDIES

Attention to spontaneous abortions in female operating room personnel began in 1967 when Vaisman noted that pregnancies in 18 of 31 anesthetists ended in spontaneous abortion (49). Several retrospective studies (49–62) have shown high rates of spontaneous abortion in operating room and dental operatory personnel, compared to women engaged in similar pursuits but in different environments. The validity of many of these studies has been questioned (47, 48, 63, 64) and a number of other studies have failed to find significant increases in spontaneous abortions in exposed personnel (65–70).

Cohen (11) reported that the length of exposure was important. Exposure of a pregnant woman during the first trimester results in only a slightly increased risk. If one added previous exposure of at least a year preceding pregnancy, the risk increased significantly. The risk returns toward normal with removal from the operating room environment.

One study of interest was that of Rosenberg and co-workers (60) who studied spontaneous abortion rates among nurses in intensive care and trauma units, anesthetic nurses, and scrub nurses. They found that the frequency of miscarriages among nurses working in intensive care units was approximately equal to that of nurses in anesthesia, suggesting that psychic and physical stress may be the causative factors.

ANIMAL STUDIES

The picture is no less confusing when animal studies are examined. All inhalation anesthetics in current use when administered to pregnant animals at anesthetic or near-anesthetic concentrations for sufficient duration can produce toxic effects in embryos. This information cannot be used to infer that similar results will follow exposure to trace concentrations.

Enflurane: Several investigations (71–75) failed to show any effects toxic to fetuses in animals exposed to concentrations as high as 10,000 ppm.

Methoxyflurane: No increase in reproductive loss has been found with exposures up to 2000 ppm (76–77).

Halothane: Investigations (76–81) have shown no lethal effects to embryos from exposures of up to 3200 ppm.

Nitrous oxide: Vieira and colleagues (82) found that exposure to 1000 ppm nitrous oxide caused fetal death and resorption, but no effect was seen when 500 ppm was used. Corbett (54) also showed an increase in fetal death in rats exposed to 1000 ppm, but not 100 ppm. It has been reported that a repeat study of nitrous oxide exposure by these authors proved negative (47). Pope (76) and Mazze and associates (83) found no increased toxicity to fetuses in rats exposed to concentrations as high as 500,000 ppm.

Mixtures: Investigations using mixtures of halothane and nitrous oxide have found no effect with concentrations as high as 1600 ppm halothane and 100,000 ppm nitrous oxide (76, 79, 84).

In summary, with the possible exception of nitrous oxide, all animal studies indicate that if a toxic threshold concentration of inhalation anesthetics causing increased spontaneous abortions exists, it is 10 to 100 or even 1000 times that commonly found in operating rooms. A finding of some interest in one study (76) was that animals stressed by experimental handling had dramatically higher fetal losses, again suggesting that stress may be at least part of the etiology.

A suggested etiological factor for spontaneous abortion is mutations in germ cells. The reader is referred to the section on mutagenesis.

Spontaneous Abortion in Spouses

Several studies (51, 62, 85–88) have shown an increased spontaneous abortion rate in wives of exposed males. Other investigators have not found this to be the case (50, 58, 61, 68).

In humans, Wyrobek and co-workers (89) found no changes in sperm concentration or morphology in male anesthesiologists working in hospitals with scavenging equipment.

In animal studies, Coate (88, 90) found significant increases in chromosomal aberrations in spermatogonial cells exposed to 10 ppm halothane and 500 ppm nitrous oxide. Similar but less marked changes were seen with lower concentrations. Changes in sperm morphology were reported by Land (91, 92) using similar concentrations. Land and colleague (91) found morphological changes in mouse spermatozoa after exposure to 12,000 ppm enflurane, but not after exposure to nitrous oxide, halothane, methoxyflurane, or isoflurane. Other studies have failed to show any adverse effect on reproductive processes of male animals (72, 93).

Involuntary Infertility

Two studies have noted higher than expected rates of involuntary infertility among exposed personnel (57, 62). Some of this data has been questioned (47, 69). Other investigators have found no effect from maternal (94) or paternal (58) exposure.

No changes in sperm count or morphology have been found in male anesthesiologists working in scavenged operating rooms (89).

Animal studies show conflicting data.

Halothane: Wharton (77) found a decrease in fertility in rats exposed to 3000, but not 1000, ppm halothane. Kennedy and colleagues (95) found exposure to 14,000 ppm halothane before mating had no effect on fertility in rats.

Enflurane: No effect on fertility in mice has been found from exposure to concentrations of enflurane up to 5000 ppm (71).

Nitrous oxide: Mazze and co-workers (83) found no change in male fertility with exposure up to 500,000 ppm.

Mixtures: Decreased ovulation and implantation in rats exposed to halothane 1 ppm and nitrous oxide 50 ppm has been demonstrated (84, 90).

Dangers to Unborn Offspring

Several studies in humans have found an increase in congenital malformations in children of exposed personnel (50, 55, 57, 62, 67, 96, 97). Some of these studies have been questioned (47, 48, 63, 64, 98) and several studies (51, 56, 58, 60, 65, 68, 87) have shown no increase. A few studies have shown low birth weights (60, 62, 67, 68). Rosenberg and associates (31) were unable to demonstrate chromosomal abnormalities in exposed nurses and Wyrobeck (89) found no changes in sperm morphology in male anesthesiologists working in scavenged operating rooms.

A pattern of specific types of defects might be expected if associated with drug toxicity. Some studies have not shown any particular system to be involved (57, 58), while others have shown an increase in cardiovascular abnormalities (67), musculoskeletal abnormalities (55, 68, 88), problems in the musculoskeletal and nervous systems (62), multifactorial abnormalities (50), and cutaneous and musculoskeletal anomalies (96). Two studies suggest an increased rate of malignancy among offspring of exposed personnel (62, 96).

Cohen (11) found that exposure of at least one year preceding pregnancy was more important than exposure during the first trimester. He also found that the rate of congenital malformation tended to return to normal after time away from the operating room.

In animal studies most, but not all, studies have found that inhalation agents in anesthetic concentrations cause increased rates of congenital anomalies in animals (95, 99, 100–103), but this cannot be used to infer that a similar effect occurs with trace concentrations.

Enflurane: Wharton and colleagues (71, 72) found no gross fetal effects in mice exposed to 5000 ppm enflurane. Pope and co-worker (74) found exposure of rats to subanesthetic concentrations of enflurane led to growth retardation, but no significant abnormalities. Chalon and associates (104) found that exposure to enflurane adversely affected the learning function of progeny and Land (91) found changes in spermatozoa after exposure to high concentrations.

Halothane: Chang and colleagues (105) found microscopic morphological changes (but no gross abnormalities) in the kidneys, livers, and brains of rats exposed to halothane 10 ppm in utero. However, the significance of these changes has been questioned (42).

Chronic exposure of rats to 10 ppm of halothane in utero has been shown to produce later deficits in learning (104, 106, 107), raising the question of learning deficits in offspring of female anesthesia personnel. However, the significance of some of this data has been questioned (47).

Several investigations have found exposure of pregnant rats to concentrations of halothane of up to 3200 ppm produced retardation of maturation and an increased incidence of skeletal developmental variants, but no effects that could be expected to result in permanent abnormalities or decreased survival (75, 76, 80, 81, 108).

Methoxyflurane: Exposure of up to 800 ppm has been found to cause a decrease in fetal weight and slight developmental retardation, but no gross abnormalities (76, 103).

Nitrous oxide: Pope and co-workers (76) found exposure to 10,000 to 500,000 ppm nitrous oxide could cause a decrease in fetal weight and slight developmental retardation, but this was not accompanied by any evidence of gross abnormalities. Vieira and colleagues (82) found skeletal abnormalities in the form of rib malformation and abnormal vertebral columns in fetuses exposed to 100,000 but not 50,000 ppm. Land and co-workers (109) found no evidence of mutagenesis in the sperm of mice exposed to 800,000 ppm nitrous oxide.

Mixtures: Investigations (76, 84, 90) have found decreases in fetal weight and slight developmental retardation with exposure to a mixture of nitrous oxide, 100,000 ppm, and halothane, 1600 ppm, but this was unaccompanied by any evidence of gross abnormalities.

In summary, studies of laboratory animals show that concentrations of inhalation agents that produce gross malformations are well above those found in even unscavenged operating rooms. The question of learning deficits, however, deserves more study. Since abnormalities in offspring could be related to chromosomal mutations in germ cells, the reader is referred to the section on mutagenesis.

Impairment of Skilled Performance

Operating room personnel are subjected to many stimuli which require precise, split-second, and complicated responses. Since the patient's survival depends upon the alertness and performance of the professional team, anything that interferes with their ability to perceive changes in signals and react quickly and appropriately may cause harm to a patient.

Bruce and co-workers (110) exposed volunteers to nitrous oxide, 500 ppm, with or without halothane, 15 ppm, and ran a battery of cognitive, perceptual, and motor tests before and after exposure. They found that exposure to nitrous oxide and halothane caused significant decreases in performance. Subjects exposed to nitrous oxide alone showed less effect. Similar results were found when enflurane was used in place of halothane (111). In a later study Bruce and associates (112) found decrements in performance in volunteers given 50 ppm nitrous oxide with and without 1 ppm halothane, but no effects at 25 ppm nitrous oxide and 0.5 ppm halothane.

These results have not been confirmed by others. Smith and Shirley (113), using 500 ppm nitrous oxide and 15 ppm halothane, and using the same tests employed by Bruce, were unable to demonstrate any decrease in performance. Failure to demonstrate effects on mental function by trace levels of anesthetics were reported by Cook and colleagues (114, 115) and Frankhuizen and associates (116). Allison and co-workers (117) and Cook and co-workers (115) found that the threshold concentrations of nitrous oxide, halothane, and enflurane needed to decrease performance were hundreds of times greater than the average levels found in unscavenged operating rooms. In laboratory tests, chronic exposure of adult rats to 10 ppm halothane failed to affect learning (107), although Chang and co-workers (105) found degenerative changes in cortical neurons in rats exposed to 10–500 ppm halothane.

A different approach to the problem has been to test operating room personnel at the end of the workday and compare them to similar personnel from other areas of the hospital (19, 118, 119). These studies have failed to demonstrate decreased skills in exposed personnel.

Smith and Shirley (120), in reviewing the effects of trace concentrations of anesthetics on performance, concluded that the current balance of data suggests that average levels of trace gases in the operating room have no effect on performance. This does not exclude the possibility of interactions with other factors which might impair performance or that anesthesiologists using unscavenged anesthetic circuits might be exposed to very high concentrations and conceivably suffer impairment of performance, especially when using high fresh gas flows.

Cancer

That malignancies can be caused by chronic inhalation of chemical compounds has been known for many years. Because anesthetics are known to interfere with the mitotic process and because there are similarities in structure between anesthetic agents and proven carcinogens, concern about their potential carcinogenicity has been expressed.

EPIDEMIOLOGICAL STUDIES

The possibility that cancer may result from exposure to trace anesthetic gases was raised by a report by Corbett and co-workers (121) in which it was found that the incidence of malignancies in female nurse anesthetists was more than three times the expected rate. Several aspects of this study have been criticized (46, 47, 122). A larger study (50) found no increase in cancer in exposed males but indicated that females in the operating room were at higher risk for cancer, especially leukemia and lymphoma, than nonexposed females. The significance of this data has also been questioned (47, 48). Similar results have been reported for female dental operatory assistants (55). Two epidemiological studies of dentists have shown that the incidence of cancer is not significantly different among those exposed and those not exposed to trace concentrations of anesthetics (55, 87).

MORTALITY STUDIES

There is no increased death rate from cancer in male anesthesiologists (123–126). The cancer rate among female anesthesiologists is high compared to male anesthesiologists and control groups (123, 125), but the numbers are too small to permit any strong conclusions.

It should be pointed out that the "lag time" for industrial carcinogens is 20 years. Thus, the carcinogenic effects of the halogenated agents, if any, may not yet be manifest. New therapeutic modalities have resulted in higher cancer cure rates, preventing an assessment of incidence of cancer by mortality data.

ANIMAL STUDIES

Enflurane: Mice exposed to up to 10,000 ppm enflurane have been found to have no increased risk of neoplasms (127, 128).

Isoflurane: Corbett (8) induced hepatic neoplasms in mice by exposure during gestation and early life to 1000–5000 ppm isoflurane. The validity of this study has been questioned because of defects in experimental design, and it now appears that the increased incidence of liver tumors may have been due to other factors. In a later study no evidence of increased carcinogenicity could be found in mice exposed to up to 6000 ppm isoflurane (128).

Halothane: Studies have found no evidence of increased carcinogenicity in animals exposed to up to 6000 ppm halothane (122, 128, 129).

Nitrous oxide: No evidence of increased carcinogenicity in mice has been found with exposure of up to 800,000 ppm (109, 128).

Mixtures: Coate and co-workers (90) found no increase in neoplasms in rats exposed to 10 ppm halothane and 500 ppm nitrous oxide, although cytogenic aberrations were found in bone marrow and spermatological cells.

MUTAGENICITY TESTING

Testing for carcinogenicity requires years, large numbers of animals, and a great expenditure of money and effort. A more rapid and inexpensive method is to look for an increase in mutagens in a bacterial system exposed to an inhalational anesthetic. One of the mechanisms by which environmental agents are thought to produce cancer involves mutation of DNA (130). Since the DNAs of all organisms are chemically similar, a study of mutagenic effects in a simpler organism may be helpful in predicting carcinogenicity in humans.

It has been found that mutagenicity tests have predictive value in detecting carcinogens. Lack of mutagenicity, however, does not exclude the possibility that an agent may be carcinogenic to chronically exposed operating room personnel. One must also keep in mind the possibility that an anesthetic agent could increase the risk of cancer by enhancing the carcinogenic effect of other chemical and physical factors.

HUMAN STUDIES

Baden and co-workers (131) found there was no statistical difference in urinary mutagenic activity between individuals working in scavenged and unscavenged operating rooms. Also the urines of anesthesiologists collected before and after beginning training had similar mutagenic activities. In another study (130), it was found the urine of patients anesthetized with halothane did not increase mutagenesis. Husam and colleagues (132) found no evidence of mutation of DNA material in operating room personnel (132). McCoy and co-workers (133) did find increased mutagenic activity in the urines of a small group of anesthesiologists.

ANIMAL STUDIES

Enflurane: Several investigations (134–137) were unable to demonstrate mutagenic effects induced by enflurane.

Isoflurane: Several investigations (134–136, 138) have found isoflurane was not mutagenic.

Halothane: Several investigators (130, 135, 136, 138–140) have found halothane not mutagenic. Kramers and co-workers (141) found it had produced weak mutagenic activity.

Some investigators (130, 138, 142) found no evidence of mutagenicity with halothane metabolites, but others (143–145) found halothane metabolites exhibited weak mutagenicity.

Methoxyflurane: Several investigations (134–136, 138) have found methoxyflurane not mutagenic.

Nitrous oxide: Investigations (135, 136, 146) have found nitrous oxide not to be mutagenic.

Mixtures: One investigation (139) found that halothane plus nitrous oxide did not increase mutagenesis.

Liver Diseases

EPIDEMIOLOGICAL STUDIES

The ASA National Study (50) found that both male and female operating room personnel had higher than expected rates of hepatic disease. Interpretation of this data has been questioned (48). Similar results have been reported in male dentists (55, 87) and female chairside assistants (147). A study in Great Britain also showed a higher than expected frequency of liver disease in male anesthesiologists (46). Another study failed to show evidence of an increase in liver disease in anesthesiologists (148). Studies of anesthesia personnel have failed to show evidence of hepatocellular damage (149–151). A study of delivery ward personnel showed increases in liver enzymes following exposure to low concentrations of methoxyflurane (152).

Recurrent hepatitis has been demonstrated in

a few individuals exposed to halothane (153–156) and exposure to trace anesthetic agents does enhance hepatic metabolism of some drugs (157, 158). The relevance of these facts to the effects of trace concentrations is not clear.

MORTALITY STUDIES

No increase in the death rate due to liver disease has been seen among anesthesiologists (125).

ANIMAL STUDIES

The literature on anesthetic effects on the livers of laboratory animals is conflicting (47, 159).

Renal Disease

EPIDEMIOLOGICAL STUDIES

The ASA National Study found that male and female operating room nurses and technicians and female anesthesiologists had a higher risk of kidney disease than did comparable groups outside the operating room (50). These differences were not found in male anesthesiologists. These results have been questioned (48).

Another study in Great Britain failed to find any increase in kidney disease in male anesthesiologists (46).

An early study in exposed dentists showed no increase in renal disease (87) but a later study showed an increase in both exposed dentists and female chairside assistants (55).

One study of delivery ward personnel did show alterations in renal function following exposure to methoxyflurane (152).

MORTALITY STUDIES

In mortality studies no increase in deaths due to renal disease among anesthesiologists has been found (125).

ANIMAL STUDIES

The literature of anesthetic effects on the kidney in laboratory animals is conflicting (47).

Hematological Problems

EPIDEMIOLOGICAL STUDIES

In one epidemiological study a higher than expected rate of leukemia was found in female anesthesiologists, but the small data base makes any valid conclusions difficult (50).

ANIMAL STUDIES

Enflurane: Baden and co-workers (160) found chronic intermittent exposure to 3000 ppm enflurane had no effect on hematopoiesis in mice.

Halothane: Baden and co-worker (122) found no hematological effects from exposure of mice to 500 ppm halothane.

Nitrous oxide: Cleaton-Jones and colleagues (161) found exposure to 10,000 ppm nitrous oxide caused no changes in hematopoiesis in rats (161).

Mixtures: Coate (162) found no hematological effects from exposing rats to halothane, 10 ppm, plus nitrous oxide, 500 ppm, although damage to bone marrow cells was seen in other studies (84, 90).

Alterations in the Immune Response

Studies both in vivo and in vitro have shown that in anesthetic concentrations inhalation agents may interfere with many phases of the immune response (47, 163, 164).

Beall (165), Bruce (166), and Salo and co-workers (167) found that work in operating room did not cause changes in the immune response. Pettingale (168), however, reported depressive changes.

It has been suggested that trace concentrations of anesthetics may stimulate rather than depress the immune response (169) and Mathiew and colleagues (170) found an increase in active T lymphocytes, suggesting stimulation of the cell-mediated immune system. Bardzik and co-workers (149) showed raised levels of some immunoglobulins in a group of anesthesia personnel.

Cardiac Disease

Studies have shown a greater than expected frequency of hypertension (46) and arrhythmias (61), and there is one case report of auricular fibrillation secondary to halothane exposure (171). However, mortality studies give no evidence that anesthesiologists have a higher than expected risk of dying from coronary artery disease.

Neurological Symptoms

Brodsky and co-workers (172) and Cohen and colleagues (55) found an increase in neurological symptoms (numbness, tingling, and/or muscle weakness) in dentists and female chairside assistants exposed to anesthetic gases and a questionnaire survey of dentists and dental assistants showed an increased incidence of neurological complaints in those who worked with nitrous oxide (173). Another study failed to detect any problems (174).

A non-specific polyneuropathy due to chronic exposure to nitrous oxide has been described (175–178).

In animals, high levels of nitrous oxide have not been shown to cause neuromuscular or neurological abnormalities (174).

Miscellaneous

Higher than expected incidences of bone and joint disease (46), peptic ulcer (46, 61), ulcerative colitis (61), gall bladder disease (46), and migraine (61) have been reported in anesthesiologists.

Case reports have been made of exposed personnel who developed asthmatic symptoms (179), laryngitis (180), ophthalmic hypersensitivity (181), chronic conjunctivitis (182), exacerbation of myasthenia gravis (183), and skin eruptions (184, 185). Mortality statistics show a disturbingly high incidence of suicide among anesthesiologists (123, 125).

Summary

The balance of the foregoing evidence from man and animal investigations suggests that anesthetic agents may be the causative factor or one of several causative factors in the occupational hazards reported. However many doubts there may be about the magnitude of the problem or even its reality, the evidence cannot be ignored. The benign, almost cavalier complacency that once existed about trace concentrations of anesthetics in operating room air is gone forever.

The increased hazard, if it exists, is not great. It is more properly regarded as disquieting than alarming. It is somewhat reassuring to note that two studies have shown that anesthesiologists have a mortality rate less than that expected for physicians or the general population (124, 125). However, reproductive problems such as spontaneous abortion and congenital anomalies are not reflected in mortality data and high cure rates may be responsible for the lack of increased mortality from health problems.

A cause-and-effect relationship between occupational exposure and the problems described has not been established. The cause of increased risk may be related to other factors such as mental and physical stress; fatigue, strenuous physical demands; disturbed night rest; need for constant alertness; long and inconvenient working hours often interfering with domestic life; irregular routine; exposure to transmissible infections, solvents, freon propellants, cleaning solutions, laser beams, methylmethacrylate, x-rays, radium implant procedures, microwave radiation, electrocautery, and ultraviolet light; advancing age; pre-existing health and reproductive problems; hormonal or dietary disturbances; the physical or emotional makeup of those who choose to work in operating rooms; socioeconomic factors; or some other as yet undefined factor. Causes may be multiple. Final proof that trace amounts of anesthetic gases contribute to the increased risk must await demonstration that measures to reduce their levels in operating room air also reduce the risk.

The authors of this text feel that until answers to the questions raised have been obtained, the onus of proof falls on those who would deny that pollution by trace anesthetic gases creates a health hazard, and that taking positive actions to reduce the levels of trace anesthetics in operating rooms to the lowest level consistent with reasonable cost is a rational response to the above data. The price in terms of human suffering may be quite heavy should the relationship between the hazards and trace gases later be proved and steps to reduce the levels not have been taken.

Apart from mitigating any effect on their own performance, health, and subjective well being, anesthesiologists have a responsibility to consider the welfare of others working in operating rooms. If future studies show that precautions were unnecessary how much has been lost? To insist on a level of proof beyond all reasonable doubt before taking preventive measures could raise major legal issues.

Some final words of caution are in order, however. While there is no direct evidence that trace concentrations of anesthetics are beneficial, the low mortality rates among anesthesiologists and the suggestion that anesthesiologists may be immunostimulated by trace anesthetics cannot be ignored. Further, while scavenging appears to have little benefit for the patient (other than perhaps having a healthier person administering the anesthetic), definite hazards to the patient have been created by the introduction of scavenging equipment (see section on hazards of equipment in this chapter). Only time will tell whether scavenging does more harm than good.

CONTROL MEASURES

Complete elimination of all anesthetic molecules from the operating room atmosphere is an impossible task. The goal should be to reduce the concentrations to the lowest level possible with reasonable expenditure of time, effort, and money. To achieve this goal, attention must be focused on four areas: capture and disposal of waste gases (scavenging), leaks, work techniques and the room ventilation system. If anesthetic pollution is to be effectively controlled, attention must be paid to all of these areas. None by itself is sufficient. The measures required are straightforward, impose a minimum of inconvenience and require only a modest outlay of time and capital. Most importantly, they do not require that familiar and safe anesthetic practices be modified.

Scavenging

Scavenging is defined as the collection of vented gases and subsequent removal of these gases from the operating room. The anesthesia machine is usually adjusted to deliver more anesthetic gases than the patient can utilize. In the absence of scavenging these gases escape into the operating room air. Installation of an efficient scavenging system is the most important step in reducing trace gas levels, since it will lower ambient concentrations by about 90% (34, 40, 66).

EQUIPMENT

A scavenging system, diagrammed in Figure 9.1, consists of five basic components: a gas collection assembly, which captures excess anesthetic gases at the site of emission, and delivers them to the transfer tubing; transfer tubing, which conveys them to the interface; the interface, which provides positive (and sometimes negative) pressure relief and may provide reservoir capacity; gas disposal assembly tubing, which conducts the gases from the interface to the gas disposal assembly; and the gas disposal assembly, which is the means by which the

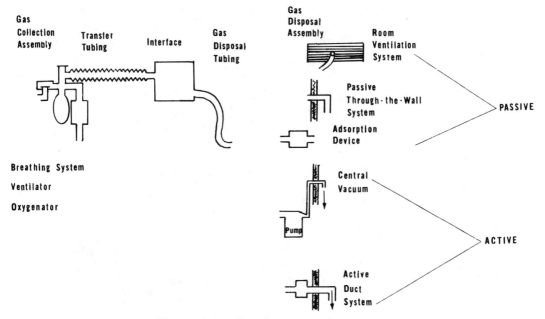

Figure 9.1. Complete scavenging system.

excess gases are ultimately eliminated. Frequently, some or all of these components are combined into a single device.

The Gas-Collecting Assembly (Gas-Capturing Assembly, Device, or Valve; Scavenging Trap or Valve; Collecting or Collection Valve; Scavenging Exhale Valve; Evacuator; Anti-Pollution Valve; Ducted Expiratory Valve; Exhaust Valve)

The gas collecting assembly collects the waste gases from their source (breathing system, ventilator or extracorporeal pump oxygenator) and delivers them to the transfer tubing. It may either attach to, or be an integral part of, the source. The ANSI standard (186) specifies that the outlet from the assembly be either a 19- or 30-mm male fitting. This is important because it should not be possible to connect components of the breathing system to the outlet. Some early assemblies had a 22-mm fitting. As a result, cases of misconnection with breathing system hoses have occurred (187, 188). Adapters are available to change these to 19 or 30 mm (189), and this should be done as soon as possible to prevent assembly errors.

If any equipment in an anesthesia department is not fitted with a gas collecting assembly, the anesthesiologist should confer with the manufacturer and either have a gas collecting assembly attached or have the equipment replaced.

Breathing Systems. *Systems Containing a Relief Valve.* The commonest route for anesthetic effluent is through the relief valve in the breathing system. It is necessary either to replace the normal relief valve with a special valve or to fit a suitable gas-tight hood to an existing valve. Numerous devices are available for attachment to, or a substitute for, the usual relief valve in the circle systems found on most older machines and other breathing systems (Fig. 9.2). Unfortunately, some of the early valves with gas collecting assemblies were far from gas-tight, but later models are more efficient.

The relief valve should still function and feel as much as possible like the valve it replaces. The screw adjustment should be easy to reach and manipulate and should have low resistance.

With the circle and Mapleson D systems, the weight of the pressure relief valve and gas collecting assembly can be supported by the anesthesia machine, a distinct advantage. With the Mapleson A, B and C systems, these must be near the patient port and the extra bulk and weight may make the systems somewhat cumbersome. Smaller sizes of some relief valves with gas collecting assemblies are available for these systems.

One disadvantage of using a relief valve

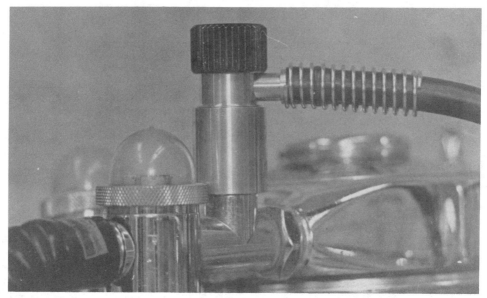

Figure 9.2. Gas collection assembly used in the circle system. (Courtesy of Boehringer Laboratories, Inc.)

equipped with with a gas collecting assembly is that because the valve is enclosed, the usual auditory signal created by the passing gas is silenced, and this prevents its use as an aid in monitoring respiration. This should not be considered a hazard, since other means of monitoring these parameters are available.

Systems Containing Non-Rebreathing Valves. A non-rebreathing valve with a scavenging adapter is commercially available. It is fairly simple to devise a means to attach transfer tubing to the exhalation port of some existing non-rebreathing valves lacking scavenging adapters without affecting valve function.

T-Piece Systems. The T-piece system is somewhat difficult to scavenge because of the absence of a relief valve. Numerous devices have been described for evacuating through the tail of the bag (2, 190–200).

With all of these it is important that there be some means for preventing occlusion of the tail due to accidental twisting and a mechanism to regulate occlusion of the tail for intermittent positive pressure. Another method has been described which utilizes a scavenging dish attached to suction. The waste gases are discharged into the dish from the open end of the bag tail. The high volume of the suction system will remove them before they are distributed throughout the room (201).

It is even more difficult to evacuate gases

when the hole is in the side of the bag, although one home-made device has been described (194).

Ventilators. Anesthesia ventilators should be equipped when new or retrofitted with a gas collecting assembly. Because of their complexity, a detailed description of these is beyond the scope of this book. However, the reader should be aware that some of the early gas collecting assembly attachments were inefficient. Many ventilators had to be totally redesigned to provide efficient scavenging. Most ventilators are now equipped with gas-tight gas collecting assemblies, and some of the newer ventilators also come with an interface and disposal system fitted.

For those ventilators with only a gas collecting assembly, it is useful to attach the outlet of the assembly to a Y that joins the effluent from the relief valve in the breathing system (196, 197) (see Fig. 9.5). Use of the Y permits all connections to be made before anesthesia is induced and reduces the possibility of pollution when switching between hand ventilation and use of an automatic ventilator during a procedure (197). With some ventilators it is necessary to have a unidirectional valve between the ventilator and the Y to prevent flow of gases back into the ventilator and into the operating room atmosphere when the ventilator is not in use.

With some ventilators the exhaust includes not only the excess circuit gases, but the driving gas as well, so that a disposal system of high capacity is required. The ventilator manufacturer should specify the requirements for effective scavenging.

Extracorporeal Pump Oxygenators. Collecting devices are available for extracorporeal pump oxygenators (202, 203), but in some cases have not been well developed (204). It is especially important to provide an effective interface with these because significant positive or negative pressure alterations at the outflow port can markedly alter oxygenator function (204).

Transfer Tubing (Exhaust Tubing)

The transfer tubing connects the gas collecting assembly with the interface. Its inlet fitting should be either 19 or 30 mm conical unless it is an integral part of the gas collecting assembly.

The transfer tubing should be as short as practical and of large enough diameter to carry a high flow of gas without a significant increase in pressure. It should be sufficiently rigid that occlusion by twisting or kinking (see Fig. 9.6) is unlikely to occur. It should be free of leaks and capable of forming gas-tight connections. It should be clearly visible to the anesthesiologist in his normal position and easy to disconnect from the collecting assembly in the event of malfunction or occlusion of the scavenging system downstream. It should be different (either by color or configuration) from the breathing system tubes to discourage misconnections.

The Interface (Balancing Valve or Device, Pressure Balancing Valve or Device, Interface System, Intermediate Site, Safety Block)

From the standpoint of patient safety, the interface is the most important component in the scavenging system. It serves to prevent harmful pressure increases or decreases in the scavenging system from being transmitted to the breathing system, ventilator, or extracorporeal pump oxygenator. Current recommendations are that the interface should limit pressures immediately downstream of the gas collecting assembly to between -0.5 and $+10$ cm H_2O (-50 and $+1000$ Pa) during normal operating conditions and up to $+15$ cm H_2O (1500 Pa) with obstruction of the scavenging system for scavenging from a breathing system or ventilator (186). For scavenging from extracorporeal oxygenators, the recommended limits are -0.25 to 0 cm H_2O (186).

The interface may be part of the gas collection assembly in a breathing system, incorporated into a ventilator, or an independent device. It should be situated as close to the gas collecting assembly as possible and where it can be observed easily by the anesthesiologist. It should be compact and not clutter up the work area. If possible, it should be off the floor.

There are three basic elements to an interface: positive pressure relief, negative pressure relief, and reservoir capacity. Irrespective of what type of disposal system is used, positive pressure relief must be provided to protect the breathing system in the event of scavenging system occlusion. If an active disposal system is used, the interface must also provide negative pressure relief to prevent subatmospheric pressure from reaching the breathing system and should have reservoir capacity to allow efficient scavenging at low removal flows. An audio device which varies in intensity with the patient's respiratory rate is incorporated into some interfaces to substitute for the sound made by a conventional relief valve.

A distensible reservoir allows monitoring of the scavenging system. This should only be used with active disposal systems. If the distensible reservoir is a bag, it should be of a different color from, and situated away from, the breathing system reservoir bag. It should be in a position where it can be easily observed by the anesthesiologist. By observing the bag, the anesthesiologist can adjust the rate of flow from the gas disposal assembly to the optimal level. If the bag is continually collapsed, the flow should be adjusted to a lower level. If the bag overdistends, the flow should be increased.

Interfaces can be divided into two types, depending on the means used to provide positive and negative pressure relief.

Open Interfaces (205, 206). An open interface is one that is open to atmosphere (allowing positive and negative pressure relief) and contains no valves. It should be used only with a disposal system that actively removes gases.

Since the discharge of waste gases is usually intermittent and flow through an active disposal assembly is continuous, a reservoir is needed to contain surges of gases that enter the interface at an inflow greater than the disposal system flow. The gases are then held in the reservoir until the disposal system removes them. The reservoir allows the flow rate in the disposal system to be kept just above the average, rather than the peak, flow rate of gases from the gas collecting assembly.

It is essential that the reservoir have adequate capacity, especially if a ventilator in which the driving gas mixes with waste gases is used. The resulting combined flow rate will be quite large and unless the reservoir is also large, the flow rate in the disposal system will have to be kept high to prevent excess gases from overflowing into room air.

T-Tube (207). An example of a simple type of open interface, known as a T-tube, is shown in Figure 9.3A. One limb of the T attaches to the transfer tubing with the side limb leading to the active disposal system. The third limb of the T is fitted with a piece of tubing that serves as a reservoir. Surges of gases flowing out of the transfer tubing flow partly into the disposal system and partly into the reservoir tubing. They can then be removed from the reservoir by the disposal system.

As long as the free end of the reservoir remains open to atmosphere there is no danger of applying significant negative or positive pressure to the breathing system. It is important that a guard or case be placed at the free end to prevent occlusion or that escape or inlet holes be provided near the end (Fig. 9.3A) so that an opening to atmosphere is still present if the end of the tubing becomes occluded.

Tube-within-a-Tube. A second type of open interface, known as the tube-within-a-tube, is shown in Figure 9.3B. It consists of two coaxial tubes. The proximal end of the inner tube is open to the outer tube and the distal end is connected to the active disposal device. The outer tube is connected to the transfer tubing proximally and the distal end is open to atmosphere. A variation of this type of interface is shown in Figure 9.3C. It has a distensible bag added so that the adequacy of scavenging can be monitored.

Another variation of this type of open interface is shown in Figure 9.3D. Anesthetic gases from the transfer tubing enter at the top and are conducted to the base where they are dispersed by copper mesh. Suction is applied to the base and this serves to remove the gases. Gases are stored in the reservoir between exhalations. The holes at the top are open to atmosphere.

With any open interface it is important that the inlet for waste gases, the disposal system connection, and the opening to atmosphere be arranged so that waste gases are removed preferentially before room air is entrained.

The open interface is simple, but is fraught with the danger of polluting the atmosphere should the reservoir not have sufficient volume to contain the boluses of waste gases. Unless there is a distensible reservoir, leakage can be reliably determined only by air monitoring.

Closed Interfaces. A closed interface is one in which the connection(s) with the atmosphere are through valve(s). A positive pressure relief valve is always required to allow release of gases into the room if there is obstruction of the scavenging system downstream of the interface. If an active disposal system is to be used, a

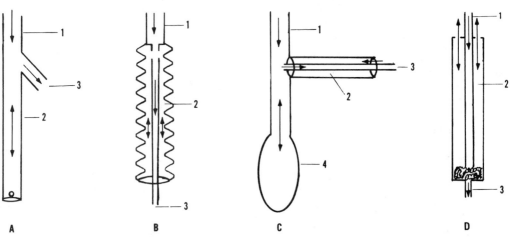

Figure 9.3. Open interfaces. *1,* transfer tubing; *2,* reservoir; *3,* active disposal system; *4,* scavenging bag. *A,* T-tube interface. Note the escape/inlet hole near the free end of the reservoir tubing. *B,* tube-within-a-tube interface. *C,* tube-within-a-tube interface with distensible bag for monitoring efficiency of scavenging. *D,* tube-within-a-tube with the escape/inlet holes at top. (Redrawn from a drawing furnished by Boehringer Laboratories, Inc.)

negative pressure relief valve (dumping valve, pop-in-valve, inlet relief valve) is necessary to allow entrainment of air when the pressure falls below atmospheric.

A reservoir is not required with a closed interface and should not be used unless an active disposal system is used, in which case a distensible bag is useful for monitoring the functioning of the scavenging system, as described above.

Positive Pressure Relief Only. This type of closed interface is used only with passive disposal systems. An example is shown in Figure 9.4A. The positive pressure relief valve is normally closed, except in case of a problem downstream of the interface. If the valve opens frequently, the scavenging system should be checked for obstructions.

Positive and Negative Pressure Relief. If it is planned to use an active disposal system a negative pressure relief valve must be present. Examples of this type of closed interface are shown in Figures 9.4B and 9.5. When a passive disposal system is used, the negative pressure relief will remain closed at all times. If an active disposal system is used, it should close during high peak

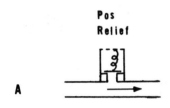

Pos
Relief

A

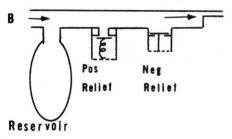

B

Pos   **Neg**
Relief   **Relief**

Reservoir

Figure 9.4. Closed interfaces. *A,* without reservoir or negative relief device. For use with passive disposal systems only. *B,* with reservoir bag and negative pressure relief valve. For use with either a passive or active disposal system. If an active disposal system is used, the bag will be collapsed except during periods of high flow from the gas collection assembly and inadequate output will be indicated by bag distention.

flow rates from the gas collecting assembly and open when the disposal system flow is greater than the flow of gases from the gas collecting assembly. If the negative pressure relief valve remains open continually, the flow in the disposal system should be adjusted to a lower level.

The rate of flow into the gas disposal assembly should be adjusted to the optimal level. This is done by observing the reservoir bag (if present) and the positive and negative relief valves. If the bag is continually collapsed or the negative pressure relief valve opens frequently, the flow should be adjusted to a lower rate. If the bag overdistends or the positive pressure relief valve functions frequently, flow should be increased.

A closed interface is less likely to result in room air pollution than an open interface and can be used with any type of disposal system. The presence of valves adds to the complexity. They must be well designed so that they do not stick or leak. Interfaces with two negative pressure relief valves are available commercially and add a margin of safety.

Gas Disposal Assembly Tubing

The gas disposal assembly tubing connects the interface to the disposal assembly (Fig. 9.1). It should be of different size and appearance from the breathing system hoses to avoid misconnections. It should be as collapse-proof as possible. The gas disposal tubing should be free of leaks. This is especially important with a passive disposal system, since the gases will be under slight positive pressure. With a passive system it is important that the hose be as short and wide as practical to minimize resistance.

Ideally, the gas disposal tubing should be run overhead to minimize the risk of occlusion and to avoid the dangers of personnel tripping over it or other apparatus becoming entangled in it (208). Should the disposal point be a significant distance from the anesthesia machine or the tubing obstruct personnel or equipment movement, it may be hidden in a false ceiling (196). If the tubing must be run across the floor, it should be routed where it is least likely to be stepped on or have equipment rolled on it. If it must pass a doorway, it should follow the door frame.

Gas Disposal Assembly (Elimination System or Route, Disposal/Exhaust Route)

The gas disposal assembly consists of the components used to remove waste gases from

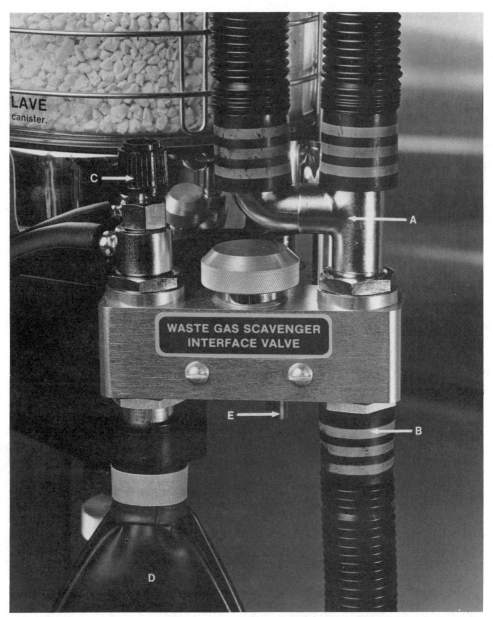

Figure 9.5. Closed interface. There are three inlet ports to accommodate evacuation from a relief valve and ventilator joined by a Y connection (*A*) and an outlet from another type of gas collection assembly such as from an other type of breathing system (*B*). A device to regulate suction flow is at *top left* (*C*). The reservoir bag at *bottom left* (*D*) allows monitoring of the scavenging efficiency and permits adjustment of suction flow to the minimum necessary. *E* and *F* permit both positive and negative pressure relief. If a passive disposal system is used, the reservoir bag is removed and the mount capped. The needle valve is closed and a tubing is attached from (*B*) to the gas disposal system. (Courtesy of Ohio Medical Products, a division of Airco, Inc.)

the operating room. With any type of disposal system it is important that the gases be vented either to atmosphere at a point where contamination of hospital air intake will not occur, or to a part of the hospital where there will be no further exposure of personnel to waste gases.

Disposal assemblies are of two types: active, in which a mechanical flow-inducing device moves the gases, and passive, in which the work of moving the gases is supplied by the patient during spontaneous ventilation, the anesthesiologist's hand during manually assisted or controlled ventilation, or the automatic ventilator when one is in use. With an active system there will be a negative pressure in the gas disposal tubing. With a passive system, the pressure in this tubing will be positive.

Active systems are usually considered more effective in keeping operating room pollution levels low, because any leaks will be inward (209, 210). They have the advantage that small bore gas disposal tubing can be used and excessive resistance is not a problem. They also aid room air exchange. They are, however, expensive in terms of energy costs. They are not automatic and must be turned on and off. If they are not turned on, air pollution will occur; if they are not turned off, there will be needless waste of energy. Active systems are more complex than passive ones. Their use requires that the interface have negative pressure relief.

Passive systems are simpler, but may not be as effective in eliminating waste gases, since the positive pressure encourages outward leaks. Excessive resistance may be a problem, especially if there is a significant distance from the gas collection assembly to the disposal system. It has been recommended that the resistance of a system not exceed 0.5 cm H_2O (50 Pa) at a flow rate of 30 liters/min (211). They are less expensive to operate than active systems.

Passive Systems. Venting to the Floor. Venting to the operating room floor is an ineffective method of disposal. It is based on the assumption that since anesthetic gases are heavier than air, they will layer along the floor and flow out of the room via the ventilation system. In reality, turbulence induced by the ventilation system and personnel movements stirs up even the heaviest agents. The result is almost equal distribution throughout the operating room (29, 212). Several investigators (2, 21, 29, 213, 214) have found that venting to the floor does not significantly reduce personnel exposure. It does, however, reduce the anesthesiologist's exposure in relation to that of other personnel.

Room Ventilation System (196, 197, 208, 215, 216). A second type of passive disposal assembly is the non-recirculating portion of the room ventilation system. Ventilation systems used in operating rooms are of two types: non-recirculating (one-pass, single pass, 100% fresh air) and recirculating.

NON-RECIRCULATING SYSTEMS. The non-recirculating system takes in exterior air and processes it by filtering, adjusting the humidity and heating or cooling. The processed air is circulated through the operating room and then all of it is exhausted to atmosphere. Non-recirculating systems typically provide 12 to 15 changes per hour. This type of system is expensive to operate and is less likely to be installed in these times of energy conservation.

If one has this type of ventilation system, it can be easily used for waste gas disposal by securing the gas disposal tubing to a convenient exhaust grille, where the sweeping effect of air flowing into the ventilation system will remove these gases from the operating room.

RECIRCULATING SYSTEMS. With a recirculating ventilation system a small amount of exterior air is taken in from atmosphere. Most of the gases exhausted from the operating room are shunted back into the intake and recirculated, while a volume of circulated air equal to the fresh air is exhausted. Recirculating systems typically provide only five fresh air exchanges per hour. In the past these systems were not used in operating rooms because of the danger of recirculating bacteria-contaminated air. With the availability of high efficiency particulate air (HEPA) filters, recirculating systems have become popular because they are more economical than non-recirculating systems due to reduced energy consumption.

With a recirculating ventilation system, waste gases must be vented beyond the point of recirculation, since venting gases upstream of this point would result in contamination of all rooms on the common manifold. Long segments of plastic tubing are suitable for this purpose (217).

The hospital engineer should be able to inform the anesthesiologist which type of ventilation system is present. If not, absence of recirculation can be determined by sampling the fresh gas inlet to see if it is free of trace gases after they have been released in another room.

An important consideration relating to the use of the room ventilation system for waste gas disposal is the increase in negative pressure downstream in the exhaust duct, away from the grille. If the waste gases are introduced at the exhaust grille, negative pressure is low and will not interfere with the breathing system (196). If waste gases are introduced at a distance downstream in the duct (as they must be with a recirculating system), negative pressure relief must be provided in the interface.

The advantages of using the room ventilation system are several. It is economical since an existing structure is used and no expenditure of energy is necessary. It is automatic, so there is no need to turn anything on or off or make adjustments. It is easy to use and safe for the disposal of flammable waste gases.

In many operating rooms the exhaust grilles are not always located close to the anesthesia machine. In these cases the disposal tubing can be extended to a wall- or ceiling-mounted disposal connection that leads to a pipe in the wall (196, 216). The pipe connects to the exhaust duct in the crawl space, preferably near the exhaust grille, to avoid excessive negative pressure. If electrical outlets are close to the gas supply standpipe and flammable agents are used, this disposal route is contraindicated because of the possibility of an explosion (196).

Passive through-the-Wall System (198, 209, 210, 218–223) (Direct Duct or Vent, Specialized Duct System, Direct Disposal Line). A passive through-the-wall system is one in which the excess anesthetic gases are vented through the wall, window, or floor to the atmosphere, using only the pressure of the gases to provide the flow. To prevent cross-flow between rooms, each room must have its own duct.

The inlet to the system in each room should be close to the anesthesia machine (222). The duct should be constructed of a material resistant to anesthetic gases. Plastic and copper are commonly used. To minimize resistance, the pipe should be at least an inch (25 mm) in diameter (211, 221, 222, 224) and as short and straight as possible. If excessive resistance is a problem, a wider bore pipe should be used. A unidirectional valve may be placed in the piping to prevent outside air from entering the operating room and to minimize the effects of wind pressure on the disposal system (222, 225). The pipe should be inclined so that water will not accumulate. There should be a cap for the opening of the pipe in the wall to use when it is not connected to the gas disposal tubing.

The discharge point on the outside should be carefully selected so that it is away from high wind pressures, ignition hazards, windows, and the inlets for the ventilation system. It may be advantageous to attach a short T-piece as a terminal (211). The open end(s) should point downward to minimize the entry of water and dirt and be fitted with fine mesh netting to prevent insects, rodents, and foreign matter from entering the pipe.

Such a disposal assembly is inexpensive, easy to use, and can be used with flammable agents, but it requires a special installation. This is best done during construction. In redesigning an existing operating room or designing a new room, construction of a separate "dedicated" anesthetic gas scavenging system should be considered. If the operating rooms are not near the outside of a building, this type of disposal assembly may not be practical.

Problems that can occur with this system include both positive and negative pressure caused by wind currents (209), obstruction from ice buildup (226) and accumulation of foreign matter at the outlet. There must be a means to determine the patency of the system. It is important to do gas monitoring under conditions of use with this system, to make sure a flow-inducing device is not needed.

Adsorption Device (227–236). Activated charcoal is produced by the actions of chemicals and/or steam on carbon. This activating process enlarges the surface area, which enables the charcoal to adsorb large amounts of toxic substances.

Activated charcoal has been used since World War I as a means of adsorbing toxic gases from the atmosphere. Its adsorption properties have found many applications in industry and during World War II it was recommended that activated carbon filters from gas masks be used to eliminate the odor and explosive hazard from ether in confined spaces such as the sick bays of destroyers in action (237).

Canisters of varying shape and capacity filled with activated charcoal have been used as waste gas disposal assemblies, by directing the gases from the gas disposal tubing through them. The effectiveness of individual canisters and various brands of charcoal vary widely (227, 229). Some can be regenerated by autoclaving (228).

Charcoal canisters have the advantages of being simple, portable and not requiring expensive installation or maintenance. They also have a number of disadvantages. At present, there is no substance available for adsorption of nitrous oxide. Diethyl ether and cyclopropane are not well adsorbed (231, 238). They are fairly expensive and effective for only relatively short periods of time. They must be replaced regularly and pose problems of storage and transport within the hospital and of disposal. Finally, a large canister may impose significant resistance (227).

It is recommended that use of these devices

be limited to situations where nitrous oxide is not being employed or where no other means of eliminating waste gases are available.

Active Systems. *Central Vacuum Systems (196, 207, 239, 240).* Use of the central vacuum system for gas disposal is the most popular method in this country. The gases must be removed by piped suction, as a free-standing electric pump will merely put the gases into the room air.

An interface with negative pressure relief must be used and a reservoir is very useful. The larger the reservoir, the lower the suction flowrate needed. With a large reservoir the flow in the suction system need be only slightly greater than the minute volume of excess gases.

The central vacuum system should be capable of providing high volume (30–40 liters/min) flow, but only slight negative pressure is needed. There should be a means to allow the user to control the suction flow (Fig. 9.5). This will conserve energy, cut down the wear and tear on the central pumps and reduce the noise level in the operating room. A restrictive orifice is often placed in the suction nipple to limit the flow (241).

Maximum convenience is achieved by mounting the suction equipment on the gas machine. All controls should be located within easy reach of the anesthesiologist.

The main advantages of using the central vacuum system is that no new equipment or installation is required and it is easy to use. There are a number of problems associated with its use.

INADEQUATE NUMBER OF OUTLETS. Many operating rooms have only two suction outlets. This is barely enough for some surgical procedures, let alone anesthesia requirements. Ideally, the anesthesiologist should have two suction outlets available, one for suctioning the airway and one for scavenging waste gases. If one has a ventilator whose scavenging system connects directly to a vacuum outlet, a third outlet is desirable.

If the suction flow is adequate, a Y may be inserted into the suction line to create two lines. Unfortunately, this may so reduce the suction flow that it is inadequate for either use.

Some anesthesiologists use a single suction line for scavenging and for removal of secretions. The suction line remains attached to the interface most of the time and is detached when needed for suctioning. Unfortunately, it is human nature to sometimes forget to reattach a line and there will be a break in the waste gas removal. There may be escape of anesthetic gases into the room while suctioning is being performed. Since most airway suctioning is done at the end of the surgical procedure, it is suggested that the anesthesiologist try to use the surgical suction line at that time. Since the surgical suction tubing will usually already be contaminated and the tubing used for scavenging clean, only the surgical suction tubing will need to be changed.

INCONVENIENT OUTLETS. If a suction outlet is not near the anesthesia machine, long suction tubings must reach across the floor. This may present the dangers of occlusion, tripping of personnel, and entanglement with other apparatus.

OVERLOAD OF THE SYSTEM. It is possible to overload the central vacuum system if too many devices are in use at once. This is especially likely with older systems which over the years have had added to them more capacity than they were designed to handle. Overcoming this problem may require a major renovation of the system. The drain can be reduced if the anesthesiologist will adjust the suction flow down to that necessary to prevent spillage of gases into the room air and turn off the suction after use.

DAMAGE TO THE SUCTION PUMP. Normal wear and tear on the suction pump can be expected to increase if the central vacuum system is used for disposal of anesthetic gases. In addition, most anesthetic agents are highly oil soluble and may collect in the pump oil. Oil dilution and gum formation may lead to failure of the pump. A few manufacturers have recommended that anesthetic gases not be evacuated through their pumps.

Widespread use of central vacuum systems for disposal of anesthetic gases and a paucity of reports of problems with pumps suggest that pump damage is not a great hazard. The massive dilution which occurs with shared suction would result in very low concentrations of anesthetic gases passing through a pump. The possibility of explosion does make this method unsuitable for disposal of flammable agents unless a special water-sealed pump is used.

PERSONNEL EXPOSURE. If the exhaust from the central vacuum pump goes to an area frequented by personnel, or is situated near an air intake, use of the system for gas disposal will result in additional exposure of personnel to waste gases. It may be necessary to relocate the pump exhaust.

INCONVENIENCE. Use of the suction system means that the tubing must be connected to the wall outlet at the beginning of each day. For energy conservation, it should be turned on just before anesthesia is begun and turned off at the termination of a procedure. For further energy conservation, the anesthesiologist should regulate the suction flow according to the volume of waste gases. These extra duties for the operating room staff and the anesthesiologist may result in their being neglected and there will be either wasted energy or operating room pollution.

Active Duct System (209, 210, 220, 224, 242–244) (Independent Blower-Operated System, Dedicated Suction or Blower System, Low Velocity Specialized Duct System). The other type of active disposal assembly is a dedicated duct system which leads to the outside and employs a flow-inducing device (fan, pump, or Venturi) to move the gases along. Each operating room is supplied with a duct, all of which are connected together to a common duct which leads to the outside. The flow-inducing device is located in the common duct and provides one-way movement of gases at a low negative pressure. The negative pressure ensures that cross-contamination between operating rooms will not occur and prevents atmospheric conditions from affecting the outflow from the system.

The flow-inducing device should provide a high volume (20–40 liters/min) flow (211, 220, 224, 242, 245), but not high vacuum. It should be situated near the outlet to atmosphere to reduce noise and clutter in the operating rooms. It has been recommended that two flow-inducing devices be provided and arranged so that if one fails to start the second one will run. Also it is recommended that there be a pilot light at the operating room control desk to indicate "Scavenging System Running."

A valve to adjust the flow and/or a flowmeter may be incorporated into the common duct. An on/off valve that can be controlled inside the operating room should be present. The outlet to atmosphere must be away from windows and air-conditioning intakes.

The advantages of this system are that resistance is not a problem and one need not worry about the effects of wind currents on the system. However, it requires a special installation, which is best done during construction. Installation of such a system should be considered during renovation or in the design of a new operating room.

Disadvantages include those of any active system: added complexity and the need for a negative pressure relief and reservoir capacity in the interface. The flow-inducing device must be housed somewhere and an energy supply provided. The flow-inducing device means added energy consumption. It must be switched on whenever anesthesia is being given, which is inconvenient, or left on permanently, which is very wasteful of energy. It requires regular attention, lubrication, etc., by the engineering staff. Flammable agents cannot be disposed of by this route unless the flow-inducing device is made spark-proof (196).

Choice of Disposal System (246). No single type of disposal system will prove ideal for all institutions. The following points should be considered before making a choice:

1. Simplicity. It should be easy to operate and maintain.

2. Efficiency. It should be capable of removing all of the waste gases from the operating room.

3. Automatic. It is desirable to keep the number of connections and adjustments made by the anesthesiologist and other operating room personnel to a minimum.

4. Convenience. If possible, bulky parts should be off the floor, out of the way, and not obstruct operating room traffic. Controls should be within easy reach.

5. Safety of Operating Room Personnel. Tubings running across the floor should be kept to a minimum.

6. Compatibility with Flammable Agents. If one plans to use flammable anesthetic agents, certain types of disposal systems cannot be used.

7. Economy. The cost should be as low as is consistent with efficiency. Consideration should be given to the expense both of installation and operation. Often, one may need to be weighed against another. Current physical facilities and future construction plans should be considered. Active disposal systems and non-recirculating ventilation systems are expensive to operate, and this cost may increase rapidly in the future. Specialized duct systems are expensive to install except in new construction where the cost should be minimal. Modification of the central vacuum system to add more capacity or outlets for scavenging is also expensive, but may prove

more economical than converting the air conditioning system to a non-recirculating type.

HAZARDS OF SCAVENGING EQUIPMENT

Pressure Alterations in the Breathing System

In essence the scavenging system extends the anesthesia breathing system all the way to the disposal point. When a scavenging system malfunctions or is misused, pressure alterations can be transferred to the breathing system, markedly altering its performance with potential harm to the patient.

Safety measures to prevent these untoward incidents include awareness and vigilance on the part of anesthesiologists toward problems occurring downstream of the breathing system or ventilator, incorporation of positive and negative pressure relief mechanisms in the interface (and regular checking of these for proper functioning), use of transfer tubing that is resistant to occlusion by kinking or twisting and that can be easily disconnected, use of pressure monitors

(see Chapter 5) and possibly a pressure-limiting valve (247) in the breathing system.

Positive Pressure Buildup. Positive pressure can result from several causes. Tubings that run across the floor may become occluded by the wheels of an anesthesia machine or other apparatus (188, 248, 249). A passive through-the-wall system can become occluded by ice (226), insects, or other foreign matter. Misassembly of the connection to the exhaust grille (250) and failure to include an opening between the inner and outer tube of a tube-within-a-tube system (251) have been reported. Excessive resistance in scavenging equipment with a passive disposal assembly or inadequate flow in an active assembly will cause increased pressure. These malfunctions will not result in a pressure buildup if a positive pressure relief mechanism is incorporated into the interface. However, obstruction of the transfer tubing may occur (Fig. 9.6) (252). Since this is on the patient side of the interface, disconnection of the transfer tubing from the gas collection assembly is necessary to prevent a dangerous increase in pressure.

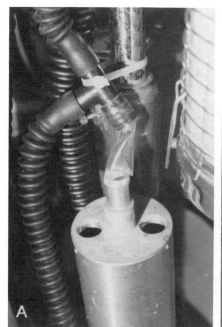
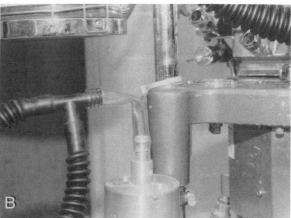

Figure 9.6.   Twisting (*A*) or kinking (*B*) of the transfer tubing can cause pressure buildup in the scavenging system that may be transmitted to the anesthesia breathing system. Occlusion at this site is particularly dangerous since it is upstream of the interface. Rapid disconnection of the tubing from the gas collection device must be performed to relieve the pressure buildup. A leak between the transfer tubing and the interface is also demonstrated in *A*.

Negative Pressure. In systems utilizing an active disposal assembly, there is the danger that subambient pressure will be applied to the breathing system or ventilator.

Cases have been reported in which a malfunction of the negative pressure relief mechanisms occurred. In one case the valve disc became stuck in the closed position (253). In another case the mechanism became covered by a plastic bag so that air could not be entrained (254). In still another case the opening to atmosphere of an open interface was taped over (255). Excessive resistance to air flow through some negative pressure relief mechanisms may result in vacuum flow exceeding waste gas plus air entrainment flow (256). Abramowitz and co-workers (241) pointed out that with some scavenging systems utilizing central vacuum, a restrictive orifice is incorporated into the vacuum hose fitting to limit the evacuation of gas, regardless of the pressure applied by the central vacuum source. Should this restrictive orifice be omitted or become damaged, full vacuum would be applied to the interface and the capacity of the negative pressure relief mechanisms could be exceeded.

The consequences of subambient pressure being applied to the breathing system will depend on the type of relief valve in the system. Sharrock and colleagues (257) found that relief valves with a spring-loaded disc allowed negative pressure to be transmitted to the breathing system in varying degrees, depending on the opening of the valve. When negative pressure was applied to a relief valve with a diaphragm, the diaphragm was drawn against the exhaust port, sealing the valve, and preventing the egress of gas from the breathing system.

Prevention of these problems include provision of at least two negative relief mechanisms (258) and protection of the openings to atmosphere from accidental external occlusion.

Misassembly of Components

The additional, sometimes complex, equipment that scavenging adds provides additional opportunities for misconnections of components. Connection of a circle system hose to the outlet of the relief valve has been reported (187, 188, 259). Use of an outlet connection of either 19 or 30 mm, fixing the exhaust port of the collection assembly to exit in the opposite direction to the breathing system ports, and use of transfer and gas disposal hoses of different color

and/or configuration from breathing system hoses should help to prevent this problem. However, even this will not completely prevent misconnections, since there may be other apparatus in the room which will accept 19- or 30-mm connections (260).

Loss of Means of Monitoring

Two cases have been reported in which an overdose of a potent anesthetic occurred and recognition of the ensuing cardiac arrest was not made promptly in part because the strong odor of the anesthetic was concealed by the scavenging equipment (252, 261).

It has already been pointed out that conversion of pressure relief valves to gas collecting assemblies has the effect of silencing them, thereby removing one means of monitoring a patient's ventilation. The sounds emitted by a mechanical ventilator can be appreciably altered when scavenging lines are attached (252).

Alterations of Work Practices (1, 59, 242, 245)

The manner in which anesthesia is administered can significantly affect trace gas levels. A number of work practices that allow anesthetic gases to bypass the scavenging system have been identified. Most cause only transient (but significant) elevations of trace gas concentrations, although a poor mask fit can cause high levels to persist throughout a case.

Lack of attention to these practices can completely nullify the most effective gas scavenging system. In many cases a lack of awareness or concern on the part of the anesthesia personnel may be present and some education may be necessary. Continuous trace gas monitoring can be of great value in showing anesthesia personnel the effects of certain practices on trace gas levels.

Adherence to the following suggested practices will significantly reduce contamination of operating room air. Obviously they must be of secondary importance when patient safety is in question. Most of the time they can be followed without compromising safety and some of them are beneficial to the patient.

PROPER MASK FIT

A good mask fit is critical, especially during assisted or controlled ventilation, when the higher pressures in the breathing system will magnify the leak between the patient and the mask. Investigators have found it very difficult to keep trace anesthetic levels within safe limits unless the face mask was strapped extremely tightly (262, 263). Often a very small change in mask angle can mean the difference between a good and bad fit. Several types and sizes of masks should be available. The aim should be to achieve a tight fit with minimal pressure. If it is difficult to obtain a tight fit, the advantages and disadvantages of intubation should be weighed against the potential hazards imposed by high trace gas levels.

AVOIDANCE OF UNSCAVENGEABLE TECHNIQUES (OPEN DROP OR INSUFFLATION)

Fortunately, the open drop technique has been nearly abandoned. Insufflation techniques in which an anesthetic mixture is introduced into the patient's respiratory system and delivery is accomplished upon inhalation are still widely used in laryngoscopy and bronchoscopy. High flow rates are required because of dilution of the anesthetic with room air and result in a high flow of anesthetic gases into the room. Reduction in room levels can be achieved by placing an active scavenging device near the leak site (264).

PREVENTION OF FLOW FROM THE BREATHING SYSTEM INTO ROOM AIR

One should avoid turning on the nitrous oxide or a vaporizer at the beginning of an anesthetic until the mask is fitted to the patient's face or the patient is intubated and connected to the breathing system. If it is preferred to turn on agents before induction, the patient port may be covered (perhaps by the circulating nurse) and the relief valve opened so that the gases enter the scavenging system.

After anesthesia has begun, accidental disconnections can be prevented by making certain that all connections are tight. Use of a pressure monitor (see Chapter 5) will help in early detection of a disconnection. Nonessential disconnections for such activities as taping the endotracheal tube or positioning the patient on the operating table should be avoided.

Flow of anesthetic gases into the room during intubation, extubation, and suctioning can be avoided if the bag is first emptied (gradually rather than violently dumping it) into the scavenging system and the anesthetic agents are turned off. Alternately, the patient port can be occluded and the relief valve opened so that the gases will enter the scavenging system.

Contamination of room air during removal of the reservoir bag prior to connecting a ventilator hose can be avoided if the bag is first emptied into the scavenging system and the anesthetic agents turned off. Use of an absorber-mounted selector valve (see Fig. 8.12) is also effective.

WASHOUT OF ANESTHETIC GASES AT THE END OF A CASE

At the end of an anesthetic, 100% oxygen (or air and oxygen) should be administered as long as possible before extubation or removal of the mask, so the scavenging system can eliminate the majority of washed-out anesthetic agents. This practice benefits the patient and keeps contamination to a minimum.

PREVENTION OF LIQUID AGENT SPILLAGE

It is easy to spill some of the agent when filling a vaporizer, so care should be exercised. Use of a pin-indexed vaporizer (see Chapter 4) will reduce spillage. The bottle should be capped immediately after filling or draining a vaporizer.

CHECKING THE SCAVENGING SYSTEM BEFORE USE

Before starting an anesthetic, the scavenging system should be checked to see that it is connected to the disposal system and that the disposal system is turned on if an active system is used.

PROPER USE OF TRACHEAL TUBES

Cuffed tracheal tubes should always be used in adults and the cuff inflated until there is no leak. Only small leaks should be permitted around uncuffed tubes in pediatric patients. Reduction of operating room contamination with an uncuffed tube can be achieved by placing a suction catheter in the mouth (265) and using a throat pack with dental cases (266).

DISCONNECTION OF NITROUS OXIDE SOURCES

Nitrous oxide and oxygen pipeline hoses leading to the machine should be disconnected at the end of the operating schedule. The disconnection should be made as close to the wall outlet as possible and not at the back of the anesthesia machine, so that if there is a leak in the hose, no gases will escape to room air while the hose is disconnected. This will result in lower levels of nitrous oxide in the operating room when the hoses are reconnected and will conserve gases.

When cylinders are used, the cylinder valve should be closed at the end of the operating schedule. Gas remaining in the machine should be "bled out" and evacuated through the scavenging system.

USE OF LOW FRESH GAS FLOWS (43, 267–270)

Use of low fresh gas flows has been suggested as a means of reducing the volume of anesthetic gases added to the room. Without any question, this will reduce the magnitude of pollution resulting from disconnections in the breathing system and from inefficient scavenging. With use of good work practices and proper scavenging, use of lower flows should have little influence on trace gas concentrations. Use of low flows and even a closed system does not make scavenging unnecessary, since high flows must still be used at times (see Chapter 8). It does allow the anesthesiologist to use lower removal flows with active disposal assemblies, resulting in energy conservation and reduced wear and tear on the disposal device.

Control of Leakage (1, 2, 198, 245, 262, 271–274)

Adding a scavenging system and correcting work practices will reduce trace gas concentrations markedly, but are still not enough to keep them at acceptable levels. Leakage of gases from equipment which has been reported to account for 2.5–87% of total contamination (272) must be controlled. Some leakage is inevitable, but it can be minimized.

Most anesthesia machines are under contract to undergo servicing by a manufacturer's representative at 4-month intervals. At these times the anesthesia machine and breathing systems should be examined and leaks corrected. Unfortunately, experience has shown that these routine visits do not always identify or correct all leak points (204). In addition, leakage in some equipment develops fairly frequently so that quarterly servicing is not sufficient. In-house monitoring and maintenance are necessary to minimize leakage. It has been suggested that a non-polluting anesthesia machine, ventilator and pipeline hoses be available to replace leaking equipment that requires servicing by a manufacturer's representative (275).

Initially, elimination of significant leakage will take a fair amount of time and effort, but following this anesthesia equipment can usually be maintained in an acceptably leak-free state with a minimum of effort. It is recommended that one individual supervise leakage control. In a small department this may be the same person who monitors the trace gas levels. In a larger department more than one person may be involved, but there should be close communication between them.

PRESSURE TERMINOLOGY

Some confusion exists in the literature as to the terminology of various pieces of anesthesia equipment. Some literature on scavenging has referred to all equipment upstream of the flow control valves as the high-pressure system and all equipment between the flow control valves and the patient plus the scavenging equipment as the low-pressure system (245, 276). However, older terminology established by the National Fire Protection Association defines high pressure as over 200 psig (277–279).

In this book, the high-pressure system refers to those components which contain gas whose pressure is normally above 50 psig. This includes the components of the machine between the cylinder and the regulator. The intermediate pressure system includes components normally subjected to a pressure of approximately 50 psig. This includes the hospital pipeline pipes and hoses and the components of the machine between the regulators or pipeline inlets and the flow control valves. The low-pressure system consists of components downstream of the flow control valves to the patient, plus the scavenging system. Pressures in this system will vary somewhat due to use of the oxygen flush valve and pressure variations in the breathing system, but will seldom exceed 40 cm H_2O.

IDENTIFICATION OF LEAK SITES

Once it has been determined that significant leakage exists, there are several techniques for precisely locating the leak sites.

A continuous infrared nitrous oxide analyzer

can be used. The equipment under test is pressurized with nitrous oxide and the sampling probe directed at suspected leak sites. The meter reading indicates the presence or absence of leakage. This will identify most leaks. An exception would be leakage in a vaporizer. Use of an infrared analyzer is the only way to find leakage in complicated pieces of equipment such as ventilators.

Leak sites can also be identified by application of a soap solution made by mixing 50% liquid soap and 50% water or a commercial leak test solution to a piece of equipment under pressure. Application may be facilitated by using a cotton-tipped applicator or a squeeze bottle. Leakage will be revealed by bubbling.

Leaks in smaller pieces of equipment such as bags, hoses, and even absorbers can be localized by pressurization to 30 cm H_2O, immersion in water and observation of bubbling. It is important to maintain pressure in immersed pieces at all times to prevent water from entering. Overpressurization should be avoided and pressure gauges should not be immersed. Pipeline hoses can also be pressurized and tested for leaks by immersion.

Leak sites can be detected by trial and error. The total leak rate for a system is determined, after which a component of the system is excluded and the leak rate redetermined. The difference is the leak rate for that piece of equipment.

THE HIGH-PRESSURE SYSTEM

To test for leakage in the high-pressure system, the pipeline hoses should be disconnected and the flow control valves closed. The valve on a nitrous oxide cylinder should be opened fully, the pressure recorded and the cylinder valve closed. One hour later the pressure should be recorded again. If little or no pressure drop has occurred, there is no significant leakage. If it falls, the high-pressure system is not tight. The test should be repeated with the other nitrous oxide cylinder if there is a double yoke.

If significant leakage is found, the most common site is the yoke and application of a leak test solution will demonstrate a poor seal. Merely tightening the cylinder in its yoke will often seal off the leak. Other easily correctible causes include double, absent, or deformed washers. If found, these should be replaced. If remedying these problems does not cause the pressure to hold, the leak is inside the machine or at the flow control valve and must be corrected by a manufacturer's service representative.

Since leakage in this area does not occur often, checking every 2 to 4 months and after a cylinder has been changed should be sufficient (1, 2, 245, 280). A form for recording this testing is shown in Figure 9.7.

THE INTERMEDIATE PRESSURE SYSTEM

Leakage in these components can be determined by measuring the nitrous oxide concentrations in the operating room when no anesthesia is being given (245). All rooms can be surveyed quickly at the one time using a continuous infrared analyzer. The survey should be begun at least 2 hr after all anesthesia has been completed, the flow control valves closed, the pipeline hoses disconnected, and cylinder valves closed.

Control measurements should be obtained in each room. The pipeline hoses should then be connected, but the flow control valves left

Figure 9.7. High-pressure leakage test form.

| Date | Room | Machine No. | N$_2$O Pressures | | Comments |
			Initial	After 1 Hour	

closed. After 1 hr, nitrous oxide concentrations should be measured in each room. Both surveys should result in concentrations of nitrous oxide of less than 5 ppm in the air (1, 204).

A high initial pressure indicates a leak somewhere in the nitrous oxide pipes leading to the operating rooms or in a station outlet and should be reported to the hospital engineer. An increase after the pipeline hoses are connected indicates a leak in the intermediate pressure system.

The pipeline hoses are the most frequent source of leaks in this system. Common problems include worn wall connections, loose high-pressure hose connections (especially quick-connects), deformed compression fittings, and holes in the hoses. These should be corrected or the hoses replaced. Leaks inside the anesthesia machine require correction by a service representative.

If one does not have a continuous infrared monitor, one should make sure that monitoring of trace gas levels includes determinations before anesthesia has begun or two hours after it was finished, as described above. If elevated levels are found, nitrous oxide hoses and station outlets should be checked by application of a leak test solution.

Once leakage is corrected, it is suggested that testing of the intermediate pressure system be performed every 2–4 months (1, 2, 204, 245, 280). The form for recording the testing is shown in Figure 9.8.

LOW-PRESSURE SYSTEM

This portion of the system develops leaks more frequently than other parts. It is unfortunate that the usual test for leaks in the breathing system, described in Chapter 14, is sufficient for the safe conduct of anesthesia, yet can miss leaks that emit large amounts of anesthetic gases into room air.

The procedure for quantifying leakage in the low-pressure system is shown in Figure 9.9. The breathing system is assembled as for clinical use. Equipment such as an oxygen analyzer that is normally used should be present in its usual position. The patient port is connected to an endotracheal tube connector which is occluded. The bag is removed and the bag mount plugged or occluded. This is necessary because the bag's compliance makes it hard to quantitate low leak rates. The bag should be tested separately for leaks by pressurization. The vaporizers to be used on the anesthesia machine should be turned on. The relief valve should be fully open and the scavenging system occluded upstream of the interface.

A flow control valve is now opened sufficiently to establish and maintain a steady pressure of 30 cm H_2O on the pressure gauge in the breathing system. Caution is necessary to avoid damage to the pressure gauge from overpressurization. If the machine is equipped with a built-in vaporizer such as the Copper Kettle, the flow control valve associated with this vaporizer should be opened. If these vaporizers are not present the oxygen flowmeter should be used. If the machine is not equipped with a low-range flowmeter, a T connection can be inserted into the fresh gas line and a low-range non-pressure-compensated flowmeter connected.

The flow necessary to maintain 30 cm H_2O pressure is the leak rate and should be less than 100 cc/min. Leakage of this magnitude will be of little importance in a well-ventilated operat-

Figure 9.8.   Intermediate pressure leak test form.

Date	Room No.	Machine No.	Nitrous Oxide Concentrations		Comments
			Before Connecting Pipeline Hoses	After Connecting Hoses	

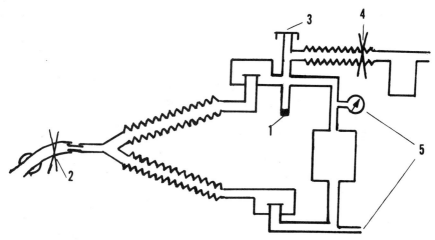

Figure 9.9. Test for quantifying low-pressure leakage. *1,* remove reservoir bag and occlude mount (with cork or hand); *2,* attach endotracheal tube connector and occlude connector or endotracheal tube; *3,* open relief valve; *4,* occlude transfer tubing just upstream of interface; *5,* adjust and maintain oxygen flow sufficient to maintain a pressure of 30 cm H_2O on pressure gauge in breathing system.

ing room. If the leak rate exceeds 100 cc/min but is considered compatible with safe anesthesia, the anesthesiologist might proceed with the case but mark the machine for servicing at the end of the work day. If the leak rate is greater than 1 liter/min the machine should not be used.

If the leak rate exceeds 100 cc/min, the relief valve should be closed and the leak rate redetermined. The difference is the leak rate in the scavenging system.

The remaining leakage can be divided into that associated with the machine and that associated with the breathing system by attaching the fresh gas line to a sphygnomanometer bulb and determining the oxygen flow necessary to achieve and maintain a pressure of 22 mm Hg. This is the portion of the low-pressure leakage contributed by the machine. The machine leakage can be further divided by turning off the vaporizers and redetermining the leak rate.

Problems in the scavenging system may be as simple as a hole in a tubing (especially where it gets kinked) or a poor connection. Valves in the closed interface frequently leak (281).

If it has been determined that a vaporizer is leaking, a search should be made for loosened parts. Correction of most leaks requires servicing by a manufacturer's representative.

Other parts of the machine low-pressure system that frequently leak are connections along the back bar. Leaks here can often be corrected by tightening and application of lubricant be-

tween the metal-to-metal fittings. Another frequent leak site is the fresh gas outlet. This is usually a metal-to-metal fitting. Often the metal part attached to the fresh gas line gets dropped and becomes deformed. This should be replaced by a plastic component. The fresh gas line itself may have been punctured or become cracked with age, especially near the ends.

The breathing system is the most common location of significant low pressure leakage and the most common site in the breathing system is the absorber. Important causes include defective gaskets or seals, improper closure, inadequate tightening and open or leaky drain cocks. Absorbent spilled on the gasket can prevent a tight seal. Many of these problems can be easily corrected. Complicated repairs should be done by the manufacturer's representative.

All rubber or plastic tubings, including the bypass tubing on the absorber, can be punctured or become cracked with time. These should be replaced.

Valve covers over unidirectional valves may become cracked or loose and should be replaced or tightened. Fittings for oxygen analyzer sensors that leak should be replaced.

Cottrell and co-workers (147) and Hovey (263) found that swivel-type disposable circle systems had high leak rates, so a significant reduction in leakage may result from using ones without swivel Y-pieces.

Berner (272) found high leakage rates at the

junction of the Y-piece and endotracheal tube connector. The Y-piece is frequently dropped on the floor and metal ones may become deformed. These should be replaced with plastic ones that are more resistant to deformation.

Considerable controversy exists as to how often the low-pressure system should be tested for leakage. Suggested intervals vary from daily (1, 204), to every other week (245, 280) to monthly (2). It should be repeated with new equipment and when the absorbent is changed. A suggested form is shown in Figure 9.10.

Room Ventilation System (29, 33, 212, 282)

An effective room ventilation system serves as an important adjunct to trace gas control by removing anesthetic gases resulting from leaks, errors in technique and scavenging system malfunctions.

Classically, ventilation system function is described in room air turnovers per hour. Ten turnovers is probably the minimal acceptable number (221).

The effect of the ventilation system on gas removal can be calculated using the following formula (29, 218, 282–285)

$C = (60 \times L \times 10)/NV(1 - r)$ where
C is the concentration of gases in the operating room in parts per million;
L is the rate at which anesthetic gases are released into room air in liters per minute;
N is the number of air changes per hour;
V is the volume of the room in liters; and
r is the fraction of air that is recirculated.

A rule of thumb is that in a typical operating room with ten fresh air exchanges per hour,

every 100 ml/min leak of gas leads to approximately 5 ppm in the atmosphere (198).

Recirculating systems are less effective in removing trace gases than non-recirculating systems because of the lower dilution rate (196). A downward displacement ventilation system is more effective in eliminating trace gases than a turbulent flow system (40, 212).

The anesthesiologist can help to assure proper functioning of the room ventilation system by contacting the hospital engineers and urging them to keep the filters and grilles clean and the flows balanced (204).

Placing the anesthesia machine in the main flow channel from the inflow to the exit grille is an aid in eliminating spilled gases. The anesthesia machine should be placed as close to the exhaust grille as possible (59). This will assure maximum removal of gases by the ventilation system plus make it easy to use the ventilation system as the disposal system. This should be taken into consideration when constructing a new operating room or renovating an older one.

MONITORING TRACE GASES
Rationale

All the control measures discussed thus far cannot ensure acceptably low levels of trace gases. This can only be realized if monitoring of the levels is performed.

Monitoring is the final and most important assessment of a pollution control program's effectiveness. It reflects how well leaks and technique errors are being controlled plus the efficiency of the scavenging and room ventilation systems and documents trace levels for medicolegal purposes.

The necessity for a monitoring program seems

Figure 9.10. Form for low-pressure leakage.

Date	Machine No.	Total Leak Rate	Scavenging System Leak Rate	Machine Leak Rate	Machine Leak Rate with Vaporizers Off	Leak Sites and Corrections

inescapable. A scavenging system that appears adequate in design may perform inefficiently in use. Leaks in the intermediate pressure system may be impossible to detect without monitoring. Even relatively large leaks may be inaudible. Nitrous oxide is odorless and the threshold for smelling potent agents such as halothane varies from 5 to 300 ppm (17, 228, 286, 287). However, the threshold for methoxyflurane is 0.1 to 2 ppm (287). Without a monitoring program the operating room personnel may be unaware that atmospheric contamination is at unacceptable levels. A properly conducted air monitoring program provides a subtle constructive method of reminding the anesthesiologist to avoid careless work habits and to make consistent use of available scavenging equipment.

While such a program will increase a hospital's operating expense slightly, it will help to reduce the institution's liability exposure by refuting workers' compensation or liability claims related to alleged overexposure to waste gases. Also correction of leakage in nitrous oxide lines will result in a savings to the hospital.

In-House Monitoring Versus Commercial Laboratory

The monitoring program should be directed by an interested and qualified person, preferably from the anesthesia department. The method chosen will vary with the size of the institution, the money available and the objectives. Generally desirable features in a monitoring program are simplicity, reliability, economy, and immediacy. It should disrupt the operating room routine as little as possible.

In a large hospital with many operating rooms, the expense of sending multiple samples to a commercial laboratory makes in-house equipment more economically feasible. In a teaching hospital a continuous monitor is useful for demonstrating the effects of technique errors on trace gas levels.

A smaller hospital might periodically lease an instrument or share one with other hospitals in the area rather than purchase its own analyzer. Another alternative is to use a commercial agency that both performs preventive maintenance and does air monitoring at the same time.

A third option is to obtain air samples from the operating rooms and send them to a commercial laboratory. Such a laboratory can supply all the necessary sampling equipment. A serious disadvantage of this method is the delayed reporting of results. The precise circumstances of sampling are likely to be forgotten and the effect of corrective measures cannot be immediately assessed. In addition, analysis of a large number of samples is expensive.

Techniques for Determining Trace Gas Concentrations

INFRARED ANALYZERS (1, 274, 276, 288–291)

Each anesthetic gas has a unique spectrum of absorption peaks in the infrared (IR) spectrum. In an infrared analyzer, a light beam of the proper wavelength is passed through a cell containing the sample to be analyzed. The concentration of the gas can be determined by measuring the amount of light absorbed. Air can be passed directly through portable IR instruments, through tubes to remote instruments or samples can be collected in suitable containers and then analyzed.

These monitors are the most practical for the average hospital because they are reliable, relatively inexpensive, and easy to use. They give continuous measurements so that exposed workers and those responsible for air monitoring are given an immediate indication of system efficiency. When operated on battery power, a number of locations can be sampled quickly. They are very useful for tracing and pinpointing of leaks. A recording attachment may be useful.

These instruments are most often used for monitoring nitrous oxide concentrations. Unfortunately, carbon dioxide and water vapor in high concentrations will interfere with the analysis. This can be avoided by sampling 6–10 inches away from personnel (276, 290). End-tidal concentrations cannot be measured by this method. Analyzers with variable filters are available which are capable of measuring the halogenated anesthetics, but analysis of these agents is fraught with technical difficulties and alcohols and other substances in the operating room cause interference (10, 288, 292).

IONIZING LEAK DETECTOR (2, 284, 293, 294) (LEAKMETER)

The leakmeter, an instrument designed for the detection of low concentrations of volatile halogenated hydrocarbons in industry, is suitable for detecting low concentrations of volatile halogenated anesthetic agents. It consists of three components: an electron capture detector housed within a handpiece and fitted with a probe; a control unit which processes the signal from the detector and displays the output on a meter; and an argon carrier gas supply. The instrument is compact, relatively inexpensive, portable, and can be operated on batteries.

It is suitable for measuring low concentrations of halogenated agents. However, there may be interference from other halogenated agents in the area, including antibiotic and skin-protection sprays. It is not useful for nitrous oxide detection. It is somewhat unstable in use, requiring frequent zeroing and recalibration (2, 29).

MASS SPECTROSCOPY (34)

The mass spectrometer, discussed in Chapter 5, is capable of measuring very low concentrations accurately and quickly and can be specific for any particular agent. It can be used for end-tidal samples (34). At present, however, the equipment is probably too complicated and expensive for the average hospital to use for monitoring trace gas concentrations.

GAS CHROMATOGRAPHY (1, 2, 14, 30, 38, 214, 295–297)

In gas chromatography the components of a sample are separated and their concentrations measured. This method is accurate and reliable for measuring halogenated agents but nitrous oxide determinations are fraught with difficulty (59, 297). It can be used for measuring end-tidal and blood samples.

The equipment is expensive and requires highly trained personnel. The machines are bulky and not suitable for most in-theater use (284). They do not permit continuous monitoring, although short analysis time allows determinations to be made at frequent intervals. This equipment is most suitable for commercial laboratories and research institutions.

Sampling Methods

INSTANTANEOUS SAMPLING (204, 276) (GRAB, SINGLE SHOT, PERIODIC, SNATCH)

Instantaneous sampling is performed by first drawing a sample of air into a container and then measuring the trace gas concentration either in house or by a commercial laboratory using one of the techniques described above. The

container must not adsorb or absorb the contaminant or leak. Nylon bags are the preferred storage container when nitrous oxide levels are to be measured (298). Glass and plastic syringes are unsatisfactory unless concentrations can be determined immediately after sampling.

This method is relatively inexpensive, simple to perform, quickly accomplished and does not involve taking bulky equipment into the operating room. It has some serious disadvantages. One is the delay in reporting of results. A long interval between sampling and reporting makes it difficult to remember the precise circumstances that were in effect when the sample was taken and the effect of corrective measures cannot be immediately assessed. It is of limited value in determining leak sites and assessing correction of leaks. Another serious disadvantage is that because of variations in trace gas concentrations with time, the sample may be taken at the peak or valley of the situation. Beynen and co-workers (36) found that gradients in operating rooms were sufficiently large to invalidate estimation of personnel exposure from instantaneous samples. This disadvantage can be decreased by taking multiple samples, but this increases the expense.

The instantaneous sample is probably best employed for analysis of steady-state contamination, i.e., sampling prior to starting anesthesia for intermediate pressure leaks or where an equilibrium has been achieved (22). If good techniques are employed and leakage has been controlled, trace gas levels tend to rise in a fluctuating pattern during the early part of an anesthetic, then roughly equilibrate, reaching a level that represents the net effects of leaks, air conditioning flow, inflow gas rate, scavenging efficiency and personnel movement (36). Under these circumstances an instantaneous sample 30–45 min after induction is probably a good index of the average trace gas levels (22, 36, 204). If poor techniques are employed and/or no attempt has been made to eliminate leakage, pollution levels will vary markedly and instantaneous samples may be quite misleading. If unacceptably high levels are found, one cannot be sure whether the cause is a leak, poor technique or a fault in the scavenging system.

When an instantaneous sample is taken, it is important to record the date and time of sample collection, the work practices (breathing system, fresh gas flow rate, use of mask or endotracheal tube, use of ventilator, spontaneous or manually controlled ventilation), location of sample, and the person administering anesthesia.

TIME-WEIGHTED AVERAGE SAMPLING (276) (INTEGRATED PERSONNEL, TIME-INTEGRATED)

The potential toxicity of trace gases is probably a function of both dose and exposure time. Hence a sampling method that gives an average exposure level during the sampling period (an integrated sample) is of interest.

Time-weighted average (TWA) sampling may be performed by pumping ambient air continuously at a low flow rate into a gas-tight inert container (2, 10, 12, 17, 276, 291, 299–301) or a tube or other device filled with a substance that adsorbs anesthetic agents (1, 10, 303–309) over a period of time.

The container, badge, or tube may be worn by a person in the operating room or may be placed at a fixed site. The gases thus collected are analyzed to obtain the average trace gas concentration over the time period. Sampling should cover the entire workday or at least a significantly representative sample.

Other ways of obtaining a time-weighted average are to average the results for many instantaneous samples, take the average of concentrations measured at equal time intervals throughout the recorded tracing of a continuous analyzer or to integrate the output of a continuous analyzer (302).

By eliminating the potential for errors due to temporal fluctuations in trace gas levels, time-weighted average sampling reflects personnel exposure better than instantaneous sampling. It requires only a modest capital investment and there is a considerable savings of time and labor compared with taking and analyzing multiple instantaneous samples.

There are several disadvantages to this method. It is cumbersome in terms of time required to set up the apparatus and subsequently to wash out and evacuate the bag completely before making further collections (276, 302). A serious disadvantage is that it does not assist in improving work techniques or in leak detection. Delayed results make it difficult to correlate with activities at the time of collection. If concentrations in excess of those recommended are found, one cannot tell whether the problem is technique errors, leaks, or inadequate scavenging.

CONTINUOUS MONITORING (2, 22, 59, 276)

Continuous monitoring is carried out using an infrared analyzer or leakmeter. Use of a battery-powered instrument allows for easy movement about a room and from room to room. Time is saved by eliminating the need for attaching the power cord and warming up the instrument each time it is moved.

The continuous monitor allows one to check trace gas concentrations at various sites in the room. If a writer is attached and the analyzer is run over a period of time, a time-weighted average sample is obtained (302).

The continuous monitor can be used to detect leaks by probing about the machine, pipelines, wall sockets, etc., with the sampling hose. One can also determine if a leak has been successfully corrected.

If a continuous analyzer is operated during anesthesia, it will demonstrate to the anesthesiologist the effects of improper work practices on trace levels and the results of modifying or improving those practices.

Patient safety may be enhanced by use of a continuous analyzer. One of the earliest warnings of a disconnection in the breathing system may be observation of a rise in the room concentration of a trace gas (198, 276).

The convenience and immediate feedback of continuous monitoring are distinct advantages over instantaneous or time-weighted average sampling. When high readings are obtained the causes can usually be determined immediately and corrective measures taken.

One disadvantage of continuous monitors is that they are somewhat expensive, so that in a small hospital the time and expense required to maintain a continuous monitor may make it uneconomical. In such circumstances, several hospitals might consider sharing an instrument or a manufacturer's service representative might utilize one during his routine quarterly maintenance calls. Sampling with them tends to disrupt the operating room routine more than instantaneous or time-weighted average sampling. Finally, rapidly changing concentrations are difficult to interpret in terms of personnel exposure unless integration over time is employed.

END-TIDAL SAMPLING (4, 5, 17, 19, 27, 28, 34, 36, 39, 41, 301, 310)

End-tidal samples of gases may be taken from exposed personnel after a period of exposure.

They are inherently time-weighted and show less scatter than time-weighted average samples (297). This method is most suitable for potent halogenated agents. Nitrous oxide is so rapidly absorbed and excreted that its level in end-tidal gas reflects only the most recent exposure of the subject. To obtain meaningful data on average nitrous oxide exposure multiple end-tidal samples must be taken (301).

Disadvantages of this method include the fact that an infrared analyzer cannot be used because carbon dioxide and water vapor interfere with nitrous oxide analysis. Collecting end-tidal samples is disruptive to operating room personnel (although less so than taking of blood samples) performing their duties. With high levels of agents in the atmosphere, some agent may be detectable in the morning from the previous day's exposure (4, 28, 34, 39, 295, 310).

VENOUS BLOOD SAMPLING (17, 19, 27, 28, 31, 38–40, 310, 311, 312)

Samples of venous blood can be drawn from exposed personnel at the end of an exposure period and be analyzed.

In personnel exposed to high concentrations of potent agents, a detectable amount may be present in morning samples, so that these individuals are constant carriers of the agent (28, 310).

Agent(s) to Be Monitored

Ideally all gases employed in the conduct of an anesthetic should be measured. Analyzers are available which can scan the infrared spectrum and are programmable to distinguish individual inhalation anesthetics. Likewise, mass spectrometry and gas chromatography can be used to measure all agents. However, it is simpler to monitor a single gas. But which gas?

If one agent were clearly more toxic than others, it would be logical to monitor that agent. In the light of present knowledge, it cannot be stated that nitrous oxide is either more or less toxic than the more potent agents (290). The NIOSH criteria document (1) does not require monitoring of all anesthetic agents, but only the one most frequently used.

NITROUS OXIDE

Many people feel that nitrous oxide is the most logical agent to monitor because it is administered more frequently and in larger quan-

tities than other agents, is easy to measure, and is more likely to be subject to occult leakage than potent agents (276).

Since nitrous oxide and other agents are not separated by buoyancy effects (2, 29), they will be present in a room in the same ratio in which they are introduced. Because of this, many people feel that nitrous oxide can serve as an indicator or tracer of other agents administered with it to a degree of accuracy sufficient for routine appraisal of occupational exposure (313).

This tracer concept holds best under conditions of steady-state anesthesia and tightly controlled equipment leakage. It does not apply while a vaporizer is being filled or drained or during the induction and recovery phases of anesthesia. These phenomena are transient. It does not hold when there is a nitrous oxide leak or a leak in a vaporizer.

POTENT AGENTS

Monitoring of other agents can be beneficial (314, 315). Leakage of other agents does not always occur in the same proportions as delivered with nitrous oxide. Volatile halogenated agents can leak independently of nitrous oxide. Since a leak in a vaporizer is a potential source of contamination with fully saturated vapor, even a small leak can cause very high levels. Air contamination with potent agents independent of nitrous oxide also occurs when a vaporizer is filled or drained.

Sites to Monitor

PERSONNEL MONITORING

Sampling the breathing zone of exposed personnel (especially anesthesia personnel) is usually considered the preferred method. The anesthesiologist is the most important person to monitor since he usually inhales higher concentrations than other operating room personnel and is more apt to remain in the room for the entire duration of anesthesia administration. NIOSH recommends that all locations with a potential for worker exposure be sampled (1). Personnel monitoring is especially preferred in poorly ventilated rooms (316). Recommended sites include the lateral aspect of the neck (11), mid-clavicle (217, 291, 301), or attached to the eyeglasses frame or headlight (291), the shoulder (276), attached to the anesthesiologist's scrub suit or gown (10, 304, 306), or behind the neck (2). Beynen and co-workers (36) found that samples collected behind the head of the person administering anesthesia were not representative of true inspired gas. Sampling directly in the pathway of the subject's expired air must be avoided if nitrous oxide analysis by infrared spectroscopy is to be used. Fixed sites near the anesthesiologist may be used to estimate exposure (317) but if high levels are found, additional sampling is warranted.

One problem with personnel monitoring is that it requires the cooperation of personnel. Scrubbed personnel may be disturbed by the risk of accidental contact with the sampling equipment. The analyzer operator must be thoroughly familiar with sterile technique in the operating room and should be known to and accepted by the operating team.

AREA SAMPLING (2, 22, 276) (ROOM SAMPLING)

Area sampling is justifiable only when it has been clearly demonstrated that gases are evenly distributed. This requires analysis of multiple samples in each room (198), which can be easily accomplished with a portable analyzer. In the operating room where all leakage is under effective control, gas concentrations are apt to be similar throughout the room. In this event, area sampling is appropriate (198).

The exhaust grill of the air conditioning system or the open door will be representative of average personnel exposure if it has been determined that gases are evenly distributed in the room. Piziali and co-workers (29) and others have found "hot spots" where trace gas concentrations are 10 to 15 times the room average. Such hot spots may surround the head of any person in the operating room with high concentrations of anesthetic gases with increased exposure of personnel. Hot spots are related to air conditioning flow rates and other variables such as the position of the anesthesia machine, furniture, movement of personnel, locations of ventilation ducts relative to the anesthesia machine, and opening and closing of doors. The magnitude of their effects is not predictable. In general, an operating room having more than 15 air changes per hour will have few hot spots and sampling at the exhaust grille or door will be quite satisfactory (29, 86). If the room has fewer than 15 changes per hour, readings at other locations should be taken. Area sampling is less disruptive to the operating room routine and less disturbing to personnel than personal monitoring. It requires no cooperation of personnel

and does not interfere with activities in the room.

RECOVERY ROOMS (24, 25, 28, 35, 45, 310)

Bruce and co-workers (35) measured concentrations 24 inches over the patient's head. A more elaborate method was used by Berner (45). Samples were taken at 50 cm above the patient's thorax, at the foot end of the bed, and 2 m from the foot end of the bed, both at 180 cm above floor level. The concentrations were then multiplied by how long personnel remained in the different areas. Berner suggested that concentrations be measured during the "peak load period" when there are a maximum number of patients exhaling gases.

Frequency of Monitoring

The ideal frequency of monitoring depends on the experience of each suite. At the initiation of a waste gas control program frequent monitoring (at least weekly) under actual working conditions will be necessary. As experience is gained and equipment is maintained leak-tight, the frequency can be decreased. The minimum should be every 3 months (276). However, whenever concentrations higher than acceptable are found, new equipment is installed or old equipment modified, monitoring should be repeated.

Time-weighted average monitoring of each member of the staff for a short period, such as a week, repeated on a 6-month basis has been suggested (10).

The monitoring should be scheduled so that the work of each group of anesthesia personnel and of each operating room is checked while using a mask and an endotracheal tube and while using an automatic ventilator. Monitoring should also proceed during spontaneous, manually assisted, and manually controlled ventilation. The results of the monitoring should be analyzed and compared with previous results and discussed with all parties concerned. A form recording the results and sampling conditions is shown in Figure 9.11.

ROLE OF THE FEDERAL GOVERNMENT AND THE JOINT COMMISSION ON ACCREDITATION OF HOSPITALS (318–321)

Two federal government agencies are concerned with the issue of trace gases: the National

Figure 9.11.   Total room survey.

Room	Machine No.	Ventilator No.	Anesthesiologist	V/C/A/S	M/E	N₂O/O₂	Breathing System	Nitrous Oxide Readings				Comments
								Sample 1	Sample 2	Sample 3	Sample 4	

C, manually controlled ventilation
V, mechanically controlled ventilation
A, assisted ventilation
S, spontaneous ventilation
M, mask
E, endotracheal tube
N₂O/O₂ flows in liters/minute
Breathing system: circle, Mapleson D, T-piece, non-rebreathing valve, etc.
Sample 1, anesthesiologist's breathing zone
Sample 2, exhaust vent
Sample 3, door
Sample 4, other site (specify)

Date _____

Time of Day _____

Institute for Occupational Safety and Health (NIOSH), an agency of the Department of Health and Human Services; and the Occupational Safety and Health Administration (OSHA), an agency of the Department of Labor. Although both agencies were created by the Occupational Safety and Health Act of 1970, their duties differ.

NIOSH has three major mandates: (a) to fund and conduct research for determining the effects of chronic low-level exposure; (b) to educate employers and employees about preventing occupational illnesses; and (c) to develop criteria for recommended standards and transmit these to OSHA.

Research activities undertaken so far by NIOSH have included the following: (a) providing funding to the American Society of Anesthesiologists for a national health survey of operating room personnel and dentists (50); (b) a questionnaire survey of 1200 hospitals to obtain information concerning anesthesia practices; (c) awarding of contracts to study potential effects of trace anesthetics on behavioral performance (112), methods for eliminating waste gas exposure (2) and controlling exposure to nitrous oxide in dental offices (290); (d) awarding of contracts to conduct studies on the effects of inhalation anesthetic agents on laboratory animals.

After gathering information from these and various other sources, NIOSH prepared a criteria document which was published and transmitted to OSHA in 1977 (1). Important aspects of this document are as follows:

1. Although NIOSH considered that a safety level of exposure to waste anesthetic gases could not be defined, maximum concentrations to which a worker should be exposed were recommended. For halogenated agents used alone this concentration was 2 ppm time-weighted average collected during anesthesia administration. When halogenated agents are used in combination with nitrous oxide the concentrations were 25 ppm nitrous oxide and 0.5 ppm of the halogenated agent. The Ad Hoc Committee of the American Society of Anesthesiologists has sug-

gested that less than 180 ppm is satisfactory with mask techniques (204).

2. Air monitoring is recommended in all areas with potential for worker exposure on a quarterly basis and whenever any equipment is modified. Breathing zone or immediate work area samples are most desirable.

3. Results of monitoring and corrective measures are to be maintained and retained for 20 years.

4. Recommendations were made regarding scavenging, ventilation systems, leak testing, and work practices aimed at minimizing employee exposure.

5. Comprehensive pre-employment medical histories are required. Annual physical examinations are recommended. Medical records are to be maintained for the period of employment plus 20 years.

6. Employees are to be informed of the possible health effects of exposure to trace anesthetics, especially possible effects on reproduction.

OSHA has as its major responsibilities the following:

1. Encouragement of reduction of hazards in the workplace;

2. Establishment of separate but dependent responsibilities and rights for employers and employees for achievement of better health conditions;

3. Establishment of record-keeping procedures to monitor job-related illnesses;

4. Development, promulgation and enforcement of mandatory health standards. To date no permanent standard has been issued.

The Joint Commission on the Accreditation of Hospitals, which inspects most hospitals in the United States in its 1979 Accreditation Manual for Hospitals, recommended, but did not require, that each anesthesia machine be equipped with a gas scavenging device. It does now recommend that a monitoring program be performed but does not as yet require a method.

MEDICO-LEGAL CONSIDERATIONS (321)

Because the NIOSH document does not constitute a promulgated OSHA standard, employers are not obligated to comply with its recommendations. However, it is still possible for OSHA to conduct inspections in facilities that use inhalation anesthetics and to cite and penalize (usually fine) employers and other parties, especially anesthesiologists. In addition to re-quiring compliance with specific standards, OSHA imposes upon employers the broad general duty of providing a place of employment free from recognized hazards. The Act gives each employee the right to request an OSHA inspection if the employee feels he or she is in imminent danger from a hazard or OSHA standards are being violated. Several inspections in response to employee complaints have been carried out with resultant citations and fines to both hospital administration and the anesthesiologists involved, on the position that exposure of employees to high levels of waste anesthetics is in violation of OSHA's general duty clause (320, 322).

All states have enacted workers' compensation laws that provide a scheme of employer liability without fault to injured employees. Individuals suffering occupational diseases can collect workers' compensation benefits from their employer. It is immaterial whether or not the employer's negligence caused the employee's injury. It is possible that a workers' compensation case could arise from an operating room employee suffering from one of the problems described in the first section of this chapter, provided the employee could show that the illness was work connected and that employment in the operating room subjected him or her to special risk in excess of those experienced by the general public. In most states workers' compensation laws preclude private lawsuits by an employee against his or her employer.

Unfortunately, the exclusivity of workers' compensation proceedings applies only to actions by employees against their employers. An employee, in addition to making a claim for workers' compensation against the employer, is free to bring civil suit for damages against a third party whom the employee claims caused injury. An operating room employee would not be precluded by workers' compensation laws from bringing an action against an anesthesiologist on the basis that the anesthesiologist's work practices increased the levels of waste anesthetics. Similarly, an injured anesthesiologist would not be precluded from bringing an action against the hospital where he or she practices on the basis that inadequate monitoring, equipment maintenance, or scavenging devices were provided by the hospital.

The authors of this text feel that each anesthesia department has a moral (but not necessarily legal) obligation to notify operating room personnel that a potential health hazard may exist consequent to employment in the operating room, that every effort is being made to limit their exposure to trace gases, and that they have the option of working in another area where they will not be exposed to trace levels of anesthetic gases. A sample notice has been published (323). It is suggested that these notices be acknowledged and that a record be kept of these acknowledgments.

References

1. *Criteria for a Recommended Standard. Occupational Exposure to Waste Anesthetic Gases and Vapors.* DHEW (NIOSH) Publication No. 77-140, 1977.
2. *Development and Evaluation of Methods for the Elimination of Waste Anesthetic Gases and Vapors in Hospitals.* DHEW (NIOSH) Publication No. 75-137, 1975.
3. Corbett TH, Ball GL: Chronic exposure to halothane: possible occupational hazard to anesthesiologists. Scientific Papers, American Society of Anesthesiologists Annual Meeting, 1971, pp 151-152.
4. Corbett TH: Retention of anesthetic agents following occupational exposure. *Anesth Analg* 52:614-618, 1973.
5. Corbett TH, Ball GL: Respiratory excretion of halothane after clinical and occupational exposure. *Anesthesiology* 39:342-345, 1973.
6. Corbett TH: Anesthetics as a cause of abortion. *Fertil Steril* 23:866-869, 1972.
7. Corbett TH: Inhalation anesthetics—more vinyl chloride? *Environ Res* 9:211-214, 1975.
8. Corbett TH: Cancer and congenital anomalies associated with anesthetics. *Ann NY Acad Sci* 271:58-66, 1976.
9. Davenport HT, Halsey MJ, Wardley-Smith B, Bateman PE: Occupational exposure to anaesthetics in 20 hospitals. *Anaesthesia* 35:354-359, 1980.
10. Campbell D, Davis PD, Halliday MM, MacDonald I: Comparison of personal pollution monitoring techniques for use in the operating room. *Br J Anaesth* 52:885-892, 1980.
11. Cohen EN: *Anesthetic Exposure in the Workplace.* Littleton, Mass., PSG Publishing, 1980.
12. Davenport HT, Halsey MJ, Wardley-Smith FB, Wright BM: Measurement and reduction of occupational exposure to inhaled anaesthetics. *Br Med J* 2:1219-1221, 1976.
13. Duvaldestin P, Mazze RI, Hazebrouck J, Nivoche Y, Cohen SE, Desmonts J: Halothane biotransformation in anesthetists. *Anesthesiology* 51:41-46, 1979.
14. Gelbicova-Ruzickova J, Novak J, Janak J: Application of the method of chromatographic equilibration to air pollution studies. The determination of minute amounts of halothane in the atmosphere of an operating theatre. *J Chromatogr* 64:15-23, 1972.
15. Gothe CZ, Ovrum P, Hallen B: Exposure to anesthetic gases and ethanol during work in operating rooms. *Scand J Work Environ Health* 2:96-106, 1976.
16. Gotell P, Sundell L: Anaesthetists' exposure to halothane. *Lancet* 2:424, 1972.
17. Hallen B, Ehrner-Samuel H, Thomason M: Measurements of halothane in the atmosphere of an operating theatre and in expired air and blood of the personnel during routine anaesthetic work. *Acta Anaesth Scand* 14:17-27, 1970.
18. Knights KM, Armstrong RF, Strunin L: Halothane 1 ppm—is it practical? *Br J Anaesth* 48:815-816, 1976.
19. Korttila K, Pfaffli P, Linnoila M, Blomgren E, Hanninen H, Hakkinen S: Operating room nurses' psychomotor and driving skills after occupational exposure to halothane and nitrous oxide. *Acta Anaesth Scand* 226:33-39, 1978.
20. Linde HW, Bruce DL: Occupational exposure of anesthetists to halothane, nitrous oxide and radiation. *Anesthesiology* 30:363-368, 1969.
21. Lane JR: Anaesthetic pollution and its prevention. *Proc R Soc Med* 67:992-994, 1976.
22. Lecky JH, Neufeld GR: Approaches to operating room pollution control. Exhibit, ASA Meeting, 1975.
23. Mehta S, Cole WJ, Chari J, Lewin K: Operating room air pollution: influence of anaesthetic circuit, vapour concentration, gas flow and ventilation. *Can Anaesth Soc J* 22:265-274, 1975.
24. Nikki P, Pfaffli K, Ahlman K, Ralli R: Chronic exposure to anaesthetic gases in the operating theatre and recovery room. *Ann Clin Res* 4:266-272, 1972.
25. Nicholson JA, Sada T, Aldrete JA: Residual halothane: patient and personnel exposure. *Anesth Analg* 54:449-454, 1975.
26. Nicholson JA: How much are we exposed to? *J Ky Med Assoc* 73:98-116, 1975.
27. Pfaffli P, Nikki P, Ahlman K: Concentrations of anaesthetic gases in recovery rooms. *Br J Anaesth* 44:230, 1972.
28. Pfaffli P, Nikki P, Ahlman K: Halothane and nitrous oxide in end-tidal air and venous blood of surgical personnel. *Ann Clin Res* 4:273-277, 1972.
29. Piziali RL, Whitcher C, Sher R, Moffat RJ: Distribution of waste anesthetic gases in the operating room air. *Anesthesiology* 45:487-494, 1976.
30. Ramanthan PS, Srivastava OP, Venkateswarlu CH, Walvekar AP: Study of anaesthetic vapour concentrations in operation theatres by gas chromatography. *Indian J Med Res* 67:656-661, 1978.
31. Rosenberg PH, Kallio H: Operating-theatre gas pollution and chromosomes. *Lancet* 2:452-453, 1977.
32. Smith WDA: Pollution and the anesthetist. In Hewer CL, Atkinson RS (eds): *Recent Advances in Anaesthesia and Analgesia.* Edinburgh, Churchill Livingstone, 1976, pp 131-175.
33. Usubiaga L, Aldrete JA, Fiserova-Bergerova V: Influence of gas flows and operating room ventilation on the daily exposure of anesthetists to halothane. *Anesth Anals* 51:968-974, 1972.
34. Whitcher CE, Cohen EN, Trudell JR: Chronic exposure to anesthetic gases in the operating room. *Anesthesiology* 35:348-353, 1971.

35. Bruce DL, Linde HW: Halothane content in recovery room air. *Anesthesiology* 36:517–518, 1972.

36. Beynen FM, Knopp TJ, Rehder K: Nitrous oxide exposure in the operating room. *Anesth Analg* 57:216–223, 1978.

37. Corbett TH, Ball GL: Chronic exposure to methoxyflurane: a possible occupational hazard to anesthesiologists. *Anesthesiology* 34:532–537, 1971.

38. Krapez JR, Hackett H, Hinds CJ, Saloojee Y, Cole PV: Blood concentrations of nitrous oxide in theatre personnel. *Br J Anaesth* 51:64P, 1979.

39. Korttila K, Pfaffli P, Ertama P: Residual nitrous oxide in operating room personnel. *Acta Anaesth Scand* 22:635–639, 1978.

40. Krapez JR, Saloojee Y, Hinds CJ, Hackett GH, Cole PV: Blood concentrations of nitrous oxide in theatre personnel. *Br J Anaesth* 52:1143–1148, 1980.

41. Mehta S, Burton P, Simms JS: Occupational exposure to inhaled anaesthetics. *Br Med J* 1:507, 1977.

42. Ross WT Jr: Are effects of halothane on hepatocytes "pathologic"? *Anesthesiology* 47:76, 1977.

43. Virtue RW, Escobar A, Modell J: Nitrous oxide levels in operating room air with various gas flows. *Can Anaesth Soc J* 26:313–318, 1979.

44. Yanagida H, Kemi C, Suwa K, Yamamura H: Nitrous oxide content in the operating suite. *Anesth Analg* 53:347–350, 1974.

45. Berner O: Concentration and elimination of anaesthetic gases in recovery rooms. *Acta Anaesth Scand* 22:55–57, 1978.

46. Spence AA, Knill-Jones RP: Is there a health hazard in anaesthetic practice? *Br J Anaesth* 50:713–719, 1978.

47. Ferstandig LL: Trace concentrations of anesthetic gases: a critical review of their disease potential. *Anesth Analg* 57:328–345, 1978.

48. Walts LF, Forsythe AB, Moore G: Critique: Occupational disease among operating room personnel. *Anesthesiology* 42:608–611, 1975.

49. Vaisman AI: Working conditions in surgery and their effect on the health of anesthesiologists. *Eksp Khir Anestesiol* 3:44, 1967.

50. Ad Hoc Committee on the Effects of Trace Anesthetics on the Health of Operating Room Personnel, American Society of Anesthesiologists: Occupational disease among operating room personnel: a national study. *Anesthesiology* 41:321–340, 1974.

51. Askrog VF, Harvald B: Teratogen effekt of inhalatiosanaestetika. *Nord Med* 83:498–500, 1970.

52. Bussard DA: Congenital anomalies and inhalation anesthetics. *J Am Dent Assoc* 93:606–609, 1976.

53. Cohen EN, Bellville JW, Brown BW: Anesthesia, pregnancy and miscarriage: a study of operating room nurses and anesthetists. *Anesthesiology* 35:343–347, 1971.

54. Corbett TH, Cornell RG, Endres JL, Millard RI: Effects of low concentrations of nitrous oxide on rat pregnancy. *Anesthesiology* 39:299–301, 1973.

55. Cohen EN, Brown BW, Wu ML, Whitcher CE, Brodsky JB, Gift HC, Greenfield W, Jones TW, Driscoll EJ: Occupational disease in dentistry and chronic exposure to trace anesthetic gases. *J Am Dent Assoc* 10:21–31, 1980.

56. Mirakhur RK, Badve AV: Pregnancy and anaesthetic practice in India. *Anaesthesia* 30:18–22, 1975.

57. Knill-Jones RP, Rodrigues LV, Moir DD, Spence AA: Anaesthetic practice and pregnancy. *Lancet* 1:1326–1328, 1972.

58. Knill-Jones RP, Newman BJ, Spence AA: Anaesthesia practice and pregnancy. *Lancet* 2:807–809, 1975.

59. Lecky JH: Chronic exposure to anesthetic trace levels. Ninth Annual Anesthesiology Symposium, Naval Regional Medical Center, Portsmouth, Va., 1978, No. 105.

60. Rosenberg P, Kirves A: Miscarriages among operating theatre staff. *Acta Anaesth Scand (Suppl)* 53:37–42, 1973.

61. Spence AA, Cohen EN, Brown BW, Knill-Jones RP, Himmelberger DU: Occupational hazards for operating room-based physicians. Analysis of data from the United States and the United Kingdom. *JAMA* 238:955–959, 1977.

62. Tomlin PJ: Health problems of anaesthetists and their families in the West Midlands. *Br Med J* 1:779–784, 1979.

63. Ferstandig LL: Trace concentrations of anesthetics are not proved health hazards. In Eckenhoff JE (ed): *Controversy in Anesthesiology.* Philadelphia, W. B. Saunders, 1979.

64. Rushton DI: Anaesthetics and abortions. *Lancet* 2:141, 1976.

65. Ericson A, Kallen B: Survey of infants born in 1973–1975 to Swedish women working in operating rooms during their pregnancies. *Anesth Analg* 58:302–305, 1979.

66. Nikki P, Pfaffli P, Ahlman K, Ralli R: Chronic exposure to anaesthetic gases in the operating theatre and recovery room. *Surv Anesthesiol* 17:464–465, 1973.

67. Pharoah POD, Alberman E, Doyle P: Outcome of pregnancy among women in anaesthetic practice. *Lancet* 1:34–36, 1977.

68. Rosenberg PH, Vanttinen H: Occupational hazards to reproduction and health in anaesthetists and paediatricians. *Acta Anaesth Scand* 22:202–207, 1978.

69. Spence AA, Knill-Jones RP, Newman BJ: Studies of morbidity in anaesthetists with special reference to obstetric history. *Proc R Soc Med* 67:989–990, 1974.

70. Wharton RS, Baden JM, Hitt BA, Mazze RI: Fertility and embryolethality in mice chronically exposed to halothane. Abstracts of Scientific Papers, American Society of Anesthesiologists Annual Meeting, 1976, pp 143–144.

71. Wharton RS, Mazze RI: Reproductive safety of enflurane in female mice. *Anesthesiology* 51:S261, 1979.

72. Wharton RS, Mazze RI, Wilson AI: Reproduction and fetal development in mice chronically exposed to enflurane. *Anesthesiology* 54:505–510, 1981.

73. Strout CD, Nahrwold ML, Taylor MD, Zagon IS: Effects of subanesthetic concentrations of enflurane on rat pregnancy and early development. *Environ Heath Perspect* 21:211–214, 1977.

74. Pope WDB, Persaud TVN: Foetal growth retardation in the rat following chronic exposure to the inhalation anaesthetic enflurane. *Experientia* 34:1332–1333, 1978.

75. Halsey MJ, Green CJ, Monk SJ, Dore C, Knight JF, Luff NP: Maternal and paternal chronic exposure to enflurane and halothane: fetal and histological changes in the rat. *Br J Anaesth* 53:203–215, 1981.

76. Pope WDB, Halsey MJ, Phil HD, Lansdown ABG, Simmonds A, Bateman PE: Fetotoxicity in rats following chronic exposure to halothane, nitrous oxide, or methoxyflurane. *Anesthesiology* 48:11–16, 1978.

77. Wharton RS, Mazze RI, Baden JM, Hitt BA, Dooley JR: Fertility, reproduction and postnatal survival in mice chronically exposed to halothane. *Anesthesiology* 48:167–174, 1978.

78. Bruce DL: Murine fertility unaffected by traces of halothane. *Anesthesiology* 38:473–477, 1973.

79. Corbett TH, Beaudoin AR, Endres J, Mellinehamp A, Nathan J: Teratogenicity studies with halothane (100 ppm) and halothane (100 ppm) + nitrous oxide (0.5%). Abstracts of Scientific Papers, American Society of Anesthesiologists Annual Meeting, 1976, pp 139–140.

80. Pope WDB, Halsey MJ, Lansdown ABG, Bateman PE: Lack of teratogenic dangers with halothane. *Acta Anaesthesiol Belg* 26(supp):169–173, 1975.

81. Lansdown ABG, Pope WDB, Halsey MJ, Bateman PE: Analysis of fetal development in rats following maternal exposure to subanesthetic concentrations of halothane. *Teratology* 13:299–303, 1976.

82. Vieira E, Cleaton-Jones P, Austin JC, Moyes DG, Shaw R: Effects of low concentrations of nitrous oxide on rat fetuses. *Anesth Analg* 59:175–177, 1980.

83. Mazze RI, Wilson AI, Rice SA, Baden JA: Effects of nitrous oxide on fetal development and male fertility in mice. *Anesthesiology* 55:A188, 1981.

84. Coate WB, Kapp RW Jr., Ulland BM, Lewis TR: Toxicity of low concentration long-term exposure to an airborne mixture of nitrous oxide and halothane. *J Environ Pathol Toxicol* 2:209–231, 1979.

85. Furuhyelm M, Janson B, Lagergren GG: The quality of human semen in spontaneous abortion. *Int J Fertil* 7:17–21, 1961.

86. *Draft Report on Anesthetic Waste Gas Scavenging for Ministry of Health,* Province of Ontario, Canada, October 1977.

87. Cohen EN, Brown BW, Bruce DL, Cascorbi HF, Corbett TH, Jones TW, Whitcher CE: A survey of anesthetic health hazards among dentists. *J Am Dent Assoc* 90:1291–1296, 1975.

88. Cohen EN, Brown BW, Wu L, Whitcher CE, Brodsky JB, Gift HC, Greenfield W, Jones TW, Driscoll EJ: Occupational disease in dentistry and chronic exposure to trace anesthetic gases. *J Am Dent Assoc* 101:21–31, 1980.

89. Wyrobek AJ, Brodsky J, Gordon L, Moore DH, Watchmaker G, Cohen EN: Sperm studies in anesthesiologists. *Anesthesiology* 55:527–532, 1981.

90. Coate WB, Kapp RW Jr., Lewis TR: Chronic exposure to low concentrations of halothane-nitrous oxide: reproductive and cytogenetic effects in the rat. *Anesthesiology* 50:310–318, 1979.

91. Land PC, Owen EL, Linde HW: Morphologic changes in mouse spermatozoa after exposure to inhalational anesthetics during early spermatogenesis. *Anesthesiology* 54:53–56, 1981.

92. Land PC: Halothane plus $N_2O:O_2$ increases sperm abnormalities in mice. *Anesthesiology* 55:A196, 1981.

93. Baden JM, Land PC, Egbert B, Kelley M, Mazze RI: Lack of toxicity of enflurane on male reproductive organs in mice. *Anesth Analg* 61:19–22, 1982.

94. Cohen EN, Brown BW, Wu, M: Anesthetic health hazards in dental operatory. *Anesthesiology* 51:S254, 1979.

95. Kennedy GL Jr., Smith SH, Keplinger ML, Calandra JC: Reproductive and teratologic studies with halothane. *Toxicol Appl Pharmacol* 35:467–474, 1976.

96. Corbett TH, Cornell RG, Endres JL, Leiding K: Birth defects among children of nurse-anesthetists. *Anesthesiology* 41:341–344, 1974.

97. Tomlin PJ: Pollution by anaesthetic gases. *Lancet* 2:142, 1976.

98. Cote CJ: Birth defects among infants of nurse anesthetists. *Anesthesiology* 42:514–515, 1975.

99. Basford AB, Fink BR: The teratogenicity of halothane in the rat. *Anesthesiology* 29:1167–1173, 1968.

100. Fink BR, Shepard TH, Blandau RJ: Teratogenic activity of nitrous oxide. *Nature* 214:146–148, 1967.

101. Lane GA, Nahrwold ML, Tait AR, Taylor MD, Beaudoin AR, Cohen PJ: Nitrous oxide is teratogenic: xenon is not! *Anesthesiology* 51:S260, 1979.

102. Smith BE, Gaub ML, Moya F: Investigations into the teratogenic effects of anesthetic agents: the fluorinated agents. *Anesthesiology* 26:260–261, 1965.

103. Wharton RS, Sievenpiper S, Mazze RI: Developmental toxicity of methoxyflurane in mice. *Anesth Analg* 59:421–425, 1980.

104. Chalon J, Tang C, Ramanathan S, Eisner M, Katz R, Turndorf H: Exposure to halothane and enflurane affects learning function of murine progeny. *Anesth Analg* 60:794–797, 1981.

105. Chang LW, Katz J: Pathologic effects of chronic halothane inhalation: an overview. *Anesthesiology* 45:640–653, 1976.

106. Quimby KL, Katz J, Bowman RE: Behavioral consequences in rats from chronic exposure to 10 ppm halothane during early development. *Anesth Analg* 54:628–633, 1975.

107. Quimby KL, Aschkenase LJ, Bowman RE, Katz J, Chang LW: Enduring learning deficits and cerebral synaptic malformation from exposure to 10 ppm of halothane per million. *Science* 185:625–627, 1974.

108. Wharton RS, Wilson AI, Mazze RI, Baden JM, Rice SA: Fetal morphology in mice exposed to halothane. *Anesthesiology* 51:532–537, 1979.

109. Land PC, Owen EL, Murphy NL: Nitrous oxide does not alter spermatogenesis in the mouse. *Anesthesiology* 53:S255, 1980.

110. Bruce DL, Bach MJ, Arbit J: Trace anesthetic effects on perceptual cognitive and motor skills. *Anesthesiology* 40:453–458, 1974.

111. Bruce DL, Bach MJ: Psychological studies of human performance as affected by traces of enflurane and nitrous oxide. *Anesthesiology* 42:194–196, 1975.

112. Bruce DL, Bach MJ: Effects of trace anaesthetic gases on behavioural performance of volunteers. *Br J Anaesth* 48:871–875, 1976.

113. Smith G, Shirley AW: Failure to demonstrate effect of trace concentrations of nitrous oxide and halothane on psychomotor performance. *Br J Anaesth* 49:65–70, 1977.

114. Cook TL, Smith M, Winter PM, Starkweather JA, Eger EI: Effect of subanesthetic concentrations of enflurane and halothane on human behavior. *Anesth Analg* 57:434–440, 1978.

115. Cook TL, Smith M, Starkweather JA, Winter PM, Eger EI: Behavioral effects of trace and subanesthetic halothane and nitrous oxide in man. *Anesthesiology* 49:419–424, 1978.

116. Frankhuizen JL, Vlek CAJ, Burm AGL, Rejger V: Failure to replicate negative effects of trace anaesthetics on mental performance. *Br J Anaesth* 50:229–234, 1978.

117. Allison RH, Shirley AW, Smith G: Threshold concentration of nitrous oxide affecting psychomotor performance. *Br J Anaesth* 51:177–180, 1979.

118. Gamberale F, Svensson G: The effect of anesthetic gases on the psychomotor and perceptual functions of anesthetic nurses. *Work Environ Health* 11:108–113, 1974.

119. Gambill AF, McCallum RN, Henrichs TF: Psychomotor performance following exposure to trace concentrations of inhalation anesthetics. *Anesth Analg* 58:475–482, 1979.

120. Smith G, Shirley AW: A review of the effects of trace concentrations of anaesthetics on performance. *Br J Anaesth* 50:701–712, 1978.

121. Corbett TH, Cornell RG, Lieding K, Enders JL: Incidence of cancer among Michigan nurse anesthetists. *Anesthesiology* 38:260–262, 1973.

122. Baden JM, Mazze RI, Wharton RS, Rice SA, Kosek JC: Carcinogenicity of halothane in Swiss/ICR mice. *Anesthesiology* 51:20–26, 1979.

123. Bruce DL, Eide KA, Smith NJ: A prospective survey of anesthesiologist mortality, 1967–1971. *Anesthesiology* 41:71–74, 1974.

124. Doll R, Peto R: Mortality among doctors in different occupations. *Br Med J* 1:1433–1436, 1977.

125. Lew EA: Mortality experience among anesthesiologists, 1954–1976. *Anesthesiology* 51:195–199, 1979.

126. Linde HW, Mesnick PS, Smith NJ: Causes of death among anesthesiologists 1930–1946. *Anesth Analg* 60:1–7, 1981.

127. Baden JM, Egbert B, Mazze RI: Carcinogen bioassay of enflurane in mice. *Anesthesiology* 56:9–13, 1982.

128. Eger EI II, White AE, Brown CL, Biava CG, Corbett TH, Stevens WC: A test of the carcinogenicity of enflurane, isoflurane, halothane, methoxyflurane and nitrous oxide in mice. *Anesth Analg* 57:678–694, 1978.

129. Linde HW, Bruce DL: Effects of chronic exposure of rats to trace of halothane. In *Proceedings of the Fourth World Congress of Anesthesiologists*, London, 1968. Amsterdam, Excerpta Medica Foundation, 1970, p 923.

130. Baden JM, Brinkenhoff M, Wharton RS, Hitt BA, Simmon VF, Mazze RI: Mutagenicity of volatile anesthetics: halothane. *Anesthesiology* 45:311–318, 1976.

131. Baden JM, Kelley M, Cheung A, Mortelmans K: Lack of mutagens in urines of operating room personnel. *Anesthesiology* 53:195–198, 1980.

132. Husum B, Wulf HC: Sister chromatid exchanges in lymphocytes in operating room personnel. *Acta Anaesth Scand* 24:22–24, 1980.

133. McCoy EC, Hankel R, Rosenkranz HS, Giuffrida JG, Bizzari DV: Detection of mutagenic activity in the urines of anesthesiologists: a preliminary report. *Environ Health Perspect* 21:221–223, 1977.

134. Baden JM, Kelley M, Wharton RS, Hitt BA, Simmon VF, Mazze RI: Mutagenicity of halogenated ether anesthetics. *Anesthesiology* 46:346–350, 1977.

135. White AE, Takehisa S, Eger EI, Wolff S, Stevens WC: Sister chromatid exchanges induced by inhaled anesthetics. *Anesthesiology* 50:426–430, 1979.

136. Stevens WC, White AE, Takehisa S, Eger EI, Wolff S: Sister chromatid exchanges induced by inhaled anesthetics. Abstracts, American Society of Anesthesiologists Annual Meeting, 1977, pp 495–496.

137. Sturrock JE: No mutagenic effect of enflurane on cultured cells. *Br J Anaesth* 49:777–779, 1977.

138. Waskell L: A study of the mutagenicity of anesthetics and their metabolites. *Mutat Res* 57:141–153, 1978.

139. Sturrock J: Lack of mutagenic effect of halothane or chloroform on cultured cells using the azaguanine test system. *Br J Anaesth* 49:207–210, 1977.

140. Basler A, Rohrborn G: Lack of mutagenic effects of halothane in mammals in vivo. *Anesthesiology* 55:143–147, 1981.

141. Kramers PGN, Burm AGL: Mutagenicity studies with halothane in Drosophila melanogaster. *Anesthesiology* 50:510–513, 1979.

142. Waskell L: Lack of mutagenicity of two possible metabolites of halothane. *Anesthesiology* 50:9–12, 1979.

143. Edmunds HN, Baden JM, Simmon VF: Mutagenicity studies with volatile metabolites of halothane. *Anesthesiology* 51:424–429, 1979.

144. Garro AJ, Phillips RA: Mutagenicity of the halogenated olefin, 2-bromo-2-chloro-1,1-difluoroethylene, a presumed metabolite of the inhalation anesthetic halothane. *Environ Health Perspect* 21:65–69, 1977.

145. Sachdev K, Cohen EN, Simmon VF: Genotoxic and mutagenic assays of halothane metabolites in Bacillus subtilis and Salmonella typhimurium. *Anesthesiology* 53:31–39, 1980.

146. Baden JM, Kelley M, Mazze RI, Simmon VF: Mutagenicity of inhalation anesthetics: trichlorethylene, divinyl ether, nitrous oxide, and cyclopropane. *Br J Anaesth* 51:417–421, 1979.

147. Cottrell JE, Chalon J, Turndorf H: Faulty anesthesia circuits: a source of environmental pollution in the operating room. *Anesth Analg* 56:359–

362, 1977.

148. Knill-Jones RP: Comparative risk of hepatitis in doctors working within hospitals and outside hospitals. *Digestion* 10:359–360, 1974.

149. Bardzik J, Przezdziak J, Bardzik I: Immunoglobulins in persons with long-term exposure to halothane. *Anaesth Resusc Intensive Ther* 3:285–290, 1975.

150. Bardzik J, Bardzik I, Kryszewski A, Suchorzewska J: Serum enzyme levels in anaesthetic personnel. *Anaesth Resusc Intensive Ther* 3:291–295, 1975.

151. Nunn JF, Sharer N, Royston D, Watts WE, Purkiss P, Worth HG: Serum methionine and hepatic enzyme activity in anaesthetists exposed to nitrous oxide. *Br J Anaesth* 54:593–597, 1982.

152. Dahlgren BE: Hepatic and renal effects of low concentrations of methoxyflurane in exposed delivery ward personnel. *J Occup Med* 22:817–819, 1980.

153. Belfrage S, Ahlgren I, Axelson S: Halothane hepatitis in an anaesthetist. *Lancet* 2:1466–1467, 1966.

154. Johnston CI, Mendelsohn F: Halothane hepatitis in a laboratory technician. *Aust NZ J Med* 2:171–173, 1971.

155. Klatskin G, Kimberg DV: Recurrent hepatitis attributable to halothane sensitization in an anesthetist. *N Engl J Med* 280:515–522, 1969.

156. Lund I, Skulberg A, Helle I: Occupation hazard of halothane. *Lancet* 2:528, 1974.

157. Ghoneim MM, Delle M, Wilson WR, Ambro JJ: Alteration of warfarin kinetics in man associated with exposure to an operating-room environment. *Anesthesiology* 43:333–336, 1975.

158. Harman AW, Russell WJ, Frewin DB, Priestly BG: Altered drug metabolism in anaesthetists exposed to volatile anaesthetic agents. *Anaesth Intensive Care* 6:210–214, 1978.

159. Stevens WC, Eger EI, White A, Halsey M, Munger W, Gibbon RD, Dolan W, Shorgel R: Comparative toxicities of halothane, isoflurane, and diethyl ether at subanesthetic concentrations in laboratory animals. *Anesthesiology* 42:408–419, 1975.

160. Baden JM, Egbert B, Rice SA: Enflurane has no effect on haemopoiesis in mice. *Br J Anaesth* 52:471–474, 1980.

161. Cleaton-Jones P, Austin JC, Banks D, Vieira E, Kagan E: Effect of intermittent exposure to a low concentration of nitrous oxide in haemopoiesis in rats. *Br J Anaesth* 49:223–226, 1977.

162. Coate WB, Ulland BM, Lewis TR: Chronic exposure to low concentrations of halothane-nitrous oxide. *Anesthesiology* 50:306–309, 1979.

163. Duncan PG, Cullen BF: Anesthesia and immunology. *Anesthesiology* 45:522–538, 1976.

164. Lecky JH: Anesthesia and the immune system. *Surg Clin N Am* 55:795–799, 1975.

165. Beall GN, Nagel EL, Matsui Y: Immunoglobulins in anesthesiologists. *Anesthesiology* 42:232, 1975.

166. Bruce DL: Immunologically competent anesthesiologists. *Anesthesiology* 37:76–78, 1972.

167. Salo M, Vapaavuori M: Peripheral blood t- and b-lymphocytes in operating theatre personnel. *Br J Anaesth* 48:877–880, 1970.

168. Petingale KW, Al-Affas N, Tee DEH, Strunin L: Immunosuppression among anaesthetists. *Br J Anaesth* 50:73–74, 1978.

169. Rosenbaum KJ: Are anesthesiologists immunostimulated? *Anesthesiology* 38:200, 1973.

170. Mathieu A, Mathieu D, Kerman R: T lymphocyte function and PMN chemotaxis in anesthesiologists and other OR personnel. *Anesthesiology* 53:S29, 1980.

171. Lattey M: Halothane sensitization. A case report. *Can Anaesth Soc J* 17:648–649, 1970.

172. Brodsky JB, Cohen EN, Brown BW, Wu ML, Whitcher CE: Occupational exposure to nirous oxide and neurologic disease. *Anesthesiology* 53:S367, 1980.

173. Brodsky JB, Cohen EN, Brown BW, Wu ML, Whitcher CE: Exposure to nitrous oxide and neurologic disease among dental professionals. *Anesth Analg* 60:297–301, 1981.

174. Dyck P, Grina A, Lambert EH, Calder CS, Oviatt K, Rehder K, Lund BA, Skau KA: Nitrous oxide neurotoxicity studies in man and rat. *Anesthesiology* 53:205–208, 1980.

175. Anonymous: Nitrous oxide hazards. *FDA Drug Bull* 10:15–16, 1980.

176. Layzer RB, Fishman RA, Schafer JA: Neuropathy following abuse of nitrous oxide. *Neurology* 28:504–506, 1978.

177. Layzer RB: Myeloneuropathy after prolonged exposure to nitrous oxide. *Lancet* 2:1227–1230, 1978.

178. Nevins MA: Neuropathy after nitrous oxide abuse. *JAMA* 244:2264, 1980.

179. Schwettmann RS, Casterline CL: Delayed asthmatic response following occupational exposure to enflurane. *Anesthesiology* 44:166–169, 1976.

180. Pitt EM: Halothane as a possible cause of laryngitis in an anaesthetist. *Anaesthesia* 29:579–580, 1974.

181. Boyd CH: Ophthalmic hypersensitivity to anaesthetic vapours. *Anaesthesia* 27:456–457, 1972.

182. Dadve AV, Mirakhur RK: Ophthalmic hypersensitivity to anaesthetic vapours. *Anaesthesia* 28:338–339, 1973.

183. Elder BF, Beal H, DeWald W, Cobb S: Exacerbation of subclinical myasthenia by occupational exposure to an anesthetic. *Anesth Analg* 50:383–387, 1971.

184. Bodman R: Skin sensitivity to halothane vapour. *Br J Anaesth* 51:1092, 1979.

185. Soper LE, Vitez TS, Weinberg D: Metabolism of halogenated anesthetic agents as a possible cause of acneiform eruptions. *Anesth Analg* 52:125–127, 1973.

186. *American National Standard for Anesthesia Gas Pollution Control.* Z79.11, American National Standards Institute, 1430 Broadway, New York, N.Y. 10018, 1982.

187. Flowerdew RMM: A hazard of scavenger port design. *Can Anaesth Soc J* 28:481–483, 1981.

188. Tavakoli M, Habeeb A: Two hazards of gas scavenging. *Anesth Analg* 57:286–287, 1978.

189. Nott MR: Resistance of anti-pollution circuits. *Anaesthesia* 32:917–918, 1977.

190. Brinklov MM, Andersen PK: Gas evacuation from paediatric anaesthetic systems. *Br J Anaesth* 50:305, 1978.

191. Cestone KJ, Ryan WP, Loving CD: An anes-

thetic gas scavenger for the Jackson-Rees system. *Anesthesiology* 55:881–882, 1976.

192. Emralino CQ, Bernhard WN, Yost L: Overflow-gas scavenger for Jackson-Rees anesthesia system. *Resp Care* 23:178–179, 1978.

193. Keneally JP, Overton JH: A scavenging device for the T-piece. *Anaesth Intensive Care* 5:267–268, 1977.

194. Karski J, Sych M: A simple device designed to protect operating theatres against atmospheric pollution by volatile anaesthetics. *Anaesth Res Intensive Ther* 4:61–64, 1976.

195. Maver E: Extractors for anaesthetic gases. *Anaesth Intensive Care* 3:348–350, 1975.

196. Whitcher C: Waste anesthetic gas scavenging—indications and technology. ASA Refresher Course No. 126, 1974.

197. Whitcher C: Control of waste anesthetic gases. In *Handbook of Hospital Facilities for the Anesthesiologist*, ed 2. American Society of Anesthesiologists, 515 Bussie Highway, Park Ridge, Ill. 60068, 1974.

198. Whitcher CE: Control of occupational exposure to inhalational anesthetics—current status. ASA Refresher Courses No. 205, 1977.

199. Weng J, Smith RA, Balsamo JJ, Gooding JM, Kirby RR: A method of scavenging waste gases from the Jackson-Rees system. *Anesth Rev* 7:35–38, 1980.

200. Flowerdew RMM: Coaxial scavenger for paediatric anaesthesia. *Can Anaesth Soc J* 26:367–368, 1979.

201. Hatch DJ, Miles R, Wagstaff M: An anaesthetic scavenging system for paediatric and adult use. *Anaesthesia* 35:496–499, 1980.

202. Muravchick S: Scavenging enflurane from extracorporeal pump oxygenators. *Anesthesiology* 47:468–471, 1977.

203. Annis JP, Carlson DA, Simmons DH: Scavenging system for the Harvey blood oxygenator. *Anesthesiology* 45:359–360, 1976.

204. Ad Hoc Committee on Effects of Trace Anesthetic Agents on Health of Operating Room Personnel, American Society of Anesthesiologists: Waste gases in operating room air: a suggested program to reduce personnel exposure. 1981. American Society of Anesthesiologists, 515 Busse Highway, Park Ridge, Ill. 60068.

205. Anonymous: New pollution-free anaesthesia system from Medishield. Anaesthesia Equipment and Technology, Sept. 1976, pp 10–11.

206. Meyers EF: An effective low-cost scavenging system. *Anesthesiology* 52:277, 1980.

207. Enderby DH, Booth AM, Churchill-Davidson HC: Removal of anaesthetic waste gases. An inexpensive antipollution system for use with pipeline suction. *Anaesthesia* 33:820–826, 1978.

208. Bruce DL: A simple way to vent anesthetic gases. *Anesth Analg* 52:595–598, 1973.

209. Asbury AJ, Hancox AJ: The evaluation and improvement of an anti-pollution system. *Br J Anaesth* 49:439–446, 1977.

210. Armstrong RF, Kershaw EJ, Bourne SP, Strunin L: Anaesthetic waste gas scavenging systems. *Br Med J* 1:941–943, 1977.

211. Vickers MD: Pollution of the atmosphere of operating theatres. Important notice. *Anaesthesia* 30:697–699, 1975.

212. Langley DR, Steward A: The effect of ventilation system design on air contamination with halothane in operating theatres. *Br J Anaesth* 46:736–741, 1974.

213. McIntyre JWR, Pudham JT, Jhsein HR: An assessment of operating room environment air contamination with nitrous oxide and halothane and some scavenging methods. *Can Anaesth Soc J* 25:499–505, 1978.

214. Strunin L, Strunin JM, Mallios CC: Atmospheric pollution with halothane during outpatient dental anaesthesia. *Br Med J* 4:459–460, 1973.

215. Bethune DW, Collis JM: Anaesthetic practice. Pollution in operating theatres. *Biomed Eng* 9:157–159, 1974.

216. Oulton JL: Operating-room venting of trace concentrations of inhalation anesthetic agents. *Can Med Assoc J* 116:1148–1151, 1977.

217. Whitcher C: Control of occupational exposure to inhalational anesthetics. ASA Refresher Courses in Anesthesiology, vol 6, 1978.

218. Asbury AJ, Hancox AJ: Theatre pollution control. *Anaesthesia* 31:802–803, 1976.

219. Enderby GEH: Gas exhaust valve. *Anaesthesia* 27:334–337, 1972.

220. Lack JA: Theatre pollution control. *Anaesthesia* 31:259–262, 1976.

221. McInnes IC: Practical considerations in prevention of anaesthetic agent pollution of theatre air. Anaesthesia Equipment and Technology, Nov. 1975, pp 6–7.

222. Mehta S, Behr G, Chari J, Kenyon D: A passive method of disposal of expired anaesthetic gases. *Br J Anaesth* 49:589–593, 1977.

223. McInnes IC: Experience with use of a passive anti-pollution system. *Anaesth Intensive Care Equipment*, July/Aug. 1978, pp 9–15.

224. Parbrook GD, Mok IB: An expired gas collection and disposal system. *Br J Anaesth* 47:1185–1193, 1975.

225. Mehta S: Terminal gas-exhaust valve for a passive disposal system. *Anaesthesia* 32:51–52, 1977.

226. Hagerdal M, Lecky JH: Anesthetic death of an experimental animal related to a scavenging system malfunction. *Anesthesiology* 47:522–523, 1977.

227. Alexander KD, Stewart NF, Oppenheim RC, Brown TCK: Adsorption of halothane from a paediatric T-piece circuit by activated charcoal. *Anaesth Intensive Care* 5:218–222, 1977.

228. Capon JH: A method of regenerating activated charcoal anaesthetic adsorbers by autoclaving. *Anaesthesia* 29:611–614, 1974.

229. Enderby DH, Bushman JA, Askill S: Investigations of some aspects of atmospheric pollution by anaesthetic gases. II. Aspects of adsorption and emission of halothane by different charcoals. *Br J Anaesth* 49:567–573, 1977.

230. Hawkins TJ: Atmospheric pollution in operating theatres. *Anaesthesia* 28:490–500, 1973.

231. Kim BM, Sircar S: Adsorption characteristics of volatile anesthetics on activated carbons and performance of carbon canisters. *Anesthesiology* 46:159–165, 1977.

232. Murrin KR: Atmospheric pollution with halothane in operating theatres. A clinical study us-

ing activated charcoal. *Anaesthesia* 30:12–17, 1975.

233. Maggs FAP, Smith ME: Adsorption of anaesthetic vapours on charcoal beds. *Anaesthesia* 31:30–40, 1976.

234. Murrin KR: Adsorption of halothane by activated charcoal. Further studies. *Anaesthesia* 29:458–461, 1974.

235. Vaughan RS, Mapleson WW, Mushin WW: Prevention of pollution of operating theatres with halothane vapour by adsorption with activated charcoal. *Br Med J* 1:727–729, 1973.

236. Vaughan RS, Willis BA, Mapleson WW, Vickers MD: The Cardiff Aldavac anaesthesic-scavenging system. *Anaesthesia* 32:339–343, 1977.

237. Epstein HG: Removal of ether vapor during anaesthesia. *Lancet* 1:114–116, 1944.

238. Cundy JM: Adsorption of ether by activated charcoal. *Anesthesiology* 48:77, 1978.

239. Kolman LP: Anesthesia waste evacuation by central vacuum pipelines. *Items Topics* 21:6–7, 1975.

240. Wright BM: Vacuum pipelines for anaesthetic pollution control. *Br Med J* 1:918, 1978.

241. Abramowitz M, McGill WA: Hazard of anesthetic scavenging device. *Anesthesiology* 51:276, 1979.

242. Ilsley AH, Crea J, Cousins MJ: Assessment of waste anaesthetic gas scavenging systems under simulated conditions of operation. *Anaesth Intensive Care* 8:52–64, 1980.

243. Jorgensen S, Thomsen A: A transportable ejector flowmeter. *Acta Anaesth Scand* 20:405–408, 1976.

244. Lai KM: A flow-inducer for anaesthetic scavenging systems. *Anaesthesia* 32:794–797, 1977.

245. Lecky JH: The mechanical aspects of anesthetic pollution control. *Anesth Analg* 56:769–774, 1977.

246. Mehta S: Atmospheric pollution with halothane in operating theatres. *Anaesthesia* 30:406–407, 1975.

247. Norry HT: A pressure limiting valve for anaesthetic and respirator circuits. *Can Anaesth Soc J* 19:583–588, 1972.

248. Davies G, Tarnawsky M: Letters to the editor. *Can Anaesth Soc J* 23:228, 1976.

249. Mantia AM: Gas scavenging systems. *Anesth Analg* 61:162–164, 1982.

250. Hamilton RC, Byrne J: Another cause of gas-scavenging-line obstruction. *Anesthesiology* 51:365–366, 1979.

251. Malloy WF, Wightman AE, O'Sullivan D, Goldiner PL: Bilateral pneumothorax from suction applied to a ventilator exhaust valve. *Anesth Analg* 58:147–149, 1979.

252. O'Connor DE, Daniels BW, Pfitzner J: Hazards of anaesthetic scavenging: case reports and brief review. *Anaesth Intensive Care* 10:15–19, 1982.

253. Mor ZF, Stein ED, Orkin LR: A possible hazard in the use of a scavenging system. *Anesthesiology* 47:302–303, 1977.

254. Patel KD, Dalal FY: A potential hazard of the Drager scavenging interface system for wall suction. *Anesth Analg* 58:327–328, 1979.

255. Rendell-Baker L: Hazard of blocked scavenge valve. *Can Anaesth Soc J* 29:182–183, 1982.

256. Andersen PK, Brinklov MM: Scavenging of anesthetic gases. *Anesthesiology* 49:53, 1978.

257. Sharrock NE, Leith DE: Potential pulmonary barotrauma when venting anesthetic gases to suction. *Anesthesiology* 46:152–154, 1977.

258. Milliken RA: Hazards of scavenging systems. *Anesth Analg* 59:162, 1980.

259. Mann ES, Sprague DH: An easily overlooked malassembly. *Anesthesiology* 56:413–414, 1982.

260. Stringer BW: Scavenging adaptor misconnection. *Anaesth Intensive Care* 10:169, 1982.

261. Sharrock NE, Gabel RA: Inadvertent anesthetic overdose obscured by scavenging. *Anesthesiology* 49:137–138, 1978.

262. Torda TA, Jones R, Englert J: A study of waste gas scavenging in operating theatres. *Anaesth Intensive Care* 6:215–221, 1978.

263. Hovey TC: A gas scavenger system. *J Am Assoc Nurse Anesthetists* 45:170–177, 1977.

264. Nilsson K, Stenqvist O, Lindberg B, Kjelltoft B: Close scavenging experimental and preliminary clinical studies of a method of reducing anaesthetic gas contamination. *Acta Anaesth Scand* 24:475–481, 1980.

265. Becker MJ, McGill WA, Oh TH, Epstein BS: The effect of an airway leak on nitrous oxide contamination of the operating room. *Anesthesiology* 55:A335, 1981.

266. Vickery IM, Burton GW: Throat packs for surgery. An improved design based on anatomical measurements. *Anaesthesia* 32:565–572, 1977.

267. Dunkin LJ: Polluting the atmosphere. *Anaesthesia* 27:239, 1972.

268. Mostert JW: Closed-circuit protection for anaesthetists. *Lancet* 2:758–759, 1972.

269. Millman BS: Compatibility of scavenging with low flow and closed breathing systems. In Aldrete JA, Lowe HJ, Virtue RW (eds), *Low Flow and Closed System Anesthesia*. New York, Grune & Stratton, 1979, pp 289–293.

270. Smith RM: Editorial. *Surv Anesthesiol* 19:219, 1975.

271. Albert SN, Kwan AM, Dadisman JW Jr.: Leakage in anesthetic circuits. *Anesth Analg* 56:878, 1977.

272. Berner O: Anaesthetic apparatus leakages. A possible solution. *Acta Anaesth Scand* 17:1–7, 1973.

273. Berner O: Concentration and elimination of anaesthetic gases in operating theatres. *Acta Anaesth Scand* 22:46–54, 1978.

274. Whitcher CE: Methods of control. In Cohen EN (ed): *Anesthetic Exposure in the Workplace.* Littleton, Mass., PSG Publishing Co., 1980, pp 117–148.

275. Milliken RA, Milliken GM, Marshall BJ: OR pollution can have adverse effect on safety. *Hospitals* 50:97–104, 1976.

276. Whitcher C, Piziali RL: Monitoring occupational exposure to inhalation anesthetics. *Anesth Analg* 56:778–785, 1977.

277. *Respiratory Therapy.* NFPA 56B, National Fire Protection Association, Batterymarch Park, Quincy, Mass. 02269, 1974.

278. *Inhalation Anesthetics in Ambulatory Care Facilities.* NFPA 56G, National Fire Protection Association, Batterymarch Park, Quincy, Mass. 02269, 1980.

279. *Pressure Regulators, Gauges, and Flow Metering Devices for Medical Gas Systems.* CSA Z305.3–

M1979, Canadian Standards Association, 178 Rexdale Blvd., Rexdale, Ontario, Canada, M9W 1R3.

280. Lecky JH, Springstead JM, Neufled GR: In-house manual for the control of anesthetic gas contamination in the operating room. University of Pennsylvania, Dept. of Anesthesia.

281. Brinklov MM, Andersen PK, Jorgensen S: The negative pressure relief valve: pressure-flow relationships. *Br J Anaesth* 50:1025–1029, 1978.

282. Male CG: Theatre ventilation. A comparison of design and observed values. *Br J Anaesth* 50:1257–1263, 1978.

283. Aldrete JA, Virtue RW: Maintaining low levels of waste anesthetics in the operating room. In Cohen EN (ed): *Anesthetic Exposure in the Workplace.* Littleton, Mass., PSG Publishing Co., 1980, p 121.

284. Holmes CM: Pollution in operating theatres. Part 2. The solution. *N Z Med J* 87:50–53, 1978.

285. Neufeld GR, Flemming DC, Lecky JH: Evaluation of operating room clearance of trace anesthetic gases. ASA Scientific Papers, pp 371–372, 1975.

286. Neufeld GR, Lecky JH: Trace anesthetic exposure. Consequences and control. *Surg Clin N Am* 55:967–973, 1975.

287. Halsey MJ, Chand S, Dluzewski AR, Jones AJ, Wardley-Smith BS: Olefactory thresholds: detection of operating room contamination. *Br J Anaesth* 49:510–511, 1977.

288. Ilsley AH, Crea J, Cousins MJ: Evaluation of infrared analysers used for monitoring waste anaesthetic gas levels in operating theatres. *Anaesth Intensive Care* 8:436–440, 1980.

289. Lane GA: The measurement of low concentrations of nitrous oxide and halothane by infrared spectroscopy. *Br J Anaesth* 48:274, 1976.

290. Whitcher CE, Zimmerman DC, Piziali RL: Control of occupational exposure to nitrous oxide in the dental operatory. DHEW (NIOSH) Publication No. 77-200, 1977.

291. Whitcher CE, Zimmerman DC, Tonn EM, Piziali RL: Control of occupational exposure to nitrous oxide in the dental operatory. *J Am Dent Assoc* 95:763–776, 1977.

292. Halliday MM, Carter KB, Davis PD, MacDonald I, Collins L, McCreaddie G: Survey of operating room pollution with an N.H.S. district. *Lancet* 1:1230–1232, 1979.

293. Knights KM, Strunin JM, Strunin L: Measurement of low concentrations of halothane in the atmosphere using a portable detector. *Lancet* 1:727–728, 1975.

294. Knights KM, Strunin JM, Strunin L: Measurement of low concentrations of halothane in the atmosphere using a portable detector. *Br J Anaesth* 47:635–636, 1975.

295. Anonymous: Workshop on anesthetic pollution. *Anesthesiol Rev* 4:25–34, 1977.

296. Robinson JS, Thompson JM, Barratt RS, Belcher R, Stephen WI: Pertinence and precision in pollution measurements. *Br J Anaesth* 48:167–177, 1976.

297. Salamonsen LA, Cole WJ, Salamonsen RF: Simultaneous trace analysis of nitrous oxide and halothane in air. *Br J Anaesth* 50:221–227, 1978.

298. Austin JC, Shaw R, Crichton R, Cleaton-Jones PE, Moyes D: Comparison of sampling techniques for studies of nitrous oxide pollution. *Br J Anaesth* 50:1109–1112, 1978.

299. Austin JC, Shaw R, Moyes D, Cleaton-Jones PE: A simple air sampling technique for monitoring nitrous oxide pollution. *Br J Anaesth* 53:997–1003, 1981.

300. Lecky JH, Andrews R, Springstead J: Intraoperative monitoring of anesthetic trace gas levels. ASA Papers, 1978, pp 415–416.

301. Mehta S, Burton P, Simms JS: Monitoring of occupational exposure to nitrous oxide. *Can Anaesth Soc J* 25:419–423, 1978.

302. Mcgill WA, Rivera O, Howard R: Time-weighted average for nitrous oxide: an automated method. *Anesthesiology* 53:424–426, 1980.

303. Burm AG, Spierdijk J: A method for sampling halothane and enflurane present in trace amounts in ambient air. *Anesthesiology* 50:230–233, 1979.

304. Burm AG, Spierdijk J: Personal sampling of halothane in operating room air. *Anesthesiology* 51:S355, 1979.

305. Carter KB, Halliday MM: A personal air sampling pump for hospital operating staff. *J. Med Eng Technol* 2:310–312, 1978.

306. Dupressoir CAJ: A practical apparatus for measuring average exposure of operating theatre personnel to halothane. *Anaesth Intensive Care* 3:345–347, 1975.

307. Choi-Lao AT: Trace anesthetic vapors in hospital operating-room environments. *Nurs Res* 30:156–161, 1981.

308. Hunter L: An occupational health approach to anaesthetic air pollution. *Med J Aust* 1:465–468, 1976.

309. Halliday MM, Carter KB: A chemical adsorption system for the sampling of gaseous organic pollutants in operating theatre atmospheres. *Br J Anaesth* 50:1013–1018, 1978.

310. Nikki P, Pfaffli P, Ahlman K: End-tidal and blood halothane and nitrous oxide in surgical personnel. *Lancet* 2:490–491, 1972.

311. Cole P: Occupational exposure to inhaled anaesthetics *Br Med J* 4:1563, 1976.

312. Hillman KM, Saloojee Y, Brett II, Cole PV: Nitrous oxide concentrations in dental surgery. Atmospheric and blood concentrations of personnel. *Anaesthesia* 36:257–262, 1981.

313. Whitcher C: Correspondence. *Anesthesiol Rev* 3:41–42, 1976.

314. Milliken RA: A plea for monitoring both halogenated and non-halogenated anesthetic agents in the operating room. *Anesthesiol Rev* 3:29–31, 1976.

315. Milliken RA: Correspondence. *Anesthesiol Rev* 3:42, 51, 1976.

316. Lecky JH: Trace anesthetic exposure. *Audio Digest* 18: No. 13, 1976.

317. Kaarakka P, Malischke PR, Kreul JF: Alternative sites for measuring breathing zone N_2O levels. *Anesthesiology* 55:A139, 1981.

318. Geraci CL Jr: Operating room pollution: governmental perspectives and guidelines. *Anesth Analg* 56:775–777, 1977.

319. Geraci CL: Role of federal government. In Cohen

EN (ed): *Anesthetic Exposure in the Workplace.* Littleton, Mass., PSG Publishing Co., 1980.

320. Mazze RI: Waste anesthetic gases and the regulatory agencies. *Anesthesiology* 52:248–256, 1980.

321. Mondry GA: Medical-legal implications. In Cohen EN (ed): *Anesthetic Exposure in the Workplace.* Littleton, Mass., PSG Publishing Co., 1980.

322. Anonymous: OSHA inspections of hospital operating rooms. ASA Newsletter, Dec. 1980, p 7.

323. Lecky JH: Anesthetic pollution in the operating room: a notice to operating room personnel. *Anesthesiology* 52:157–159, 1980.

CHAPTER 10

Hazards of Anesthesia Machines and Breathing Systems

Accidents, both trivial and common, involving anesthesia machines and breathing systems continue to occur all too often. This chapter will examine these hazards as viewed from the end result. In addition, there will be some discussion of accident investigation and prevention.

It is impossible to list every conceivable hazard, so only the more common and serious will be covered. Many involve older types of equipment or peculiar situations which have been eliminated or modified by the manufacturer. They are included here because some of the older apparatus is still in use.

HYPOXIA

Hypoxia is a greatly feared complication because the consequences to the patient frequently are brain damage or death. Damage depends on the degree of hypoxia and the length of time it exists. Neither blood pressure nor heart rate is a reliable indicator of hypoxia (1).

Oxygen Supply Problems

In a study in Britain between 1964 and 1973, oxygen failure was the leading cause of cardiac arrest (2) and it is still responsible for a number of deaths.

PIPELINE PROBLEMS

Most hospitals have piping systems for nitrous oxide and oxygen. These are usually quite dependable and this may cause personnel to take it for granted that these gases will always be available. In a survey of hospitals in 1976, 31% reported difficulties with the pipeline systems and the most common malfunction was insufficient oxygen pressure (3).

Some of the causes for low or absent oxygen pressure are damage during construction, debris left in the line following installation, unan-nounced system shutdowns, regulator malfunction, bulk tank damage due to adverse weather (4), spontaneous closure of an isolation valve (5, 6) the reserve system not being properly filled, jammed shutoff valve on the reserve supply, and the reserve alarm being turned off when the tank is filled and not activated after filling has been completed. Low-pressure alarms can fail and personnel who hear an alarm may not know what to do when the alarm sounds (7). It is possible for someone to turn off the supply to the operating room (8–10).

Inside the operating room, a station outlet may not accept a quick connect (11) or may become blocked (12). The connections on the hoses which connect the anesthesia machine to the piping system may hold together but fail to pass an adequate gas flow (9, 13–16). One may forget to attach the hoses (16) or inadvertently disconnect a hose during anesthesia (15). Hose connections may spontaneously detach from the station outlet or the machine (17, 18).

A hose may develop a leak (19), become plugged (12, 20) or develop a kink which obstructs the flow to the machine (21).

In departments where the pipeline system terminates in a movable ceiling column, retractable reel, or sliding tract, a hose is incorporated in the ceiling or column to allow movement. These hoses will deteriorate with time and movement. Since these hoses are not seen and are inspected infrequently (if at all) this deterioration can go unnoticed until a leak either reduces or terminates oxygen delivery. Oxygen source failure due to pipeline problems can be prevented by making certain that routine inspection and maintenance of the piping system is carried out.

Pipeline pressure gauges should be checked before starting and during anesthesia. On some machines the pipeline pressure gauges are connected in such a way that they register pressure if the cylinder supply is turned on (22, 23).

Cylinder valves should be remain closed when a pipeline system is in use so the operator will know whether or not the pipeline is supplying the machine. The presence of functional emergency oxygen cylinders should always be verified before starting a case so that if the pipeline supply fails, there will be no delay in supplying oxygen to the patient.

An effective emergency hospital response to the loss of piped oxygen should be organized. This should include communication, conservation of supplies and remedial action to correct the fault or damage. All clinical areas likely to be affected and all staff involved with gas supplies need to be notified. Areas using oxygen should reduce their utilization as much as possible and bring in reserve cylinders. If necessary, additional supplies should be ordered from suppliers or other hospitals to meet the expected duration of the emergency. Particular attention should be paid to the recovery room. Should pipeline failure occur, it may be advisable to take an anesthesia machine not in use to the recovery room to supply oxygen until the pipeline problem can be solved.

CYLINDER PROBLEMS

Empty Oxygen Cylinder

Pipeline System Not in Use. When a pipeline system is not used, cylinders are the source of oxygen and oxygen source failure will occur if they empty (13, 24).

A machine with a double yoke for oxygen should be used so that a full tank can be kept in reserve while the other tank is in use. When one cylinder becomes exhausted, the valve should be closed, the valve on the reserve cylinder opened and the exhausted cylinder immediately replaced. While some people have advocated keeping both cylinder valves open (25), this practice should be discouraged, since the user may fail to notice that transfer to the reserve cylinder has occurred and he may then run out of oxygen and have none in reserve (26–30).

Partially filled and empty cylinders may be delivered marked full (31). It is important to check the pressure of cylinders before starting an anesthetic and when a new cylinder is installed on a machine.

Pipeline System in Use. When pipeline systems are in use, the oxygen cylinder pressure should be checked before beginning anesthesia to make certain the tank is full or nearly so and

the cylinder valve closed. The cylinder valve should not be left open, since the cylinder could then empty. The reason for this is that on most anesthesia machines the oxygen regulator is set to deliver gas at a pressure below the usual pipeline inlet pressure so that oxygen from the piping system is preferentially used. If the pipeline inlet pressure falls below the regulator pressure and the cylinder valve is open, gas will flow from the cylinder until the pipeline inlet pressure exceeds the regulator pressure.

Many people rationalize leaving a cylinder valve open while the pipeline is in use by pointing out that if the pipeline system fails oxygen will automatically be supplied by the cylinder. This reasoning is dangerous for two reasons. First, if the pipeline system fails, one needs to be aware of this so one can make arrangements to obtain additional cylinders. Secondly, if the pipeline supply fails, the oxygen in the cylinder will be used and soon there will be no reserve oxygen available (15, 32).

If a case is begun with cylinder oxygen and moved to a location where piped gases are to be used, or if a cylinder is opened to supply gas when moving the anesthesia machine from one location to another, it is important to turn off the cylinder valve as soon as the switch to pipeline oxygen is made (8).

On many older machines the pipeline inlet pressure gauges indicate the higher of either pipeline pressure or machine circuit pressure (distal to the cylinder regulator). This means that during operation of the machine from a cylinder source, the pipeline pressure gauge will register near-normal pressure. A hazard can arise if the user does not understand this. With the cylinder valve open but the pipeline not connected or pressurized, the operator may incorrectly conclude that the unit is operating from the pipeline source. Only when the cylinder empties will the pipeline inlet gauge indicate a loss of pressure. The cylinder normally reserved for emergency situations will be empty. The machine standard requires the pipeline pressure gauge to be downstream of the check valve to prevent it from registering a pressure if the pipeline is not connected.

Inability to Use a Cylinder

No Handle. The mere fact that a full cylinder is present on an anesthesia machine does not always mean that there will be oxygen available when needed. First, there must be a means of opening the cylinder. A good practice is to chain a cylinder handle to each machine (Fig. 10.1). Often a cylinder handle is borrowed for opening a portable cylinder or some other purpose and not returned. If the handle is permanently attached to the machine it will always be there when it is needed.

Improper Installation. Before a cylinder can be used it must be correctly installed on the machine. Frequently the most inexperienced person in the operating room is told, without any instructions, to replace an empty cylinder. He may fail to crack the valve; install it without a washer, with a damaged washer or with two washers; fail to remove the dust protection cap (Fig. 10.2); or fail to check to see that the cylinder is full. Another error is screwing the retaining screw of the yoke into the port of the safety relief device on the cylinder (33–35). Responsibility for proper installation of cylinders should be that of the person using the machine. Personnel involved in the everyday handling of cylinders should receive instructions regarding safe use.

It is sometimes possible to spot an incorrectly placed cylinder simply by looking at it. A cylinder improperly installed may hang at an angle instead of parallel to the machine and perpendicular to the floor (Fig. 10.3).

Cylinder Valve Problems. A full cylinder may fail to deliver oxygen because of a problem with the valve. A report has been made where a portion of a cylinder valve seat extruded and blocked the exit (31).

Loose valve assemblies and the inability to open a cylinder valve have been reported (7, 31).

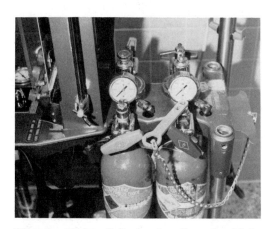

Figure 10.1. Cylinder handles should be chained to the machine so they will be available when needed.

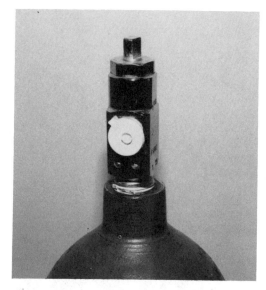

Figure 10.2. Failure to remove the dust protection cap from a cylinder before installing it on a machine caused a portion of the cap to be pushed into the cylinder valve port and this blocked the exit of gas from the cylinder.

Cylinders with inoperable valve assemblies may be delivered (31).

Marginal opening of an oxygen cylinder valve may result in failure to deliver gas when the cylinder pressure has fallen only slightly. Lethal anoxia resulting from this error has been reported (13, 36).

MACHINE PROBLEMS

In any machine where the components are connected by rubber tubing, there is a possibility that one of these hoses may become kinked. If it is the oxygen hose, oxygen source failure will result (37).

USER PROBLEMS

The oxygen failure safety valve and oxygen alarm are two devices that warn the operator of oxygen source failure. They were discussed in Chapter 3, but are included here because they have certain limitations which, if not fully understood, constitute hazards.

Oxygen Failure Safety Valve

The oxygen failure safety valve (36) is designed to interrupt the flow of anesthetic gases if the oxygen pressure falls. The presence of this device may impart a false sense of security to

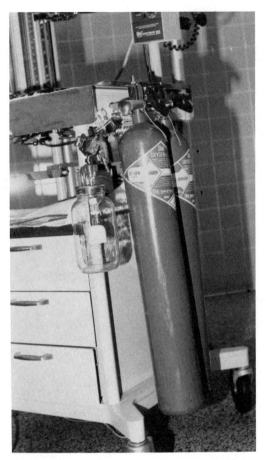

Figure 10.3. A sure sign that a cylinder is not correctly fitted in its yoke is that it hangs ·at an angle to the machine rather than perpendicular to the floor.

the user. In no way does it guarantee that the mixture of gases issuing from the machine contains an adequate amount of oxygen. All the valve needs to function is oxygen *pressure.* Oxygen *flow* need not be present (38). The device will not protect the patient if oxygen is turned off or if there is loss of oxygen through or distal to the flowmeter. Also these valves can malfunction. On some machines closing the valve on an oxygen cylinder part way will cause the oxygen flowmeter indicator to fall and remain at a low level without activating the oxygen failure safety valve (15). Therefore, while this device does provide a measure of protection from certain occurrences, its limitations must be appreciated by all who use anesthesia machines.

Alarm Devices

Oxygen alarms provide an audible and often a visible signal when the oxygen pressure falls below a predetermined minimum. Some of these devices are not permanently connected to the machine or breathing system. Like the oxygen failure safety valve they monitor oxygen pressure, not flow. Some offer the disadvantage that they can be turned off (39). The batteries may fail on electronic devices. Devices powered by oxygen pressure have the disadvantage that additional oxygen is lost through the whistle, and when the oxygen is depleted the whistle will cease to function. Devices that are powered by an anesthetic gas require a supply of that gas to give warning (40, 41). Simultaneous failure of both oxygen and the anesthetic gas or failure to turn on the gas will result in no warning being given (13). Audible alarms can be turned off or otherwise put out of action when, as is bound to happen, they give a false alarm (42). Some warning devices will fail when used in conjunction with certain ventilators that provide a sustained pressure (13, 43–46).

Nitrous Oxide Supply Pressure Variations

Pressure surges in the pipeline system may occur and can cause hypoxia by increasing the flow of nitrous oxide in relation to oxygen (47). Since the nitrous oxide regulator in the machine only affects the pressure of gas coming from a cylinder, it will be of no value in controlling surges in pipeline pressure. When cylinder supplies are used, a regulator could malfunction and deliver a higher than normal pressure of nitrous oxide.

Incorrect Agent Delivered

Each year there are several reports of brain damage or death resulting from a gas other than oxygen being supplied in its place.

PIPING SYSTEM ERROR

Crosses between oxygen and other gases may occur anywhere in a piped system. Oxygen storage tanks have been mistakenly filled with nitrogen (48, 49). More commonly, the error occurs in the piping itself (3, 8, 13, 50–57). Frequently the crossover is made when an addition or remodeling is done. Following construction or repair, pipelines may remain full of air or nitrogen rather than oxygen (13, 50, 58, 59).

Inside the operating room, incorrect wall outlets may be installed (60). An incorrect connection may be placed on a hose (14, 61–66) or on the pipeline inlet of the anesthesia machine (2, 61, 64, 66–68). Quick connect fittings may be damaged or poorly designed so that an incorrect connection can be made (69–71). Finally, connections between piped gases can occur in peripheral equipment (72, 73) including an anesthesia machine (74) and this can lead to the oxygen pipeline being filled with another gas.

MACHINE CROSSOVERS

Crossovers between oxygen and other gases inside an anesthesia machine have been reported (64, 66, 74, 75).

WRONG CONTENTS IN OXYGEN CYLINDER

It is possible for a cylinder labeled oxygen to contain a gas other than oxygen (14). It is also possible that a cylinder may be improperly labeled or painted. The cylinder may be exposed to such prolonged handling and adverse weather that the label cannot be read (7, 31). A cylinder may be painted a color other than that normally used (31). Particular care should be taken with cylinders in other countries, since there are four internationally used colors for oxygen (74).

ATTACHMENT OF WRONG CYLINDER TO OXYGEN YOKE

The Pin Index Safety System was discussed in Chapter 1. Although it has worked well, it is not foolproof and provides only partial protection against placing a cylinder on the wrong yoke (76–79).

The system can be overridden and an incorrect cylinder placed on a yoke in a number of ways. Cases still occur where a valve for a gas other than that contained is placed on a cylinder (7, 31). It is possible to remove pins (80) or the pins may be of inadequate length (54). Two or more washers over the nipple will build it out so that the pins do not meet the cylinder holes.

Pins can be bent or completely broken by a strenuous attempt to incorrectly seat a cylinder (54). One of the pins may be pushed deeper into the hole in the yoke. Breakage of one of the pins or forcing it into its seating hole reduces the indexing from a two-pin to a one-pin system.

Some yoke blocks may be inserted upside

down, thereby causing the incorrect gas to be delivered (81, 82).

Measures to prevent an incorrect agent being delivered through the pipelines, cylinders, or machines are described in Chapters 1–3. Hypoxia due to this can be detected easily if a properly functioning oxygen analyzer calibrated on room air is used. The anesthesiologist should always remember that his patient's survival depends on his acknowledging the possibility that crossing of supplies can take place. One should always think of transposition of gases when a patient becomes cyanotic with 100% oxygen. When the cause of progressive cyanosis is not immediately obvious, the patient should be disconnected from all apparatus and ventilated with room or expired air.

Flowmeter Problems

ERRONEOUS SELECTION AND/OR MANIPULATION OF FLOW CONTROL VALVE

Hypoxia may be caused by simply closing, partly or fully, the flow control valve for oxygen while allowing the nitrous oxide flow to continue (83–88). This is most likely to occur at the conclusion of the case when the operator means to turn off the nitrous oxide.

This hazard arises partly because of a lack of standardization of the position of the oxygen flow control valve in relation to those of other gases. Newer machines in the United States and Canada have the oxygen flow control valve to the right of the flowmeter head. Some older machines have it in other positions and confusion may result, especially if both types of machine are present in the same department.

Calverly (89) recommended that the oxygen flow control knob have projections for positive touch identification and all other flow control knobs remain round. This suggestion has been incorporated into the ANSI anesthesia machine standard. This increases the ability of the anesthesiologist to distinguish the oxygen flow control knob from other knobs, but is not a substitute for looking at the flow control valve.

Oxygen flow can be inadvertently lowered (or nitrous oxide flow increased) if a flow control knob is bumped by a chart or other item on the surface below or when hoses or wires are allowed to drape over the flow control valves (Fig. 10.4). With some flowmeters, in and out movement of the flow control valve, such as might be pro-

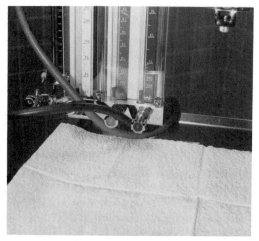

Figure 10.4. Wires and hoses should be kept away from the flow control knobs as they may cause alterations in flow.

duced by accidental contact with the knob, can change the flow significantly (90). Someone helping to move the machine could move a flow control valve knob and change the flow (Fig. 10.5). Some manufacturers provide a guard over the flow control valves to help prevent inadvertent flow alterations (Fig. 10.6).

Hypoxia due to erroneous selection and/or manipulation of flow control valves may be pre-

vented by special devices designed to provide a minimum oxygen concentration (see Chapter 3). These devices sometimes malfunction (91). An important part of the anesthesiologist's routine should be to frequently monitor the flowmeter settings.

INCORRECT FLOWMETER READING

Observing the incorrect flowmeter scale is a possible cause of hypoxia (14, 16, 92).

The accidental use of a low flow of oxygen when a high one is intended is a hazard whenever two oxygen flowmeter assemblies, one for low flows and one for high flows, are present (8, 14, 88, 89, 93). Flowmeters in series controlled by a single flow control knob are safer than separate flowmeters, although they are not entirely without the hazard of reading the wrong scale.

When the same flowmeter contains high and low oxygen flow graduations it is always possible for milliliters to be misread for liters.

In some machines, the flowmeter indicator can disappear from view at the top of the tube when the flow of gas exceeds the maximum scale calibration. Such a flowmeter is very similar in appearance to one with the indicator resting at the bottom of the tube (94). If the gas is nitrous oxide, a hypoxic mixture may result.

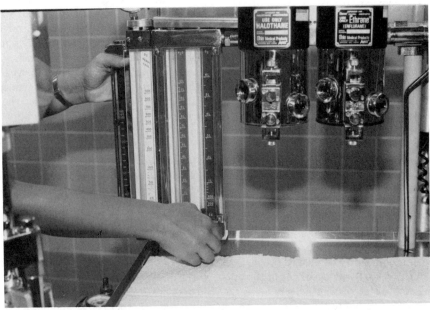

Figure 10.5. A dangerous practice. The flow control knob may look like a good thing to grab to someone moving an anesthesia machine. The flows may be altered in the process.

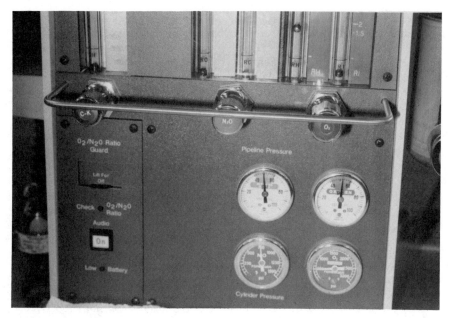

Figure 10.6. The guard bar in front of the flow control knobs serves to prevent inadvertent alterations in flows.

LEAKS

If an oxygen flowmeter tube is cracked or chipped or a loose connection develops at the top (95, 96) oxygen will be preferentially lost (97, 98). The position of the flowmeter indicator will not be affected, since the leak is downstream. Cracks and chips are sometimes produced when the user pounds on the tube to dislodge a sticking indicator. Often a crack cannot be seen until the tube is disassembled (95).

Other leakage around flowmeters can cause hypoxia, the magnitude of which will depend on the size of the leak, the location of the oxygen flowmeter (downstream or upstream) and the pressure developed in the breathing system (99).

The importance of the sequence of flowmeter placement was discussed in Chapter 3. If the oxygen flowmeter tube is not closest to the outlet, oxygen may be preferentially lost through any leak upstream of the flowmeter head outlet (16, 29, 89, 100, 101). If the oxygen flowmeter is closest to the outlet, anesthetic gas will be preferentially lost and a hypoxic mixture will not be produced.

Possible cause of leaks are retrograde flow through an empty yoke (133, 95, 102), a loose connection downstream of a flow control valve (103), a cracked flowmeter tube (16, 104) and a worn sealing washer at the top of a flowmeter (105).

Leakage in a machine can be detected by doing a pre-use check, as outlined in Chapter 14. It is important to use a yoke plug in any yoke not containing a cylinder (102). If this is not done, oxygen may leak out in retrograde fashion if a flow control valve is left open.

INACCURATE FLOWMETERS

If a flowmeter is not accurate, anesthetic gas may be delivered in excess of or oxygen delivered at less than the indicated flow.

Flowmeter inaccuracies are common and can occur in machines covered by preventive maintenance contracts even though recently serviced (106, 107). Accuracy is usually less at low flows (107–109).

Some causes of inaccurate flowmeter readings are dirt, grease or oil which has entered the system, sticking or damaged indicator (13, 110–112), misalignment of the tube, static electricity (113–119), improper calibration (120), the stop at the top of the flowmeter tube to prevent the indicator from obstructing the gas outflow falling down onto the indicator, and transposition of indicators, scales, or tubes (88, 121–123).

Oxygen Shunted from the Machine

The type I vaporizer circuit control valve described in Chapter 3 may be a source of hypoxia if all or a substantial part of the patient's oxygen requirement is provided by the vaporizer carrier gas instead of through the usual oxygen flowmeter (124–125). This is usually done when it is necessary to vaporize an agent of low volatility. If the vaporizer circuit control valve is turned to the OFF position, the flowmeter will indicate flow, but the flow will be vented into atmosphere (88). Unless adequate oxygen is supplied in the diluent flow, hypoxia will result. The new ANSI anesthesia machine standard requires that all gas flows shown on the flowmeters be delivered to the common gas outlet.

Air Leak into the System

When ventilators, especially those which generate a negative pressure during exhalation, are used, air leaking into the ventilator or breathing system may cause a diminution in the inspired oxygen if they are not adjusted properly and there are leaks (126, 127). In one case known to the authors, the filler cap of a vaporizer became loose and all the fresh gas flow from the machine escaped to atmosphere. The ventilator entrained room air and the patient suffered fatal hypoxia. Ventilators powered by air may allow air to enter the system through a leak in the bellows.

Hypoxia Secondary to Rebreathing

Rebreathing was discussed in Chapter 5. One of its effects is a lowered inspired oxygen concentration (128). Oxygen is continually removed from the breathing system by the patient. If a sufficient volume is not added in the fresh gas flow, hypoxia will result.

Inadequate fresh gas flow caused by leaks in the machine or fresh gas line can cause hypoxia secondary to rebreathing (129–131). For this reason, use of an oxygen analyzer is especially important when low fresh gas flows are used. Other causes of rebreathing are problems with unidirectional and non-rebreathing valves and are discussed in the section on hypercarbia.

The logical method of preventing hypoxia is to include an oxygen analyzer in each breathing system. Unfortunately, early models had many problems and it was difficult to keep them functioning properly. Although problems still exist, they have become dependable. Like any complicated piece of equipment, they need some care. Careful maintenance and calibration as prescribed for each analyzer should provide the user with a reliable instrument.

The authors feel that a properly calibrated and functioning oxygen analyzer should always be used when general anesthesia is administered so that hypoxia can be detected early enough to prevent serious complications. In some areas, professional liability insurance carriers require their use.

HYPERCARBIA

Hypercarbia can occur in spite of adequate ventilation if removal of carbon dioxide from the inspired gases is inadequate. Neither blood pressure nor heart rate is a reliable indicator of hypercarbia (1). Fortunately excessive concentrations of carbon dioxide usually take more than a few minutes to accumulate and produce adverse effects (132).

Absorber or Absorbent Failure

If the absorber is not properly packed, low resistance passages called channels may form (133–135) and the absorbent along these channels becomes exhausted quickly. Indicator color change occurring along the channels may not be seen from the outside of the absorber.

Hypercarbia can occur if the absorbent becomes exhausted. Cases have been reported in which color change did not take place because the absorbent did not contain an indicator (136, 137).

Hypercarbia can occur if a false channel which allows gases to bypass the absorbent develops within the absorber (138–139).

Bypassed Absorber

Many absorbers are fitted with a bypass mechanism that allows some or all of the gases to bypass the absorber. A bypass can be used to change the absorbent during a case or to deliberately elevate the inspired carbon dioxide concentration.

Not infrequently the bypass is left on at the conclusion of a case and the next anesthesiologist begins a case without turning it off. The partial bypass on the Ohio 20–21 absorber is located on the side of the absorber opposite from where the user normally stands (Fig. 10.7). It is easy to miss seeing that the valve is in the bypass position unless a special effort to check this is made.

Addition of Carbon Dioxide

On anesthesia machines with a carbon dioxide flowmeter, the possibility exists of the flowmeter

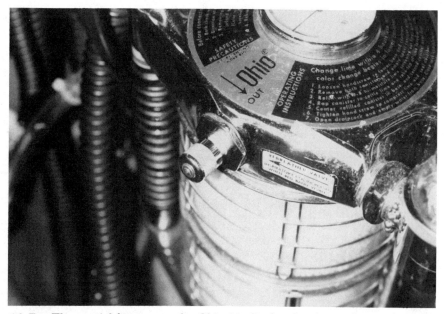

Figure 10.7. The partial bypass on the Ohio 20–21 absorber is on the opposite side of the absorber from where the anesthesiologist normally stands and is not easily seen.

being accidentally turned on and not being noticed (98, 99, 140–144). Often when this occurs the flowmeter indicator is at the top of the tube.

One case has been reported where the nitrous oxide hose was connected to the carbon dioxide station outlet (71).

Rebreathing

UNIDIRECTIONAL VALVE PROBLEMS

Correct movement of gases in a circle system is dependent upon proper functioning of the unidirectional valves. If they do not function properly, the patient will rebreathe varying amounts of carbon dioxide (145–148).

Incompetent Valves

Since a permanently open valve offers less resistance to flow than a closed valve, respiration will take place primarily through the incompetent valve.

The leaflet in a unidirectional valve may become sticky or damaged so that it will not seat properly (146, 149). Condensed moisture may cause it to adhere to the dome unless a guard prevents the disc from reaching the dome or the disc is not wettable (13, 16). The seat may be damaged during maintenance or cleaning. Foreign material may prevent proper seating of the leaflet. Finally, a defective leaflet may be re-

placed with an incorrect leaflet which is too large or small to function properly (149).

Absent Valves

Leaflets might not be replaced if they are removed for cleaning or servicing. Also it is possible to assemble a system with no unidirectional valves (150) (Fig. 10.8). This is most likely to occur if a department has both absorber-mounted unidirectional valves and unidirectional valves in Y-pieces.

NON-REBREATHING VALVE PROBLEMS

If a non-rebreathing valve allows significant back leak of exhaled gases hypercarbia may occur (151). The amount of hypercarbia will depend on the total fresh gas flow and the amount of back leak.

Improper assembly of some non-rebreathing valves can lead to partial or total rebreathing if the exhalation port is obstructed and the inhalation port is incompletely occluded during exhalation (152).

INADEQUATE FRESH GAS FLOW

In systems without carbon dioxide absorption such as the Mapleson systems, a low fresh gas flow can result in dangerous rebreathing with

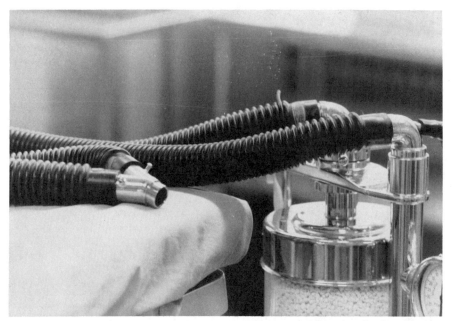

Figure 10.8. Circle system assembled with no unidirectional valves.

hypercarbia. A low fresh gas flow could be caused by the flows being set too low, a leak or obstruction in the machine (16, 99, 153), obstruction of the fresh gas delivery hose, an empty cylinder (154), a leak in the fresh gas line, as in a humidifier (155), or use of the Bain system with an intermittent (demand) flow anesthesia machine (156, 157).

PROBLEMS WITH THE INNER TUBE OF THE BAIN SYSTEM

Hypercarbia can occur with the Bain modification of the Mapleson D system (Fig. 10.9). If the inner tube becomes avulsed or kinked at the machine end, if there is a leak in the inner tube at the machine end, or if the inner tube is omitted or does not extend to the patient port, the entire length of the outer tube from the patient port to the defect becomes dead space (Fig. 10.9) (158–167). Some of these may be caused by stretching the circuit after washing. All can be detected by checking the system before use, as outlined in Chapter 14.

IMPROPER ASSEMBLY

The Bain System

In one reported case, the fresh gas inflow line from the machine was connected by mistake to the nipple of a pressure manometer of a respirator while the manometer was connected to the inflow orifice of the Bain tube (168). The entire hose became dead space and fresh gas escaped through the relief valve. In another case the Bain system was assembled without the inner tube (163). In still another case the relief valve was connected to the inspiratory limb (169).

Magill System

A problem with the Magill system was reported when a pressure-limiting bag was used in place of the usual reservoir bag. Gas was relieved through the bag rather than the relief valve.

A recent development in anesthesia is increasing use of exhaled carbon dioxide monitoring (see Chapter 5). Although somewhat expensive, these monitors provide a wealth of information and their use will result in early detection of hypercarbia. The authors of this book support the increased use of end-tidal carbon dioxide monitoring.

HYPOVENTILATION

Problems with equipment can result in less than adequate ventilation of the patient, leading to carbon dioxide retention and hypoxia. Adverse effects can appear within a few minutes. Inadequate ventilation can be of varying degrees and is not necessarily due to malfunction of equipment.

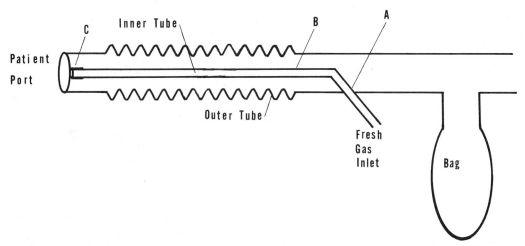

Figure 10.9. Possible problems with the inner tube of the Bain system that can result in hypercarbia. *A*, the tube carrying the fresh gas to the inner tube can become detached; *B*, the inner tube can become kinked or develop a leak; *C*, the inner tube may not extend to the patient port.

Early detection of hypoventilation is essential, but it is often missed. Monitoring of vital signs does not always detect the effects of inadequate ventilation promptly enough to avoid complications (171). Frequent observation of chest motion is helpful, but cannot always be used. Neither the sound nor the bellows movement of a ventilator may be altered appreciably even though a significant fraction of the intended tidal volume is lost into the room. Although a precordial or esophageal stethoscope is a direct, reliable link to the patient, in lengthy or tiring cases or in the presence of excessive background noise, it is far from foolproof (171). The most satisfactory means of assessing the adequacy of ventilation are blood gas analysis, exhaled carbon dioxide monitoring and measurement of exhaled volumes (172).

Blockage of Both Inspiration and Expiration

This is most commonly caused by obstruction of the endotracheal tube or its connector, but may be due to a malfunction of a non-rebreathing valve (152). In two reported cases the patient connector was obstructed by a membrane which totally occluded the lumen (173, 174).

Inadvertently Low Tidal Volume

Not all of the volume of gas discharged by a ventilator or leaving the reservoir bag during controlled or assisted ventilation will enter the patient's lungs. The increased pressure during inspiration may result in some gas remaining in the system or leaving the system through the relief valve or leaks. The discrepancy is particularly important when small patients are being anesthetized, since even small losses can be significant. The discrepancy between the volume delivered by the bag or ventilator and that inflating the patient's lungs will be increased by decreased patient compliance and increased airway and tracheal tube resistance.

WASTED VENTILATION

If, instead of entering the patient's lungs, some gas remains in the breathing system during inspiration, it is lost to the patient. The fresh gas flow will tend to make the volume entering the patient higher, but there are two factors that cause the volume to be lower. These are compression of gases in the system and distension of system components (175).

The volume lost due to compression of gases will increase as the volume of the system and the peak pressure attained increase. Systems vary considerably in volume, with most circle systems having higher volumes than other systems. Equipment such as humidifiers can increase the volume (172).

The volume lost due to distension of components will depend on the compliance of the various components, their volume and the pressures during inspiration. Usually the breathing tubes are the most distensible components. Plastic tubes have a low compliance compared to rubber tubes, so there is less volume loss with their use (176).

RELIEF VALVE NOT PROPERLY ADJUSTED

When manually controlled or assisted ventilation is used, gas is vented from the system during inspiration (unless a closed system technique is used). Compressing the bag creates a difference in pressure between the bag and the patient's lungs and also between the bag and the relief valve, which permits escape of gas. Part of the gas displaced from the bag goes to the patient and part of it escapes. The person squeezing the bag may find it difficult to estimate how much gas is entering the patient and how much is escaping to atmosphere. Frequent adjustment of the relief valve may be necessary to achieve the desired level of ventilation. A hazard is created if there is an illusion of adequate ventilation when in reality most or all the gas is being vented. Complete airway obstruction may not be diagnosed until cardiac arrest occurs (10, 177).

Another cause of inadequate ventilation is leaving a relief valve open when using an automatic, volume-controlled ventilator. Some absorber-mounted selector valves now available cause the relief valve to be excluded from the system when the switch to the ventilator mode is made (see Chapter 8).

LEAKS

Leaks also reduce the amount of gas entering the patient's lungs. Most leaks are too small to be of clinical significance, but occasionally are large enough that the volume entering the patient is inadequate. Leaks are best detected by a fall in tidal volume registered on a respirometer placed in the expiratory limb or by monitoring exhaled carbon dioxide. Most ventilators are not equipped to give an indication of a leak unless it is a very large one.

Anesthesia Machine

If the machine has a check-valve, leaks upstream of the check valve will reduce the fresh gas flow but will not affect the tidal volume. Leaks downstream of any check valves will cause a reduction in the tidal volume. They may occur in any location in a machine. Some of the more common sites are given below.

Leaks are particularly a problem with the Ohio DM 5000 machine, which has a pressurizing valve at the machine outlet that keeps the machine circuitry above atmospheric pressure. This increases the flow through leak sites so that the entire fresh gas flow may be lost through a relatively small leak.

Vaporizers. Leaks may occur at a loose connection at the vaporizer inlet or outlet (129, 130, 178), a loose or absent vaporizer filler cap (179, 180), a defect in the vaporizer (181) or a problem with a vaporizer selector valve (182).

Some machines have mechanisms which allow vaporizers to be placed in parallel (see Fig. 4.46). If a connection becomes loose or disconnected, all the fresh gas flow can be lost. Other machines are designed so that when a vaporizer is removed, a manifold cap must be placed where the vaporizer was situated. Failure to do this will result in a major leak if the vaporizer selector switch is turned to divert gases to the empty vaporizer position.

It is important to check the anesthesia machine for leaks with a vaporizer turned on, as described in Chapter 14. Otherwise a leak associated with a vaporizer may be missed.

Flowmeter Leaks. A leaking flowmeter tube (104, 105) or an open flow control valve with an opening to atmosphere upstream (95, 103) will result in loss of gas.

Connections Downstream of the Flowmeters. Connections downstream of the flowmeters usually include slip-on fitting hoses and metal-to-metal connections which are susceptible to leaks. Connections between the vaporizers on the back bar are quite susceptible to leaks.

A potential leak site in one machine was caused by the weight of the table and cylinders placing weight on the tubing which carries the gases from the flowmeters and vaporizers to the plumbing below the table top (183).

Breathing System

Absorber. The most common location for leaks in the circle system is the absorber. If the canisters do not fit together properly or the top and bottom do not seal well, large leaks can result.

In-System Vaporizers. Leaks in in-system vaporizers can occur around a loose filler cap or bottle, or through the base of the vaporizer if no bottle is present and the control dial is in the on position (Fig. 10.10). When not in use, these vaporizers should always have the bottle attached to prevent leaks should the control han-

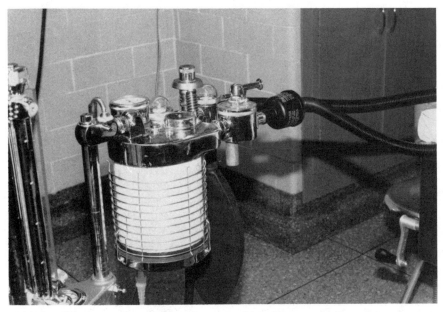

Figure 10.10. In-system vaporizers such as the Ohio No. 8 vaporizer shown here should not have the bottle removed. Opening the control dial at the top will allow a leak from the breathing system. If further use of the vaporizer is not anticipated, it should be removed completely.

dle be inadvertently turned on. If these vaporizers are no longer being used, they should be removed from the machine.

Other Components. If a non-rebreathing valve is used, during inflation a portion of the volume delivered may escape from the exhalation port of the valve, producing a forward leak (151, 152). Breathing tubes, bags, and Y-pieces may develop leaks (184–188). Humidifiers are a common source of leaks. A case of breakage of a reservoir bag mount has been reported (189). Connectors for oxygen analyzers and other monitors often develop cracks.

Ventilator Leaks

Leaks may occur either in the ventilator itself (190–191), in the attachment to the breathing system (192–193), or in a selector valve (194–195). Leaks in a ventilator are often due to improper seating of the outside housing. Leaks in the bellows may or may not result in a loss of gas from the breathing system.

When a leak is suspected, a systematic search of the machine and breathing system should be made, following the route of gas travel. All connections should be examined, using leak detection fluid, soapy water or a nitrous oxide trace gas analyzer (see Chapter 14).

VENTILATOR PROBLEMS

Hypoventilation can be caused by a ventilator accidentally being turned off (196), failing to cycle (197) or delivering a minute ventilation less than that preset (198, 199).

FAILURE OF THE FRESH GAS FLOW

A basic function of an anesthesia machine is to produce a flow of respirable gases with which to inflate the patient's lungs. Failure of the fresh gas flow can result in hypoventilation.

One cause is the oxygen failure safety valve cutting off the flow of gases when the oxygen pressure falls. Another cause is obstruction to gas flow inside the machine. In one reported case the leaflet from a check valve became dislodged and trapped within the piping of the machine, resulting in occlusion (99).

Problems with the hose that runs between the common gas outlet of the machine and the breathing system can cause failure of the fresh gas flow. The hose can become detached (126, 200) or occluded (201). In one case the inflow into the system was obstructed by the addition of a connection between the T-piece and the endotracheal tube connector (202). The inner tube of the Bain system, which carries the fresh gas flow, can be obstructed by kinking (164) or torsion (166).

DISCONNECTIONS

A disconnection is an unintended separation of components in a breathing system that causes gas intended to ventilate a patient to escape into the atmosphere. Most breathing system connections are slip fittings that relay on friction to hold them together. They will come apart if sufficient tension is applied. Disconnections are the most frequent ventilation hazard and the most likely to result in mortality or morbidity.

Disconnections can occur anywhere in the breathing system. The most frequent site is between the breathing system and endotracheal tube connector (Fig. 10.11) (30, 171, 203). This is particularly a problem during head and neck surgery, when the patient's head is covered by drapes and some movement of the head is likely.

Disconnections can be avoided by making secure connections. Anti-disconnect devices are available (204–210), and may be useful at some places in the breathing system. Many clinicians believe, however, that they should not be used at the connection between the endotracheal tube connector and the breathing system. It is reasoned that it is safer for such a joint to come apart under inadvertent tension than for the tracheal tube to be pulled out of the patient

(211). In addition, it may be necessary to make an intentional disconnection rapidly at this point for suctioning or to relieve a high pressure in the breathing system.

Disconnections are hazardous when they are not detected immediately. This is most likely during mechanically controlled ventilation, unless a disconnect alarm, a change in the ventilator sounds or tidal volume, or absence of breath sounds or exhaled carbon dioxide warns of the problem.

Some mechanical ventilators react to a disconnection with a different sequence of sounds or a collapsing bellows, but others show no change. Ventilators which allow a negative pressure to be generated in the bellows during exhalation can entrain room air through the point of disconnection (212). There may be no visible deflation of the bellows or activation of the low pressure alarm.

BLOCKAGE OF INSPIRATORY PATHWAY

Partial or complete blockage between the reservoir bag or ventilator and the patient can prevent generation of sufficient pressure to ventilate a patient.

Cases have been reported where the reservoir bag was connected improperly to the absorber support tube (213) or the inspiratory valve port

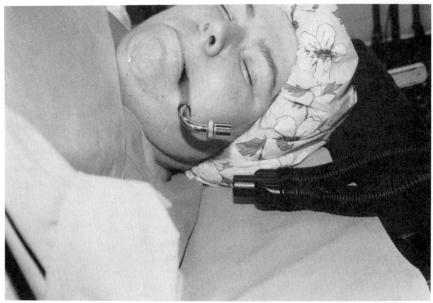

Figure 10.11.   Disconnections occur most commonly between the breathing system and the endotracheal tube.

(214). A bag can become obstructed at the neck (Fig. 10.12). Breathing tubes can become kinked (184) (Fig. 10.13). An obstructed ventilator tubing has been reported (215). Unidirectional valves can be crossed if a circle system is assembled with unidirectional valves both in the Y-piece and at the absorber (see Chapter 8). Obstruction resulting from the seals on a disposable absorbent package not being removed (216) (Fig. 10.14) or a clogged absorber screen will result in blockage of the inspiratory pathway if the bag is upstream of the absorber.

SUCTION APPLIED TO THE SYSTEM

A popular way of removing excess gases from the operating room is to utilize the hospital central vacuum system (see Chapter 9). If the inlet valve of the interface becomes stuck or blocked or the interface is inadvertently omitted, a subatmospheric pressure may be transmitted across the relief valve (217–221). Should this occur, the transfer tubing should immediately be disconnected from the relief valve. One case has been reported where a gastric suction tube incorrectly placed in the trachea caused evacuation of the breathing system (222).

If there is a delay in diagnosing hypoventilation, the patient will be put in danger. There are a variety of means of detecting problems. Monitoring of breathing system pressures, described in Chapter 5, is desirable. These provide a high degree of safety. However, there are a number of problems with them and they cannot be totally relied upon (196, 197, 212, 223–230).

Respiratory meters, especially if equipped with an alarm device, are useful. However, they cannot be used with ventilators having a de-

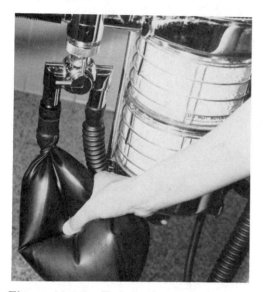

Figure 10.12. Twisting has caused this bag to become obstructed. Many bags have a guard in the neck to prevent this.

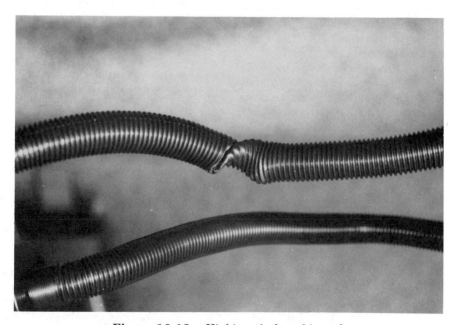

Figure 10.13. Kinking of a breathing tube.

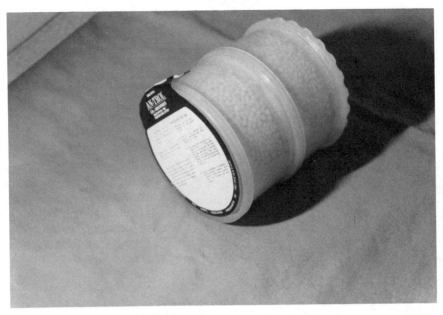

Figure 10.14.   Pre-packed absorbent container. Failure to remove the label from the top and/or bottom will result in obstruction to flow through the absorber.

scending bellows during expiration. Such bellows would continue to draw room air into the bellows in the event of a disconnect and thus "fool" the meter.

A ventilator that changes sound with a disconnect should be used. Monitoring of chest wall movements, deflections of the pressure gauge in the breathing system, breath sounds, and exhaled carbon dioxide (preferably using a monitor with an alarm) will increase the chances of a problem being discovered early.

A resuscitation bag should always be readily available in every operating room and if sufficient pressure to ventilate a patient cannot be generated, no more than 1 minute should be spent trying to diagnose or correct the problem. If it is possible to obtain fresh gas from the machine, the fresh gas line should be attached to the inlet of the resuscitation bag and the patient ventilated while the problem is corrected or a replacement machine brought into the room. Even if fresh gas flow cannot be obtained, ventilation with room air for a few minutes will usually avert serious damage.

HYPERVENTILATION

A hole in the bellows (231–234) or misassembly (235) can cause hyperventilation by increasing the tidal volume beyond the preset level. One investigator found that when nitrous oxide

was the main gas going through a ventilator, the volume of gas delivered increased dramatically (236).

EXCESSIVE PRESSURE

A number of cases of high pressure in the breathing system transmitted to the patient's respiratory tract during anesthesia have been reported (237, 238). In addition to interfering with ventilation, a high pressure can cause barotrauma and adverse effects on the cardiovascular system. Neurological changes, possibly secondary to cerebral air embolism, have been reported (239). Irreversible damage may be produced in a matter of seconds.

Modifying Factors

The rate and extent of the pressure rise are important and will be modified by a number of factors, including the reservoir bag, the volume of the system, the compliance of the tubings and use of a cuffed or uncuffed tube (241). The most important of these is the bag.

One of the functions of the reservoir bag is to buffer increases in volume in the system so that excessive pressure is not produced. The pressure in the breathing system is normally limited to 50 cm H_2O by the reservoir bag (241). Although a distended bag prevents spontaneous ventilation, the pressurized bag is usually readily apparent and the anesthesiologist should be able to release the pressure quickly enough to prevent damage.

Exclusion of the bag from the breathing system removes the buffering capacity and allows dangerously high pressures to be attained rapidly when there is coincidental obstruction to the outflow of gases from, or high inflow into, the circuit. Unfortunately, this situation is commonly compounded by operation of the oxygen flush valve (238). An anesthesiologist who finds a reservoir bag that is not filled may incorrectly assume that there is a large leak in the system and operate the oxygen flush in an attempt to compensate.

The most common cause of exclusion of the bag is obstruction of the expiratory limb upstream of the bag (see below). It is possible to omit the bag from the system (238, 242, 243). Older versions of the bag mount allowed it to be closed off with a tap (238). The bag may be obstructed by kinking of its neck (241) (Fig. 10.12).

Causes

HIGH INFLOW

Failure of regulators to reduce cylinder pressure has been reported (16). The ANSI machine standard requires that regulators be equipped with a safety relief valve or be designed so that the diaphragm will rupture if the pressure is too high. Gas at high pressure can be delivered by the hospital piping system (244).

Too high an inflow of gas into the breathing system may occur if the oxygen flush valve sticks in the on position. Some older anesthesia machines had oxygen flush valves which could be locked in the flush position. Oxygen flush valves on most newer machines are designed to close automatically.

With some oxygen flush valves, it is possible for the anesthesiologist to accidentally push them with his body. A case has been reported where a thermometer box fell onto a vertically mounted oxygen flush valve, jamming it (245). The new ANSI machine standard (246) requires that the flush valve be designed to minimize inadvertent operation by equipment or personnel accidentally pressing against it (Fig. 10.15).

Automatic ventilators may lock in the inspiratory position (247). Fortunately, most ventilators now have devices to limit the maximum pressure developed.

LOW OUTFLOW

Inadvertent buildup of pressure will occur when there is obstruction to the outflow of gases during a continuous flow of gases into the system (238). Defects that limit or prevent exhalation

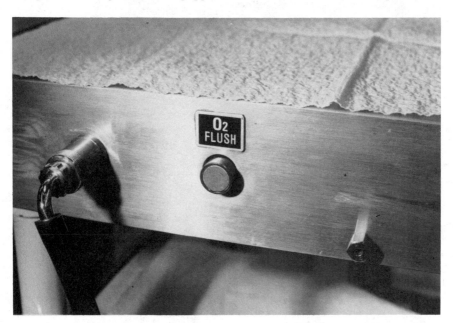

Figure 10.15. This oxygen flush valve has a protective ring around it to prevent accidental activation.

can result in a "stacking" of breaths as the ventilator delivers successive tidal volumes (248).

Obstruction to Expiratory Limb

As noted above, exclusion of the bag from the breathing system results in loss of its buffering capacity. Thus obstruction of the expiratory limb is particularly hazardous if it occurs upstream of the bag.

Causes of obstruction include an obstructed bacterial filter in the expiratory limb (173, 243, 249, 250) or in a ventilator tube (251, 252), a circle system with two inspiratory valves but no expiratory valve (8) interchange of the expiratory tube and bag (243, 253), and a bushing in the absorber bypass control inserted in reverse (8).

Misconnections involving ventilator-mounted selector valves were discussed in Chapter 8. If the hose to the breathing system is connected incorrectly to the bag mount and the valve is placed in the ventilator mode, there will be no outlet for gas (unless the relief valve in the system is open), and no bag to buffer the pressure increase (254–258).

Another case involved use of a system with unidirectional valves at both the absorber and Y-piece with the valves opposed to each other. Use of the oxygen flush caused herniation of the leaflet of the opposed valve on the inspiratory side of the Y-piece. However, the expiratory side was blocked by the other unidirectional valve in the Y-piece (239).

Another case involved a machine that had separate common gas outlets for the Magill and circle systems. The expiratory hose of the circle system became detached and was accidentally reinserted not into the port from which it had come but into the common gas outlet for the Magill circuit (8).

Kinking of tubes can cause obstruction of the expiratory limb of a circle or Mapleson system (259, 260). Obstruction of the outlet of a T-piece circuit by the anesthesiologist's finger has been reported (261).

Another cause of expiratory limb obstruction is misconnection of parts of the scavenging apparatus with the breathing system, usually by connecting one of the breathing tubes to the exit port of the collection device (262–264) (Fig. 10.16). The new ANSI standard (246) on scavenging requires that this port be 19 or 30 mm (and therefore incompatible with the 15- and

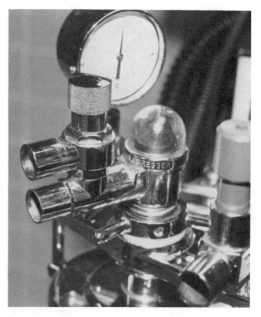

Figure 10.16. Some older relief valves had 22-mm connections on the collection device. It is easy to see how a breathing tube could be connected to the collection device by mistake.

22-mm fittings used for breathing system components). It is recommended that older equipment with scavenging connectors of 15 or 22 mm be replaced or modified (265). Other measures that help to prevent this are pointing the exhaust port from the relief valve away from the inlets to the unidirectional valves and making scavenging hoses distinctive from other hoses by using a different color hose or placing colored bands on the connecting end.

Foreign bodies can find their way into a breathing system. Two cases have been reported where the leaflet from a unidirectional valve was lost during servicing (266, 267). It was found later obstructing the connection to the bag mount. It allowed gas to enter the system, but during exhalation gas could not reach the ventilator.

Obstruction at the Relief Valve

Sticking, omission or malfunction of a relief valve is not uncommon (238, 241, 268), so its function should always be checked prior to starting anesthesia. The anesthesiologist may fail to open the relief valve (241), especially when switching from controlled to spontaneous ventilation (257). Ventilator relief valves may malfunction or become obstructed (257, 269–272).

Obstruction in the Scavenging System

The scavenging apparatus is essentially an extension of the breathing system. Obstruction between the relief valve (either in the breathing system or in the ventilator) and the interface will prevent gas from leaving the breathing system (273–276). For this reason it is suggested that the transfer tubing be as incompressible and unkinkable as possible. It should also be situated where it can be easily seen and be easy to disconnect from the relief valve.

Obstruction will also occur if the interface is omitted or if there is a problem such as that shown in Figure 10.17. With certain relief valves application of subambient pressure from active

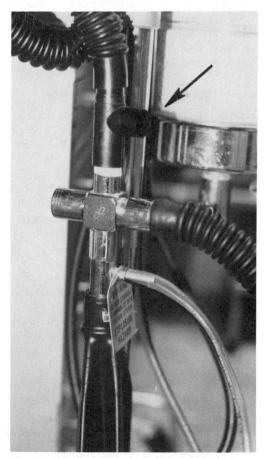

Figure 10.17. The transfer tubing has been placed over the positive pressure relief valve of the interface. It should have been placed over the T connection just above the interface (*arrow*). The transfer tubing will be obstructed and gas cannot exit from the breathing system through the relief valve.

scavenging will cause the valve to close, preventing the egress of gas from the breathing system (221, 275, 277, 278). It is important that active scavenging systems have negative pressure relief.

Problems with Non-rebreathing Valves

A sudden high inflow of gas (as may occur on flushing oxygen into the breathing system) may build up sufficient pressure to "lock" a non-rebreathing valve in the inspiratory position. A squeeze or bump on the bag may have the same effect (279). This may also occur when changing abruptly from controlled to spontaneous ventilation, when apnea or hypoventilation may persist for several minutes. Unless the pressure in the reservoir bag is decreased to release the locked valve, inflow will cause a continuous rise in pressure (10, 242, 280).

Incorrect assembly or malfunction of a non-rebreathing valve may cause an obstruction to exhalation (152, 281–286).

PREVENTION

The most important step in preventing the buildup of excessive pressure is to conscientiously follow the checking procedures in Chapter 14 before starting a case.

It has been suggested that each breathing system incorporate a pressure-limiting device and/or an audible alarm to warn the operator when a high pressure is reached (287).

Norry (255) and others (186, 238, 288, 289) have described pressure-limiting devices. This type of device will not protect against stacking of breaths, only very high pressures. Use of a device of this type could cause hypoventilation if the peak inspiratory pressure needed to ventilate the patient exceeded the pressure at which it released gas (290).

A number of low-pressure relief valves have been described which vent excess gas at a low pressure (150, 291–295). Some are described in Chapter 5. Other approaches have been to modify the reservoir bag to release pressure (170, 238, 296–300), or to create a compressible exhalation tunnel (301). These may be useful in preventing excessive pressure due to low outflow.

Use of these devices has not been widespread. Most are difficult to use with closed systems, some seal inadvertently with high pressures and some are not available with satisfactory collection devices for scavenging. Some require adjustment when going from controlled to spontaneous ventilation. Proper functioning of these devices should not be taken for granted and attention must be paid to pressures in the breathing system at all times.

MONITORING

When an automatic ventilator is used, it is essential that the anesthesiologist pay as much attention to the patient's ventilation as if he were inflating the lungs by hand. A ventilator which signals when it delivers a high pressure, changes sound with stacked breaths and limits the maximum pressure developed to 60 cm H_2O should be used (231). Monitoring of chest wall motion, deflections on the pressure gauge in the breathing system and breath sounds is essential.

Vigilance aids described in Chapter 5 are also useful. A respirometer placed on the expiratory limb gives confirmation that ventilation is occurring. Exhaled carbon dioxide monitoring is very useful for detecting problems. Pressure alarm systems that warn of a very high pressure in the breathing system and "stacking" of breaths due to low outflow are available (248).

TREATMENT

If there is a positive pressure buildup in the system, the anesthesiologist should immediately make a disconnection at the endotracheal tube connector. Ventilation can be carried on with a resuscitation bag until the problem is diagnosed and corrected.

ASPIRATION OF FOREIGN SUBSTANCES

Absorbent Dust

Inhalation of absorbent dust can cause wheezing, bronchospasm, laryngospasm, cough, and decreased compliance (302, 303).

Absorbent dust originates in the canister and travels down the inspiratory tubing. This can occur when the bag is on the expiratory side, since a bag squeeze will push gas at high velocity through the absorber. Overdistension of the bag and sudden release of pressure at the Y-piece when checking the circle system for leaks can force a cloud of dust into the breathing system (304–306). The design of certain circle systems which have the fresh gas inlet at the bottom of the absorber may contribute to the problem (302).

Inhalation of dust is less likely with large diameter canisters, since the larger cross-section lowers the flow velocity so there is less turbulence (10).

The problem can be avoided by placing a filter on the inspiratory side of the circle system, placing the reservoir bag on the inspiratory limb, releasing the pressure at the relief valve when checking for leaks (306), and shaking the canister to remove the dust before it is put into use.

Ethylene Oxide and Glycol

If equipment sterilized with ethylene oxide is not aerated adequately, residual ethylene oxide will diffuse into the breathing system and be inhaled.

When non-disposable equipment is cleaned, water may remain on it unless special care is taken to ensure it is dry. If wet equipment is sterilized with ethylene oxide, ethylene glycol will be formed and subsequently inhaled.

Piping System Contaminants

One of the problems in opening new hospitals or remodeled sections of older ones is that there may be particulate matter and gaseous contaminants inside the new pipelines (307, 308).

Oil mist contamination of piped air supplies can be a problem (309). If the air inlet is poorly situated the air may have other contaminants. A situation was reported where a halogenated hydrocarbon was used to clean air compressor filters. This resulted in contamination of the compressed air system (310).

Water coming out of a new pipeline installation as a result of a leaky joint allowing seepage of water into the pipe has been reported (311).

A fire in a ventilator traceable to contaminants in the pipeline has been reported (7).

Cylinder contents can also have contaminants (31, 312).

Metallic Flaking

Some manufacturers have adopted the practice of plating the inside surfaces of anesthetic equipment. This metal may flake off and be inhaled by the patient (313–315).

Bacteria

Bacteria and other organisms can be inspired from contaminated anesthesia equipment. This problem is discussed more fully in Chapter 15.

Breakdown Products of Anesthetic Agents

Volatile metabolites of anesthetic agents can be isolated in exhaled gases. Sharp and co-workers (316) isolated a halothane degradation product from patients who had received halothane through a circle system. They were not able to detect it in patients who had been anesthetized using a non-rebreathing system. The significance of this has been questioned (317). There is evidence that halothane can decompose when exposed to a heated humidifier (318).

Other substances that have been detected include methane, acetone, and carbon monoxide (319, 320).

ANESTHETIC AGENT OVERDOSE

An overdose of anesthetic agent can result in hypotension, cardiac arrest, or dysrhythmias. The extent of danger depends on how high a concentration the patient is exposed to and for how long. If liquid anesthetic agent gets into the fresh gas line or the breathing system a lethal situation may result.

Overfilled Vaporizer

This is primarily a problem with vaporizers that are filled from the top, such as older models of the Copper Kettle (Fig. 10.18) (88, 321). In a dimly lit room it is difficult to see the top of the liquid. A full vaporizer may appear empty. If additional fluid is added, liquid anesthetic can be pushed into the outflow tube. This problem can occur with other vaporizers which fill from the top.

To solve this problem, most modern vaporizers (including newer models of the Copper Kettle and sidearm Verni-Trol) have side filling ports so that the level in the vaporizing chamber cannot exceed the height of the opening. Top-filling models of these vaporizers should be replaced to eliminate this hazard.

Older model Verni-Trol and the sidearm Verni-Trol vaporizers are capable of delivering liquid anesthetic when the flow control valve is turned several turns past the point where the flowmeter indicator is at the top of the tube and the vaporizer filled to the top (322–324). A flow-limiting valve was added to the sidearm Verni-Trol circuit by the manufacturer. These vaporizers should not be filled to more than ¾ capacity. The sight tubes on newer models show the

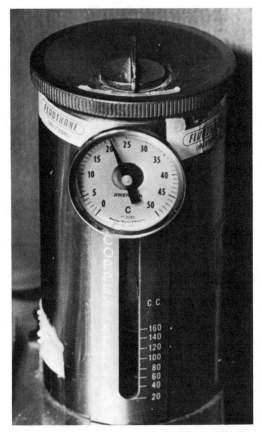

Figure 10.18. Copper Kettle vaporizer. Older version with filling port at the top. This carries the danger of overfilling and should be replaced by a model with a side-filling funnel.

maximum safe capacity at this level, but older ones show the maximum safe level near the top.

Tipping of a Vaporizer

Only a few vaporizers have design characteristics that isolate the vaporizing chamber from the outflow tract, thereby preventing liquid agent from getting into other parts of the apparatus if the vaporizer is tipped. The result of tipping or agitating a vaporizer charged with liquid may be that a very high concentration of agent is delivered when the vaporizer is first turned on (325, 326).

Some machines feature mechanisms that allow vaporizers to be easily removed from the machine. It is important to remember that easy removal allows more opportunities for tipping.

Vaporizers with first generation keyed fillers (two ports) had a minor problem. The filling device (two-port design) extended below the base of the vaporizer. The manufacturer supplied a base secured to the base of the vaporizer to lower its bottom, allowing the vaporizer to be set on a table (Fig. 10.19). These bases sometimes did not remain with the vaporizer, so that the vaporizer could not be set on a table top. Replacement bases can be ordered from the manufacturer to correct this problem.

The hazard of tipping a vaporizer can largely be avoided by mounting vaporizers securely in an erect position permanently attached to the machine. If a vaporizer must be detached, it should first be drained of all liquid agent. During transport it should be maintained in a vertical position. After being reinstalled on the machine, a high flow of oxygen should be run through it for a few minutes to clear any agent which may have entered the outflow tract.

Incorrect Calculation

Calculations are required with measured-flow vaporizers to determine the concentration delivered. Whenever calculations are made, the potential for errors exists. Various devices are available to simplify the calculations, but these are not always handy and can be misread.

The flowmeters for the measured-flow vaporizers on the Ohio DM 5000 machine are calibrated in cubic centimeters of saturated vapor. The flowmeters for most other measured-flow vaporizers are calibrated in cubic centimeters of carrier gas. If an operator accustomed to the calculations for a Verni-Trol or Copper Kettle applied them to the Ohio DM 5000, more anesthetic agent than anticipated would be delivered.

Incorrect Flowmeter Readings

If a flowmeter associated with a measured-flow vaporizer indicates lower flows than are actually occurring, or if the diluent flowmeters indicate more flow than is actually occurring, an anesthetic overdose will result. In one reported case, a vaporizer flowmeter was replaced but the calibration was not checked by the repairman. The replacement flowmeter delivered approximately six times the flow indicated (120).

Some measured-flow vaporizers are supplied with different flowmeters, depending on what agent it is anticipated will be used. For example, if it is anticipated that a vaporizer will be filled with methoxyflurane, a flowmeter that allows high flows may be supplied. If it is anticipated that the vaporizer will be filled with an agent of lower volatility, a flowmeter with much lower

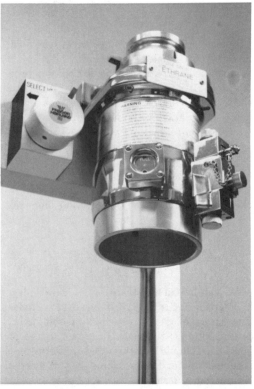

Figure 10.19. Vaporizers fitted with the pin safety system for filling cannot be set upright on a flat surface unless the filling block extends over the edge. Fitting such a vaporizer with an extender ring, as shown above, allows it to be set upright.

flows will be supplied. Accidents have occurred when an operator accustomed to one flowmeter sets the flow on a different vaporizer. If he does not read the flow, but simply sets the flow at the usual level, gross overdosage may result.

Inadvertent Administration

Even small amounts of agent can be harmful in a sensitized patient or one susceptible to malignant hyperpyrexia.

VAPORIZER INADVERTENTLY TURNED ON

Not infrequently a vaporizer is turned on without the knowledge of the operator (327). The previous use of the machine by a colleague or servicing by a technician can lead to the control knob being left in the on position. Someone who is helping to move the machine may grasp a control dial, inadvertently turning it on.

The older Fluomatic vaporizer is easy to turn on because the dial is at the top and does not have a lock. Another vaporizer which is easy to turn on inadvertently is the Ohio No. 8 bottle. The control lever is on the top and may be bumped by the anesthesiologist or equipment.

To prevent these problems, always check the vaporizers on a machine before using it to determine that they are in the OFF position. Be watchful of people touching your machine and encourage a "hands off" policy. It should not be allowed to become a leaning rail for personnel. Take time to instruct the operating room personnel about safe places to grasp the machine when it is to be moved and be especially watchful during and after the move that vaporizers are not turned on or the concentration dial altered. In-system vaporizers should be drained immediately after use and the bottle replaced to prevent leaks. Some of the newer vaporizers have a release button that must be depressed before a vaporizer can be turned on. Also some machines have mechanisms to prevent more than one vaporizer being turned on at a time (see Chapter 4).

CROSS-CONTAMINATION BETWEEN VAPORIZERS

Another cause of inadvertent administration is cross-contamination between vaporizers. When this occurs, the downstream vaporizer will contain some upstream agent. Both agents will then be delivered when the downstream vaporizer is turned on (328–330). The results are unpredictable. There are several devices on the market that prevent this problem by keeping vaporizers in parallel or by preventing simultaneous use (see Chapter 4).

VAPORIZER LEAKS

Inadvertent administration can result from anesthetic vapor coming from a vaporizer which has been turned off (331–336). These problems can be minimized by using exclusion devices such as those described in Chapter 4.

If a vaporizer circuit control valve is left in the on position, use of the oxygen flush may cause delivery of vapor (337).

DIFFUSION OF AGENT

Inadvertent administration can result from vapor coming from equipment other than a vaporizer. After an anesthesia machine and breathing system have been used to administer a volatile agent, they may contain enough of that agent to deliver a substantial amount to successive patients. Rubber goods especially will absorb anesthetic agent (331, 338–340). Anesthetic agent can be taken up by absorbent, especially if dry (341–343).

Other sources of contamination include metallic surfaces, elastomeric seals, and certain rigid plastics within anesthetic apparatus (331, 335, 340, 344, 345). Changing the absorbent and rubber goods reduces the concentration, but does not eliminate it.

CONDENSATION INSIDE THE BREATHING SYSTEM

It has been reported that liquid halothane or enflurane can condense inside the fresh gas delivery tubing if the flow control valve to a measured-flow vaporizer is turned on for an extended period of time with no accompanying diluent flow.

THE PUMPING EFFECT

The pumping effect was discussed in Chapter 4. In some vaporizers back pressure can cause an increased volume of unsaturated gas from the diluent flow to come into contact with the liquid and pick up vapor. More anesthetic than anticipated will be administered. Back pressure may be created by ventilation or by use of the oxygen flush valve (346). The pumping effect has been largely eliminated with newer vaporizers and newer machines.

Incorrect Agent

Vaporizers may inadvertently be filled with the wrong agent, particularly if this task is delegated to inexperienced personnel and/or the vaporizers are similar in external configuration (347).

If an agent-specific vaporizer designed for an agent of low volatility is filled with an agent of high volatility, anesthetic overdosage may result (13, 125, 349). Keyed filling devices (350) are a means of preventing the wrong agent being put into the vaporizer but are not foolproof (351, 352).

Intentional filling of agent-specific vaporizers with an incorrect agent is a dangerous practice. This is occurring with Forane and halothane. Two potential problems exist. The first is the impression by the user that when the vaporizer is drained and the sight window is empty that there is no agent remaining in the vaporizer. Agent-specific vaporizers utilize wicks which retain approximately 35 ml of agent. Addition of a different agent results in an unknown mixing of agents. The second problem deals with incompatible materials. Anesthetic agents attack various materials, resulting in corrosion and deterioration. Agent-specific vaporizers are designed for only one agent. Introducing a different agent may result in damage to the vaporizer (348).

Multiple-agent vaporizers should always be labeled as to their contents. If a multiple-agent vaporizer is filled with more than one agent, there is no way that anesthesia can be administered safely (88, 321). If the user is unsure of the contents, the vaporizer should be drained. Smell cannot be depended upon to identify the contents of a vaporizer, since the odor of one agent can mask that of another (353).

Loss of Diluent Gas

A leak in a machine downstream of the flowmeters and upstream of the point where the diluent flow and the output of a measured-flow vaporizer meet can cause anesthetic overdosage, since only diluent gas will be lost (178). Leaks which occur downstream of where the vaporizer output and diluent flow join will not cause an increase in vapor concentration, because both vapor and diluent flow will be lost.

Rebreathing with In-System Vaporizers

As discussed in Chapter 4, rebreathing will increase the output of an in-system vaporizer. A circulator can change an in-circuit vaporizer into a potentially lethal device (354).

Inaccurate Vaporizer

Dial settings of vaporizers are frequently not accurate (333, 355–359). The concentration of vapor delivered by a vaporizer may be influenced by factors such as the fresh gas composition (360, 361), fresh gas flows (358, 362, 363), and accumulation of preservative in the vaporizing chamber. Accuracy will be increased by following the manufacturer's suggested schedule for cleaning and recalibration.

It occasionally happens that a vaporizer's accuracy deteriorates slowly and the anesthesiologist accommodates to the change, which is so imperceptible that he is not conscious of it. After the vaporizer is recalibrated, the user may be surprised at the depth of anesthesia resulting from use of the vaporizer.

Foaming

Foam can form inside a bubble-through vaporizer when methoxyflurane, trichlorethylene, chloroform, and, under certain circumstances, halothane come into contact with a silicone lubricant, sealant, or leak detection fluid (88, 364–367). Only trace amounts of these may cause the agent to foam (367). If the foam enters the outflow tubing an overdose will result. Foaming does not occur with flow-over vaporizers (367).

Incorrect Vaporizer Installation

If an in-system bubble-through vaporizer is connected backwards, liquid anesthetic may be delivered into the breathing system (88, 368). Fatalities from this hazard have occurred.

If a direct-reading vaporizer is connected with the flow reversed, the concentration of vapor coming from the vaporizer may increase considerably (368). This is most likely to occur if the vaporizer is connected in the delivery hose between the machine outlet and the breathing system. Mounting the vaporizer on the machine between the flowmeters and the common gas outlet will avoid this error.

Vaporizer Control Knob Turned the Wrong Way

Clockwise rotation of the control on the top of most modern vaporizers reduces the concentration of agent or turns it off. On some older vaporizers this requires counterclockwise rotation (367, 369). If both types of vaporizers are in the same department, and especially if they are on the same machine, an error can easily be made. The new ANSI machine standard requires that all vaporizer control knobs rotate counterclockwise to increase the concentration.

Discharge of Liquid Agent into the Fresh Gas Line

This can be caused by overfilling or tipping. With certain older Verni-Trol and sidearm Verni-Trol vaporizers, if the vaporizer circuit control valve was turned on and the flow control valve was open, occlusion and sudden release of the fresh gas flow could create sufficient turbulence to deliver liquid anesthetic (370). To prevent this, the manufacturer will install a pressure relief valve on the machine.

Overdosage of anesthetic agent can usually be avoided by exercising reasonable care in checking, using, and monitoring equipment and having it serviced regularly. The patient's vital signs should always be closely monitored so that the effects of overdosage can be detected early. Smelling cannot be relied upon to detect overdosage because use of scavenging devices will conceal the odor (275, 371).

When an overdose of anesthetic agent is suspected, the patient should be disconnected from the breathing system and ventilated using other means (preferably a resuscitation bag). If it is determined that the fresh gas flow does not contain anesthetic agent, a high flow of oxygen can be used to ventilate the patient. If anesthetic agent can be smelled in the fresh gas flow, the patient should be ventilated using room air.

ANESTHETIC AGENT UNDERDOSAGE

Not delivering enough anesthetic agent can be as serious as delivering too much, or at the very least, quite embarrassing.

Failure of the Nitrous Oxide Supply

Pipeline supplies of nitrous oxide are not foolproof. Leaks, freezing of regulators, and depletion of a system too small to meet demand have all been reported (3). Cylinder supplies can also fail. Jammed cylinder pressure gauges have given the impression that gas was present after depletion had occurred (311).

Contamination of Nitrous Oxide with Oxygen

If a connection between the nitrous oxide and oxygen sources occurs, either in the pipeline system or in the anesthesia machine, with the oxygen pressure being higher than the nitrous oxide pressure, oxygen will flow into the nitrous oxide line and less than 100% nitrous oxide will be delivered to the nitrous oxide flowmeter. One case has been reported in which a defect in the diaphragm of an oxygen failure safety valve allowed the nitrous oxide upstream of the flow control valve to become contaminated with oxygen, causing patient awareness (372).

Leaks
ANESTHESIA MACHINE

When a leak occurs in an anesthesia machine upstream of the flowmeter head outflow, nitrous oxide or carrier gas flow to a measured-flow vaporizer may be preferentially lost, so that the delivered concentration is less than expected. In one reported case there was an oxygen leak into the anesthesia machine between the oxygen flush valve and the machine outlet (373). This caused a reduced anesthetic concentration to be delivered to the breathing system.

VAPORIZERS

A leak in a vaporizer caused by a loose or absent filler cap or a defect in the inflow or outflow connections can cause an unexpectedly low concentration of vapor (129, 178, 374, 375).

BREATHING SYSTEM

Admission of air into a breathing system through a leak or disconnection in the breathing system can be a cause of patient awareness. If the patient is breathing spontaneously, the negative pressure generated during inspiration may cause significant air entrainment. Air entrainment can also occur if a mechanical ventilator which has a negative pressure phase is used (376) or when a ventilator is used as part of a non-rebreathing system and the fresh gas flow is less than the minute volume (127).

VENTILATOR

Mechanical ventilators may leak and draw in driving gas (oxygen or air) if there is a hole in the bellows (127, 232, 234, 235, 260, 376–379) or the bellows is improperly connected.

Repeated Use of Oxygen Flush

Repeated use of the oxygen flush in order to keep the reservoir bag filled when there was failure of the fresh gas flow or a leak has led to patient awareness (200).

Inaccurate Flowmeter

If the nitrous oxide flowmeter indicates more flow than is actually occurring (or the oxygen flowmeter indicates less), the concentration will be less than expected (122, 123).

If the flowmeter associated with a measured-flow vaporizer indicates more flow than is actually occurring (or the diluent flow less) a lower anesthetic concentration than expected will result.

Vaporizer Turned Off

Most anesthesiologists who have used a vaporizer which has a vaporizer circuit control valve associated with it, such as the Copper Kettle or Verni-Trol, have at least once made the error of not turning the valve to the ON position at the beginning of the case, or after activating the oxygen flush in those machines which have both functions in the same valve.

Empty Vaporizer

An occasional cause of underdosage is a vaporizer that has been emptied and not refilled or runs empty during a case. Some vaporizers have a small vaporizing chamber and will empty during a long case, especially if high flows of carrier gas are used. It is important to check the liquid level before beginning a case, adding more if necessary.

Miscalculations

With any of the vaporizers that require calculations to determine the delivered concentration, an error may be made and the result may be an underdose.

Incorrect Agent

If a vaporizer designed for use with a highly volatile agent is filled with one of low volatility, the patient will fail to receive the expected concentration (349). For example, if a halothane vaporizer were filled with methoxyflurane, sub-anesthetic concentrations would result.

Incorrect Dial Setting

An incorrect setting of a vaporizer control knob or flowmeter can be a cause of underdosage. It is important to check settings frequently during a case, as a setting can be altered without the operator's knowledge. Also it is imporant to observe the concentration dial whenever a change in setting is made.

FIRES AND EXPLOSIONS

The idea that a fire or explosion could occur in the operating room is usually dismissed by those who do not use flammable anesthetic agents. Unfortunately, this complancency is unwarranted. Fires and explosions can and do still occur.

Factors

Three things must be present for a fire or explosion to occur: a gas to support combustion, a source of ignition, and a flammable substance (380–383).

GAS TO SUPPORT COMBUSTION

Air will support combustion, since it contains oxygen. High concentrations of oxygen make any conflagration that occurs more violent than it otherwise would be and may render some materials flammable (380, 384). Nitrous oxide will support combustion and in the process will release the energy of its formation, providing increased heat (382, 385, 386).

Fire hazards are especially acute during surgery of the head and neck because oxygen and nitrous oxide tend to build up beneath the surgical drapes or in the oropharyngeal cavity, creating an "enriched" atmosphere.

SOURCE OF IGNITION

The source of ignition is most commonly an electrosurgical unit. The high current density at the tip causes local heating. The tip may remain hot for a short time after the switch has been released. Ignition can result from contact of this hot tip with flammable substances as well as arcing at the surgical site. In addition, the current from an improperly grounded electrosurgical unit may find a pathway to ground through an anesthesia circuit, causing an explosion or fire (387–390).

There are other sources of ignition in the operating room. A laser used in microsurgery of the larynx and trachea can cause an unprotected tracheal tube to catch fire. This will be discussed more fully in Chapter 13. The operating room light was the source of ignition in at least one fire when the heat from it weakened an oxygen hose, causing it to burst (19). Defective electrical equipment and static electricity can also be the source of ignition (380, 383, 391, 392). A fiberoptic light source can transmit sufficient heat to ignite substances (392).

Adiabatic compression of gases can generate sufficient heat to cause ignition. Opening a cylinder valve causes an inrushing of gas at high pressure. Subsequent recompression in a small space causes heat to be produced. This can ignite combustible substances such as grease or oil.

A COMBUSTIBLE SUBSTANCE

A number of articles used in or near the patient can become the flammable material. Endotracheal and tracheostomy tubes (381, 384, 393, 394); adhesive tape, especially plastic (19, 382, 395); breathing tubes and bags (387, 389, 396, 397); gauze pads and sponges (19, 382, 398); eye patches; oxygen catheters (383); masks; airways; paper products; ointments; blood pressure and tourniquet cuffs; gloves; stethoscope tubing; patient hair; gastrointestinal tract gases; surgical drapes (385, 399), gowns, masks, hoods, etc., may catch on fire.

Agents used by the surgeon and other operating room personnel including cleaning agents such as alcohol, acetone, and ether (400–403), prep solutions such as tincture of benzalkonium (402, 404), and aerosol or liquid adhesives such as tincture of benzoin (405, 406) may become sources of combustion.

Prevention

1. Open a cylinder valve before attaching it to the machine or regulator to blow out dust particles. Always open cylinders slowly to minimize recompression heat (407).

2. Moisten gauze to be used in the oral cavity with water or saline. Never use a flammable liquid such as alcohol (398, 404).

3. Avoid insufflation techniques or leaks around the tracheal tube if electrosurgery is used in the oropharynx.

4. Use water-based prep solutions, or, if alcohol-based solutions must be used, delay draping until vapor dissipation has occurred.

5. Handle flammable liquids and sprays in such a way that pooling or saturation of patient drapes is avoided.

6. Make hair near the operative site nonflammable by coating it thoroughly with a water-soluble lubricating jelly (392).

7. Try to prevent oxygen and oxygen-nitrous oxide mixtures from being vented near the source of ignition or where they will be trapped under drapes. This can be accomplished by using a cuffed or tight-fitting endotracheal tube and scavenging to remove gases.

8. When the electrosurgery is used while oxygen is being administered nearby (as during eye procedures done under local anesthesia), antic-ipate the use of electrosurgery by at least 1 minute and discontinue oxygen administration to the patient (392).

9. Make certain that the electrosurgical unit is functioning properly and has a proper dispersive (ground plate) circuit. This may shorten the required duty cycle and minimize extra heating of the tip (408).

Action in Case of a Fire

1. Keep a means for extinguishing a fire readily available. If a fire occurs, disconnect the fresh gas flow and extinguish the fire.

2. Make sure personnel know about shutoff valves and test them periodically.

3. If a fire occurs, sound the alarm and shut off gas flow to the area where the fire is located.

4. If a cylinder is connected to, but is some distance away from, an apparatus involved in a fire and it is safe to do so, the valve should be turned off and if possible, the cylinder removed from the area. Cylinders that cannot be reached and removed safely may burst due to excessive heat. Therefore the immediate area must be evacuated.

ACCIDENT INVESTIGATION

Whenever a patient appears to have suffered harm, one of the first concerns should be to find the cause. A frequent (and often initially overlooked) cause is the equipment used when the problem occurred. The medicolegal literature contains many unfortuante examples where two or more patients in succession suffered injury or death when defective equipment continued to be used after an accident had occurred because the equipment was not suspected. Any time a patient has an unexplained problem, equipment malfunction should be suspected and the equipment not used again until this has been disproved. Appropriate personnel and the manufacturer should be notified in order to prevent harm to other patients.

Numerous photographs of the operating room where the accident occurred should be taken. This may answer questions which arise at a later date when memories have faded. These pictures should be taken from various angles, including wherever the personnel present at the time were located. All pieces of equipment should be situated where they were at the time the problem occurred.

After pictures have been taken, all equipment

which is suspected to have contributed to the problem should be put in a safe place to prevent modification before it is examined by an expert.

It is important that the anesthesiologist contact his professional liability insurance carrier at once. The insurance company will have an important interest in subsequent investigations.

An impartial expert should be chosen to investigate a suspected equipment problem. This should be a person knowledgeable about the various pieces of equipment as well as the patient problem. If possible, all parties, including the anesthesiologist, patient, hospital, surgeon, equipment manufacturers, and service representative should agree on the expert. In the absence of such agreement each party can bring his own expert.

The investigation should be scheduled at a time when all the interested parties and/or their representatives can be present. The procedure for the investigation should be agreed upon beforehand.

The investigator needs to have certain information before he comes to the scene. This includes the name, model, serial number, servicing information, and hospital and anesthesia department records for each piece of equipment which may have been involved. The anesthesia record and any pertinent information from the patient's chart and anesthesia records for cases using the equipment prior to the accident should be made available. If any equipment was moved into the room just before the case, the records of the preceding cases in that room and in the room from which the equipment was obtained should be available.

The following questions need to be answered:

1. What was the date and approximate time of the problem?

2. Had the patient had uneventful anesthetics in the past?

3. What was the surgical procedure being performed?

4. What was the first indication that there was a problem?

5. At what time did this occur?

6. Who first noted the problem?

7. What signs did the patient exhibit?

8. In what room or area did the problem occur?

9. Had there been any recent modifications to the electrical or gas pipelines to that area?

10. Was this a newly opened area of the hospital?

11. Was this the first case performed in that room that day?

12. Was there a problem with previous cases performed in the room that day or the previous day?

13. Were there any unusual occurrences in the other operating rooms that day or the previous day?

14. Was any equipment moved from another room? Were there any problems noted in the room where it was previously used?

15. What checks were made of the anesthesia machine, breathing system, and ventilator before use?

16. Who last filled the vaporizers on the machine?

17. Was the vaporizer attached to the machine just before the case began?

18. If the vaporizer was just attached to the machine, were there any precautions taken to prevent liquid from being spilled into the outflow tract?

19. Was an electrosurgical machine used?

20. When was the line isolation monitor last checked?

21. What monitors were being used during the case?

22. On what values were the alarms on the monitors set?

The investigation itself should consist of interviews with eyewitnesses of the accident and an in-depth examination of the equipment similar to the checking procedures described in Chapter 14. Vaporizers should be calibrated, checked to determine if vapor is delivered in the OFF position and an analysis made of their contents.

If a problem with the equipment is found, an attempt should be made to reconstruct the accident if this can be done without danger to anyone and the equipment should again be locked up until any litigation involving the case is settled. If the investigation reveals no problems, the equipment can be returned to service with the consent of all parties.

Following the investigation a report should be made in clear and concise language detailing all facts, analyses, and conclusions.

ACCIDENT PREVENTION

Prevention of accidents in which anesthesia equipment plays a part is a vital but difficult task. Checking and maintenance of equipment and use of vigilance aids are all important, but other measures are necessary.

Selection of proper equipment is essential. Reliability, safety, and cost should all be considered. Equipment should be evaluated in a clinical setting under conditions similar to those expected during use. Standardization of equipment, both within the anesthesia department and with other hospital areas, will help to decrease mishaps.

Replacement of obsolete equipment is a necessary ongoing process. Unfortunately, a piece of equipment that appears to be the best available at one time may become inferior as improved apparatus becomes available.

Proper communication among members of the department is important. A large number of accidents associated with equipment occur because the user was not familiar with it. It is essential that all members of the department receive sufficient instruction to use new equipment safely and properly. Initial close supervision can protect both the patient and the apparatus from harm. Instructions for setting up and calibration, together with appropriate warnings, should be clearly and permanently attached to specific pieces of equipment. Manuals that come with equipment should be reviewed periodically by department members. Information about equipment modifications and problems should be conveyed to each member of the department.

It is important that accidents and near accidents be discussed, as they usually indicate that something is wrong. Frequently steps can be taken to prevent such occurrences in the future.

Another very important factor in accident prevention is attention to the human element. Human errors caused by preoccupation, mental lapses, or carelessness can be identified in nearly all equipment-related accidents. Unfortunately, vigilance aids and safety devices tend to instill a false sense of security in the user. It should not be forgotten that equipment is only as good as the person who operates it. The anesthesiologist must remain at all times alert to any suspected or obvious malfunction and investigate it immediately. Nothing can take the place of the watchful eye of an alert anesthesiologist.

References

1. Manninen P, Knill RL: Cardiovascular signs of acute hypoxaemia and hypercarbia during enflurane and halothane anaesthesia in man. *Can Anaesth Soc J* 26:282–287, 1979.
2. Anonymous: There, but for the grace of God. *Lancet* 1:231, 1975.
3. Feeley TW, Hedley-Whyte J: Bulk oxygen and nitrous oxide delivery systems: design and dangers. *Anesthesiology* 44:301–305, 1976.
4. Johnson DL: Central oxygen supply versus Mother Nature. *Resp Care* 20:1043–1044, 1975.
5. Gibson OB: Another hazardous pipeline isolator valve. *Anaesthesia* 34:213, 1979.
6. MacWhirter GI: An anaesthetic pipeline hazard. *Anaesthesia* 33:639, 1978.
7. Hedley-Whyte J: Mechanical failures leading to hypoxia. *Audio Digest* 19, No. 14, July 18, 1977.
8. Wyant GM: *Mechanical Misadventures in Anaesthesia.* Toronto, University of Toronto Press, 1978.
9. Newson AJ, Dyball LA: A visual monitor for piped oxygen supply systems to anaesthetic machines. *Anaesth Intensive Care* 6:146–148, 1978.
10. Eger EI, Epstein RM: Hazards of anesthetic equipment. *Anesthesiology* 25:490–504, 1964.
11. Anonymous: Hospital negligent in supply of oxygen. *J Legal Med* 3:12–13, 1975.
12. Morrison AB: Medical gas station outlets and connectors. Health Protection Branch, Health and Welfare, Canada, Jan. 14, 1981.
13. Ward CS: The prevention of accidents associated with anaesthetic apparatus. *Br J Anaesth* 40:692–701, 1968.
14. Mazze RI: Therapeutic misadventures with oxygen delivery systems: the need for continuous in-line oxygen monitors. *Anesth Analg* 51:787–792, 1972.
15. Meyer JA: Guest discussion. *Anesth Analg* 51:790–791, 1972.
16. Eger EI, Epstein RM: Hazards of anesthetic equipment. *Anesthesiology* 25:490–504, 1964.
17. Anonymous: Wall oxygen adapters. *Health Devices* 2:179, 1973.
18. Anonymous: Chemetron (NCG) outlet station adapters. *Health Devices* 3:124, 1974.
19. Anderson EF: A potential ignition source in the operating room. *Anesth Analg* 55:217–218, 1976.
20. Janis KM: Sudden failure of ceiling oxygen connector. *Can Anaesth Soc J* 25:155, 1978.
21. Muir J, Davidson-Lamb R: Apparatus failure—cause for concern. *Br J Anaesth* 52:705–706, 1980.
22. Craig DB, Longmuir J: Anaesthetic machine pipeline inlet pressure gauges do not always measure pipeline pressure. *Can Anaesth Soc J* 27:510–511, 1980.
23. Wilson AM: The pressure gauges on the Boyle International anaesthetic machine. *Anaesthesia* 37:218–219, 1982.
24. Anonymous: Judge awards $219,000 in oxygen equipment case. *Biomed Safety Standards* 10:42, 1980.
25. Sniper W: Ensuring the oxygen supply. *Br J Anaesth* 39:608–609, 1967.
26. Hill EF: Another warning device. *Br J Anaesth* 28:228–229, 1956.
27. McInnes IC: Safety of oxygen supplies. *Br J Anaesth* 45:1221, 1973.
28. Dornette WHL: A plea. *Anesthesiology* 17:503, 1956.

29. Eger EI, Epstein RM: Hazards of anesthetic equipment. *Anesthesiology* 25:490–504, 1964.

30. Cooper JB, Newbower RS, Long CD, McPeek B: Preventable anesthesia mishaps: a study of human factors. *Anesthesiology* 49:399–406, 1978.

31. Feeley TW, Bancroft ML, Brooks RA, Hedley-Whyte J: Potential hazards of compressed gas cylinders: a review. *Anesthesiology* 48:72–74, 1978.

32. Meyer JA: Guest discussion. *Anesth Analg* 51:790–791, 1972.

33. Fox JWC, Fox EJ: An unusual occurrence with a cyclopropane cylinder. *Anesth Analg* 47:624–626, 1968.

34. Milliken RA: An explosion hazard due to an imperfect design. *Arch Surg* 105:125–127, 1972.

35. Milliken RA: Correspondence. *Anesth Analg* 50:775, 1971.

36. Epstein RM, Rackow H, Lee ASJ, Papper EM: Prevention of accidental breathing of anoxic gas mixtures during anesthesia. *Anesthesiology* 23:1–4, 1962.

37. Lack JA, Honan M: Oxygen supply hazard. *Br J Anaesth* 47:1234, 1975.

38. Levin MJ, Balasaraswathi K: "Fail Safe"? Unsafe! *Anesthesiology* 48:152–153, 1978.

39. Anonymous: Doctors cleared of perjury. *Br Med J* 3:302–303, 1973.

40. Dawkins M: Anaesthetic safety devices. *Br Med J* 4:299, 1973.

41. Cartwright FF: Warning of an empty oxygen cylinder. *Lancet* 2:407, 1963.

42. Davenport HT, Wright BM: Anaesthetic safety devices. *Br Med J* 4:357, 1973.

43. Fraser-Jones J, Jenkins AV, Thomas E: Intermittent positive pressure respirators and the "Bosun" oxygen warning device. *Anaesthesia* 20:95–96, 1965.

44. Fraser-Jones J, Jenkins AV, Thomas E: Dangerous anaesthetic device. *Br Med J* 4:1396, 1964.

45. Howells TH: Dangerous anaesthetic devices. *Br Med J* 4:1659, 1964.

46. Hurter DG, Williams D: The Bosun device. *Lancet* 2:480, 1964.

47. Finlay J, Pelton DA: Needed: error prevention. *Hospitals* 45:64–66, 1971.

48. Sprague DH, Archer GW: Intraoperative hypoxia from an erroneously filled liquid oxygen reservoir. *Anesthesiology* 42:360–363, 1975.

49. Anonymous: O_2-N_2O mix-up leads to probe into deaths of two patients. *Biomed Safety Standards* 11:123–124, 1981.

50. Anonymous: Hospital death probe continues. *Am Med News* August 15, 1977, p 26.

51. Ayres SM: Clean air therapy. *Resp Care* 17:54–57, 1972.

52. Anonymous: Installation of oxygen system probed in N_2O death suit. *Biomed Safety Standards* 10:41–42, 1980.

53. Wylie WD: There, but by the grace of God . . . *Ann R Coll Surg Engl* 56:171–180, 1975.

54. Goebel WM: Failure of nitrous oxide and oxygen pin-indexing. *Anesth Prog* 27:188–191, 1980.

55. Meyer JA: Crossed gas supplies: a preventable accident. ASA Newsletter, Nov, 1977, p 3.

56. LeBourdais E: Nine deaths linked to cross connection: Sudbury General Inquest makes hospital history. *Dimens Health Serv* 51:10–12, 1974.

57. DeVore DT: How to check for proper installation of anesthetic equipment. *J Oral Surg* 35:955, 1977.

58. Anonymous: Emergency room mixup, deaths linked. *Am Med News* Aug 8, 1971, p 3.

59. Anonymous: Editorial. *Anaesthesia* 22:543–544, 1967.

60. Anonymous: Old-style Chemetron central gas outlets. *Health Devices* 10,9:222–223, 1981.

61. Anonymous: The Westminster inquiry. *Lancet* 2:175–176, 1977.

62. Cundy JM: A safety feature for piped gas supplies. *Anaesthesia* 31:109–110, 1976.

63. Davis PD, Shaw A: Anaesthetic machine safety. *Lancet* 2:357–358, 1977.

64. McCormick JM: National fire protection codes—1968. *Anesth Analg* 47:538–547, 1968.

65. Robinson JS: A continuing saga of piped medical gas supply. *Anaesthesia* 34:66–70, 1979.

66. Spurring PW, Shenolikar BK: Hazards in anaesthetic equipment. *Br J Anaesth* 50:641–645, 1978.

67. Hunter AR: Pipe-line accident. *Br J Anaesth* 49:281–282, 1977.

68. Anonymous: Nitrous-oxide asphyxia. *Lancet* 1:848, 1974.

69. Wolff JDP, Lionarons HB, Mesdag MJ: A failure of the pin-index system of anesthetic gas tube connections. *Arch Chir Neerl* XXII-IV, 1970.

70. Lane GA: Medical gas outlets—a hazard from interchangeable "quick connect" couplers. *Anesthesiology* 52:86–87, 1980.

71. Klein SL, Lilburn JK: An unusual case of hypercarbia during general anesthesia. *Anesthesiology* 53:248–250, 1980.

72. Bageant RA, Hoyt JW, Epstein RM: Error in a pipeline gas concentration. An unanticipated consequence of a defective check valve. *Anesthesiology* 54:166–169, 1981.

73. Ziecheck HD: Faulty ventilator check valves cause pipeline gas contamination. *Resp Care* 26:1009–1010, 1981.

74. Rendell-Baker L: Problems with anesthetic gas machines and their solutions. In *Problems with Anesthetic and Respiratory Therapy Equipment.* Boston, Little Brown, 1982.

75. Kalra AN, Doughty AG: The wrong gas (correspondence). *Anaesthesia* 18:234–236, 1963.

76. Hogg CE: Pin-indexing failures. *Anesthesiology* 38:85–87, 1973.

77. MacMillan RR, Marshall MA: Failure of the pin index system on a Cape Waine ventilator. *Anaesthesia* 36:334–335, 1981.

78. Mead P: Hazard with cylinder yoke. *Anaesth Intensive Care* 9:79–80, 1981.

79. Youatt G, Love J: A funny yoke. Tale of a unscrewed pin. *Anaesth Intensive Care* 9:178, 1981.

80. Saposnick AB: Maintenance and repair of gas, humidity, and aerosol equipment. *Resp Care* 20:938–941, 1975.

81. Steward DJ, Sloan IA: Additional pin-indexing failures. *Anesthesiology* 39:355, 1973.

82. Rawstron RE, McNeill TD: Pin index system. *Br J Anaesth* 34:591–592, 1962.

83. Anonymous: Oxygen deprivation alleged in $2.5 million negligence suit. *Biomed Safety Standards* 11:53, 1981.

84. Brown FN, Hilton JHB: Inadvertence in anaesthesia leading to disaster. Seventy-Sixth Annual Report, Canadian Medical Protective Association, 1977. In Wyant GM: *Mechanical Misadventures in Anaesthesia.* Toronto, University of Toronto Press, 1978, pp 15–18.

85. McGarry PMF: Anaesthetic machine standard. *Can Anaesth Soc J* 25:436, 1978.

86. Wear JO: Documentation for preventive maintenance. AAMI 13th Annual Meeting, Washington, D.C., March 28–April 1, 1978, p 289.

87. Wyant GM: Some dangers in anaesthesia. *Can Anaesth Soc J* 25:71–72, 1978.

88. Rendell-Baker L: Some gas machine hazards and their elimination. *Anesth Analg* 55:26–33, 1976.

89. Calverley RK: A safety feature for anaesthetic machines—touch identification of oxygen flow control. *Can Anaesth Soc J* 18:225–229, 1971.

90. Linton RAF, Foster CA, Spencer GT: A potential hazard of oxygen flowmeters. *Anaesthesia* 37:606–607, 1982.

91. Malone BT: Failure of a new system to prevent delivery of hypoxic gas mixture. *Anesthesiology* 54:436–437, 1981.

92. Rendell-Baker L: Audience participation. *Anesth Analg* 51:792, 1972.

93. Mazze RI: Therapeutic misadventures with oxygen delivery systems: the need for continuous in-line oxygen monitors. *Anesth Analg* 51:787–792, 1972.

94. Cooper JB, Newbower RS: The anesthesia machine—an accident waiting to happen. In Pickett and Triggs (eds): *Proceedings of the NATO Symposium on Human Factors in Health Care*, Lisbon, 1974. Lexington, Mass., Lexington Books, 1975, pp 345–358.

95. Liew PC, Ganendran A: Oxygen failure: A potential danger with air-flowmeters in anesthetic machines with controlled needle valves. *Br J Anaesth* 45:1165–1168, 1973.

96. Powell J: Leak from an oxygen flow meter. *Br J Anaesth* 53:671, 1981.

97. Chung DC, Jing QC, Prins L, Strupat J: Hypoxic gas mixtures delivered by anaesthetic machines equipped with a downstream oxygen flowmeter. *Can Anaesth Soc J* 27:527–530, 1980.

98. Edwards G, Morton HJV, Park ER, Wylie WD: Deaths associated with anaesthesia. *Anaesthesia* 11:194–220, 1956.

99. Chang JL, Larson CE, Bedger RC, Bleyaert AL: An unusual malfunction of an anesthetic machine. *Anesthesiology* 52:446–447, 1980.

100. Rendell-Baker L: Anesthetic accident caused by unusual leakage of rotameter. *Br J Anaesth* 48:500, 1976.

101. Eger EI, Hylton RR, Irwin RH, Guadagni N: Anesthetic flowmeter sequence—a cause for hypoxia. *Anesthesiology* 24:396–397, 1963.

102. Liew RPC: Oxygen loss down the third flowmeter. *Anaesthesia* 28:579, 1973.

103. Katz D: Recurring cyanosis of intermittent mechanical origin in anesthetized patients. *Anesth Analg* 47:233–237, 1968.

104. Bishop C, Levick CH, Hodbson C: A design fault in the Boyle apparatus. *Br J Anaesth* 39:908, 1967.

105. Gupta BL, Varshneya AK: Anaesthetic accident caused by unusual leakage of rotameter. *Br J Anaesth* 47:805, 1975.

106. Sadov MS, Thomason RD, Thomason CL, Ries M: An evaluation of flowmeters. *J Am Assoc Nurse Anesthetists* 44:162–165, 1976.

107. Saunders RJ, Calkins JM, Gooden TM: Accuracy in rotameters and linear flowmeters. *Anesthesiology* 55:A116, 1981.

108. Waaben J, Stokke DB, Brinklov MM: Accuracy of gas flowmeters determined by the bubble meter method. *Br J Anaesth* 50:1251–1256, 1978.

109. Waaben J, Brinklov MM, Stokke DB: Accuracy of new gas flowmeters. *Br J Anaesth* 52:97–100, 1980.

110. Mazzia VDB, Mark LC, Binder LS, Crawford EJ, Gade H, Henry EL, Marx G, Schrier RI: Oxygen and the anesthesia machine. *NY State J Med* 62:2845–2846, 1962.

111. Bracken A: Deposits in cyclopropane flowmeter tubes. *Br J Anaesth* 48:52, 1976.

112. Battig CG: Unusual failure of an oxygen flowmeter. *Anesthesiology* 37:561–562, 1972.

113. Clutton-Brock J: Static electricity and rotameters. *Br J Anaesth* 44:86–90, 1972.

114. Clutton-Brock J: Static electricity and rotameters. *Br J Anaesth* 45:304, 1973.

115. Dobb G: Electrical conductivity of flowmeter tubes. *Br J Anaesth* 50:1270, 1978.

116. Greenbaum R, Hesse GE: Electrical conductivity of flowmeter tubes. *Br J Anaesth* 50:408, 1978.

117. Hagelsten J, Larsen OS: Static electricity in anaesthetic flowmeters eliminated by radioactive pistol. *Br J Anaesth* 37:799–800, 1965.

118. Hagelsten JO, Larsen OS: Inaccuracy of anaesthetic flowmeters caused by static electricity. *Br J Anaesth* 37:637–641, 1965.

119. Hodge EA: Accuracy of anaesthetic gas flowmeters. *Br J Anaesth* 51:907, 1979.

120. Kelley JM, Gabel RA: The improperly calibrated flowmeter—another hazard. *Anesthesiology* 33:467–468, 1970.

121. Chadwick DA: Transposition of rotameter tubes. *Anesthesiology* 40:102, 1974.

122. Walts LF, Inglove H: Malfunction of a new anesthetic machine. *Anesthesiology* 25:867, 1964.

123. Slater EM: Transposition of rotameter bobbins. *Anesthesiology* 41:101, 1974.

124. Horn B: Correspondence. *Anesth Analg* 43:150–151, 1964.

125. Nagel EL: Equipment hazards in anesthesia. In Saidman LJ, Moya F (eds): *Complications of Anesthesia*. Springfield, Ill., Charles C Thomas, 1970, pp 266–281.

126. Liston AJ: Coaxial breathing circuits. Medical Devices Alert, No. 40, October 1, 1981. Health Protection Branch, Health and Welfare, Canada.

127. Waters DJ: Factors causing awareness during surgery. *Br J Anaesth* 40:259–264, 1968.

128. Sykes MK: Rebreathing circuits. *Br J Anaesth* 40:666–674, 1968.

129. Mulroy M, Ham J, Eger EI: Inflowing gas leak,

a potential source of hypoxia. *Anesthesiology* 45:102–104, 1976.

130. Capan L, Ramanathan S, Chalon J, O'Meara JB, Turndorf H: A possible hazard with use of the Ohio Ethrane vaporizer. *Anesth Analg* 59:65–68, 1980.

131. Comm G, Rendell-Baker L: Back pressure check valves a hazard. *Anesthesiology* 56:327–328, 1982.

132. Dyer ED, Maxwell JG, Peterson DE, Mitchell CR: Disposable fiberglass filter to counter bacterial contamination of intermittent positive pressure breathing equipment. *Anesth Analg* 49:140–147, 1970.

133. Bracken A, Sanderson DM: Some observations on anaesthetic soda lime. *Br J Anaesth* 27:422–427, 1955.

134. Brown ES, Elam JO: Practical aspects of carbon dioxide absorption. *NY State J Med* 23:3436–3442, 1955.

135. Elam JO: Channeling and overpacking in carbon dioxide absorbers. *Anesthesiology* 19:403–404, 1958.

136. Barasch ST, Booth S, Modell J: Hypercapnia during cyclopropane anesthesia: a case report. *Anesth Analg* 55:439–441, 1976.

137. Detmer MD, Chandra P, Cohen PJ: Occurrence of hypercarbia due to an unusual failure of anesthetic equipment. *Anesthesiology* 52:278–279, 1980.

138. Owen SB: Defective carbon dioxide absorption in anesthetic machine. *Anesthesiology* 17:829–830, 1956.

139. Whitten MP, Wise CC: Design faults in commonly used carbon dioxide absorbers. *Br J Anaesth* 44:535–537, 1972.

140. Esplen JR: A device giving warning of impending failure of the nitrous oxide or oxygen supply. *Br J Anaesth* 28:226–227, 1956.

141. Trubuhovich RV: Carbon dioxide cylinders on anaesthetic machines. *Br J Anaesth* 39:607–608, 1967.

142. Prys-Roberts C, Smith WDA, Nunn JF: Accidental severe hypercapnia during anaesthesia. *Br J Anaesth* 39:257–267, 1967.

143. Ross EDT: Accidental hypercapnia and rotameter bobbins. *Br J Anaesth* 40:45, 1968.

144. Dinnick DP: Accidental severe hypercapnia during anaesthesia. *Br J Anaesth* 40:36–45, 1968.

145. Orton RH: Carbon dioxide accumulation. *Anaesthesia* 7:211–216, 1952.

146. Kerr JH, Evers JL: Carbon dioxide accumulation: Valve leaks and inadequate absorption. *Can Anaesth Soc J* 5:154–160, 1958.

147. Schultz EA, Buckley JJ, Oswald AJ, VanBergen FH: Profound acidosis in an anesthetized human: report of a case. *Anesthesiology* 21:285–291, 1960.

148. Schweitzer SA, Babarczy AJ: An unexpected hazard of the Boyles machine. *Anaesth Intensive Care* 4:72–73, 1976.

149. Fogdall RP: Exacerbation of iatrogenic hypercarbia by PEEP. *Anesthesiology* 51:173–175, 1979.

150. Smith RH, Volpitto PP: Volume ventilation valve. *Anesthesiology* 20:885–886, 1959.

151. Loehning RW, Davis G, Safar P: Rebreathing with "nonrebreathing" valves. *Anesthesiology* 25:854–856, 1964.

152. Wisborg K, Jacobsen E: Functional disorders of Ruben and Ambu-E valves after dismantling and cleaning. *Anesthesiology* 42:633–634, 1975.

153. Mullin RA: Letter to the Editor. *Can Anaesth Soc J* 25:248–249, 1978.

154. Dunn AJ: Empty tanks and Bain circuits. *Can Anaesth Soc J* 25:337, 1978.

155. Nimocks JA, Modell JH, Perry PA: Carbon dioxide retention using a humidified "nonrebreathing" system. *Anesth Analg* 54:271–273, 1975.

156. Anonymous: Hazard with "Bains" type circuits. *Anaesth Equip Technol* Nov 1976, page 7.

157. Sugg BR: Misuse of co-axial circuits. *Anaesthesia* 32:293–294, 1977.

158. Salt R: A test for co-axial circuits. *Anaesthesia* 32:675–676, 1977.

159. Seed RF: A test for co-axial circuits. *Anaesthesia* 32:676–677, 1977.

160. Breen M: Letters to the Editor. *Can Anaesth Soc J* 22:247, 1975.

161. Hannallah R, Rosales JK: A hazard connected with re-use of the Bain's circuit: a case report. *Can Anaesth Soc J* 21:511–513, 1974.

162. Naqvi NH: Torsion of inner tube. *Br J Anaesth* 53:193, 1981.

163. Peterson WC: Bain circuit. *Can Anaesth Soc J* 25:532, 1978.

164. Mansell WH: Bain circuit: "The hazard of the hidden tube." *Can Anaesth Soc J* 23:227, 1976.

165. Fukunaga AF: Torsion and disconnection of inner tube of coaxial breathing circuit. *Br J Anaesth* 53:1106–1107, 1981.

166. Inglis MS: Torsion of the inner tube. *Br J Anaesth* 52:705, 1980.

167. Wildsmith JAW, Grubb DJ: Defective and misused co-axial circuits. *Anaesthesia* 32:293, 1977.

168. Paterson JG, Vanhooydonk V: A hazard associated with improper connection of the Bain breathing circuit. *Can Anaesth Soc J* 22:373–377, 1975.

169. Cundy J, Baldock GJ: Safety check procedures to eliminate faults in anaesthetic machines. *Anaesthesia* 37:161–169, 1982.

170. Waters DJ: Use and misuse of a pressure-limiting bag. *Anaesthesia* 22:322–325, 1967.

171. Newbower RS, Cooper JB, Long CD: Failure analysis—the human element. In Gravenstine JS, Newbower RS, Rean AK, Smith NT (eds): *Essential Noninvasive Monitoring in Anesthesia.* New York, Grune & Stratton, 1980, pp 269–281.

172. Cote CJ, Ryan JF, Wood JB, Robinson MA, Vacanti FX, Welch JP: Wasted ventilation with eight anesthetic circuits used on children. *Anesthesiology* 55:A334, 1981.

173. Grundy EM, Bennett EJ, Brennan T: Obstructed anesthetic circuits. *Anesthesiol Rev* 3:35–36, 1976.

174. Poulton TJ: Potentially fatal complication with a T-adapter. *Crit Care Med* 7:324–325, 1979.

175. Mushin WW, Rendell-Baker L, Thompson PW, Mapleson WW: *Automatic Ventilation of the Lungs,* ed 3. Oxford, Blackwell Scientific Publications, 1980.

176. Verheecke G, Gilbertson A: Compliance of the tubing compartment of lung ventilators. *Intensive Care Med* 7:309–310, 1981.

177. Clinical Anesthesia Conference: Semiclosed anesthesia. *NY State J Med* 63:2124–2125, 1963.
178. Eldrup-Jorgensen S, Sprissler GT: Gas leaks in anesthesia machines. *Anesthesiology* 46:439, 1977.
179. Dolan PF: Vaporizer leak. *Anesthesiology* 49:302, 1978.
180. Anonymous: Medical equipemnt alert: gas leaks in anesthesia machine circuitry. *Items Topics*, April, 1973, p 8.
181. Rosenberg M, Solod E, Bourke DL: Gas leak through a Fluotec Mark III vaporizer. *Anesth Analg* 58:239–240, 1979.
182. Childres WF: Malfunction of Ohio Modulus anesthesia machine. *Anesthesiology* 56:330, 1982.
183. Dedrick DF, Mieras CD: Hazard associated with new Foretrend anesthesia machine. *Anesthesiology* 51:483, 1979.
184. Cottrell JE, Bernhard W, Turndorf H: Hazards of disposable rebreathing circuits. *Anesth Analg* 55:743–744, 1976.
185. Cottrell JE, Chalon J, Turndorf H: Faulty anesthesia circuits: a source of environmental pollution in the operating room. *Anesth Analg* 56:359–362, 1977.
186. Carden E: A new pressure relief (safety) valve. *Anaesthesia* 25:411–417, 1970.
187. Anonymous: Pediatric anesthesia circuit from Bard: limited recall in progress. *Biomed Safety Standards* 11:86, 1981.
188. Mantia AM: Faulty Y-piece. *Anesth Analg* 60:121–122, 1981.
189. Stevenson PH, McLeskey CH: Breakage of a reservoir bag mount, an unusual anesthesia machine failure. *Anesthesiology* 53:270–271, 1980.
190. Higgs BD, Garrett CP: A possible hazard with the Manley ventilator. *Anaesthesia* 34:680–681, 1979.
191. Freeman MF: A hazard of the East Radcliffe respirator. *Anaesthesia* 30:825–826, 1975.
192. Rolbin S: An unusual cause of ventilator leak. *Can Anaesth Soc J* 24:522–524, 1977.
193. Wolf S, Watson CB, Clark P: An unusual cause of leakage in an anesthesia system. *Anesthesiology* 55:83–84, 1981.
194. Warren PR, Gintautas J: Problems with Dupaco ventilator valve assembly. *Anesthesiology* 53:524–525, 1980.
195. Cooper JB: Prevention of ventilator hazards. *Anesthesiology* 48:299–300, 1978.
196. Ciobanu M, Meyer JA: Ventilator hazard revealed. *Anesthesiology* 52:186–187, 1980.
197. Sarnquist FH, Demas K: The silent ventilator. *Anesth Analg* 61:713–714, 1982.
198. Simionescu R: Sticking valve on East-Radcliffe ventilator. *Br J Anaesth* 43:1065, 1971.
199. Jorgensen S: An expired gas collection and disposal system. *Br J Anaesth* 48:502–503, 1976.
200. Longmuir J, Craig DB: Misadventure with a Boyle's gas machine. *Can Anaesth Soc J* 23:671–673, 1976.
201. Dolan PF: Connections from anesthetic machine to circle system unsatisfactory. *Anesthesiology* 51:277, 1979.
202. Haley FC: Letters to the Editor. *Can Anaesth Soc J* 22:628–629, 1975.
203. Utting JE, Gray TC, Shelley FC: Human misadventure in anaesthesia. *Can Anaesth Soc J* 26:472–478, 1979.
204. Condon HA: An antidisconnexion device. *Anaesthesia* 37:103–104, 1982.
205. Dolan PF: A simple safety device. *Br J Anaesth* 48:499, 1976.
206. Gilston A: Safety clip for Tunstall paediatric connections. *Anaesthesia* 35:1119, 1980.
207. Knell PJW: Accidental disconnection of anaesthetic breathing systems. *Anaesthesia* 35:825–826, 1980.
208. Malloy WF, Poznak AV, Artusio JF: Safety clip for endotracheal tubes. *Anesthesiology* 50:353–354, 1979.
209. Pogulanik J: An easily contrived device for preventing disconnection. *Anaesthesia* 35:826–827, 1980.
210. Star EG: A simple safety device. *Br J Anaesth* 47:1034, 1975.
211. Dinnick OP: Reducing the hazard of disconnected tubes. *Anaesthesia* 32:922, 1977.
212. Morrison AB: Failure to detect anaesthetic circuit disconnections. Medical Devices Alert, Health and Welfare, Canada, Health Protection Branch, January 15, 1981.
213. Cobcroft MD: More misconnected Boyle circuit tubings. *Anaesth Intensive Care* 6:170–171, 1978.
214. Baraka A: Misconnection of Boyle circuit tubings. *Anaesth Intensive Care* 3:260–261, 1975.
215. Cozanitis DA, Takkunen O: Aneurysm of ventilator tubing. A warning. *Anaesthesia* 26:235–236, 1971.
216. Feingold A: Carbon dioxide absorber packaging hazard. *Anesthesiology* 45:260, 1976.
217. Abramowitz M, McGill WA: Hazard of an anesthetic scavenging device. *Anesthesiology* 51:276, 1979.
218. Morr ZF, Stein ED, Orkin LR: A possible hazard in the use of a scavenging system. *Anesthesiology* 47:302–303, 1977.
219. Mostafa SM, Sutciffe AJ: Antipollution expiratory valves. A potential hazard. *Anaesthesia* 37:468–469, 1982.
220. Patel KD, Dalal FY: A potential hazard of the Drager scavenging interface system for wall suction. *Anesth Analg* 58:327–328, 1979.
221. Sharrock ME, Leith DE: Potential pulmonary barotrauma when venting anesthetic gases to suction. *Anesthesiology* 46:152–154, 1977.
222. Stirt JA, Lewenstein LN: Circle system failure induced by gastric suction. *Anaesth Intensive Care* 9:161–162, 1981.
223. Anonymous: Tubing connector kit or ventilator alarm involved in class I recall by Puritan-Bennett. *Biomed Safety Standards* 12:98–99, 1982.
224. Anonymous: Canadian government issues alert on Monaghan/Hospal 703 ventilator alarm. *Biomed Safety Standards* 10:135, 1980.
225. Anonymous: Hazard: Bunn Model 65 ventilation alarm. *Technol Anesth* 2:1, 1981.
226. Anonymous: Breathing circuit alarms. Health Devices Alert, vol. 4, No. 22, Nov 21, 1980. p 1.
227. Mazza N, Wald A: Failure of battery-operated alarms. *Anesthesiology* 53:246–248, 1980.
228. McEwen JA, Small CF, Saunders BA, Jenkins

LC: Hazards associated with the use of disconnect monitors. *Anesthesiology* 53:S391, 1980.

229. Lahay WD: Defective pressure/flow alarm. *Can Anaesth Soc J* 29:404–405, 1982.

230. Morrison AB: Failure to detect anesthetic circuit disconnections: Canadian "Medical Devices Alert" issued by HPB. *Biomed Safety Standards* 11:28, 1981.

231. Anonymous: Anesthesia ventilators. *Health Devices* 8:151–164, 1979.

232. Baraka A, Muallem M: Awareness during anaesthesia due to a ventilator malfunction. *Anaesthesia* 34:678–679, 1979.

233. Longmuir J, Craig DB: Inadvertent increase in inspired oxygen concentration due to defect in ventilator bellows. *Can Anaesth Soc J* 23:327–329, 1976.

234. Waterman PM, Pautler S, Smith RB: Accidental ventilator-induced hyperventilation. *Anesthesiology* 48:141, 1978.

235. Love JB: Misassembly of a Campbell ventilator causing leakage of the driving gas to a patient. *Anaesth Intensive Care* 8:376–377, 1980.

236. Jones CS: Gas viscosity effects in anesthesia. *Anesth Analg* 59:192–196, 1980.

237. Newton NI: Safety in the operating theatre: the meaning of excessive airway pressure. *Br J Hosp Med* 25:504–509, 1981.

238. Newton NI, Adams AQ: Excessive airway pressure during anesthesia. *Anaesthesia* 33:689–699, 1978.

239. Dogu TS, Davis HS: Hazards of inadvertently opposed valves. *Anesthesiology* 33:122–123, 1970.

240. Tate N: Excessive airway pressure during anaesthesia. *Anaesthesia* 34:212, 1979.

241. Thompson PW: Prevention of the hazard of excessive airway pressure. *Anaesthesia* 34:593, 1979.

242. Davenport HT, Keenleyside HB: Interstitial emphysema and pneumothorax associated with the use of a modified non-rebreathing valve. *Can Anaesth Soc J* 4:126–130, 1957.

243. Ringrose NH: Design of the Boyle Absorber. *Anaesth Intensive Care* 2:269–271, 1974.

244. Feeley TW, McClelland KJ, Malhotra IV: The hazards of bulk oxygen delivery systems. *Lancet* 1:1416–1418, 1975.

245. Anderson CE, Rendell-Baker L: Exposed O_2 flush hazard. *Anesthesiology* 56:328, 1982.

246. *American National Standard for Anesthesia Gas Pollution Control.* A79.11,1982, American National Standards Institute, 1430 Broadway, New York, NY, 10018.

247. Collis JM, Bethune DW, Tobias MA: Miniature ventilators: an assessment. *Anesthesiology* 24:81–89, 1969.

248. Anonymous: Ventilation alarms. *Health Devices* 10:204–220, 1981.

249. Escobar A, Aldrete JA: Bacterial filters for anesthesia apparatus. Review and case report. *Anesthesiol Rev* 4:25A–25B, 1977.

250. Loeser EA: Water-induced resistance in disposable respiratory-circuit bacterial filters. *Anesth Analg* 57:269–271, 1978.

251. Anonymous: Ventilator breathing circuits. *Health Devices Alerts* 5:2, 1981.

252. Mason J, Tackley R: An acute rise in expiratory resistance due to a blocked ventilator filter. *Anaesthesia* 36:335, 1981.

253. Gartrell P: Design of Boyle absorber. *Anaesth Intensive Care* 3:160–161, 1975.

254. Morrow DH, Dixon WM, Townley NT, Hebert CL: A safety modification of the Air-Shields ventimeter ventilator. *Anesthesiology* 26:361–362, 1965.

255. Norry HT: A pressure limiting valve for anaesthetic and respirator circuits. *Can Anaesth Soc J* 19:583–588, 1972.

256. Sears BE, Bocar ND: Pneumothorax resulting from a closed anesthesia ventilator port. *Anesthesiology* 47:311–313, 1977.

257. Sellery GR: Hazards of artificial ventilation in the operating room. *Can Med Assoc J* 107:421–423, 1972.

258. Turndorf H, Capan L, Kessel JW: Prevention of misconnection of the Air-Shields ventimeter-ventilator. *Anesth Analg* 53:342–343, 1974.

259. Taylor C, Stoelting VK: A modified Ayre's T-tube technic—anesthesia for cleft lip and palate surgery. *Anesth Analg* 42:55–62, 1963.

260. Lynch CGM: The tail of a bag: a hazard. *Anaesthesia* 31:803–804, 1976.

261. Arens JF: A hazard in the use of an Ayre T-piece. *Anesth Analg* 50:943–946, 1971.

262. Flowerdew RMM: A hazard of scavenger port design. *Can Anaesth Soc J* 28:481–483, 1981.

263. Mann ES, Sprague DH: An easily overlooked malassembly. *Anesthesiology* 56:413–414, 1982.

264. Tavakoli M, Habeeb A: Two hazards of gas scavenging. *Anaesth Analg* 57:286–287, 1978.

265. Milliken RA: Safe anesthetic gas pollution control. *Anesthesiology* 57:543, 1982.

266. Anonymous: Disk misplacement in anesthesia exhalation check valve. *Technol Anesth* 34:1–2, 1982.

267. Dean HN, Parsons DE, Raphaely RC: Case report: bilateral tension pneumothorax from mechanical failure of anesthesia machine due to misplaced expiratory valve. *Anesth Analg* 50:195–198, 1971.

268. Dinnick OP: Hazards of respiratory circuits. *Ann R Coll Surg Engl* 52:349–354, 1973.

269. Duckett JE, Hice C, Smith TC: Hazard of a ruptured exhalation mushroom diaphragm. *Crit Care Med* 8:750–751, 1980.

270. Henzig D: Insidious PEEP from a defective ventilator gas evacuation outlet valve. *Anesthesiology* 57:251–252, 1982.

271. Sia RL: Accidental closure of the expiratory outlet in the Engstrom Ventilator (200) during anaesthesia. *Can Anaesth Soc J* 19:101–104, 1972.

272. Wrigley FRH: Letter to the Editor. *Can Anaesth Soc J* 21:434, 1974.

273. Davies G, Tarnawsky M: Letters to the Editor. *Can Anaesth Soc J* 23:228, 1976.

274. Mantia AM: Gas scavenging systems. *Anesth Analg* 61:162–164, 1982.

275. O'Conner DE, Daniels BW, Pfitzner J: Hazards of anaesthetic scavenging: case reports and brief review. *Anaesth Intensive Care* 10:15–19, 1982.

276. Hagerdal M, Lecky JH: Anesthetic death of an experimental animal related to a scavenging

system malfunction. *Anesthesiology* 47:522–523, 1977.

277. Malloy WF, Wrightman AE, O'Sullivan D, Goldiner PL: Bilateral pneumothorax from suction applied to a ventilator exhaust valve. *Anesth Analg* 58:147–149, 1979.

278. Rendell-Baker L: Hazard of blocked scavenging valve. *Can Anaesth Soc J* 29:182–183, 1982.

279. Potter GJ: Some clinical aspects of the nonrebreathing valve. *Anesth Analg* 38:114–117, 1959.

280. Holland R: Special committee investigating deaths under anaesthesia: memorandum on the dangers of non-rebreathing valves. *Med J Aust* 2:46–47, 1970.

281. Dolan PF, Shapiro S, Steinbach RB: Valve misassembly—manually operated resuscitation bag. *Anesth Analg* 60:66–67, 1981.

282. Anonymous: Hazard: Ambu Baby resuscitator. *Health Devices* 2:249, 1973.

283. Grogono AW, Porterfield J: Ambu valves: danger of wrong assembly. *Br J Anaesth* 42:978, 1970.

284. Kelly MP: Ventilation equipment. *Br Med J* 2:176, 1968.

285. Klick JM, Bushnell LS, Bancroft ML: Barotrauma, a potential hazard of manual resuscitators. *Anesthesiology* 49:363–365, 1978.

286. Pauca AL, Jenkins TE: Airway obstruction by breakdown of a non-rebreathing valve: how foolproof is foolproof? *Anesth Analg* 60:529–531, 1981.

287. Anonymous: Anaesthetic deaths in South Australia. *Med J Aust* 1:4, 1976.

288. Goddard PJ, Becket AJ: A simple safety valve for infant resuscitator and ventilator gas circuits. *Lancet* 2:584, 1971.

289. Wright BM: A safe expiratory valve for anaesthesia and artificial ventilation. *Lancet* 1:854–855, 1979.

290. Hirschman AM, Kravath RE: Venting vs ventilation. A danger of manual resuscitation bags. *Chest* 82:369–370, 1982.

291. Lee S: A new pop-off valve. *Anesthesiology* 25:240–242, 1964.

292. Maxwell DC, Grant GC: An inflating spill valve for controlled respiration in a semiclosed circuit. *Br J Anaesth* 32:616–618, 1960.

293. Rusz T, Duncalf D: A safe controlled pop-off valve. *Anesthesiology* 33:459–461, 1970.

294. Steen SN, Lee ASJ: Prevention of inadvertent excess pressure in closed systems. *Anesth Analg* 39:264–266, 1960.

295. Searle JB: Inflating valve. *Anaesthesia* 13:345–346, 1958.

296. Horn B: Valve for assisted or controlled ventilation. *Anesthesiology* 21:83, 1960.

297. Lee S: A universal valve for anaesthetic circuits. *Br J Anaesth* 36:318–321, 1964.

298. Lee S: A modified nonrebreathing system. *Anesthesiology* 25:238–239, 1964.

299. Linker GS, Holaday DA, Waltuck B: A simply constructed automatic pressure relief valve. *Anesthesiology* 32:563–564, 1970.

300. Lee ST: Volume controlled breathing. *Anesth Analg* 45:212–219, 1966.

301. Lee S: Exhalation tunnel for nonrebreathing techniques. *Anesthesiology* 25:716–717, 1964.

302. Lauria JI: Soda-lime dust contamination of breathing circuits. *Anesthesiology* 42:628–629, 1975.

303. Davis R: Soda lime dust. *Anaesth Intensive Care* 7:390, 1979.

304. Debban DG, Bedford RF: Overdistention of the rebreathing bag, a hazardous test for circle system integrity. *Anesthesiology* 42:365–366, 1975.

305. Amaranath L, Boutros AR: Circle absorber and soda lime contamination. *Anesth Analg* 59:711–712, 1980.

306. Ribak B: Reducing the soda lime hazard. *Anesthesiology* 43:277, 1975.

307. Eichhorn JH, Bancroft ML, Laasberg LH, du Moulin GC, Saubermann AJ: Contamination of medical gas and water pipelines in a new hospital building. *Anesthesiology* 46:286–289, 1977.

308. Tingay MG, Ilsley AH, Willis RJ, Thompson MJ, Chalmers AH, Cousins MJ: Gas identity hazards and major contamination of medical gas system of a new hospital. *Anaesth Intensive Care* 6:202–209, 1978.

309. Bushman JA, Clark PA: Oil mist hazard and piped air supplies. *Br Med J* 3:588–590, 1967.

310. Lackore LK, Perkins HM: Accidental narcosis. *JAMA* 211:1846, 1970.

311. Thompson PW: Safety of anaesthetic apparatus. *Int Anesthesiol Clin* 16,1:199–223, 1978.

312. Herlihy WJ: Report: Contamination of medical oxygen. *Anaesth Intensive Care* 1:240–241, 1973.

313. Austin TR: Metallic flaking: a further hazard of anaesthetic apparatus. *Anaesthesia* 27:92–93, 1972.

314. Anonymous: Ohio Medical Products recalls "old style" distal sensing tees. *Biomed Safety Standards* 10:27, 1980.

315. Gold MI: Defect in a T-fitting connection. *Anesthesiology* 52:184, 1980.

316. Sharp JH, Trudell JR, Cohen EN: Volatile metabolites and decomposition products of halothane in man. *Anesthesiology* 50:2–8, 1979.

317. Eger EI: Dragons and other scientific hazards (editorial). *Anesthesiology* 50:1, 1979.

318. Karis JH, O'Neal F, Weitzner SW: Alteration of halothane in heated humidifiers. *Anesth Analg* 59:518, 1980.

319. Middleton V, Poznak AV, Artusio AF, Smith SM: Carbon monoxide accumulation in closed circle anesthesia systems. *Anesthesiology* 26:715–719, 1965.

320. Morita S, Latta W, Hambro K, Snider MT: Accumulation of methane, acetone, and nitrogen in the inspired gas during closed circuit anesthesia. *Anesth Analg* 60:267–268, 1981.

321. Marx LC, Marx GF, Erlanger H, Joffe S, Kepes ER, Ravin MB: Improper filling of kettle-type vaporizers. *NY State J Med* 65:1151–1152, 1965.

322. Kopriva CJ, Lowenstein E: An anesthetic accident: cardiovascular collapse from liquid halothane delivery. *Anesthesiology* 30:246–247, 1969.

323. Rendell-Baker L, Milliken RA: Vaporizer overflow, a preventable hazard. *Anesthesiology* 50:478, 1979.

324. Sharrock NE, Gabel RA: Inadvertent anesthetic overdose obscured by scavenging. *Anesthesiology* 49:137–138, 1978.

325. Long GJ, Marsh HM: A danger—insecure positioning of anaesthetic vaporizers. *Med J Aust* 1:1108, 1969.

326. Munson WM: Cardiac arrest: a hazard of tipping a vaporizer. *Anesthesiology* 26:235, 1965.

327. Austin TR: A warning device for the 'Fluotec' Mark II and III. *Anaesthesia* 26:368, 1971.

328. Dorsch SE, Dorsch JA: Chemical cross-contamination between vaporizers in series. *Anesth Analg* 52:176–180, 1973.

329. Murray WJ, Zsigmond EK, Fleming P: Contamination of in-series vaporizers with halothane-methoxyflurane. *Anesthesiology* 38:487–490, 1973.

330. Wickett RE, Jenking LC, Root LS: Downstream contamination of in-series vapourizers. *Can Anaesth Soc J* 21:114–116, 1974.

331. Robinson JS, Thompson JM, Barratt RS: Inadvertent contamination of anaesthetic circuits with halothane. *Br J Anaesth* 49:745–753, 1977.

332. Lewis JJ, Hicks RG: Malfunction of vaporizers. *Anesthesiology* 27:324–325, 1966.

333. Noble WH: Accuracy of halothane vaporizers in clinical use. *Can Anaesth Soc J* 17:135–144, 1970.

334. Cook TL, Eger EI, Behl RS: Is your vaporizer off? *Anesth Analg* 56:793–800, 1977.

335. Ellis FR, Clarks IMC, Modgill EM, Appleyard TN, Dinsdale RCW: New causes of malignant hyperpyrexia. *Br Med J* 1:575, 1975.

336. Hunter L: Leaking halothane vaporizers. *Med J Aust* 2:716, 1974.

337. Greenhow DE, Barth RL: Oxygen flushing delivers anesthetic vapor—a hazard with a new machine. *Anesthesiology* 38:409–410, 1973.

338. Lowe HJ, Titel JH, Hagler KJ: Absorption of anesthetics by conductive rubber in breathing circuits. *Anesthesiology* 34:283–289, 1971.

339. Murray WJ, Fleming P: Patient exposure to halothane retained in anesthesia machine circuits. *Clin Pharmacol Ther* 13:148, 1972.

340. Samulksa HM, Ramaiah S, Noble WH: Unintended exposure to halothane in surgical patients: halothane washout studies. *Can Anaesth Soc J* 19:35–41, 1972.

341. Grodin WK, Epstein RA: Halothane adsorption by soda lime. *Anesthesiology* 51:S317, 1979.

342. Grodin WK, Epstein MAF, Epstein RA: Enflurane and isoflurane adsorption by soda lime. *Anesthesiology* 55:A124, 1981.

343. Grodin WK, Epstein RA: Halothane adsorption complicating the use of soda-lime to humidify anaesthetic gases. *Br J Anaesth* 54:555–559, 1982.

344. Dykes MHM, Chir B, Laasberg LH: Clinical implication of halothane contamination of the anesthetic circle. *Anesthesiology* 35:648–649, 1971.

345. Robinson JS, Thompson JM, Barratt RS, Belcher R, Stephen WI: Pertinence and precision in pollution measurements. *Br J Anaesth* 48:167–177, 1976.

346. Zimmerman BL, Lord J: Contamination of an anesthesia system with liquid halothane. *Anesthesiology* 52:512–513, 1980.

347. Karis JH, Menzel DB: Inadvertent change of volatile anesthetics in anesthesia machines. *Anesth Analg* 61:53–55, 1982.

348. Personal communication; Ronald J. Luich, Ohio Medical Products, a division of Airco, Inc.

349. Munson ES: Hazards of agent-specific vaporizers. *Anesthesiology* 34:393, 1971.

350. Anonymous: Editorial. *Can Anaesth Soc J* 22:123, 1975.

351. McBurney R: Letters to the Editor. *Can Anaesth Soc J* 24:417–418, 1977.

352. Klein SL, Camenzind T: Hazards of bottle adaptors for vaporizers. *Anesth Analg* 57:596–597, 1978.

353. Paull JD, Sleeman KW: An anaesthetic hazard. *Br J Anaesth* 43:1202, 1971.

354. Morris LE: Revell circulator and vapor concentration measurements. In Aldrete JA, Lowe HG, Virtue RW (eds): *Low Flow and Closed System Anesthesia*. New York, Grune & Stratton, 1979, pp 273–276.

355. Morgan M, Lumley J: Reliability of halothane vaporizers. *Anaesthesia* 23:440–445, 1968.

356. Hill DW: Halothane concentrations obtained with a Fluotec vaporizer. *Br J Anaesth* 30:563–567, 1958.

357. Murray WJ, Fleming P: Fluotec Mark 2 halothane output: nonlinearity from "Off" to 0.5 percent dial settings. *Anesthesiology* 36:180–181, 1972.

358. Adner M, Hallen B: Reliability of halothane vaporizers. *Acta Anaesth Scand* 9:233–239, 1965.

359. Bluth M, Gelb EJ, Steen SN: A new concept for the continuous monitoring of anesthetic gases. *Anesthesiology* 33:449–451, 1970.

360. Diaz PM: The influence of carrier gas on the output of automatic plenum vaporizers. *Br J Anaesth* 48:387–391, 1976.

361. Stoelting RK: The effect of nitrous oxide on halothane output from Fluotec Mark 2 vaporizers. *Anesthesiology* 35:215–218, 1971.

362. Latto IP: Administration of halothane in the 0–0.5% concentration range with the Fluotec Mark 2 and Mark 3 vaporizers. *Br J Anaesth* 45:563–569, 1973.

363. Paterson GM, Hulands GH, Nunn JF: Evaluation of a new halothane vaporizer: the Cyprane Fluotec Mark 3. *Br J Anaesth* 41:109–119, 1969.

364. DeGuzman CM, Cascorbi HF: An unusual hazard of methoxyflurane. *Anesthesiology* 36:305, 1972.

365. Larsen ER: Foaming in halogenated anaesthetics—the chemistry of modern inhalation anaesthetics. In Chenoweth MB (ed): *Modern Inhalation Anaesthetics*. New York, Springer-Verlag, 1972, p 29.

366. Sweatman F: Foaming of methoxyflurane contaminated with silicone. *Anesthesiology* 38:407, 1973.

367. Rendell-Baker L: Equipment standards in anesthesia practice: eliminating the hazards. *Clin Trends Anesthesiol* 7(No. 2): May–June, 1977.

368. Marks WE, Bullard JR: Another hazard of free-standing vaporizers, increased anesthetic concentration with reversed flow of vaporizing gas. *Anesthesiology* 45:445–446, 1976.

369. Wyant GM: Some dangers in anaesthesia. *Can Anaesth Soc J* 25:71–72, 1978.

370. Ricco MF: Urgent: medical device alert, February

13, 1976. Ohio Medical Products, 3030 Airco Drive, Madison Wis.

371. Sharrock NE, Gabel RA: Inadvertent anesthetic overdose obscured by scavenging. *Anesthesiology* 49:137–138, 1978.

372. Craig DB, Longmuir J: An unusual failure of an oxygen fail-safe device. *Can Anaesth Soc J* 18:576–577, 1971.

373. Anonymous: Internal leakage from anesthesia unit flush valves. *Health Devices* 10:172, 1981.

374. Morris LE: Problems in the performance of anesthesia vaporizers. *Int Anesthesiol Clin* 12:199–219, 1974.

375. Morris LE: Vaporizer malfunction. In Aldrete JA, Lowe HJ, Virtue RW (eds): *Low Flow and Closed System Anesthesia.* New York, Grune & Stratton, 1979.

376. Bookallil MJ: Entrainment of air during mechanical ventilation. *Br J Anaesth* 39:184, 1967.

377. Hillyer KW, Johnston RR: Unsuspected dilution of anesthetic gases detected by an oxygen analyzer. *Anesth Analg* 57:491–492, 1978.

378. Hough VJ: Prevention of ventilator accident. *Anesthesiology* 49:226–227, 1978.

379. Marsland AR, Solomos J: Ventilator malfunction detected by O₂ analyser. *Anaesth Intensive Care* 9:395, 1981.

380. Vickers MD: Fires and explosions. *Ann R Coll Surg Engl* 52:354–357, 1973.

381. Boyd CH: A fire in the mouth. *Anaesthesia* 24:441–445, 1969.

382. Perry LB, Gould AB Jr, Leonard PF: Discussion. *Anesth Analg* 54:153–154, 1975.

383. Perel A, Mahler Y, Davidson JT: Combustion of a nasal catheter carrying oxygen. *Anesthesiology* 45:666–667, 1976.

384. ASA Committee on Flammable Hazards and Electrical Equipment: A question of safety. ASA Newsletter, May, 1974.

385. Cameron BGD, Ingram GS: Flammability of drape materials in nitrous oxide and oxygen. *Anaesthesia* 26:281–288, 1971.

386. Neufeld GR: Physical hazards in the operating room. *Surg Clin North Am* 55:959–966, 1975.

387. Summers FW: Fire with nonflammable anesthetic agents. *Anesthesiology* 22:498–499, 1961.

388. Leonard PF: Correspondence. *Anesth Analg* 53:293–294, 1974.

389. Bergner R, Theis C: Case report—operating room fire. *Anesthesiology* 17:751, 1956.

390. Bruner JMR: Correspondence. *Anesth Analg* 53:290–293, 1974.

391. May TW: Explosion during halothane anesthesia. *Br Med J* 1:692–693, 1976.

392. Anonymous: Fires during surgery of the head and neck area. *Health Devices Alerts* 4:3–4, 1980.

393. Snow JC, Norton ML, Saluja TS, Estanislao AF: Fire hazard during CO₂ laser microsurgery on the larynx and trachea. *Anesth Analg* 55:146–147, 1976.

394. Goldman L: Questions and answers. *Anesth Analg* 55:652, 1976.

395. Anonymous: Case history number 82: "Nonflammable" fires in the operating room. *Anesth Analg* 54:152–154, 1975.

396. Bracken A, Wilton-Davies CC: Explosion risk in a non-flammable system. *Anaesthesia* 18:439–445, 1963.

397. Schettler WH: Correspondence. *Anesth Analg* 53:288–289, 1974.

398. Gupte SR: Gauze fire in the oral cavity: a case report. *Anesth Analg* 51:645–646, 1972.

399. Anonymous: Maker of surgical drape liable to burned patient. Am Med News, Oct 8, 1982, p 12.

400. Bruner JMR: Questions and answers. *Anesth Analg* 54:210–211, 1975.

401. Leonard PF: Questions and answers. *Anesth Analg* 54:210–211, 1975.

402. Walter CW: Questions and answers. *Anesth Analg* 54:211, 1975.

403. Walter CW: Anesthetic explosions: a continuing threat. *Anesthesiology* 25:505–514, 1964.

404. Nicholson MJ: Comments. *Anesth Analg* 51:646, 1972.

405. Plumlee JE: Operating-room flash fire from use of cautery after aerosol spray: a case report. *Anesth Analg* 52:202–203, 1973.

406. Shah SC, Savant NS: Correspondence. *Anesth Analg* 53:288, 1974.

407. Czajka RJ: Cylinder caution: open slowly to minimize recompression heat. *Anesthesiology* 49:226, 1978.

408. Dorsch SE: Fires in presence of non-flammable anesthetics. ASA Newsletter, July, 1977, pp 6–8.

CHAPTER 11

Face Masks and Airways

No skill is more important to the anesthesiologist than the ability to maintain an open airway and ventilate the patient. Masks and airways are therefore among the most important and frequently used pieces of equipment.

FACE MASKS

Purpose

The face mask enables the anesthesiologist to administer gases from the breathing system to the patient without introducing any apparatus into the trachea. Face masks are most often used when spontaneous or assisted ventilation is employed but may be used with controlled respiration if airway maintenance is adequate.

General Description

Face masks are constructed of rubber or of various types of plastic (1, 2). Transparent masks allow the anesthesiologist to observe for vomitus, secretions, blood, lip coloration and condensation of exhaled moisture. They may be better accepted by conscious patients.

A face mask consists of three parts: the body, the seal, and the connector.

THE BODY

This constitutes the main part of the mask. It gives structure to the mask and prevents it from collapsing. Frequently, it can be bent or molded to obtain a better fit or to reduce dead space.

THE SEAL

The seal (rim) is the part of the mask which comes in contact with the face. It may be detachable from but usually forms one piece with the body. It provides a means of preventing the escape of gas from between the mask and the face.

Two general types of seals are used. The more commonly used one consists of a cushion (rim pad). This is usually inflated with air but may be filled with materials which can be molded. The second type of seal is a rubber or plastic flange which is an extension of the body and is not inflated.

THE CONNECTOR

The connector, or orifice, is at the opposite end of the body from the seal and serves to connect the mask to the breathing system. It consists of a thickened fitting with an internal diameter of 22 mm. Often it has retaining hooks for attachment to a mask strap.

Equipment manufacturers have developed a wide variety of masks. Some are shown in Figures 11.1 through 11.9. Most are available in a variety of sizes. An assortment of different face masks should be kept readily available, since none will fit every face well.

The anatomical mask (Fig. 11.1) is the most frequently used mask for adults. The malleable body is made of a firm material and can be widened or narrowed to fit the face. It is offered in a variety of sizes from infant to large adult.

The Trimar mask (Fig. 11.2) is similar to the

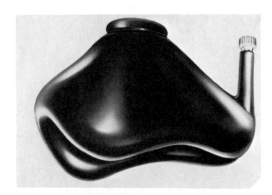

Figure 11.1. Anatomical mask (Connell mask, B.O.C., Form-It). (Courtesy of Ohio Medical Products, a division of Airco, Inc.)

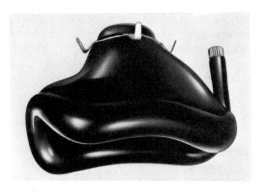

Figure 11.2. Trimar mask. (Courtesy of Ohio Medical Products, a division of Airco, Inc.)

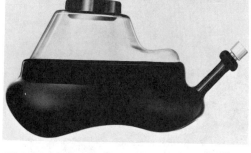

Figure 11.5. Ambu transparent mask. (Courtesy of Ambu International.)

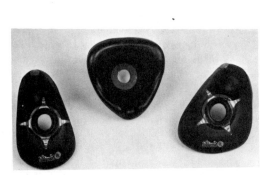

Figure 11.3. SCRAM (Selective Contour Retaining Anatomical Mask). (Courtesy of Ohio Medical Products, a division of Airco, Inc.)

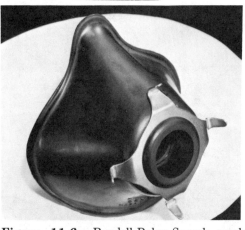

Figure 11.6. Rendell-Baker-Soucek mask. (Courtesy of Ohio Medical Products, a division of Airco, Inc.)

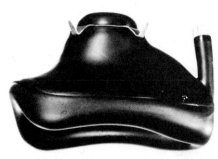

Figure 11.4. Bridgeless mask. (Courtesy of Ohio Medical Products, a division of Airco, Inc.)

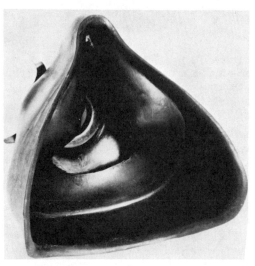

Figure 11.7. Flotex Antistatic face mask (Flotex multi-fitting face mask). (Courtesy of Harris-Lake, Inc.)

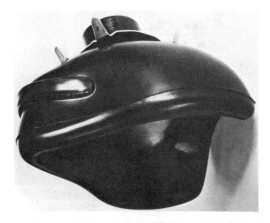

Figure 11.8. The Fleximask. (Courtesy of Harris-Lake, Inc.)

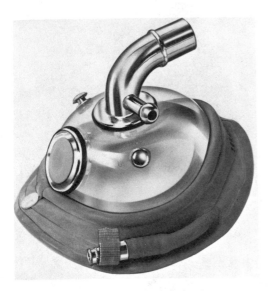

Figure 11.9. The Stephen-Slater non-rebreathing mask. (Courtesy of Air Products and Chemicals, Inc.)

anatomical mask but has a shallower body and less dead space.

The SCRAM (Selective Contour Retaining Anatomical Mask) (Fig. 11.3) is designed for difficult to fit patients. The seal is a cushion filled with plastic. The entire mask body and seal can be molded to any specific shape.

The bridgeless mask (Fig. 11.4) is designed for the face with flat features or little or no nose bridge. It has an air-filled cushion. The nose notch is eliminated. The body is shallow and the curvature of the seal is flatter than that on the anatomical mask.

The Ambu transparent mask (Fig. 11.5) is clear plastic, which allows the patient's nose and mouth to be seen. Clouding on the plastic surface indicates ventilation. The seal consists of a pneumatic cuff attached to the body. There is a thumb rest built into the body.

The Rendell-Baker-Soucek mask (Fig. 11.6) is designed to fit the pediatric patient. It is made of rubber or clear plastic. The body is not malleable. The mask fits the face well so that no special seal is necessary. The dead space is reported to be 4 cc in the size 1 and 8 cc in the size 2 when used with a divided mask adaptor (3).

The Flotex Antistatic face mask (Fig. 11.7) incorporates a rubber flange instead of a pneumatic cushion. The flange is extended so that it covers the chin and part of the cheeks. It is designed to be placed under the chin and conforms closely to facial contours (4).

The Fleximask (Fig. 11.8) is a one-piece molded conductive mask available in three sizes. It has a built-in malleable bridge to provide a close fit on all faces. In place of the conventional inflating pad, the mask incorporates a face flap.

The Stephen-Slater non-rebreathing mask (Fig. 11.9) (5), which is usually used for pediatric anesthesia, is a combination non-rebreathing valve and face mask. It has an inflatable cushion. There is an inhalation valve at the inlet to the mask. An exhalation flap is built into the side of the body. It is in such a position that the upper finger of the hand holding the jaw may close off the valve intermittently. Respiration can be assisted or controlled by closing the exhalation valve at the same time that the reservoir bag is squeezed.

Mask Fit

A good mask fit is essential for inhalation anesthesia and is not difficult with most patients, but can be a difficult and vexing problem. Considerable manual stength and dexterity are often necessary to achieve a leak-tight seal and at the same time maintain the jaw extended to prevent airway obstruction. A poor mask fit requires the anesthesiologist to maintain steady pressure. This may lead to cramped hands and tired forearms and limits his freedom to do other things. Failure to obtain a tight fit with spontaneous respirations will result in air dilution. This can be compensated for by increasing the fresh gas flow, but this is wasteful; moreover, the reservoir bag no longer serves as an adequate means of monitoring ventilation. With assisted or controlled respiration, a poor mask fit will not allow adequate positive pressure to be developed (6).

Mask fit is influenced by variables involving the mask, the patient's face and the anesthesiologist's technique of holding the mask.

MASK SELECTION

The best fit is obtained by selecting a mask and testing it before induction of anesthesia. The smallest mask that will do the job is the most desirable because it will cause the least increase in dead space and be easier to hold.

THE PATIENT'S FACE

The mask rests on the skin over the nasal and maxillary bones above and the mandible below (7). The buccinator muscle forms out the cheeks and helps to create a seal in the area between the maxilla and the mandible.

A variety of faces will be encountered in clinical practice. Infants' faces are fairly uniform in configuration, but considerable differentiation takes place in the progress to adult life and the difficulties of tailoring a mask to fit a fairly wide variety of faces—fat, emaciated, edentulous, those with prominent nares, burns, very flat noses, receding jaws, beards, or drainage tubes in the mouth or nose—increases.

The edentulous patient presents the most common problem. There is a loss of bone of the alveolar ridge, causing a loss of distance between the points where the mask rests on the mandible and nose. This loss of vertical dimensions of the face makes a gas-tight fit difficult. Inserting an oral airway will increase the distance by opening the mouth. Also in edentulous patients, the buccinator muscle loses its tone. The cheeks sag, allowing large gaps between them and the mask seal. Alveolar process resorption results in a shrinking of the corners of the mouth. Packing the cheek with gauze sponges may make up for the loss of bone structure and cheek tone (2). In some cases it may be desirable to leave the patient's dentures in place.

HOLDING THE MASK

There are several different methods of holding a mask to maintain an open airway and a tight seal. The method most commonly used is a one-hand grip using the left hand. Figure 11.10 illus-

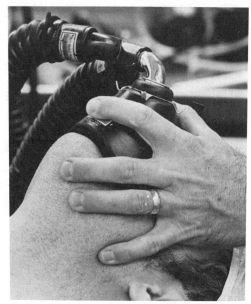

Figure 11.10. Holding the mask with one hand.

trates this method. The thumb and index finger are placed on the body of the mask on opposite sides of the connector. These fingers push downward to hold the mask to the face and prevent leaks. Additional downward pressure can be exerted by the anesthesiologist's chin on the top of the mask. The distal phalanges of the middle and ring fingers are placed on the ridge of the mandible. They pull the jaw backward and extend the neck. The fifth finger is placed under the angle of the jaw. It pulls upward on the jaw to displace the tongue forward, away from the pharynx. If an airway is in place, this action of the fifth finger may not be necessary.

A second method can be used to open any but the most difficult airways and obtain a tight fit. It is cumbersome in that it requires two hands to accomplish and a second person is necessary if assisted or controlled respiration is used. Figure 11.11 illustrates this method. Both thumbs are placed on the body of the mask on either side of the connector. The index finger is placed under the angle to the jaw. The jaw is pulled upward by the index fingers and the head is extended by both fingers. If a leak still occurs, downward pressure on the mask can be increased by using the anesthesiologist's chin.

In applying the mask, compression of the eyes and excessive pressure on the face must be avoided. If excessive pressure on the face must

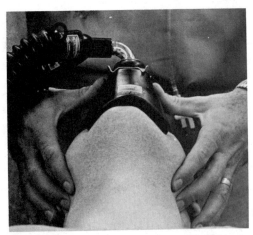

Figure 11.11. Holding the mask with two hands.

be exerted or there is extreme difficulty in maintaining an airway, endotracheal intubation should be considered. Anterior displacement of the jaw can exert pressure on the lingual and chorda tympani nerves (8). This can result in loss of taste and numbness of the tongue.

Dead Space

In any apparatus involving their use, the face mask and its adaptor contribute the major proportion of increased dead space, provided the fresh gas flow is adequate (9). This is of greatest significance in small patients where the increase in dead space in relationship to tidal volume is greatest. Added mechanical dead space will lead to a fall in alveolar ventilation, so it should be kept to a minimum.

The dead space of various masks varies considerably (9, 10). Masks with a pneumatic cushion have the greatest dead space, whereas those such as the molded Rendell-Baker-Soucek tend to have the least. Dead space may be decreased by increasing the pressure on the mask, decreasing the volume of the cushion, or using a smaller mask.

The entire volume of the face mask may not constitute dead space. Clarke (10) suggests channeling of air currents may reduce the actual dead space.

A variety of methods and devices has been designed to wash out the volume of the mask (11–14). Most utilize an adaptor with separation of the inspiratory and expiratory channels or have a means whereby a jet of fresh gas is blown into the mask.

Mask Straps (Inhaler Retainer, Head Strap, Mask Harness, Mask Retainer, Headband, Head-Restraining Strap)

Mask straps serve to hold the mask firmly to the face. A typical mask strap consists of thin rubber strips arranged as a circle with four projections, two on either side. The head rests in the circle and the straps attach around the connector of the mask. Special mask straps have been designed (15–22). Some have combined mask straps and tubing or chin supports.

The straps at the jaw may pull it backward, tending to obstruct the airway. Crossing the two lower straps under the chin may result in a better fit and counteract the pull of the upper straps so that there is less tendency for the mask to creep up above the bridge of the nose (15).

Care must be taken not to draw the straps too tight because they can be a source of pressure damage either by themselves or by the mask (7, 23–25). The straps should be kept as loose as possible and released periodically.

Another danger of mask straps is that should vomiting or regurgitation occur, it takes a longer time to remove the mask.

Complications

CONTACT DERMATITIS

Chemical or gas sterilization can leave a residue which can cause a dermatitis after contact with the skin (26–29). An allergic dermatitis may result in the patient who is allergic to the material from which the mask is formed (29–31). The pattern of the dermatitis follows the area of contact between the mask and skin.

PRESSURE

When a face mask is applied, the pressure of the seal and straps against the skin will be transmitted to underlying structures.

Excessive pressure must be avoided because it may cause injury to branches of the trigeminal or facial nerves (7). Pressure on the medial angles of the eyes and supraorbital margins may result in edema of the eyelids, chemosis of the conjunctiva, pressure on the supraorbital and supratrochlear nerves, corneal injury and possibly temporary blindness due to acutely increased intraocular pressure (15).

Proper mask fit should be attained by proper mask selection and not by forceful application. The mask should be removed from the face occasionally and readjusted to make certain that sustained pressure is not applied to one area of the face.

VOMITING AND ASPIRATION

Assisting or controlling respiration with a mask may allow air to enter the stomach. This increases the chances of regurgitation and aspiration. This may be more easily noticed by using a clear mask. Vomitus cannot readily escape from a tight-fitting mask.

AIRWAYS

Purpose

Maintenance of a patent airway is a basic principle in administration of general anesthesia. It is unnecessary to enumerate the serious

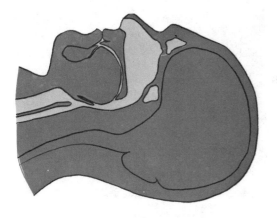

complications resulting from obstruction to breathing.

Figure 11.12, *top*, shows the normal unobstructed airway in a supine patient. The air passage has a rigid posterior wall supported by the cervical vertebrae and a collapsible anterior wall consisting of the tongue and epiglottis. Figure 11.12, *bottom*, shows the most common cause of airway obstruction. The muscles of the floor of the mouth and the pharynx supporting the tongue relax and the tongue and epiglottis fall back into the posterior pharnyx, occluding the airway. Frequently, changing the position of the head and/or jaw will relieve the obstruction. When this is unsuccessful, an airway may be employed. When in place, an airway lifts the posterior aspect of the tongue and the epiglottis from the posterior pharyngeal wall and prevents them from obstructing the space above the larynx. Insertion of an airway does not guarantee a free airway, however. Usually it is still necessary to support the mandible and/or extend the head. In addition, airways facilitate suctioning.

Techniques have been devised in which an airway is modified to accept the connection to the breathing system (32–39).

Types

OROPHARYNGEAL AIRWAYS (ORAL AIRWAYS)

Figure 11.13 shows an oropharyngeal airway in place. It extends from the lips to the pharynx, fitting between the lips and teeth and over the

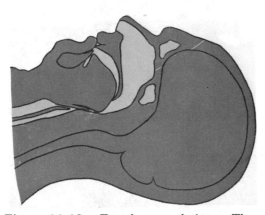

Figure 11.12. *Top*, the normal airway. The tongue and other soft tissue are forward, allowing an unobstructed air passage. *Bottom*, the obstructed airway. The tongue and epiglottis fall back to the posterior pharyngeal wall, occluding the airway. (Drawings courtesy of Vance Robideaux, M.D.)

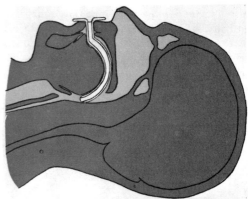

Figure 11.13. Oropharyngeal airway in place. The airway follows the curvature of the tongue, pulling it and the epiglottis away from the posterior pharyngeal wall and providing a channel for air passage. (Drawing courtesy of Vance Robideaux, M.D.)

curve of the tongue. The pharyngeal end rests on the posterior wall of the oropharynx, between it and the base of the tongue. The curved portion of the oropharyngeal airway separates the tongue from the posterior pharyngeal wall and, by pressure along the base of the tongue, pulls the epiglottis slightly forward.

Oropharyngeal airways are sometimes used to prevent a patient from biting and occluding an endotracheal tube inserted through the mouth and to alter the shape of the face for a better mask fit.

General Description

An oropharyngeal airway is shown in Figure 11.14. It is made of metal, plastic, or elastomeric materials. Metal airways have frequently been associated with trauma, especially to the teeth. Oropharyngeal airways usually have a flange at the buccal end. This prevents the airway from falling back into the mouth and possibly becoming an obstruction itself. It also may serve as a means to fix the airway in place. The flange may or may not rest on the patient's lips, depending on whether the particular oral airway being used is the correct size.

The bite portion of the airway is straight and fits between the teeth or gums. It must be firm enough that the patient cannot close the air channel by biting hard. The air channel should be as large as possible. The curved portion extends upward and backward to correspond to the shape of the tongue and palate.

Specific Airways

Below are described some of the oropharyngeal airways available commercially. They come in a variety of lengths. Some manufacturers refer to the sizes by numbers. Unfortunately, these numbers differ from manufacturer to man-

ufacturer, so there is no fixed correlation between a number and length. It has been proposed that these arbitrary numbering systems should be replaced with a system in which airways are designated by a number giving the length expressed in centimeters.

Guedel Airways. The Guedel airway is perhaps the most frequently used oropharyngeal airway. It has a large flange at the oral end, a supported bite area and a gentle curve that follows the contour of the tongue. There is a tubular channel for air exchange and suction. It

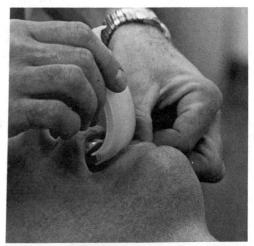

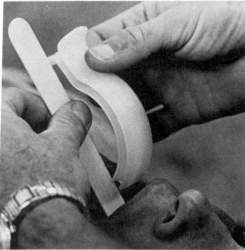

Figure 11.15. (*Top*) Insertion of oral airway. Airway is turned 180 degrees from final resting position.

Figure 11.16. (*Bottom*) Alternative method of inserting an oral airway. A tongue blade is used to displace the tongue forward.

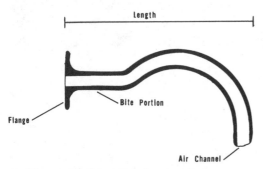

Figure 11.14. Oropharyngeal airway.

is manufactured in various types of plastic and black rubber. Disposable airways are available.

Connell Airway. The Connell airway is similar to the Guedel with two exceptions. It is made of metal and there are holes in the sides near the pharyngeal end.

Waters Airway. The Waters airway is the same as the Connell with the addition of a right or left nipple at the flange for attachment of an oxygen or suction line. (In British catalogues this is referred to as a Waters airway with a nipple.)

Berman Airway (40). The Berman airway (Figs. 11.15 and 11.16) has no enclosed air channel. The sides are open and there is a support through the center. The open sides allow a suction catheter to pass, in addition to providing air channels. The center may have openings in it to permit suction if the airway becomes lodged sideways. There is a flange at the oral end.

This airway is easier to clean than the preceding three types and is less likely to become obstructed by foreign bodies or mucus.

Insertion

Smooth anesthesia often is disturbed by a premature attempt to use an airway. It is advisable to wait until pharyngeal and laryngeal reflexes are depressed before inserting an airway. It is usually wise to wet or lubricate the airway to facilitate insertion.

To insert an oral airway, the operator stands at the patient's head. The jaw is opened with the left hand. The teeth are separated by pressing the thumb against the lower teeth or gum and the index or third finger against the upper teeth or gum. This crossed finger and thumb give the anesthesiologist leverage to separate moderately clenched teeth.

Oral airways may be inserted in two ways. One method is shown in Figure 11.15. The airway is inserted 180 degrees from the final position to avoid displacing the tongue backward into the hypopharynx. When the tip has passed the uvula, the airway is rotated through 180 degrees, so that the tip lies posterior to the tongue and is directed toward the larynx. This prevents the tongue from being pushed into the pharynx and causing further obstruction during insertion.

An alternate method of inserting an oral airway is shown in Figure 11.16. A tongue blade may be used to depress the tongue. The airway is inserted holding it in the position in which it will rest and slid along the roof of the mouth to avoid displacing the tongue back into the hypopharynx.

The criteria for proper size and position of the airway is unobstructed breathing.

NASOPHARYNGEAL AIRWAYS (NASAL AIRWAYS)

The nasopharyngeal airway offers an alternative to the oropharyngeal airway in providing an open airway. There are occasions when the mouth cannot be opened or when an oral airway does not provide relief from obstruction. The nasal airway is better tolerated in the semiawake patient than is the oral airway. A nasal airway may be preferred if the patient's teeth are loose or in poor condition, or with trauma or pathology of the oral cavity. Nasopharyngeal airways have been used as aids in pharyngeal surgery (41) for applying continuous positive airway pressure to facilitate tracheal suctioning (42), to reduce trauma when passing a flexible fiberoptic bronchoscope, and in the management of Pierre Robin syndrome (43).

Contraindications to the use of a nasopharyngeal airway include hemorrhagic disorders; use of anticoagulants; and pathology, sepsis, or deformities of the nasopharynx. Care should be exercised in using one in a child since trauma to the adenoid tissues may occur.

A nasopharyngeal airway is shown in position in Figure 11.17. The airway extends from the nose to the pharynx, with the pharyngeal end just above the epiglottis and below the base of

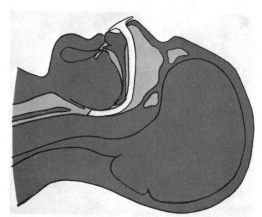

Figure 11.17. The nasopharyngeal airway in place. The airway passes through the nose and ends at a point just above the epiglottis. (Drawing courtesy of Vance Robideaux, M.D.)

the tongue. Nasopharyngeal airways may be placed in both nostrils, but one usually suffices to relieve obstruction.

General Description

There are several nasopharyngeal airways available. They may be made of plastic or rubber and resemble a shortened endotracheal tube. All have flanges at the nasal end. The tubes curve to fit the curvature of the nasopharynx. The length of airway needed for a patient can be estimated as the distance from the tragus of the ear to the tip of the nose plus 1 inch (44) or the distance from the tip of the nose to the meatus of the ear (45)

Specific Airways

Bardex Airway. The Bardex airway (Fig. 11.18) is made of soft neoprene rubber. The pharyngeal end has a bevel and there is a large flange at the nasal end.

Saklad Airway (46). The Saklad airway (Fig. 11.18) is made of plastic. It has a small flange at the nasal end. A safety pin inserted through the wall will prevent it from entering the nose completely. The pharyngeal end is blunted. There are two orifices, one on either side near the pharyngeal end. The larger hole is near the tip and has a steep shelf. It is for a suction catheter. The smaller hole is higher on the tube and serves as an air passage. These airways come as left and right sided for insertion into the corresponding nostril. They can be

identified by the site of the larger hole, which faces the midline.

Rusch Airway. The Rusch nasal airway (Fig. 11.18) is made of soft red rubber. It has a firm adustable flange at the nasal end. The pharyngeal end has a bevel.

Insertion

A nasal airway should always be lubricated thoroughly along its entire length before insertion. Although the use of vasoconstrictors before insertion of the airway has been advocated, their use may not always be beneficial. Insertion should always be done gently to prevent epistaxis.

The nasopharyngeal airway should be inserted as shown in Figure 11.19 (*top*). The airway is held in the hand on the same side as it is to be inserted and is pointed perpendicularly. If resistance is encountered during insertion, the

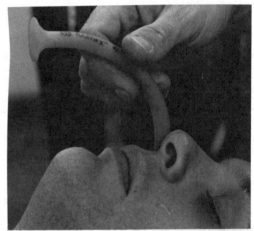

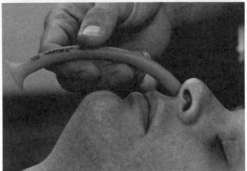

Figure 11.19. Insertion of a nasal airway. *Top*, correct. The airway is inserted perpendicularly, in line with the nasal passage. *Bottom*, incorrect. The airway is being pushed away from the air passage and into the turbinates.

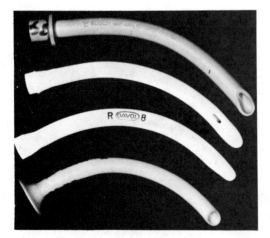

Figure 11.18. Nasopharyngeal airways. From *bottom* to *top*, Bardex, Saklad right and left, and Rusch.

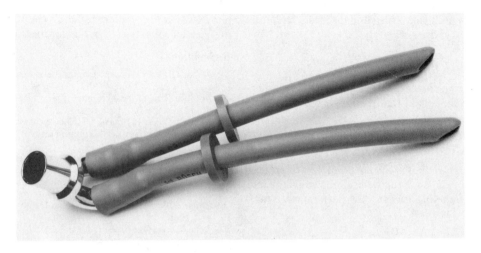

Figure 11.20.   The binasal airway. (Courtesy of Rusch.)

airway should be redirected. If excessive resistance is encountered, the other nostril or a smaller airway should be used. Figure 11.19 (*bottom*) shows an incorrect method for inserting the airway. The airway is being pushed into the turbinates and away from the nasopharynx.

The nasopharyngeal airway may be adjusted to fit the pharynx by sliding it in or out. If the tube is too long, laryngeal reflexes will be stimulated; if too short, airway obstruction will not be relieved.

The Binasal Airway Technique

A technique of anesthesia using a binasal airway has been described (47–56). The airway consists of two airways joined together by a connection which has an adaptor for connection to the anesthesia breathing system (Fig. 11.20). After the airway is inserted, the soft tissues usually seal the hypopharynx, permitting assisted or controlled respirations. Excessive inflations cause gas to overflow through the mouth. The tube is positioned so that the distal tips are near the larynx, just below the tip of the epiglottis.

BITE BLOCKS

A bite block (gag) is placed between the teeth or the jaws in edentulous patients to prevent them from clamping shut. A bite block is used to prevent external compression of an oral endotracheal tube and during electroconvulsive therapy and in unconscious individuals to prevent the patient from biting his tongue and/or lips.

Oral airways may be used as bite blocks, but are not entirely satisfactory as they do not offer protection for the teeth (57). The use of an oral airway is less desirable than a bite block when an endotracheal tube is left in the mouth for an extended period of time because the curved pharyngeal portion of the airway may be irritating (58) and may cause necrosis of the tongue (59).

Many types of bite blocks have been developed, from a variety of materials (58, 60–62). A bite block should be tough but not rigid. Some have channels incorporated into them for air passage.

Placement of a bite block for molar rather than canine compression may result in greater safety to dentition (58).

Complications
AIRWAY OBSTRUCTION

If too large an airway is used, the tip can press the epiglottis against the posterior pharyngeal wall and cover the laryngeal aperture. The oropharyngeal airway may push the tongue into the posterior pharynx, obstructing the airway if inserted incorrectly or if too small an airway is used.

Airways with tubular air channels may have foreign bodies and other material lodged inside the channel (63).

EPISTAXIS

Epistaxis can develop from the insertion of too large a nasal airway or traumatic insertion. This is usually self-limiting but can present a serious problem in bleeding disorders and anti-coagulated patients.

INFECTION

Inserting a nasal airway into a patient draining cerebrospinal fluid (CSF) or blood may induce infection.

UVULAR EDEMA

A case of uvular edema secondary to entrapment of the uvula between the hard palate and an oropharyngeal airway has been reported (64).

DENTAL DAMAGE

Teeth can be cracked or avulsed if the patient bites an airway, especially one of the metal types. Oral airways should be avoided if possible if there is evidence of periodontal disease, teeth weakened by dental caries, pronounced degrees of proclination (the front teeth having a forward inclination and overlapping the lower front teeth) and the presence of isolated teeth (65). It should be noted that with increasing years teeth become brittle and thus more likely to fracture. In these cases, use of a nasopharyngeal airway or placement of packs or props between the back teeth may be preferable.

LIP DAMAGE

When an oral airway is in place, the lip may be caught between the teeth and the airway. This may go unrecognized if a mask is in place. The airways and lips should be inspected frequently during a long case.

LARYNGOSPASM AND COUGHING

A long nasopharyngeal or oropharyngeal airway can stimulate laryngospasm if it touches the epiglottis or vocal cords. This is more likely to occur with the oral airway. It is usually caused by insertion of the airway before establishment of adequate depth of anesthesia.

ULCERATION

Ulceration of the nose or pharynx can occur if the airway remains in place for long periods of time. This is especially true in infants with a strong sucking reflex who "tongue" the airway.

NECROSIS OF THE TONGUE

Pressure necrosis of the tongue has been re-ported when an oropharyngeal airway was left in place for an extended period of time (59).

References

1. James CDT: A disposable anaesthetic face mask. *Br J Anaesth* 42:740, 1970.
2. Boulton TB: Disposable anaesthetic masks. *Anaesthesia* 22:313, 1967.
3. Rendell-Baker L, Soucek DH: New paediatric face masks and anaesthetic equipment. *Br Med J* 1:1690, 1962.
4. Binning R: The development of a new face mask. *Anaesthesia* 20:491–493, 1965.
5. Stephen CR, Slater HM: A nonrebreathing mask. *Anesthesiology* 13:226–228, 1952.
6. Cohen DD: A new mask. *Anesthesiology* 29:111–112, 1965.
7. Dornette WHL: *Anatomy for the Anesthesiologist.* Springfield, Ill., Charles C Thomas, 1964, pp 49–51.
8. James FM: Hypesthesia of the tongue. *Anesthesiology* 42:359, 1975.
9. Harrison GG, Ozinsky J, Jones CS: Choice of an anaesthetic facepiece. *Br J Anaesth* 31:269–273, 1959.
10. Clarke AD: Potential deadspace in an anaesthetic mask and connectors. *Br J Anaesth* 30:176–181, 1958.
11. Brown ES, Hustead RF: Dead space in pediatric equipment. *Items and Topics* (available from Ohio Medical Products) 13:1–3, 1967.
12. Brown ES, Hustead RF: Rebreathing in pediatric anesthesia systems. *Anesthesiology* 28:241–242, 1967.
13. Vale RJ: A modified semi-open system for children's anaesthesia. *Br J Anaesth* 30:182–187, 1958.
14. Revell DG: A circulator to eliminate mechanical dead space in circle absorption systems. *Can Anaesth Soc J* 6:98–103, 1959.
15. Chandler S: A new head strap. *Anesth Analg* 59:457–458, 1980.
16. Jeal DE: Head strap modification. *Anesth Analg* 59:809–810, 1980.
17. Buck HA: Design for an anaesthetic face mask. *Anaesthesia* 9:211–212, 1954.
18. Satterfield R: Fastener for head-retaining strap. *J Am Assoc Nurse Anesthetists* 21:117, 1953.
19. Langley DR: A new dental harness. *Br J Anaesth* 43:715, 1971.
20. Magill IW: Flexible facepiece connexion for closed circuit anaesthesia. *Lancet* 2:701, 1943.
21. Nichol H: A combined harness and tubing support. *Br Med J* 2:651, 1945.
22. Smith JM: A useful addition to the Clausen harness. *Br Med J* 2:820, 1944.
23. Keats AS: Post-anaesthetic cephalagia. *Anaesthesia* 11:341–343, 1956.
24. Morton HJV: Paralysis after anaesthesia. *Br Med J* 1:951, 1951.
25. Barron DW: Supra-orbital neurapraxia. *Anaesthesia* 10:374, 1955.
26. Anonymous: The physician and the law. *Anesth Analg* 49:889, 1970.
27. Birmingham DJ: Inhalation anesthesia mask and contact dermatitis. *JAMA* 193:987–988, 1965.
28. Potgieter SV, Mostert JW: A hazard associated

with the use of a face mask: case report. *S Afr Med J* 33:989–990, 1959.

29. Anonymous: Irritation of the skin from anesthetic or mask. *JAMA* 120:249, 1942.

30. Begenau VG: Allergic dermatitis due to rubber: report of a case. *Anesthesiology* 12:771–772, 1951.

31. Douglas BL, Fishman IM, Kresberg H: Contact dermatitis from rubber tubing. *Oral Surg* 12:92, 1952.

32. Consiglio RVA: An airway for direct coupling to the anaesthetic circuit. *Br J Anaesth* 44:1117, 1972.

33. Keeri-Szanto M: Anesthesia by nasopharyngeal tube: an improvement over the mask technique. *Anesth Analg* 38:142–145, 1959.

34. Keep PJ, Crewe TC: An airway for the edentulous adult. *Anaesthesia* 29:601–602, 1974.

35. Livingston M: Oropharyngeal airway combining molded flange and slipjoint. *Anesth Analg* 48:373–374, 1969.

36. Lieberman SL: Correspondence. *Anesth Analg* 51:568–569, 1972.

37. Suppan P: An anaesthetic airway. *Anaesthesia* 28:84–85, 1973.

38. Potter CFF: Combined airway and mouthpiece for anaesthesia. *Anaesthesia* 18:396–397, 1963.

39. Welsh BE: A non-endotracheal airway for surgery of the head in outpatients. *Anesthesiology* 40:298–299, 1974.

40. Berman RA, Lilienfeld SM: Correspondence. *Anesthesiology* 11:136–137, 1950.

41. Stallings JO, Lines J: Use of nasopharyngeal tubes as aids to lateral port construction and maintenance of the airway in pharyngeal flap surgery. *Plast Reconstr Surg* 58:379–380, 1976.

42. Wanner A, Zighelboim A, Sackner MA: Nasopharyngeal airway: a facilitated access to the trachea for nasotracheal suction, bedside bronchofiberscopy and selective bronchography. *Ann Intern Med* 75:593–595, 1971.

43. Heaf DP, Helms PJ, Dinwiddie R, Matthew DJ: Nasopharyngeal airways in Pierre Robin syndrome. *J Pediatr* 100:698–703, 1982.

44. Collins VJ: *Principles of Anesthesiology*. Philadelphia, Lea & Febiger, 1966, pp. 137–138.

45. Monheim LM: *General Anesthesia in Dental Practice*, ed 3. St. Louis, C. V. Mosby, 1968.

46. Saklad M: A new nasopharyngeal airway. *Anesthesiology* 15:325–326, 1954.

47. Elam JO, Titel JH, Feingold A, Weisman H, Bauer RO: Simplified airway management during

anesthesia or resuscitation: a binasal pharyngeal system. *Anesth Analg* 48:307–316, 1969.

48. Weisman H, Weis TW, Elam JO: Use of double nasopharyngeal airways in anesthesia. *Anesth Analg* 48:356–361, 1969.

49. Feingold A, Runyan MJ: Experience with the latex binasal pharyngeal airway. *Anesth Analg* 52:263–266, 1973.

50. Weisman H, Bauer RO, Huddy RA, Elam JO: An improved binasopharyngeal airway system for anesthesia. *Anesth Analg* 51:11–13, 1972.

51. Komesaroff D: An unusual indication for the double nasopharyngeal airway: a case report. *Anesth Analg* 50:240–243, 1971.

52. Frumin MJ, Rockow H: Nasopharyngeal administration of nitrous oxide-oxygen anesthesia: a technical note. *Anesthesiology* 13:552–553, 1952.

53. Doctor NH: Bilateral nasopharyngeal tues for outpatient dental anaesthesia. *Anaesthesia* 32:273–276, 1977.

54. Katz H, Machida RC, Wootton DG, Amonic R: A technic of general anesthesia for blepharoplasty and rhytidectomy. *Anesth Analg* 55:165–167, 1976.

55. Katz H, Richards JA: General anesthesia without intubation for cataract surgery. *Anesthesiol Rev* 3:29–31, 1976.

56. Weiseman H, Bauer RO, Elam JO: Binasopharyngeal airways. A rediscovered system for anesthesia. *Anesth Progr* 16:101–104, 1969.

57. Pollard BJ, O'Leary J: Guedel airway and tooth damage. *Anaesth Intensive Care* 9:395, 1981.

58. Schwartz AJ, Dougal RM, Lee WK: Modification of oral airway as a bite block. *Anesth Analg* 59:225, 1980.

59. Moore MW, Rauscher L: A complication of oropharyngeal airway placement. *Anesthesiology* 47:526, 1977.

60. O'Connor DCJ: A new airway-gag. *Lancet* 1:356–357, 1958.

61. Loehning RW: Blachly bite Blok for edentulous patients. *Anesthesiology* 48:364, 1978.

62. Samra SK: Endotracheal tube in place passing through bite block. *Anesth Analg* 60:66, 1981.

63. Stoneham FJR: Asphyxia due to faulty apparatus. *Br Med J* 1:400, 1957.

64. Shulman MS: Uvular edema without endotracheal intubation. *Anesthesiology* 55:82–83, 1981.

65. Wright RB, Manfield FFV: Damage to teeth during the administration of general anaesthesia. *ASA Newsletter*, May 1974, pp 3–6.

CHAPTER 12

Laryngoscopes

A laryngoscope is used to directly view the larynx and adjacent structures. Most commonly this is done for the purpose of inserting an endotracheal tube into the trachea.

RIGID LARYNGOSCOPES

Most laryngoscopes in use today consist of two basic parts: a handle and a blade.

The Handle

The handle, which is held by the hand during use, usually has a rough surface for traction. It supplies or conducts the energy for the light source. Most often this energy comes from batteries housed in the handle. Handles with rechargeable batteries are available (1). An extra handle should always be immediately available, since laryngoscope failure can be catastrophic (2).

Handles are available in several sizes. Short handles may be advantageous for patients in whom the chest and/or breasts contact the handle during use (3).

A few handles have an additional part which when attached to a blade forms the rough configuration of a "U", rather than the usual "L". These are most often used for diagnostic purposes rather than for intubation.

The connection point between the handle and the blade is called the fitting, or hinge. Most blades form a right angle with the handle when ready for use, but acute and obtuse angles may also be formed. In the United States, a hook-on connection is most commonly used. This allows for quick and easy exchange of blades. The handle is fitted with a pin that accepts the hinge slot on the base of the blade. There is also an electrical contact point and a locking groove for the blade.

The Blade

The blade is the part of the laryngoscope which is inserted into the mouth. When blades are available in more than one size, they are numbered, with the number increasing with size. The usable length is the distance between the tip and the base (Fig. 12.1).

The blade is composed of several parts: base, tongue, flange, web, tip, and socket (Fig. 12.1). The base has a slot to engage the hinge pin of the handle, a locking mechanism to engage the groove on the handle, and an electrical contact.

The tongue (spatula) is the main shaft of the blade. It serves to compress and manipulate the soft tissues (especially the tongue) and lower jaw so that a direct line of vision to the larynx is achieved. The long axis of the tongue may be straight or curved in part or all of its length. Blades are commonly referred to as curved or straight, depending on the predominant shape of the tongue. Blades with curved and straight tongues are shown in Figure 12.1.

The flange is parallel to the tongue and connected by the web. It projects from the edge of the tongue and serves to guide instrumentation and deflect interfering tissues. The flange determines the cross-sectional shape of the blade.

The tip (beak) of the blade contacts either the epiglottis or the vallecula and directly or indirectly elevates the epiglottis. It is usually blunt and thickened to decrease trauma.

The socket will accept a light bulb and has an electrical connection to the hook-on base. When the blade is locked in place on the handle the electrical contact points complete the circuit with the power source.

In most cases, use of a laryngoscope presents little or no difficulty to the experienced laryngoscopist, but there are certain situations where laryngoscopy is difficult and where one type of blade may be particularly advantageous. This has led to the development of a large number of blades, each with its own claimed advantages and indications.

The blades discussed here are those currently available commercially in the United States. A number of other blades have been described in the literature.

CURVED
(MACINTOSH)

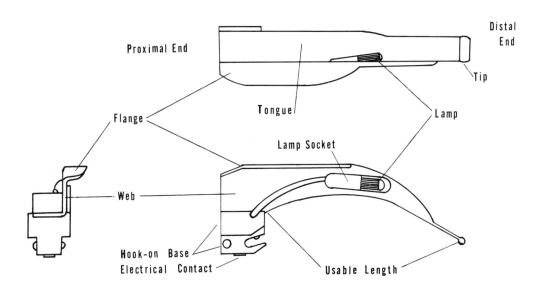

STRAIGHT
(MILLER)

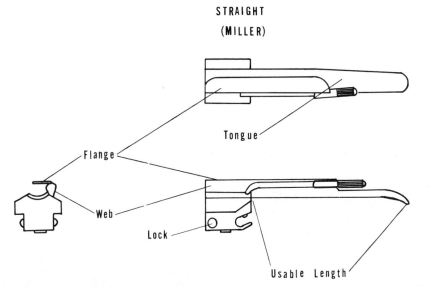

Figure 12.1. The parts of the Macintosh (*top*) and the Miller (*bottom*) are illustrated. The tip is the distal end of the blade intended for insertion into the patient. The proximal end is the part closest to the handle. (Redrawn from a drawing in *Draft Standard, Laryngoscopes for Tracheal Intubation*, Z-79 Committee, American National Standards Institute.)

MACINTOSH BLADE (4)

The Macintosh laryngoscope blade (Fig. 12.2) is one of the most popular in use today. The tongue has a smooth, gentle curve. There is a flange at the left side to push the tongue out of the way. In cross-section, the tongue, web, and flange form a reverse "Z." The blade is available in four sizes: infant, child, medium adult, and large adult. Numerous modifications have been proposed (3–14).

LEFT-HANDED MACINTOSH BLADE (15)

The left-handed Macintosh blade (Fig. 12.3) has the flange on the opposite side from the usual Macintosh blade. It is available only in the medium adult size. This blade may be useful when abnormalities of the teeth, jaws, lips, or face block the right side, for left-handed laryngoscopists, for intubating in the right lateral position, and for positioning an endotracheal tube directly on the left side of the mouth (16, 17).

POLIO BLADE

The polio laryngoscope blade (Fig. 12.4), also a modification of the Macintosh, is available only in the medium adult size. The blade is offset from the handle at an obtuse angle to allow intubation of patients in iron lung respirators, body jackets, and other difficult situations and when intubation needs to be performed after the anesthesia screen is in place (18). It is also useful for patients with obesity and mammary gland hypertrophy, kyphosis with severe barrel chest deformity, short necks, and restricted neck mobility (19).

FINK BLADE

The Fink blade (Fig. 12.5) is another modification of the Macintosh. The tongue is wider

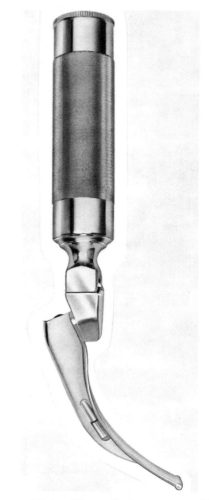

Figure 12.4. The polio laryngoscope blade. (Courtesy of Foregger, Division of Puritan-Bennett Corporation.)

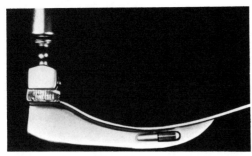

Figure 12.2. The Macintosh laryngoscope blade.

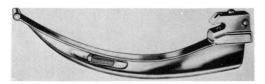

Figure 12.3. Left-handed Macintosh blade. (Courtesy of Penlon Ltd.)

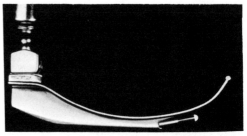

Figure 12.5. The Fink laryngoscope blade. Note that the tongue is more curved at the tip and the flange is reduced at the proximal end, in comparison with the Macintosh blade. The light bulb is placed nearer the distal end.

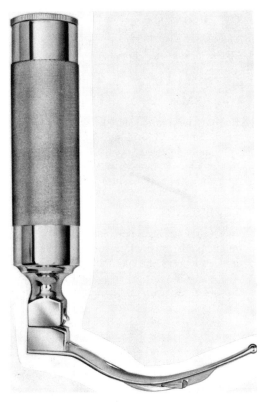

Figure 12.6. The Bizarri-Guiffrida laryngoscope blade. (Courtesy of Foregger Company, Division of Puritan-Bennett Corporation.)

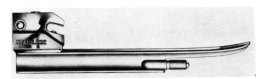

Figure 12.7. The Miller laryngoscope blade. (Courtesy of Ohio Medical Products, a division of Airco, Inc.)

and has a sharper curve at the distal end. The height of the flange is less, especially at the proximal end. The light bulb is placed further forward than on the Macintosh and is not ensheathed in metal. It is available in only one size for use in a large adult.

BIZARRI-GUIFFRIDA BLADE (20)

The Bizarri-Guiffrida laryngoscope blade (Fig. 12.6) is also a modified Macintosh. The flange has been removed, except for a small part which encases the light bulb. The absence of the

vertical component was designed to limit damage to the upper teeth, especially when the distal end must be rotated to visualize the larynx. The blade is designed particularly for patients with a limited mouth opening, prominent incisors, receding mandible, short thick neck, or anterior larynx (20). It is available in child, medium adult, and large adult sizes.

MILLER BLADE (21)

The Miller blade (Fig. 12.7) is one of the most popular blades. The tongue is straight with a slight curve near the tip. In cross-section the flange, web, and tongue form a "C" with the top flattened. Some commercial versions of the blade have the lamp socket on the tongue while other versions have it on the web. It is available in premature, infant, child, medium adult, and large adult sizes.

WISCONSIN BLADE

The Wisconsin blade (Fig. 12.8) is also a popular model. Unlike the Miller blade, the tongue has no curve. The flange is curved to form two-thirds of a circle in cross-section. The depth of the flange is small near the proximal end and flares to its largest depth about three-fourths of the way to the tip. It is available in five sizes: two infant, child, medium adult, and large adult.

WIS-FOREGGER BLADE

The Wis-Foregger is a modification of the Wisconsin blade with a straight tongue and a flange that expands slightly toward the distal end (22). The distal portion of the blade is wider and formed slightly to the right. It is available in three sizes: child, medium adult, and large adult.

WHITEHEAD MODIFICATION OF WIS-FOREGGER BLADE

This laryngoscope blade is similar to the Wis-Foregger, with the flange reduced in height and

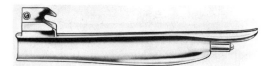

Figure 12.8. The Wisconsin laryngoscope blade. (Courtesy of Ohio Medical Products, a division of Airco, Inc.)

opened proximally and distally. It is available only in a medium adult size.

WIS-HIPPLE BLADE

The Wis-Hipple is also modified from the Wisconsin blade. The tongue is straight while the flange is large and circular. Compared to the Wisconsin blade, the flange is straighter and runs parallel to the tongue. The tip is wider. It is designed for children and is available in two sizes.

SCHAPIRA BLADE (23)

The Schapira blade is a straight blade with a tip that curves upward. There is no vertical component. The blade's curvature may facilitate intubation by cradling the tongue and pushing it to the left side of the mouth.

ALBERTS BLADE

The Alberts blade (Fig. 12.9) combines characteristics of the Miller and Wis-Hipple blades with a cutaway flange to increase visibility. There is a recess to facilitate insertion of an endotracheal tube. The blade forms a 67-degree angle with the handle. It is used for pediatrics.

MICHAELS BLADE

The Michaels blade (Fig. 12.9) differs from the Alberts blade only in that it forms a 93-degree angle with the handle.

SNOW BLADE (24)

The Snow blade (Fig. 12.10) is a hybrid blade consisting of a Miller tongue with a Wis-Foreger flange. It is available in only one adult size.

FLAGG BLADE (25)

The Flagg laryngoscope blade (Fig. 12.11) has a straight tongue. The flange has a "C" shape that gradually decreases in size as it approaches the distal end. It comes in several sizes for infants, children, and medium and large adults.

GUEDEL BLADE

The Guedel laryngoscope blade (Fig. 12.12) is a straight blade in which the tongue is set at a 72-degree angle to the handle. The flange has the shape of a "U" on its side. The light is close to the tip. It is available in infant, child, and medium and large adult sizes.

BENNETT BLADE

The Bennett laryngoscope blade (Fig. 12.13) is a modification of the Guedel blade. It also forms an acute angle with the handle. The upper part of the flange has been omitted. The available sizes differ from those of the Guedel and

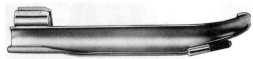

Figure 12.10. The Snow laryngoscope blade. (Courtesy of Air Products and Chemicals, Inc.)

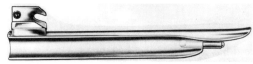

Figure 12.11. The Flagg laryngoscope blade. (Courtesy of Ohio Medical Products, a division of Airco, Inc.)

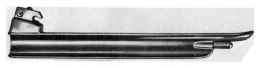

Figure 12.12. The Guedel laryngoscope blade. (Courtesy of Penlon Ltd.)

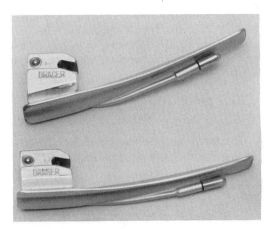

Figure 12.9. Alberts (*top*) and Michaels (*bottom*) laryngoscope blades. The Alberts blade offers a sharp 67-degree angle while the Michaels has a slight 93-degree angle. (Courtesy of North American Drager.)

are referred to as small for children and medium and large for adults.

EVERSOLE BLADE

The Eversole laryngoscope blade (Fig. 12.14)

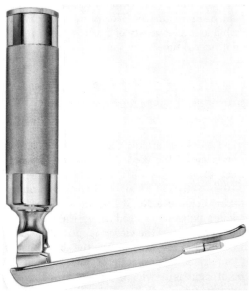

Figure 12.13. The Bennett laryngoscope blade. (Courtesy of Foregger, Division of Puritan-Bennett Corporation.)

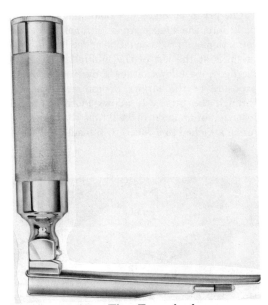

Figure 12.14. The Eversole laryngoscope blade. (Courtesy of Foregger Company, Division of Puritan-Bennett Corporation.)

has a straight tongue. The flange forms a "C" with the tongue and web near the proximal end. Midway to the tip the upper flange tapers. It is available only in a medium adult size.

SEWARD BLADE (26)

The Seward laryngoscope blade (Fig. 12.15) has a straight tongue with a curve near the tip. It has a small reverse "Z" shaped flange. It is available in only infant size and one size for children up to 5 years of age.

ROBERTSHAW BLADE (27)

This blade (Fig. 12.16) has a straight tongue with a gentle curve near the tip. It is designed to lift the epiglottis indirectly. The flange is extended to the left to allow for binocular vision and thus better depth perception. It is available in only one size for use in infants or small children.

OXFORD INFANT BLADE (28)

The Oxford infant laryngoscope blade (Fig. 12.17) has a straight tongue that curves up slightly at the tip. It has a "U" shape at the

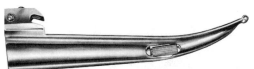

Figure 12.15. The Seward laryngoscope blade. (Courtesy of Penlon Ltd.)

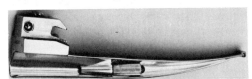

Figure 12.16. The Robertshaw laryngoscope blade. (Courtesy of Penlon Ltd.)

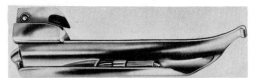

Figure 12.17. The Oxford infant laryngoscope blade. (Courtesy of Penlon Ltd.)

proximal end with the bottom limb of the "U" decreasing toward the tip. It is available in only one size. Though intended primarily for newborns it is suitable for children up to the age of four, especially those with cleft palate.

OXYSCOPE BLADE

The Oxyscope (Fig. 12.18) is a modification of the Miller blade which has a connection that allows attachment of a delivery hose. This permits delivery of oxygen or other gas mixtures during laryngoscopy (29). It is available in two infant sizes. Other laryngoscopes that allow gas administration have been described in the literature (30–32).

SIKER MIRROR BLADE (33)

The Siker mirror laryngoscope blade (Fig. 12.19) has a stainless steel mirror on the flange facing the tongue at the midpoint of the blade. The portion of the blade distal to the mirror makes an angle of 135 degrees with the proximal portion. There is only one size available. This blade is useful in patients in whom direct laryngoscopy cannot be performed because of anatomical abnormalities.

In order to use the blade, it should first be immersed in warm water for 10 min to prevent the mirror from fogging. For intubation, the blade is inserted in the mouth in the usual manner with the operator viewing the structures at the distal end by looking into the mirror. Practice is necessary for successful use of this blade, because the mirror inverts the reflected image and the user must be conditioned to look at an inverted image. Because of the curve in the blade, a curved stylet must be used in the endotracheal tube.

Accessories

HUFFMAN PRISM (34–36) AND PRISM LARYNGOSCOPE

These devices are designed to provide an indirect view of the larynx in patients in whom direct exposure is difficult. The prism (Fig. 12.20) is a block of Plexiglas shaped to fit on the proximal end of a No. 3 Macintosh blade. The ends are polished to produce optically flat surfaces; that nearest the viewer is cut at 90 degrees to the line of vision, whereas the distal face is at 30 degrees. A refraction of 30 degrees in the line of sight is provided, thereby bringing into view structures within a few millimeters of the laryngoscope tip when viewed in the normal manner at the outer end of the prism. The image is right side up. It is necessary to warm the prism before use to prevent condensation.

The prism laryngoscope blade has the prism built into the blade. An additional 20-degree refraction from right to left is added because the prism is at the left of the midline. The prism laryngoscope allows either conventional direct exposure of the larynx or indirect exposure through the prism. It allows more space for insertion of an endotracheal tube than does the prism attached to a Macintosh blade.

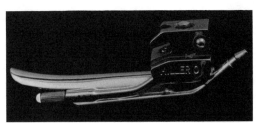

Figure 12.18. The Oxyscope. (Picture by Art Cooper, Orange Park, Fla.)

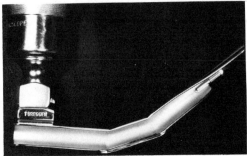

Figure 12.19. The Siker mirror laryngoscope blade.

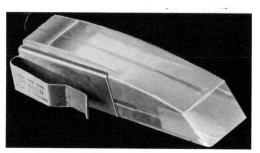

Figure 12.20. The Huffman prism. (Courtesy of Penlon Ltd.)

HOWLAND LOCK

The Howland Lock (Fig. 12.21) fits between the handle and the blade by means of hook-on connections on both the handle and the blade. Its purpose is to change the angle between the handle and the blade.

The Howland Lock has been used extensively in cases of head and neck malignancies and post-irradiation and post-radical neck surgery patients. It is advantageous in the patient with a receding mandible, anterior larynx, protruding teeth, "bull neck," facial contractures, or decreased jaw mobility. It is adaptable to all types of laryngoscope handles and blades, but it is most often used with straight blades such as the Miller.

FIBEROPTIC LARYNGOSCOPE (37–39)

The fiberoptic laryngoscope (or broncho-scope) is valuable for tracheal intubation of patients who are difficult or impossible to intubate with conventional laryngoscopes. It is also useful for verifying or reassessing endotracheal or endobronchial tube placement (40), changing endotracheal tubes (41), locating and removing secretions, examining the upper airway, assessing laryngeal or tracheal damage, and inserting nasogastric tubes when conventional techniques have failed.

Its use is associated with less trauma and fewer cardiovascular changes than use of a con-

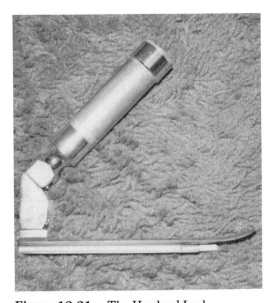

Figure 12.21.   The Howland Lock.

ventional laryngoscope (42) but it is more costly, delicate, and difficult to learn to use.

Flexible Model

The flexible fiberoptic laryngoscope (Figs. 12.22 and 12.23) is composed of several parts: light source, handle, body, flexible insertion portion, working channel, and tip cable.

LIGHT SOURCE

This includes the light and its power supply. The light and battery power supply may be contained in the handle (Fig. 12.22). This makes the instrument more portable.

An external source of light carried to the laryngoscope by a flexible cable (Fig. 12.23) provides superior illumination and is the most common source of light. Light sources for other fiberoptic instruments such as laparoscopes, bronchoscopes, and cystoscopes can be used.

HANDLE

The handle is the part held in the hand during use. It houses the batteries if they are the power source. In some scopes the handle is absent and the instrument is held by the body.

THE BODY

The body is the proximal rigid part of the laryngoscope. It includes the focusing eye piece, working channel sleeve, and the tip control knob. The eyepiece is at the proximal end. By rotating it, the image just in front of the tip of the scope can be brought into focus. The tip control knob is on the side of the body. By turning the knob the tip of the flexible portion can be flexed or extended. A full range of motion can be attained by rotating the entire instrument.

FLEXIBLE INSERTION PORTION

This consists of a bundle of image-conducting fibers, a bundle of light-conducting fibers, and a working channel which is not present with some scopes. At the distal tip of the image-conduction fibers, there is an image-forming lens.

Image-Conducting Bundle (Optic Fiber Bundle)

Optic fibers transmit the image from the lens to the eyepiece. These fibers are specially treated

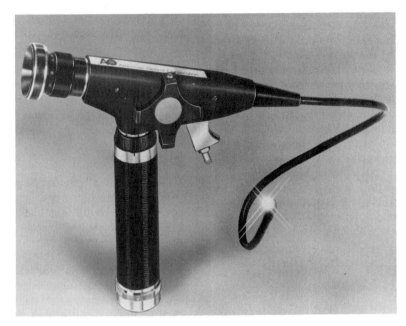

Figure 12.22.   Fiberoptic flexible laryngoscope. The power is supplied by batteries housed in the handle. (Courtesy of American Optical.)

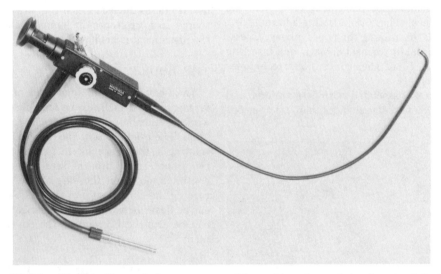

Figure 12.23.   Flexible fiberoptic laryngoscope with working channel. At the top of the body is the opening of the working channel. The light and power are supplied by an external source and connected to the laryngoscope by the cord at bottom. (Courtesy of Machida America, Inc.)

and precisely grouped so that the relationship of one fiber to the other is exactly the same at each end. This allows transmission of a clear image. Such a bundle of organized filaments is called "coherent."

Light Conducting Fiber Bundle

The light-conducting (illumination) fibers transmit the light to the tip of the scope. Glass fibers are flexible and very efficient light con-

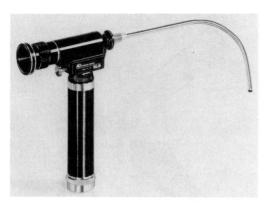

Figure 12.24. Fiberoptic stylet laryngoscope. (Courtesy of American Optical.)

ductors. A bundle of these fibers has the capability of carrying light from a powerful source without producing dangerous heating (32).

Working Channel (Optional)

Most scopes now have a working channel extending from the tip to the body (Fig. 12.23). This can be used for aspirating secretions, injection of medications, insufflation of oxygen and anesthetic gases, and passage of biopsy forceps.

Tip Cable

A cable connecting the tip to the central knob passes through the flexible insertion portion. The cable allows movement of the tip.

Stylet Laryngoscope

The stylet fiberoptic laryngoscope (Fig. 12.24) is composed of a handle, body, and stylet. The distal portion of the stylet is malleable. It can be powered by a battery or external light source.

TECHNIQUES OF USE

Laryngoscopy consists of several steps: positioning the head, inserting the laryngoscope blade, identifying the epiglottis, raising the epiglottis, and finally viewing the larynx.

The head should be positioned so that the passageway from the incisor teeth to the larynx is brought into a straight line for the best possible view of the vocal cords. The best position includes flexion of the head at the neck and extension of the head at the atlanto-occipital level, the so-called sniffing position. The head should be elevated a few inches on a low pillow

or ring (43, 44). In children, a pillow placed under the shoulder may be helpful (43, 45).

The laryngoscope handle is held in the left hand unless the operator is left-handed. Many left-handed people also hold the scope in the left hand because most blades are designed for insertion on the right side of the mouth. Moistening or lubricating the blade will facilitate insertion if the mouth is dry. If the tongue is too slippery, placement of cloth adhesive tape on the lingual surface of the blade may be helpful (46). The fingers of the right hand are used to open the mouth and spread the lips apart. Care must be taken to prevent either the lower or upper lips from becoming entrapped between the teeth and the blade. The laryngoscope is inserted between the teeth at the right side of the mouth. This reduces the likelihood that the incisor teeth will be damaged and will help push the tongue to the left out of the line of vision.

The blade is inserted toward the midline along the right dorsolateral surface of the tongue so that when it is in place the blade is in the middle of the mouth. The right hand keeps the lips from rolling between the teeth and the blade. The laryngoscope is advanced until the epiglottis comes into view.

There are two methods for elevating the epiglottis, depending on whether a straight or curved blade is being used.

Straight Blade

After exposure of the epiglottis, the blade is withdrawn slightly to scoop under the epiglottis and then lift it upward. The vocal cords should be identified. If they are not seen, an assistant is asked to push downward on the larynx. The straight blade is shown in position for intubation in Figure 12.25. It rests in the center of the mouth with the tip below the epiglottis.

If the laryngoscope is advanced too far, it will override the slanting glottis and enter the esophagus. If it is then withdrawn too far, the tip of the epiglottis will be released and will flip over the glottis.

Curved Blade

When the epiglottis is seen, the tip of the blade is advanced into the space between the base of the tongue and the epiglottis. Figure 12.26 shows the curved blade in position ready for intubation. The tip fits into the angle made

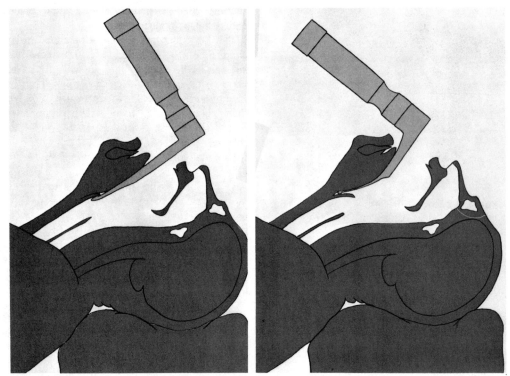

Figure 12.25. (*Left*) Intubation with a straight laryngoscope blade. The tip of the blade picks up the epiglottis. (Drawing courtesy of Vance Robideaux, M.D.)

Figure 12.26. (*Right*) Intubation with the curved laryngoscope blade. The epiglottis is below the tip of the blade. A small pillow under the head allows better visualization on the larynx. (Drawing courtesy of Vance Robideaux, M.D.)

by the epiglottis with the base of the tongue. Anatomically the relationship between the tongue and the epiglottis is such that pulling the base of the tongue forward also pulls the epiglottis forward.

After the tip is advanced the blade is lifted upward and forward along the axis of the handle to carry the base of the tongue and the epiglottis forward. The glottis should come into view. If it is not easily exposed, external pressure on the larynx may be of value. It is important for the handle to be lifted upward in the direction the handle is pointing. The upper teeth should not be used as a fulcrum to lift the epiglottis. This will cause the tip to push the larynx upward and out of sight and could cause damage to teeth or gums.

FIBEROPTIC LARYNGOSCOPY (38, 39, 47–52)

The fiberoptic laryngoscope has not yet achieved the popularity it deserves. Many anes-

thesiologists have become disenchanted when they have attempted to use it for the first time when the need to perform a difficult intubation arose and they did not meet with success. Frequently, it is used only after multiple attempts with conventional laryngoscopes. After the airway is filled with secretions or blood and compromised by edema, a high failure rate is not surprising (41).

Practice is needed to learn to handle the tip control while advancing the scope. Also the anatomy appears different from that viewed with a rigid laryngoscope. Nevertheless, facility with this instrument can be achieved without an inordinate expenditure of time or effort. As experience is gained, the average time required for intubation will decrease.

Facility should be developed first with an intubation mannequin and then with patients in whom no difficulty in intubation is anticipated, rather than making first attempts with a difficult intubation. It is preferable to use it in a spontaneously breathing patient who has received the appropriate topical anesthesia and sedation and in an unhurried atmosphere. Mechanical aids to allow administration of anesthetic mixtures during laryngoscopy have been developed (53).

Mucus, blood, and secretions will obscure the view (39) so antisialagogues should be given and gentle suctioning performed prior to starting.

FLEXIBLE MODEL

Because this instrument is expensive and delicate, great care must be taken not to damage it.

The tip should be treated with antifogging solution or placed in warm water (not saline) for several minutes before use. The light source should be connected and tested. The focus should be adjusted by viewing some small print at a distance of 2–3 cm. The outside of the flexible portion should be coated with a lubricating gel but the lubricant should not contact the lens.

The head is put in the usual position for intubation. The laryngoscopist may stand behind the patient in the conventional position, or in front of the patient whose neck is fixed in flexion.

Intubation can be accomplished either orally or nasally. The endotracheal tube is first threaded over the laryngoscope. There are two basic techniques (50). The first technique is to place the endotracheal tube over the proximal end of the flexible insertion portion, insert the flexible portion until the tip enters the larynx, then thread the endotracheal tube over the flexible portion. With the second technique, the endotracheal tube is first passed into the pharynx. The laryngoscope is passed through the tube and into the trachea. The tube is then threaded over the flexible portion. The second approach may make it difficult to expose the larynx if the endotracheal tube is not directed correctly.

The scope is held so that the index finger and thumb of one hand turn the tip control. The fingers of the other hand advance the scope.

It is important to have an air space at the end of the laryngoscope to keep it away from the tissues (51). This can be accomplished in the anesthetized patient by having an assistant pull the tongue forward out of the mouth or elevate the angle of the jaw while opening the mouth to refashion the pharyngeal space (54). Alternately, a modified surgical tongue retractor (55) or a conventional rigid laryngoscope can be used to push the tongue forward. The awake patient can be asked to stick out his tongue, which is then held gently in a gauze by an assistant.

Oral Intubation

The laryngoscope can be passed through a modified oral airway (48, 56) or bite block (50). This will protect the laryngoscope from a biting patient, guide it into the midline, and keep the tongue from falling backwards.

The laryngoscope is placed in the mouth in the midline and advanced until its tip touches the posterior wall of the pharynx. The tip is angulated acutely toward the larynx, seeking the epiglottis. Having the patient swallow and cough will elevate the larynx and clear secretions. It is important that the laryngoscope be kept in the midline as it is advanced.

When the epiglottis has been located, the laryngoscope tip is rotated downward so that it passes beneath the tip of the epiglottis and is then turned upward until the vocal cords are seen.

The tip is then passed between the vocal cords and advanced several centimeters into the trachea. For endobronchial intubation, the laryngoscope is advanced to view the carina, then threaded into the correct mainstem bronchus. The endotracheal tube is gently slipped off the scope into the trachea or bronchus. If the tube snags, pulling out on the tube and gentle rotation usually completes the intubation. The laryngoscope should be used to verify that the tip of the tube is correctly positioned, then withdrawn, leaving the tube in place.

Nasal Intubation

It is important to pass the laryngoscope through the most patent naris following use of vasoconstictors to reduce vascular congestion and the possibility of bleeding (57). Particular care should be taken not to damage the turbinates. The endotracheal tube must be large enough to pass over the laryngoscope but not too large to pass through the nose. Some endotracheal tubes are compressed in the nose so that they will not accommodate the laryngoscope, even when the tube lumen would otherwise be adequate (38). Intubation technique is similar to that of oral intubation.

STYLET MODEL (58)

Use of the stylet laryngoscope is restricted to

oral use. It is unsuitable for patients who have limited mandibular mobility.

As with the fiberoptic laryngoscope, it is preferable that the patient be awake but sedated. Topical anesthesia should be applied to the oropharynx and upper airway and, on occasion, transtracheally.

The light is checked for adequate brightness and the curve of the distal malleable portion of the stylet is adjusted as deemed appropriate for the patient's anatomy. The tip of the scope is immersed in warm water to prevent fogging. The stylet is lubricated, the tube passed over the stylet, and the outside of the tube lubricated.

The laryngoscope and tube are inserted together under direct vision in the midline of the mouth until the tips of both can no longer be seen. The laryngoscopist then directs the advance by looking through the eyepiece. The stylet is advanced behind the epiglottis to visualize the vocal cords. The tube is gently slid off the laryngoscope and into the trachea. The tip of the stylet should not pass beyond the vocal cords.

COMPLICATIONS OF LARYNGOSCOPY

Trauma

Trauma to the teeth and soft tissues of the oral and perioral areas during laryngoscopy is most frequently associated with inexperience on the part of the laryngoscopist, but in emergency situations and during difficult intubations some trauma may be inevitable. Use of a fiberoptic laryngoscope may result in less trauma than use of a rigid laryngoscope.

Local sequelae of laryngoscopy include abrasion and/or laceration of the lips, tongue, palate, pharynx, larynx and/or esophagus. The lingual nerve may be injured (59, 60). Reckless mobilization maneuvers of the head can produce dislocation of the cervical spinal column or jaw (61–64).

One of the most common complications of laryngoscopy is damage to the teeth, gums, or dental prostheses. Not only may there be cosmetic disfigurement and discomfort, but if the patient aspirates a dislodged tooth or fragment, there may be grave pulmonary complications.

A tooth or prosthetic device may be chipped, broken, or loosened. Loose teeth may be avulsed. The incisors are most often injured. This trauma usually is caused by utilization of the edge of the upper anterior teeth or gums as a fulcrum point for the laryngoscope.

The oral cavity should be carefully examined preoperatively to identify possible problems. Loose, broken, chipped, capped or diseased teeth, bridgework, and partial or complete dentures should be identified and noted on the chart. Since the anterior six teeth of both arches are most prone to trauma, emphasis should be placed on these during the examination. Anatomical variations of the mouth and pharynx that cause difficulty in exposing the larynx should be noted. The patient should be advised beforehand if dental damage is likely.

In patients in the 4–11 age range where the upper anterior region of the dental arch is in a state of relatively rapid development, the deciduous teeth are easily dislodged. Removal of such teeth before or during anesthesia may be indicated if they are noticeably loose. Orthopedic appliances should be removed if possible and protected from damage. Sutures may be placed around very loose teeth to prevent them from entering the airway should they become dislodged.

A number of mouth protectors (teeth protectors) have been created to protect both the teeth and gums (65–71). These have disadvantages. They decrease the space between the upper and lower teeth and may interfere with visualization of the larynx. They may instill a false sense of security in the laryngoscopist who may then use the covering as a fulcrum against which to pivot the blade.

If a tooth or fragment or dental appliance is broken and dislodged it must be sought. The search should start with an examination of the oral cavity and checking of the area surrounding the patient's head. X-rays must be taken if the foreign body is not found. In addition to chest x-rays, a radiograph of the neck should be taken to locate fragments obscured in the larynx (72).

Circulatory Changes

Changes in cardiac rhythm and blood pressure are common during laryngoscopy. They are less with fiberoptic laryngoscopy (42). They are best avoided by prior oxygenation, establishment of an adequate depth of anesthesia, and quick, atraumatic laryngoscopy. Topical anesthesia can also help.

Aspiration of a Foreign Body

A case has been reported where the bulb from a laryngoscope was aspirated during attempted intubation (73). Avulsed teeth have also been aspirated.

Thermal Burn

A case has been reported where a laryngoscope light was left on and contacted the patient's skin (74). A thermal burn resulted.

References

1. Binning R: The use of rechargeable batteries for laryngoscopes. *Anaesthesia* 19:451–453, 1964.
2. Anonymous: Laryngoscopes. *Technol Anesth* 3:4, 1982.
3. Datta S, Briwa J: Modified laryngoscope for endotracheal intubation of obese patients. *Anesth Analg* 60:120–121, 1981.
4. Macintosh RR: A new laryngoscope. *Lancet* 1:205, 1943.
5. Gubya R, Orkin LR: Design and utility of a new curved laryngoscope blade. *Anesth Analg* 38:364, 1959.
6. DeCiutiis VL: Modification of Mcintosh laryngoscope. *Anesthesiology* 20:115–116, 1959.
7. Dance C: Blade for lateral intubation. *Anesthesiology* 20:380–381, 1959.
8. Vellacott WH: Plastic laryngoscope. *Br Med J* 1:619, 1968.
9. Larson AG: A new laryngoscope. *Anaesthesia* 21:406–407, 1966.
10. Evans FT: Modified laryngoscope. *Lancet* 1:1161, 1951.
11. Onkst HR: Modified laryngoscope blade. *Anesthesiology* 22:846–848, 1961.
12. Ritchie JR: Modified Macintosh laryngoscope. *Anaesthesia* 11:344–345, 1956.
13. Moulden GA, Wynne RL: Post-anesthesia granuloma of the larynx. *Br J Anaesth* 23:92–102, 1951.
14. Lisman SR, Shepherd NJ, Rosenberg M: A modified laryngoscope blade for dental protection. *Anesthesiology* 55:190, 1981.
15. Pope ES: Left handed laryngoscope. *Anaesthesia* 15:326–328, 1960.
16. McComish PB: Left sided laryngoscopes. *Anaesthesia* 20:372, 1965.
17. Lagade MRG, Poppers PJ: Use of the left-entry laryngoscope blade in patients with right-sided oro-facial lesions. *Anesthesiology* 58:300, 1983.
18. Weeks DB: A new use of an old blade. *Anesthesiology* 10:200–201, 1974.
19. Lagade MRG, Poppers PJ: Revival of the polio laryngoscope blade. *Anesthesiology* 57:545, 1982.
20. Bizarri DV, Guffrida JG: Improved laryngoscope blade designed for ease of manipulation and reduction of trauma. *Anesth Analg* 37:231–232, 1958.
21. Miller RA: A new laryngoscope. *Anesthesiology* 2:317–320, 1941.
22. Portzer M, Wasmuth CE: Endotracheal anesthesia using a modified Wis-Foregger laryngoscope blade. *Cleve Clin Q* 26:140–143, 1959.
23. Schapira M: A modified straight laryngoscope blade designed to facilitate endotracheal intubation. *Anesth Analg* 52:553–554, 1973.
24. Snow JC: Modification of laryngoscope blade. *Anesthesiology* 23:394, 1962.
25. Flagg P: Exposure and illumination of the pharynx and larynx by the general practitioner. A new laryngoscope designed to simplify the technique. *Arch Laryngol* 8:716–717, 1928.
26. Seward EH: Laryngoscope for resuscitation of the newborn. *Lancet* 2:1041, 1957.
27. Robertshaw FL: A new laryngoscope for infants and children. *Lancet* 2:1034, 1962.
28. Bryce-Smith R: A laryngoscope blade for infants. *Br Med J* 1:217, 1952.
29. Todres ID, Crone RK: Experience with a modified laryngoscope in sick infants. *Crit Care Med* 9:544–545, 1981.
30. Wung J, Stark RI, Indyk L, Driscoll JM: Oxygen supplement during endotracheal intubation of the infant. *Pediatrics* 59:1046–1048, 1977.
31. Hencz P: Modified laryngoscope for endotracheal intubation of neonates. *Anesthesiology* 53:84, 1980.
32. Cork RC, Woods W, Vaughn RW, Harris T: Oxygen supplementation during endotracheal intubation. *Anesthesiology* 51:186, 1979.
33. Siker ES: A mirror laryngoscope. *Anesthesiology* 17:38–42, 1956.
34. Huffman J: The application of prisms to curved laryngoscopes: a preliminary study. *J Am Assoc Nurse Anesthetists* 35:138–139, 1968.
35. Huffman J, Elam JO: Prisms and fiber optics for laryngoscopy. *Anesth Analg* 50:64–67, 1971.
36. Huffman J: The development of optical prism instruments to view and study the human larynx. *J Am Assoc Nurse Anesthetists* 38:197–202, 1970.
37. Murphy P: A fiber-optic endoscope used for nasal intubation. *Anaesthesia* 22:489–491, 1967.
38. Murphy P: The fiberoptic laryngoscope. *Anesthesiol Rev* 8:23–27, 1981.
39. Stiles CM, Stiles QR, Denson JS: A flexible fiber optic laryngoscope. *JAMA* 221:1246–1247, 1972.
40. Whitehouse AC, Klock L: Evaluation of endotracheal tube position with the fiberoptic intubation laryngoscope. *Chest* 68:848, 1975.
41. Watson CB: Fiberoptic bronchoscopy for anesthesia. *Anesthesiol Rev* 9:17–26, 1982.
42. Ovassapian A, Yelich SJ, Dykes MHM: Blood pressure and heart rate changes during awake fiberoptic nasotracheal intubation. *Anesth Analg* 62:278, 1983.
43. Boulton TB, Cole P: Anaesthesia in difficult situations. *Anaesthesia* 21:379–399, 1966.
44. Salem MR, Mathrubhugham M, Bennett EJ: Difficult intubation. *N Engl J Med* 296:879–881, 1976.
45. Ament R: A systemic approach to the difficult intubation. *Anesthesiol Rev* 5:12–16, 1978.
46. Moynihan P: Modification of pediatric laryngoscope. *Anesthesiology* 56:330, 1982.
47. Raj PP, Forestner J, Watson TD, Morris RB, Jenkins MT: Techniques for fiberoptic laryngoscopy in anesthesia. *Anesth Analg* 53:709–714, 1974.
48. Tahir AH: Use of fiberoptic endoscope in difficult orotracheal intubation. *Anesthesiol Rev* 3:16–18, 1976.
49. Triplett WW, Ondrey JS, McDonald JS: A case report. The use of the fiberoptic laryngoscope for nasotracheal intubation. *Anesth Prog* 26:49, 1979.
50. Wang JF, Reves JG, Corssen G: Use of the fiberoptic laryngoscope for difficult tracheal intubation. *Ala J Med Sci* 13:247–251, 1976.
51. Witton TH: An introduction to the fiberoptic laryngoscope. *Can Anaesth Soc J* 28:475–478, 1981.

52. Ovassapian A, Land P, Schaffer MF, Cerullo L, Zalkind MS: Anesthetic management for surgical corrections of severe flexion deformity of the cervical spine. *Anesthesiology* 58:370–372, 1983.

53. Patil V, Stehling LC, Zauder HL, Koch JP: Mechanical aids for fiberoptic endoscopy. *Anesthesiology* 57:69–70, 1982.

54. Lamb JD: Use of the fiberoptic laryngoscope. *Can Anaesth Soc J* 29:181, 1982.

55. Childres WF: New method for fiberoptic endotracheal intubation of anesthetized patients. *Anesthesiology* 55:595–596, 1981.

56. Wang JF: Fiberoptic laryngoscope guide and protector. *Anesth Analg* 56:126–127, 1977.

57. Wright BD, Lee T: Fiberoptics for difficult intubation. In *Current Reviews in Clinical Anesthesia*, vol 1, lesson 22, 1981.

58. Kraft M: Stylet laryngoscopy for oral tracheal intubation. *Anesthesiol Rev* 9:35–37, 1982.

59. Sellars SL, Gordon MA: A modification of the Kleinsasser laryngoscope. *Br J Anaesth* 43:730, 1971.

60. Teichner RL: Lingual nerve injury: a complication of orotracheal intubation. *Br J Anaesth* 43:413–414, 1971.

61. Stauffer JL, Silvestri RC: Complications of endotracheal intubation, tracheostomy, and artificial airways. *Resp Care* 27:417–434, 1982.

62. Fisher TL: Teeth—and the anesthetist. *Can Med Assoc J* 106:602–603, 1972.

63. Nique TA, Bennett CR, Altop H: Laryngoscope modification to avoid trauma due to laryngoscopy.

Anesth Prog 29:47–49, 1982.

64. Blank VF, Trembley NAG: The complications of tracheal intubation: a new classification with a review of the literature. *Anesth Analg* 53:202–213, 1974.

65. Rosenberg M, Bolgla J: Protection of teeth and gums during endotracheal intubation. *Anesth Analg* 47:34–36, 1968.

66. Henry PJ: Mouth guards in general anaesthesia. *Med J Aust* 1:911–912, 1969.

67. Davis FO, DeFreece AB, Shroff PF: Custom-made plastic guards for tooth protection during endoscopy and orotracheal intubation. *Anesth Analg* 50:203–206, 1971.

68. Anonymous: Protector for upper teeth. *J Am Assoc Nurse Anesthetists* 17:266, 1949.

69. Agosti L: A dental protector. *Br J Anaesth* 39:895–896, 1967.

70. Hallam J: A mouth-shield for use with the bronchoscope or laryngoscope. *Br Med J* 2:571, 1948.

71. Evers W, Racz GB, Glazer J, Dobkin AB: Orahesive as a protection for the teeth during general anaesthesia and endoscopy. *Can Anaesth Soc J* 14:123–128, 1967.

72. Siek GW, Bjorkman LL: Missed pharyngeal foreign body. *JAMA* 239:722, 1978.

73. Perel A, Katz E, Davidson JT: Fiberbronchoscopic retrieval of an aspirated laryngoscope bulb. *Intensive Care Med* 7:143–144, 1981.

74. Toung TJK, Donham RT, Shipley R: Thermal burn caused by a laryngoscope. *Anesthesiology* 55:184–185, 1981.

CHAPTER 13

Endotracheal Tubes

The endotracheal tube (tracheal tube, intratracheal tube, or catheter) is one of the anesthesiologist's most important tools. Use of endotracheal tubes both inside and outside the operating room has increased steadily over the years. Although endotracheal tubes have saved many lives and made many operations which could not have been performed without them possible, they have caused a number of problems. A thorough understanding of this equipment and its hazards is essential for its safe use.

GENERAL PRINCIPLES

Resistance

FACTORS

Internal Diameter

The most important single factor in resistance associated with the endotracheal tube is the internal diameter of the tube and its connector (1). A tube with a thick wall will offer more resistance than a similar thin-walled model of the same outer diameter (2). Resistance will increase if an object such as a suction catheter or flexible bronchoscope is passed through the endotracheal tube, since this has the effect of decreasing the size of the lumen (3). Kinking also increases resistance (4).

Length

Decreasing the length decreases the resistance, but the magnitude of the effect is less than that of internal diameter. Disposable tubes are usually supplied longer than needed. These should be cut to a suitable length either before or after intubation to reduce resistance.

Configuration

Curved connectors exhibit more resistance than straight ones (5). The resistance increases with greater curvature. Abrupt changes in direction will increase resistance. A gently curved connector will have less resistance than a right-angled one. Internal smoothness also keeps resistance low.

In summary, to keep resistance to a minimum, (a) use the widest thin-walled endotracheal tube that will fit the larynx. It should, however, be kept in mind that use of too large a tube will result in increased laryngeal damage; (b) avoid using tubes which are likely to kink; (c) avoid excessively long tubes (but do not cut tubes too short because resistance cannot be greatly altered by this means); (d) use a straight connector if possible. Failing this, a gently curved connector is preferable to a right-angled one.

CLINICAL SIGNIFICANCE

Resistance is more important to the spontaneously breathing patient than one being artificially ventilated, when the added work is supplied by the ventilator or the anesthesiologist's hand. Excessively high resistance will markedly increase the work of respiration and may lead to hypoventilation. The spontaneously breathing patient will have to generate greater pressure gradients between his alveoli and the atmosphere. The alterations in alveolar pressure may have adverse effects on the cardiovascular system.

A review of recent literature shows conflicting results on the change in resistance to respiration in adults caused by endotracheal intubation. It is felt by some that use of an 8-mm endotracheal tube in adults may offer less resistance than that found in the upper airway if flow rates are not excessive (6). Other authors dispute this contention, citing the increased difficulty in weaning patients from respiratory support as evidence that endotracheal tube resistance is significant (7–9). There is evidence that the presence of an endotracheal tube stimulates reflex bronchoconstriction of the airways (10). A review of the effects of intubation on resistance to respiration in infants also yields conflicting results (1, 5, 11).

Dead Space

The endotracheal tube and connector constitute mechanical dead space, which was discussed in Chapter 5. Inasmuch as the volume of an endotracheal tube and its connector is usually less than that of the natural passages, dead space is usually reduced by intubation. In pediatrics, however, long tubes and connectors may increase the dead space beyond that normally present.

Substances Used in Endotracheal Tubes

The material from which an endotracheal tube is composed should have the following characteristics (12, 13): (a) low cost; (b) lack of toxicity; (c) transparency; (d) ease of sterilization and durability with repeated sterilizations (unless disposable); (e) nonflammability; (f) a slippery, smooth, nonwettable surface inside and outside to prevent secretion buildup, allow easy passage of a suction catheter or bronchoscope, and prevent trauma; (g) sufficient body to maintain its shape during insertion and prevent occlusion by torsion or kinking or compression by the cuff or external pressure; (h) sufficient strength to allow thin wall construction; (i) thermoplasticity to conform to the patient's anatomy when in place; and (j) nonreactivity with lubricants and anesthetic agents.

To date no substance has been found that will meet all of the above requirements. The objections to various properties of materials have led researchers to test newer materials. This section will describe some of the substances which have been used for endotracheal tubes and some of the problems encountered.

REACTIONS OF TISSUES TO ENDOTRACHEAL TUBES

Two types of reactions to endotracheal tubes by tissues should be considered: chemical and physical.

Chemical Reactions

Chemical reactions are caused by reaction of the body with the material of the tube or a substance leached from the tube into the tissues. Such reactions result in local cell death or an inflammatory reaction. They may also produce systemic symptoms. The actual manifestations of toxicity may be quite varied, depending among other things on the length of time a tube is left in place. A tube that causes mild soreness when used for a few hours may cause severe damage when used for several days.

Tissue Testing. In order to ensure the safety of a tube for use in the body, the finished tube (not the material of which it is formulated) should be subjected to tissue testing before use.

A commonly used method is that of *tissue implantation testing* (14). The tube material is cut into strips and implanted in an animal. A known positive and known negative are also implanted as controls. After a period of time, the animal is sacrificed and the implantation sites examined for evidence of tissue damage.

Another direct test is *cell culture testing* (14). Cell systems which form a monolayer under an agar layer are stained with a vital dye which is taken up by living cells but released by dead cells. A sample of the material to be tested is placed on the agar surface and incubated. Toxic materials diffuse through the agar and the cells die.

In *polymer extract testing* solvents are used to extract substances from the material. The extract is then evaluated by several methods: (a) cell culture testing; (b) administration of the extract intravenously or intraperitoneally to an animal and observing the animal; and (c) injecting the solvent intradermally and observing the injection site.

Sterility, pyrogen testing and long-term implantation to detect latent toxicity and carcinogenic activity are also performed.

Physical Reactions

Numerous studies have shown that high pressures exerted by some cuffs on the tracheal wall are responsible for serious tracheal wall damage with prolonged intubation. In addition, the surface characteristics of the cuff may be an important contributing factor in producing damage (15).

SPECIFIC SUBSTANCES

Rubber

Rubber was among the first substances used for endotracheal tubes, and endotracheal anesthesia as it is known today developed through the use of rubber endotracheal tubes. Rubber endotracheal tubes are still in widespread, although declining, use.

Rubber occurs naturally, but can also be manufactured synthetically. Numerous substances may be added to change its characteristics (16), so there is great variety in its properties.

Rubber tubes have poor resistance to kinking. They tend to become clogged by inspissated secretions more easily than plastic tubes. They do not conform to body contours well. They are deteriorated by oil- and petroleum-based lubricants and heat sterilization.

Some rubber tubes have been found to elicit a toxic response (17). Most manufacturers are currently attempting to have their products meet tissue implantation tests. When the manufacturer places "I.T." on the tube, this indicates that the product has been tested and found nontoxic. The letters "Z-79" carry the same significance.

Silicone

Silicone (polysiloxane) is a special type of synthetic rubber. "Medical grade silicone" describes a specific silicone rubber manufactured under rigidly controlled conditions (18). Medical grade silicone rubber has gained wide acceptance for prosthetic devices due to a lack of tissue reactions (16).

Silicone rubbers can be autoclaved, do not deteriorate, are not attacked by the body, do not stick to tissues, are not wetted by fluids, have relatively slick surfaces that reduce the possibility of blockage by secretions and are not attacked by the body to any great extent (18). In thousands of medical applications there have been few reports of adverse reactions to medical grade silicone rubber (18), but it should be emphasized that only medical grade silicone rubber can be used without provoking tissue reaction (19).

Teflon

Teflon is the trade name for a class of plastic materials called polytetrafluoroethylenes. Medical Teflon is essentially a pure polymer with no significant additives (18, 20) and is quite expensive.

Teflon has a slippery, nonwettable, nonadhesive surface (18). It can be sterilized by boiling or autoclaving. It evokes minimal tissue reaction in patients. Teflon endotracheal tubes are rigid, however, and tend to irritate tissues by rubbing (18, 20).

Polyethylene

Polyethylene is the generic name for a poly-

mer made from the monomer ethylene (20, 21). Polymerization is performed under a variety of conditions to produce polymers with different properties, the most important of which is density. Low-density polyethylene is flexible, but has a great tendency to kink. For this reason, most polyethylene tubes are medium or high density. Unfortunately, these tend to be rigid (20).

Most tissue reactions elicited by polyethylene tracheal tubes have been due to their rigidity (20). Tissue reactions due to impurities have been noted, but most polyethylene samples designed for medical applications have not caused adverse tissue reactions (20).

Polyvinyl Chloride (PVC)

Polyvinyl chloride is formed from the monomer vinyl chloride. A variety of substances, including stabilizers, may be added to change the properties (20). The exact combination of additives is determined by the intended use.

Stabilizers have been the source of toxicity of PVC endotracheal tubes in the past. Among the stabilizers formerly used were highly necrotizing substances known as organotin compounds. Since a warning issued by the American Society of Anesthesiologists (22), most manufacturers have deleted organotin stabilizers from their formulations (18).

PVC is the most widely used substance for plastic endotracheal tubes at present. These tubes are soft and not irritating to the tracheal mucosa. They have little tendency to kink (23). At body temperatures, they tend to mold to the curves of the upper airway. They present a smooth surface that makes passage of a suction catheter or bronchoscope easy.

PVC tracheal tubes are intended for single use. In an attempt to reduce costs, many hospitals reuse disposable PVC tubes. Because the polyvinyl chloride is thromolabile, gas sterilization is most widely used. This has the potential of causing serious toxic reactions to ethylene oxide and its reaction products. The manufacturer's instructions for cleaning and sterilization should always be followed. Tubes marked "disposable," "DO NOT REUSE," and "SINGLE USE ONLY" should not be reused.

RECOMMENDATIONS

Many materials used in the manufacture of tracheal tubes have shown evidence of tissue toxicity. Fortunately, most manufacturers now subject their products to tissue testing. The marking "IT" or "Z-79" on a tube is evidence that the tube material has been tested and no evidence of toxicity has been found. Use of such tubes is preferable.

THE TRACHEAL TUBE

The tracheal tube (endotracheal tube, intratracheal tube or catheter) is inserted through the larynx into the trachea and is used to convey gases and vapor to and from the trachea. An orotracheal tube is one designed to be inserted through the mouth into the trachea. A nasotracheal tube is designed to be inserted through the nose.

The Tube

DESCRIPTION

A typical tracheal tube is shown in Figure 13.1.

The tracheal tube standard (24) specifies a radius of curvature from 12 to 16 cm and the curves of most tubes fall within this range. The patient end of the tube may be straight. In cross-section the tube's internal and external walls should be circular. A tube whose lumen is not perfectly round but is oval or elliptical in shape is more prone to kinking.

The machine end (proximal end) receives the connector and projects from the patient. It should be possible (and is usually necessary when received from the manufacturer) to shorten this end to adjust the tube length.

The patient end (tracheal end, distal end) is inserted into the patient's trachea. It has a slanted portion called the bevel. The angle of the bevel is the angle between the bevel and the longitudinal axis of the tracheal tube.

The tracheal tube standard specifies a bevel of 38 ± 8 degrees (24). In practice bevel angles vary from 39 to 56 degrees (25). A longer bevel (smaller angle) may facilitate passage through the nares, but it increases the risk of occlusion. The opening of the bevel faces left when viewing the tube from its concave aspect. This is because most anesthesiologists are right handed and introduce the tube from the right. Having the bevel facing left facilitates visualization of the larynx as the tube is being inserted.

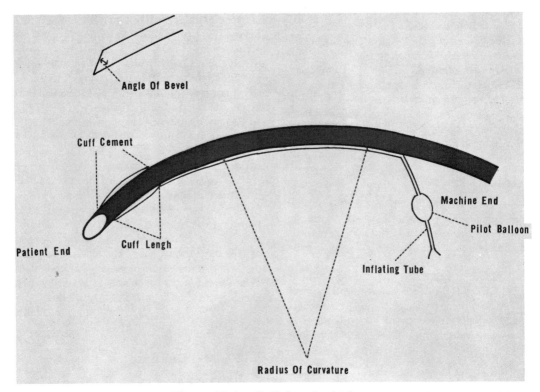

Figure 13.1.   Cuffed tracheal tube.

The tip should be rounded with no sharp points or edges. The tube shown in Figure 13.1 is commonly known as a Magill or Magill type tube. Figure 13.2 shows a tube with a hole through the tube wall near the patient end on the side opposite to the bevel. This hole is known as a Murphy eye (26) and tubes with this eye are called Murphy or Murphy type tracheal tubes. The purpose of the eye is to allow gas to pass if the bevel is occluded.

Frequently a radiopaque marker is placed at the tip or along the length of the tube to aid in determination of tube tip position after intubation.

SPECIAL TUBES

There are many tubes available. Most are familiar to the majority of anesthesiologists and do not require any special descriptions. A few have particular characteristics or purposes which deserve mention.

Cole Tube (27, 28)

The Cole tube is shown in Figure 13.3. It was designed for pediatric patients. The patient end has a smaller bore and is inserted between the vocal cords and into the trachea. The larger machine end segment has a wider bore. Cole

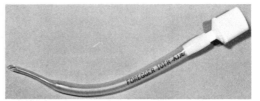

Figure 13.3. The Cole endotracheal tube.

tubes are sized according to the internal diameter of the intratracheal portion.

The flared portion near the tip provides some protection against endobronchial intubation. The tube should not, however, be inserted so far that the widened portion contacts the larynx because this will result in pressure on, and possibly dilatation of, the larynx.

Various investigators have found that the resistance offered by the Cole tube is less than that of comparable tubes of constant lumen (5, 29). Other authors have found that resistance to breathing is increased (30). The wide bore section has been found to increase dead space, but this is felt to be insignificant (29).

One disadvantage of the Cole tube is that it cannot be used nasally because the larger segment cannot pass through the infant's nares. Laryngeal dilatation has been reported with prolonged use (31).

Lindholm Tube (32)

The Lindholm endotracheal tube (Fig. 13.4) is preshaped to conform to the anatomical contours of the airway. Conventional tubes exert pressure against the posterior wall of the larynx and the anterior wall of the trachea. By reshaping the tube to fit these areas and by the addition of a 90-degree curve in the oropharynx, pressure on these points is reduced and lesions are less pronounced (32).

In a study of short-term intubations it was found that the Lindholm tube was associated with a greater incidence of sore throat than standard tubes with comparable cuffs (33). It was postulated that the greater area of contact of the tube with the mucosa might be responsible.

RAE Preformed Tracheal Tube (34)

The RAE tracheal tube is preshaped to conform to the hypopharynx and reduce posterior laryngeal pressure. There is a bend in the part of the tube that remains external to the patient.

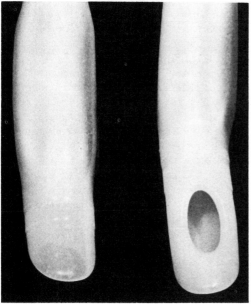

Figure 13.2. Tracheal tube tips. At *left*, Magill tube. At *right*, Murphy tube.

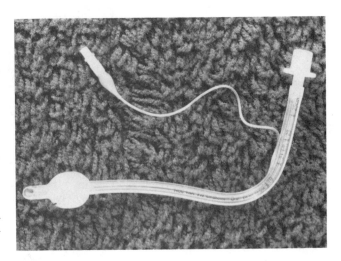

Figure 13.4. Lindholm endotracheal tube with a high-volume, low-pressure cuff.

If suctioning is desired, the curve can be straightened.

Two versions are available: one for nasal (Fig. 13.5A) and one for oral (Fig. 13.5B) use. The tube was designed for pediatric use but both the oral and nasal versions are available in adult sizes. Uncuffed versions have two ports at the tip, one on the bevel side and one on the opposite side. These are intended to provide for ventilation if the tube is advanced too far.

The oral model was designed for use during operations in the head region. It is bent at an acute angle to hold the tube in place and discourage inadvertent advancement into a bronchus. The tube is easily secured to the chin.

Tubes for nasal use are slightly longer and the preformed bend is opposite to the bend of the oral tubes so that the tube is directed over the patient's forehead. This curve helps to reduce pressure on the nares.

The linear dimensions of this tube from the bend to the distal end were determined by a series of experiments during which tubes were advanced into a main bronchus and then withdrawn until the tip entered the trachea. The maximal length to which the tube could be inserted without resulting in bronchial intubation was confirmed by x-ray and thus the appropriate length for each size tube was established. Since RAE tubes are designed to fit the average patient, users have found some tubes to be either too long or too short for certain patients. The instructions for use of RAE tubes include a statement cautioning the user to exercise special care in selecting the tube size and length.

Spiral Embedded (Flexometallic, Armored, Reinforced, Anode, Metal Spiral, Woven) Tubes

These tubes have a metal wire or nylon filament spiral embedded into the wall of the tube and covered both internally and externally with rubber, latex, or plastic (Fig. 13.6). The spiral does not extend to the distal and proximal ends.

The primary advantage of these tubes is resistance to kinking. They can withstand high external pressures without collapsing, although cases have been reported in which patients bit through the tube (35, 36). They tend to exert less pressure on the anterior trachea and interarytenoid area than other tubes. The portion of the tube outside the patient can be angled away from the surgical field.

Spiral embedded tubes are especially useful in situations where bending or compression of the tube is likely to occur, as in head or neck surgery. They are useful during laryngectomies for insertion into the tracheostomy stoma and for placement into a permanent tracheostomy.

There are a number of problems with spiral embedded tubes. Because some are floppy, forceps and/or a stylet will usually be needed for insertion. The tube may rotate on the stylet, making insertion difficult. The lack of rigidity makes use of forceps difficult. The bevel at the distal end is especially difficult to control because this area is not reinforced. Insertion through the nose is difficult and sometimes impossible. If the head is turned or the jaw moved up or down, the tip may move back between the

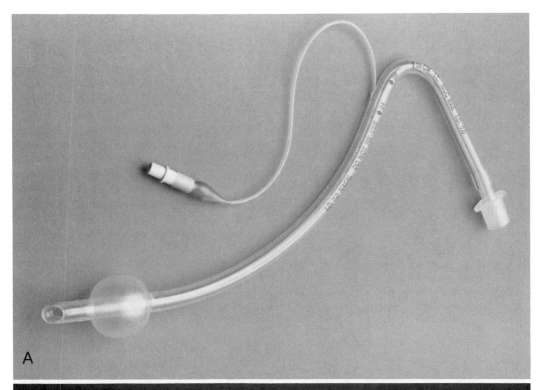

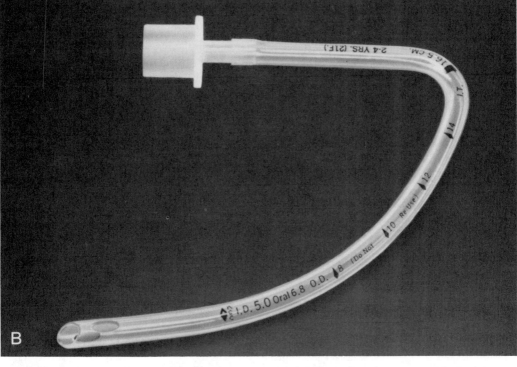

Figure 13.5. *A*, RAE nasal tracheal tube. This is the adult version fitted with a low-pressure cuff. *B*, RAE endotracheal tube, oral version. The uncuffed version has two ports at the tip, one on the bevel side and one on the opposite side. (Courtesy of NCC Division, Mallinckrodt, Inc.)

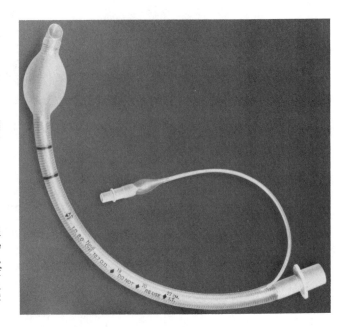

Figure 13.6. Spiral embedded endotracheal tube. This disposable tube is fitted with a high-volume, low-pressure cuff. The free end of the inflating tube is fitted with an inflating valve. (Courtesy of NCC Division, Mallinckrodt, Inc.)

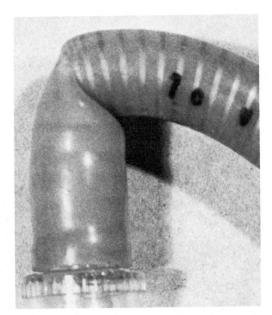

Figure 13.7. Kinking of spiral embedded tube.

vocal cords and slip out of the trachea. Because of the spiral these tubes cannot be shortened.

At either end where the layers of rubber or plastic do not enclose the coils, a possibility of obstruction exists. The soft patient end bevel can be easily pushed against the wall of the trachea or invaginated into the tube (37). Kinking can occur at the patient end if the connector

is not pushed down into the spiral (Fig. 13.7). On some tubes the connector is sealed against the reinforcing coils, reducing the possibility that the inflating tube will be occluded at this point.

The inflating tube lies inside the lumen of some spiral embedded tubes and passes outside the tube proximal to the point where the spiral ends. If the connector is then pushed into the spiral to prevent kinking, it may pinch off the inflating tube between itself and the spiral (38–40). In this case, the cuff can neither be inflated nor deflated, although the pilot balloon will inflate and deflate (39–42). This can be corrected by making a small V-shaped notch in the connector at the point where the inflation tube passes outside (39), or using a tube on which the inflating tube is attached outside the tube (40).

High temperatures that occur during boiling or autoclaving can soften the spirals of the rubber and latex so that they tend to collapse where pressure is applied to them, i.e., beneath the cuff. When the cuff is inflated, the walls of the tube bulge inward, producing obstruction (43).

Herniation of the intramural inflating tube into the lumen (41) and folding of the inner wall around the connector (43, 44) have been reported.

Rubber and latex tubes are manufactured by dipping the spiral repeatedly in solution. Air bubbles may form within the wall between the layers. During anesthesia nitrous oxide will diffuse into these bubbles causing them to expand (45–47). Tube obstruction or inability to deflate the cuff could result (48–50). This problem has not been reported with silicone or polyvinyl chloride tubes.

Latex or rubber spiral embedded tubes should not be gas-autoclaved or steam-sterilized with vacuum (51). Ethylene oxide can permeate between the layers, causing blistering and separation. The layers may also separate under vacuum. Such separations are usually invisible. During anesthesia, gases will diffuse into these areas and may cause obstruction. Manufacturers of silicone-reinforced tubes claim their tubes can be steam- or gas-sterilized without hazard.

Carden Bronchoscopy Tube

This tube is specially designed for fiberoptic bronchoscopy. The machine end is of a larger diameter than the patient end. The tube is sized by the internal diameter at the patient end. Because the diameter of the machine end is larger, the increase in resistance caused by passage of the bronchoscope is lessened. The Carden bronchoscopy tube is made of silastic and is autoclavable and reusable. A swivel adapter with a port for the bronchoscope is supplied with the tube.

Endotrol Tracheal Tube (NCC Division, Mallinckrodt, Inc.)

This tube (Fig. 13.8) provides tip control via an operator-activated ring loop. The thumb of the hand is placed against the connector and the index finger inserted into the ring loop. Pulling on the ring decreases the radius of the tube via a cable-like mechanism so that the tip moves anteriorly.

Hi-Low Jet Tracheal Tube

The Hi-Lo Jet tracheal tube (Fig. 13.9) has three lumens. The main lumen is for ventilation of the patient. The second is clear and is used for jet ventilation and administration of oxygen during suctioning and bronchoscopy. The third lumen is opaque and is used for irrigation and sampling of gases from the trachea. This lumen can be used for monitoring end-expired carbon dioxide with a withdrawal-type capnometer.

Laser-Shield Tracheal Tube

Most rubber and plastic tubes can be ignited by the laser beam used for microsurgery of the larynx. This may result in laryngeal damage. To combat this, metal tubes have been developed, but they tend to be traumatic to tissues.

The laser-shield tube (Fig. 13.10) is made of silicone impregnated with metal particles which covers the main shaft and the cuff. It is designed to withstand several impacts at the same point from a laser beam. It is recommended that the cuff be inflated with sterile saline.

TUBE SIZE

Several methods have been used in the past to size tracheal tubes. The French scale, which multiplied the external diameter in millimeters by 3, was one of the most common. Current standards designate tracheal tube size by the internal diameter in millimeters (24, 52). Most manufacturers now use this method. Often they also indicate the French scale size in catalogs and packages for those not accustomed to using the internal diameter.

Because of variations in wall thickness, tubes having the same internal diameter may have

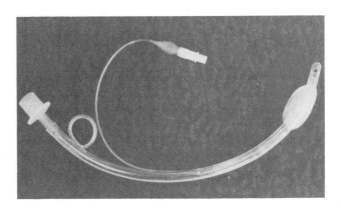

Figure 13.8. Endotrol tracheal tube. The ring is attached to the tip by a cable-like mechanism which allows the tip to be maneuvered.

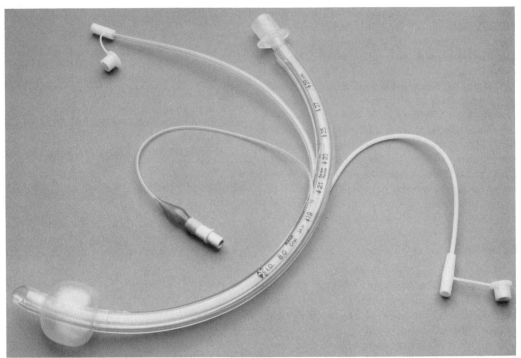

Figure 13.9. Hi-Lo Jet tracheal tube. In addition to the main lumen there are lumens for inflating the cuff, jet ventilation, and irrigation or gas sampling. (Courtesy of NCC Division, Mallinckrodt, Inc.)

quite different external diameters (25, 53, 54). The outside diameter is important, especially in children, because this is what must pass through the larynx and into the trachea. Accordingly, the tracheal tube standard specifies that tubes 6.0 and smaller show the external diameter in millimeters. Many manufacturers also mark this on larger tubes.

The choice of tube size must be a compromise among various considerations. From the standpoint of resistance, the largest tube possible should be used. Larger tubes are also associated with less risk of occlusion. However, large tubes increase the risk of excessive pressure on the larynx or trachea. Tubes of smaller diameter are easier to insert and may require a smaller reshaping force to adapt to the anatomical contours of the patient's airway (55).

Before intubation, the anesthesiologist must choose the size of endotracheal tube that he feels will be appropriate. It is important, especially in children, to be able to predict the appropriate sized tube for a patient in order to avoid trauma from trying to insert too large a tube or from reintubation if the tube is too small.

Because of anatomical variations, the optimum tube size cannot always be determined before intubation. The anesthesiologist should always have three tubes readily available: one selected by whatever method he uses, one larger, and one smaller. The correct size can then be determined by actual intubation.

In adults, an airtight fit is achieved by use of an inflatable cuff, so cuff size, not internal tube diameter, should be used to determine the best fit within the trachea (56). Ideally cuff circumference should equal tracheal lumen circumference (57). Too small a tube will lead to overinflation of the cuff, which will result in excessive cuff-tracheal wall pressure. Underinflation of too large a cuff may result in aspiration along the folds of excess cuff material and possibly tracheal erosion from the tip of the tube (57).

There is great variation in sizes and shapes of tracheas in adults (56). Subglottic transverse dimensions increase with age and tracheal dimensions are usually smaller in females, but in general correlation between age, race, height, weight, body surface area, and tracheal shape or size is poor (56, 57).

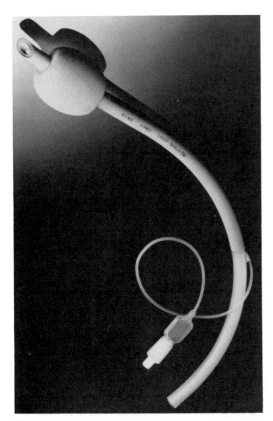

Figure 13.10. Laser-Shield endotracheal tube. (Courtesy of Xomed.)

The following recommendations should be regarded as only general guidelines for selection of tracheal tubes in adults:

Orotracheal tubes: 7.0 ID females
8.0 ID males
Nasotracheal tubes: 7.0 ID males and
females (58).

If prolonged intubation is planned, the tube should be selected on the basis of ability to achieve a cuff-to-tracheal wall pressure of 20–25 torr (25–34 cm H_2O) (92).

In children an airtight seal is achieved not by means of a cuff but by selection of the correct size of an uncuffed tube to fit the cricoid ring. There is considerable variation in subglottic size in children (59, 60).

The tube should pass easily through the larynx and should never be forced. If a tube will not gently pass the larynx, a smaller size should be tried. For prolonged intubation in children, a tube smaller than that which completely occludes the airway should be chosen. Most work-

ers feel that the tube fit is correct if a small amount of gas is heard issuing from between the tube and the trachea when 10–30 cm H_2O positive pressure is applied (61–63).

A simple formula estimating tube size for children is the following: over 6.5 years, 4.5 + age in years ÷ 4; under 6.5 years, 3.5 + age in years ÷ 3 (64, 65). In prematures the following formula has been suggested: gestational age (weeks) ÷ 10 + 0.5 (66). A simpler method is to choose a tube whose external diameter is the same width as the distal phalanx of the patient's little finger (67, 68). Another method is to use a tube the same size as the patient's ring finger.

Smaller tubes should be selected in patients with airways disease such as croup and epiglottitis (62, 69). The tube should permit adequate ventilation and suction; otherwise a tracheostomy should be performed (69).

TUBE LENGTH

Estimation of the proper length of a tube is a vexing problem. Use of too long a tube may result in increased dead space, increased likelihood of kinking in the portion external to the patient, and endobronchial intubation or impingement on the carina. Use of too short a tube may result in accidental extubation or pressure by the cuff on laryngeal structures.

Many formulas and tables to estimate the proper length of endotracheal tubes have been proposed (70–75), but none is totally satisfactory. Tube length must be tailored to the individual patient. Tubes for nasal intubation must be longer than those passed orally.

After intubation proper placement should be judged by bilateral auscultation of the peripheral lung fields and observation for symmetrical chest movement. Inflation and deflation of the cuff with palpation in the suprasternal notch may be helpful (76, 77). Whenever any doubt exists, correct placement should be confirmed by chest x-ray and/or use of a fiberoptic laryngoscope or bronchoscope (78, 79). Most workers feel that the tip of the tube should be in the middle third of the trachea with the head in a neutral position (midway between full extension and full flexion) (80, 81).

After confirmation of correct placement of the tip, the portion external to the patient should be reduced to prevent kinking. Most disposable endotracheal tubes are supplied longer than necessary so that they can be cut to the desired length after intubation (82).

TUBE MARKINGS

Typical endotracheal tube markings are shown in Figures 13.5, 13.6, and 13.9. They are situated on the beveled side of the tube above the cuff and read from the patient end to the machine end. They frequently include the following: (a) the words "ORAL" or "NASAL" or "ORAL/NASAL"; (b) tube size; (c) the external diameter; (d) the manufacturer's name or trademark (the name or trademark of the supplier may also be present); (e) "Z-79" to designate those tubes which comply with the tracheal tube standard. The terms "IT" and "Z-79/IT" have been used in the past to designate tubes which have passed tissue toxicity tests; (f) country of origin; (g) length (depth) markings in centimeters measured from the patient end; and (h) a cautionary note such as "DO NOT REUSE" or "SINGLE USE ONLY" if the tube is disposable.

Cuff Systems

A cuff system includes an optional inflating valve, an inflating lumen in the wall of the tube, an external inflation tube, an optional pilot balloon, and the cuff itself. The purpose of the cuff system is to provide a seal between the endotracheal tube and the tracheal wall to prevent or minimize leakage of gases, liquids or foreign material into or out of the trachea around the tube.

INFLATING VALVE

An inflating valve, when present, is attached to the free end of the inflating tube (Fig. 13.6). Its purpose is to prevent loss of air from the cuff system after the cuff is inflated. It has a female fitting for receiving a syringe. When a syringe is inserted into the valve, a plunger is displaced from its seat and air can be injected into the cuff. Upon removal of the syringe the valve seals and air cannot escape unless a syringe is reinserted and the air deliberately removed.

INFLATING TUBE

The inflating tube (cuff tube, pilot tube, or line) is external to the tube and attached to the tracheal tube. Its free end is fitted either with an inflating valve or a female fitting capable of accepting a standard Luer's syringe, in which case retention of air in the cuff is accomplished by placing a plug in the free end or by application of a clamp to the inflating tube.

On tubes which have embedded spirals, the inflating tube may connect to the inflating lumen just above the first spiral ring. If the connector is inserted into the tube far enough to contact the first spiral (which is desirable to prevent kinking at that point), it may impinge on the inflating tube, preventing inflation or deflation of the cuff (39, 40, 42). This can be remedied by cutting a small V in the connector and making certain that the inflating tube passes through the V. Most tubes presently available have the inflating tube outside the spirals to prevent this problem. Kinks and a crushed lumen from a clamp are other possible causes of obstruction to the inflating tube.

PILOT BALLOON

The pilot balloon (bulb) is located near the midpoint of the inflating tube or adjacent to the inflating valve. Its purpose is to give an indication of the state of inflation or deflation of the cuff.

The McGinnis balloon system (83, 84) available on certain tubes, consists of a specially designed very compliant pilot balloon inside a confining sheath with an automatic pressure-regulating valve interposed between it and the cuff. The pilot balloon serves as an indication of inflation, as an external reservoir for the cuff, and as a pressure-limiting device. It is designed to maintain an intracuff pressure of 20–25 torr at end expiration while preventing overinflation of the cuff. It also compensates automatically through the pressure control valve for increases in cuff volume and pressure caused by diffusion of nitrous oxide and other gases into the cuff (85, 86).

As air is injected, both the cuff and the balloon will be inflated in parallel. When the balloon has achieved a stretched appearance, a pressure of approximately 20–25 torr will be present in the cuff. As inflation continues, the pilot balloon fills preferentially. The intraballoon pressure remains constant and is not increased until it strikes the confining sheath. Should the trachea expand, air will flow from the balloon to the cuff. The pressure-regulating valve protects against rapid loss of cuff volume into the balloon during inhalation.

The McGinnis balloon has been found by several authors to be effective in keeping lateral tracheal wall pressure low (85, 87–89). One group of investigators found that to go from the point of tracheal occlusion to an unsafe cuff pressure required 45 ml of additional air and the pilot balloon had to be overdistended to reach a cuff pressure above 30 torr (88). Use of it eliminates the need to measure cuff pressure. However, if the patient happens to lie on the balloon or if it is compressed inadvertently by personnel, the intracuff pressure will rise (90).

INFLATING LUMEN

The inflating lumen connects the inflating tube to the cuff. It may be located either on the concave side of the endotracheal tube or within the wall of the tube.

CUFF

The cuff is an inflatable sleeve near the patient end of an endotracheal tube. Its purpose is to prevent aspiration of materials into the trachea while allowing positive pressure to be applied to the lungs. The cuff also serves to center the tube in the trachea so that the tip does not cause trauma to the mucosa.

Cuffs are usually made of the same material as the endotracheal tube. If of a different mate-rial, however, they are subject to the same tissue testing requirements as the plastic in the tube itself.

There are a large number of different cuffs available, but they can be generally classified into two categories according to their pressure-volume characteristics. Table 13.1 summarizes most of the important differences between these two types.

High-Pressure Cuff (Small Resting Diameter Cuff; Low-Compliance, High-Pressure Cuff; Low Residual Volume Cuff; Low-Volume Cuff; Small Cuff; Standard or Conventional Cuff)

Until the early 1970s all cuffs were of this type. Their use has been decreasing, especially for prolonged intubation.

Characteristics. A high-pressure cuff has a small diameter at rest, a low residual volume, and a small area of contact with the trachea. It requires a high internal pressure to obtain a seal with the trachea. All of this pressure is not exerted on the tracheal wall, however. Because of its low residual volume, the cuff is stretched—to varying degrees—when the tracheal wall is

Table 13.1.
Characteristics of High Pressure and (Idealized) Low Pressure Cuffs (90)

	High Pressure	Low Pressure
Diameter at residual volume	Small	Large (ideally approximates tracheal diameter)
Residual volume	Small (3–6 ml)	Large (usually more than 30 cc)
Area of cuff in contact with trachea with seal	Small	Large
Cuff volume-pressure relationship before seal is achieved	Linear relationship between volume and pressure	No significant pressure until seal is approached
Intracuff pressure at seal	High	Low (less than 30 torr)
Pressure exerted by cuff laterally on tracheal wall	High	Low
Relationship between intracuff pressure and pressure exerted by cuff on tracheal wall	Intracuff pressure exceeds tracheal wall pressure	Equal
Cuff behavior in relation to trachea at seal	Cuff imposes its shape on the trachea, deforming it	Cuff tends to conform to shape of trachea
Rise in cuff pressure per unit volume after seal is achieved	Steep rise	Slow rise (90)
Change of cuff pressure with airway pressure	Some rise with a rise in airway pressure, but no linear relationship (91)	Intracuff pressure automatically cycles in synchrony with airway pressure when airway pressure exceeds intracuff pressure
Cuff wall	Thick, rigid	Thin, pliable

reached. The compliance of the cuff wall itself accounts for a part of the intracuff pressure. The pressure exerted laterally on the tracheal wall will be less than intracuff pressure. The lateral wall pressure exerted by such a cuff is difficult to ascertain but has been found to be well above mucosal perfusion pressure (91–95). Ischemic damage to the tracheal mucosa could be expected to result from its prolonged use. High cuff-to-tracheal wall pressure is considered to be a fundamental cause of tracheal injury following intubation, especially if it is prolonged.

With high-pressure cuffs, the cuff pressure and the lateral pressure on the tracheal wall increase sharply as increments of air are added to the cuff (90). For this reason, use of the largest intratracheal tube possible has been advocated, so that the cuff will be minimally inflated when a seal is created (93).

Another characteristic of these cuffs is that they tend to impose their shape upon the trachea (96).

Evaluation of High-Pressure Cuffs. The most serious problem associated with high-pressure cuffs is the risk of ischemic damage to the trachea. There can be no doubt that use of high-pressure cuffs for long-term intubation is associated with a higher incidence of complications following extubation than low-pressure cuffs.

It has been alleged that these cuffs are more likely to inflate eccentrically than low-pressure cuffs (97), but this has also been observed with large-volume cuffs (98).

These cuffs do offer some advantages over low-pressure cuffs, especially for short-term intubation. Because they are usually reusable, they are less expensive to use. They usually provide better visibility during intubation, and probably offer better protection against aspiration. Several investigators have reported a lower incidence of sore throats (33, 99–105).

It is clear that for long-term intubation, use of the high-pressure cuff should be abandoned in favor of a low-pressure cuff with a means to control cuff pressure. It has been suggested that low-pressure cuffs should always be used, even for short operations, but this opinion is not universal (106, 107). As will be discussed in the next section, there are numerous potential problems associated with the use of low-pressure cuffs.

The authors of this text feel that at the present time there is no convincing evidence that high-pressure cuffs are less desirable than low-pressure cuffs for short-term intraoperative pro-

cedures and that the exercise of clinical judgment in the choice of a cuff is appropriate. If one elects to use tubes with high-pressure cuffs, one should reintubate with a low-pressure cuff if extubation is delayed beyond the normally expected postoperative recovery. If one elects to use only low-pressure cuffs, it should be done with a sound understanding of their characteristics and a preparedness to use them in such a way as to ensure optimal performance (106).

Use of High-Pressure Cuffs. After a tube with a high-pressure cuff has been inserted, the cuff should be inflated with the minimal amount of gas that will cause it to seal against the trachea at peak inspiratory pressure. Inflating until the pilot balloon is tense and/or inflating beyond seal will result in unnecessarily high cuff volume and pressure.

Listening with the unaided ear will often miss small leaks. These can be detected by palpation or auscultation of the suprasternal pretracheal area (108, 109).

Nitrous oxide and other gases diffuse into air-inflated cuffs and increase volume and pressure unless the cuff-inflating tube is open to atmosphere (110–118). During extracorporeal circulation, cuff volume and pressure may drop (112). Therefore during general anesthesia intracuff volume and pressure should be periodically readjusted. Filling the cuff with the anesthetic mixture to be used is an alternate method for maintaining the intracuff pressure constant (119).

Low-Pressure Cuff (Large Resting Diameter Cuff; Large Residual Volume Cuff; Large Cuff; High-Volume Cuff; High-Compliance, Low-Pressure Cuff; Floppy Cuff)

Because of the complications caused by high cuff-to-tracheal wall pressures, low-pressure cuffs were developed. They first became available during the first half of the 1970s and their use has increased rapidly. With their use, the frequency of significant cuff-induced complications following prolonged intubation has decreased (93, 120–123).

Some of the original low-pressure cuffs were do-it-yourself prestretched modifications of high-pressure cuffs (124). Now a wide variety of low-pressure cuffs are available commercially.

Characteristics. Most of the important attributes of a low-pressure cuff are shown in Table 13.1. It has a large residual volume prior to inflation, a large diameter and a large area of contact with the trachea.

A significant advantage of these cuffs is that the intracuff pressure closely approximates that on the wall of the trachea until the cuff wall is stretched (95, 125–129). Monitoring the intracuff pressure, therefore, gives a good idea of the pressure exerted on the tracheal wall.

During exhalation the resting intracuff (and tracheal wall) pressure can be much lower than peak airway pressure and yet provide a seal (90).

Such a cuff is floppy and easily deformed. When placed in a trachea it is easily distorted and adapts itself to the irregular surface of the trachea (93). Tracheal deformation is not observed when airway pressure is low. As intracuff pressure rises the trachea is distorted to a circular cross section (130).

In comparison with high-pressure cuffs, inflation beyond seal causes a smaller increase in the tracheal wall pressure (90, 93, 97).

With low-pressure cuffs intracuff pressure varies during the ventilatory cycle. With controlled ventilation, when airway pressure exceeds intracuff pressure (during inspiration), a positive pressure will be applied to the front face of the cuff. If the cuff wall is pliable, it will be unable to resist this pressure and will move backward. This will compress the air in the cuff until intracuff pressure equals airway pressure. During the exhalation phase the intracuff pressure will decrease until the resting pressure is reached.

With spontaneous ventilation, intracuff pressure also responds to airway pressure, but in this case it is in a negative direction on inspiration and a positive direction on exhalation (130).

It is necessary for the walls of a low-pressure cuff to be as thin and pliable as possible to allow transmission of pressure.

Unfortunately some cuffs described as low-pressure by the manufacturer are too small to fill the average adult human trachea. A large resting diameter is crucial in allowing the cuff to seal in such a way that intracuff pressure equals the pressure exerted laterally on the tracheal wall. Once residual volume is exceeded, the cuff will act like a high-pressure cuff.

Other cuffs described as low pressure have a large diameter, but the cuff wall is thick and rigid. The thicker and more rigid the wall the more the cuff will act as a high-pressure type, even if the diameter is large.

Evaluation. The main advantage of soft cuffs is that they offer protection from cuff-induced complications following prolonged intubation.

Several problems have been found to be associated with the use of the low-pressure cuffs. The incidence of sore throat has been found to be greater than when high-pressure cuffs are used unless the cuff is specially designed so that the tracheal contact area is small (33, 99, 100, 103, 104). Increased post-extubation stridor of sufficient severity to necessitate reintubation and/or tracheostomy has been reported with use of these cuffs (131).

Aspiration past low-pressure cuffs has been reported (92, 132–135). Three causes have been suggested. The first is incorrect inflation. To prevent aspiration, the cuff pressure may need to be higher than that needed for "no leak" when positive pressure is applied (92, 133). Another cause is channeling along vertical folds in the cuff (136). This can be avoided by increasing the pressure in the cuff slightly, or by using a tube with a smaller cuff. A third suggested cause is spontaneous respiration. The dilatation of the trachea and negative pressure applied to the cuff during inspiration may allow passage of fluids around the cuff (134, 135, 137).

It may be more difficult to establish the point at which a seal is just achieved during spontaneous than positive pressure ventilation (130).

These cuffs may be more difficult to insert. Even when properly deflated, the cuff provides less visibility of the tube tip than a low volume cuff. A low pressure cuff is more friable and more likely to be torn on intubation (138). Forceps should not be used on the cuff. Trauma during insertion and withdrawal may be increased. Because they are more difficult to insert, use of a stylet may be more frequent and this may increase the likelihood of trauma during insertion (131). A large cuff tends to fold on itself when fully deflated and may form wedges that cause trauma during passage through the glottis.

There appears to be a greater likelihood of spontaneous dislocation (including extubation) with these cuffs, especially with oral intubation and positive pressure ventilation (139, 140).

It has been noted that it is relatively easy to pass esophageal devices such as temperature probes and nasoenteric tubes around low-pressure cuffs (141–145). This could result in serious complications if not recognized immediately.

With large residual volume cuffs there is an increased tendency to tracheal dilatation (146, 147) the long term significance of which is unclear (106).

One of the biggest problems with use of low

pressure cuffs stems from a lack of understanding by the user. There is widespread belief that simply using these cuffs will prevent high pressures from being exerted on the wall of the trachea. If a large residual volume cuff is overinflated, dangerously high pressure can develop (148, 149).

Mucosal damage can occur with the use of these cuffs, even if the pressure is controlled (107). In comparison to the damage produced with high-pressure cuffs, erosion of the tracheal mucosa is not as deep, but is spread over a greater length of the trachea.

Use. Before a low-pressure cuff is inserted or withdrawn, it must first be emptied with a syringe until a vacuum is produced. These cuffs will not empty if the inflating tube is simply opened to atmosphere. Gently squeezing and twisting the cuff in its sterile package may aid in evacuation of the air.

Proper inflation of a low-pressure cuff is difficult because of the blind nature of the procedure. When inflating conventional cuffs, there is a certain "feel" or pressure in the inflating syringe (93). There is no such "feel" or resistance encountered when properly inflating a low-pressure cuff and if such a cuff is inflated until a certain resistance is encountered, it will be grossly overinflated.

When an endotracheal tube with a McGinnis balloon system is used, the cuff should be inflated until a seal is achieved during peak inspiration. The pilot balloon should be distended but smaller than the confining sheath.

With other low-pressure cuffs, the intracuff pressure should be measured and adjusted approximately 10 min after the cuff has been inserted (98). This delay is necessary to allow for softening of the cuff material at body temperature and for the patient to become settled, since the volume necessary for occlusion will vary with the muscle tone and state of consciousness.

The pressure should be adjusted to approximately 20–30 torr (88, 92, 148–150). This should prevent aspiration while allowing mucosal perfusion and avoid problems associated with overinflated cuffs such as herniation over the tip and compression of the tube.

Cuff pressure should be measured and adjusted when airway pressure is lowest. During positive pressure ventilation this will be at end expiration when airway pressure is atmospheric. If a low pressure cuff is adjusted to the point of just abolishing audible leakage at peak inspira-

tory pressure, the resulting intracuff pressure may not be sufficient to prevent aspiration (92, 133, 136). If any spontaneous ventilation is to be allowed, airway pressure will be lowest at peak inspiration and cuff pressure should be adjusted at this point.

Specially designed manometers are available for measuring intracuff pressure, but any manometer is suitable if the method of simultaneously inflating the cuff and manometer using either a four-way stopcock or a Y-connector is followed (151). Pressure relief valves are commercially available and can be used to ensure that during inflation, intracuff pressure does not exceed the value determined by the valve. However, variability in these devices may limit their usefulness (152).

After the cuff pressure has been adjusted, one should check to make sure there is no leak at peak inspiration. If there is a leak, the cuff is probably too small for the trachea and a tube with a larger cuff should be tried (148). If a tube with a larger cuff also requires a pressure greater than 30 torr to achieve a seal, the problem may be that leakage is occurring along longitudinal folds in the cuff and a tube with a smaller cuff should be tried.

Cuff pressure should be measured and readjusted frequently. During anesthesia, cuff pressure tends to increase unless the cuff is inflated with the gas mixture to be used. Pressure relief devices which will "bleed" the cuff when the intracuff pressure rises above a set pressure have been devised (153, 154).

The McGinnis cuff pressure regulator (Fig. 13.11) is an accessory which can be used with low pressure cuffs to prevent high intracuff pressures during positive pressure ventilation. It consists of a valve which will limit the pressure in the cuff to 20 cm H_2O during exhalation. A tube attached to the tracheal connector transmits increases in pressure from the breathing system to the cuff. This raises the cuff pressure and prevents leaks.

At the termination of anesthesia, if the tube is to remain in the trachea, the cuff should be refilled with air and the intracuff pressure readjusted.

Frequent measurement and adjustment of cuff pressure during prolonged intubation is essential since cuff pressure tends to decrease with time (155). Cuff pressure may become excessive during ascent or loss of compression, such as may occur at higher altitudes (156). Correction

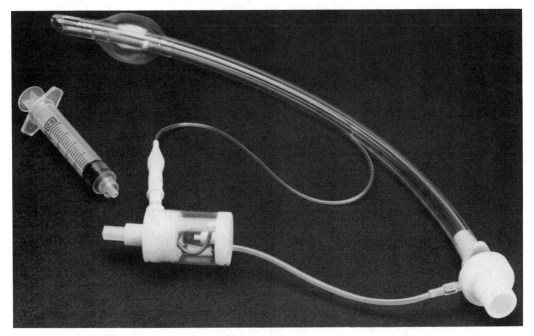

Figure 13.11. The McGinnis cuff pressure regulator. (Courtesy of Respironics, Inc.)

to the proper cuff pressure at higher altitudes may then result in insufficient seal pressure following return to ground level pressure.

Sponge Cuff (Fome Cuff, Kamen-Wilkinson Cuff)

Characteristics. The sponge cuff (157) has a large diameter and residual volume and large surface area. It is filled with polyurethane foam covered with a sheath.

Applying suction to the inflating tube causes the foam to contract. When the negative pressure is released, the cuff expands. The pressure inside the cuff will remain at atmospheric as long as the inflating tube is open to atmosphere. If the inflating tube is clamped, the cuff behaves like a low-pressure cuff.

When in place in the trachea, the degree of expansion of the foam determines the pressure exerted laterally on the tracheal wall. The more the foam is expanded, the lower the tracheal wall pressure. Thus the lateral wall pressure depends on the relationship between cuff diameter at residual volume and the diameter of the trachea. By design, the foam must be markedly compressed to exert a pressure greater than 25 torr (158). During the ventilatory cycle, the foam is alternately expanded and compressed.

Evaluation. The Foam-Cuff has been stud-ied by several workers (128, 159–161). It does provide a seal at a low tracheal wall pressure if the inflating tube is left unclamped and the relation between the cuff and tracheal diameters is optimal (90, 128, 157, 162). Tracheal dilatation has been reported to be less frequent with its use (146). Diffusion of anesthetic agents into the cuff can occur. This does not cause an increase in pressure if the inflating tube is open to atmosphere (110, 162). There is also no effect from alterations in barometric pressure as long as the inflating tube is unclamped (156).

The cuff may fail to produce no-leak ventilation and protection against aspiration when used open (87). However, if a large enough cuff is chosen and the pilot tube is clamped, it performs as a safe, low-pressure cuff. The foam may change shape with time, allowing an air leak to occur at 18–36 hr of intubation (90).

One study found a high incidence of sore throat associated with its use (33).

In one reported case (163), the inflating tube was accidentally pulled out at the point of insertion on the tube, making cuff deflation impossible. A plastic catheter was connected to the inflating tube to deflate the cuff. It has been suggested that the cuff can be removed without deflation with no untoward effects (164).

Use. The proper size needs to be selected,

since too large a tube will cause excessive pressure on the tracheal wall and too small a tube will not allow a seal if the inflating tube is unclamped. Clinically it would be difficult to insert too large a tube for in humans the diameter of the trachea at the vocal cord level is less than that below. Thus an endotracheal tube that passes the vocal cords should find room to expand in the trachea. As a general rule, in adults the 8- or 8.5-mm tube is usually suitable.

Before intubation, all the air should be removed from the cuff by aspiration. The inflating tube should then be closed or clamped off. The cuff should be inspected to make certain that it remains collapsed. If it fills, this indicates a leak, and the tube should be discarded.

After intubation has been accomplished, the inflating tube should be opened to atmosphere and the cuff allowed to fill with air. The amount of air in the cuff should be ascertained by withdrawal with a syringe. The ability to remove 2 to 3 cc from the smallest cuff or 5 to 6 cc or more from the largest cuff usually signifies that a cuff-to-tracheal wall pressure that will allow mucosal perfusion exists. If little or no air can be aspirated, the cuff may be too tight.

If an air leak is present after the cuff has been allowed to refill, wrinkles in the cuff may be present and may be straightened out by injecting 2 or 3 cc of air into the cuff then allowing it to deflate. If the leak persists, it may be desirable to reintubate with a larger tube. If this is not desirable, the inflating tube should be capped at the end of exhalation. If this is not effective, the smallest amount of air required to stop the leak should be injected and the inflating tube clamped.

For extubation the cuff should be collapsed by aspirating with a syringe or squeezing the cuff, the pilot tube clamped, and the tube removed. Several investigators have found no harmful effects from the gentle removal of the tube without prior removal of air from the cuff. This technique permits the removal of secretions that accumulate above the cuff (164).

Tracheal Tube Connectors (165)

The tracheal tube connector (union) fits directly into the tracheal tube. It serves to attach the tube to the breathing system. It may be made of plastic or metal.

The end which connects to the breathing system is called the machine or proximal end and has a 15-mm male (OD) fitting. There may be protrusions to facilitate connection and disconnection. The proximal end may be provided with lugs or other features to which elastic bands or other devices may be attached to prevent accidental disconnection from the breathing system.

The end which fits into the tube is called the patient or distal end and its size is designated by the internal diameter in millimeters. Connectors are available in 0.5-mm increments in a range of sizes.

The connector should be at least as large as the tube. This will ensure that there will be minimal reduction in lumen and that separation will be unlikely. Use of alcohol on a connector may facilitate insertion into the tube and cause bonding with the tube.

The most commonly used connectors are straight and 90-degree curved (right angle). Curved connectors have two disadvantages: (a) they cause increased resistance (5, 166, 167); (b) they must be removed from the tube when it is desired to insert a stylet or suction catheter. An advantage of a curved connector is that it exerts less weight vertically, so that displacement of the tube may be less likely. For operations around the face curved connectors can be positioned so as to interfere less with the surgical field than a straight connector.

In addition to straight and right angle connectors, a large variety of special connectors are available commercially. One is shown in Figure 13.12. Before using any of these the anesthesiologist should be certain that it will fit the breathing system to which it will be attached.

USE OF THE ENDOTRACHEAL TUBE

Checking the Tube

Before insertion, the tube and cuff should be checked for defects. If a cuff is present, it should be inflated and inspected to make certain it inflates evenly and does not cause the lumen of the tube to be reduced. The inflating tube should be clamped or the syringe removed from the inflating valve, so that the cuff remains inflated until just before intubation. This will detect slow leaks.

After the cuff is inflated, the tube should be checked for obstructions. With transparent tubes, simple observation will suffice. With

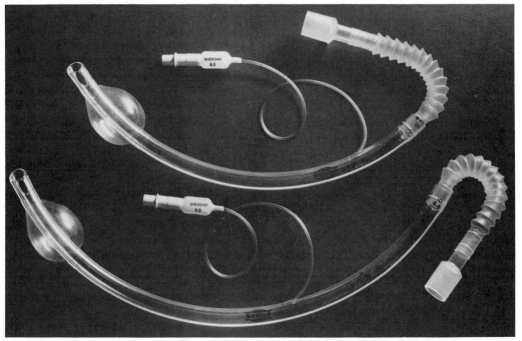

Figure 13.12. Flexible connector. (Courtesy of Sheridan Catheter Corp.)

other tubes, the anesthesiologist should look into both ends and/or insert a stylet.

Preparing the Tube

After the sterile wrapper is opened, the tube should not be handled, except at the connector end. The connector should be inserted as far as possible. Wiping the connector with alcohol may make insertion easier and cause bonding between the tube and connector.

Lubricants have been used on endotracheal tubes for many years, although their value has been questioned (168). Only sterile water-soluble lubricants should be used. For oral intubation only the distal end of the tube should be lubricated. If nasal intubation is planned, lubricant should be placed along the entire length of the tube.

Insertion of the Tube

ORAL INTUBATION

Oral intubation is generally preferred for general anesthesia and in most emergencies because it is easier, faster, and less painful than nasal intubation (169). All the nasal and paranasal complications of nasal intubation are avoided.

Disadvantages of oral intubation include the possibility of dental and oropharyngeal complications. Oral intubation is not well tolerated by the conscious patient. The patient with an oral tube has difficulty swallowing secretions.

The tube should be introduced into the right corner of the mouth and directed toward the glottis with the bevel parallel to the cords. If there is movement of the cords, the moment of greatest abduction should be chosen for insertion of the tube. The tube is passed into the larynx and trachea until the cuff is seen to disappear below the vocal cords. If no cuff is present, the tube should be inserted 3–4 cm past the vocal cords in adults, not more than 1 cm in children under 6 months and for patients up to 1 year not more than 2 cm.

A bite block, rolled gauze or small oral airway should be placed between the teeth to prevent the patient from biting down and occluding the lumen.

NASAL INTUBATION

The nasal route is often used for surgical procedures involving the oral cavity and face when an oral tube would hinder the surgeon's access to the operative field.

Intubation by the nasal route has many advantages. The tube is easier to secure, resulting in less movement. There is less tendency for spontaneous extubation (140). It may be more comfortable for patients. Oral feedings are possible during long-term intubation. Use of the nasal route eliminates the possibility of tube occlusion by biting.

Disadvantages of this route include the possibility of damage to the nasal tissues. The chances of cuff damage during intubation are increased, since forceps often must be used. Nasotracheal intubation may be associated with a higher incidence of bacteremia than orotracheal intubation. Smaller tubes must be used, resulting in increased resistance, difficulty in suctioning, and possibly making fiberoptic bronchoscopy impossible. Meteorism is seen more often (170). It has been reported that for prolonged intubations there are fewer laryngeal complications with nasal intubation than oral (171), but other studies have shown no difference (1972). This route of intubation is ill advised for patients who have undergone nasal surgery (173) and when there is nasal pathology (174) or a basilar skull fracture (8).

Before insertion of a nasotracheal tube, the nasopharynx and nostrils should be sprayed with a vasoconstrictor to increase the patency and minimize trauma to the mucosa. The patency of each nasal cavity should be assessed (175).

The patient's head should be put in the usual position for laryngoscopy (see Chapter 12). The tube should be inserted into the more patent nasal cavity. If the nares are equally patent, the initial insertion should be on the right side with the flat part of the bevel against the septum. The tip should be directed gently posteriorly until it contacts the posterior pharyngeal wall. Here the natural curve of the tube and the anterior body of the cervical spine will usually direct it anteriorly.

Resistance to passage of the tube may be met at various points along its course (175). If the tube is too large, it may be difficult to advance it through the anterior nares or past the turbinates. A deviated nasal septum can severely narrow the nasal cavity on one side and enlarged adenoids can obstruct the passage of the tube through either nasal cavity. The tube should never be forced, because this can result in perforation of the mucosa and the tube may be pushed into the submucosal tissues. Sometimes the tube will not make the bend. Plastic tubes may be stiff. Warming them in hot sterile water before insertion may make them soft enough to make the bend. Inserting a stylet with a sharp curve may help direct the tip anteriorly. Another technique is to pass a small suction catheter through the tube (176). The tip of the catheter is picked up and brought out of the mouth. A forward pull on the end of the catheter will usually bring the tip of the tracheal tube forward.

Direct

After the tube is inserted into the nasopharynx, the larynx is exposed using a laryngoscope. Lateral direction of the tube tip can usually be altered by twisting the tube. The position of the larynx relative to the tube tip may be altered by flexing or extending the neck and/or external manipulation of the larynx. If these manipulations do not allow the tube to pass into the larynx, forceps may be used to pick up and direct the tip through the vocal cords. Tubes with soft cuffs should be handled very carefully since the cuff is easily torn.

If the tip passes through the vocal cords but then encounters resistance, it is most likely because the curve of the tube is directing the tip into the anterior wall of the larynx. Withdrawing the tube slightly and flexing the neck should allow advancement. Alternately, the tube can be rotated 180 degrees, turning its concavity posteriorly before pushing it forward.

If the tube is held up at the entrance to the larynx, a suction catheter can be fed through the tube into the larynx (178). The suction tube acts as a guide for the tube. It is then removed after the tube is in place.

Blind (175)

Blind nasal intubation may be useful when direct visualization of the larynx is impossible. Its use may be associated with more trauma than intubation under direct vision.

The "classical" technique of blind nasal intubation requires a spontaneously breathing patient. Unless aspiration of gastric contents is a possibility, the nose and larynx are sprayed with a topical anesthetic or a transtracheal injection of local anesthetic may be performed. After the tube is inserted through the nostril, it is advanced blindly. The breath sounds can be heard exiting from the tube as the tip approaches the larynx. When the respiratory sounds are heard at maximal intensity, the tube will usually enter the glottis when it is pushed downward during inspiration. If the sounds suddenly cease but the patient continues to breathe, the tube has passed into a position other than the trachea. Flexion or extension of the head or manipulation of the larynx by external pressure may line up the tube and larynx. The tube tip may be rotated by twisting at the connector end (179).

A visual technique for blind intubation has been described for use if the patient is not breathing (175). Certain landmarks on the front of the neck (hyoid bone, notch of the thyroid cartilage and the cricoid cartilage) are observed. As the tube moves anteriorly, the landmarks are moved by the tip of the tube. The object is to move the tip to the midline at the thyroid angle where it should enter the larynx. If the tip is above the thyroid cartilage, flexion of the head on the neck will move the tip more caudad. If the tip is seen below the thyroid cartilage, extension of the neck will move it cephalad. If the tube tip is observed resting laterally, the tube should be withdrawn and twisted to direct the tip toward the midline or the neck turned laterally. If the tube tip passes the laryngeal inlet, but impinges on the anterior trachea, increasing cervical flexion or rotating the tube through 180 degrees while exerting forward pressure on the tube may cause it to pass into the trachea.

Translaryngeal

For difficult intubations when a fiberoptic laryngoscope or bronchoscope is not available, translaryngeal techniques have been described (180–186). Most involve passage of a catheter through the cricothyroid membrane and retrograde through the larynx where it can be recovered through the mouth or nose and used as a guide for the tracheal tube.

INFLATING THE CUFF

The cuff should be inflated as described under the three types of cuffs. The inflating tube should then be clamped between the pilot balloon and the free end (unless an inflating valve is present or a sponge cuff is used).

CHECKING TUBE POSITION

After the tube has been inserted, its position should be checked. This is done by first watching for chest movements. The lateral aspects of the thorax and the epigastrium should be auscultated. Palpation of the cuff in the sternal notch is also useful (76, 187). Tube tip position can be determined most reliably by using a fiberoptic bronchoscope or laryngoscope or x-ray of the chest.

If there is any question as to the possibility of the tube being in a bronchus, the cuff should be deflated, the tube withdrawn 1 to 2 cm, and the checking procedure repeated.

If doubt exists as to possible esophageal placement, the larynx should be visualized or the tube completely withdrawn and reinserted. Detection of carbon dioxide in the exhaled gases is proof the tube is not in the esophagus, but cannot be relied upon to detect an endobronchial intubation.

FIXING THE TUBE

Fixation of the tube to the patient is important but can be quite vexing. If a tube is not well fixed, there is increased danger of either extubation or advancement into one of the bronchi. Movement of the tube within the airway will be increased.

Each practitioner has his own idea of the best method for securing the tube. Various body positions and the need not to intrude upon the surgical field may require some innovation. Most commonly the tube is fastened to facial skin by adhesive tape which encircles the tube. Use of an adhesive spray such as tincture of benzoin on the tube and skin may make a better surface for the tape to adhere to. If the tube is inserted nasally, the tape should be applied in such a way as to pull the tube away from the nasal alae (188). The tape may encircle the head.

Numerous other techniques of fixation have been described (189–201). The variety suggests that the perfect method has not been found.

A means to prevent traction on the tube is highly desirable.

REMOVING THE TUBE

When the time for extubation arises, the mouth and pharynx should be carefully suctioned and the tape or other fixation device removed. The cuff should be deflated while applying positive pressure to the airway to blow secretions collected above the cuff into the mouth and pharynx, which should then be suctioned again. The pilot balloon should be checked to verify that it is deflated. The tube should be removed at the peak of inspiration. If the tube cannot be removed easily, the inflating tube should be checked for an obstruction distal to the pilot balloon, especially where the tape was used to hold the tube in place.

A tracheal tube should never be removed with a suction catheter inside it. This will deplete the lungs of oxygen and is not effective in preventing aspiration.

COMPLICATIONS ASSOCIATED WITH USE OF TRACHEAL TUBES

No procedure is without problems and the use of an endotracheal tube is no exception. Complications after short-term intubation are usually mild in nature. As the length of intubation increases, so do the incidence and severity of complications (202). The incidence of severe complications following prolonged intubation can be decreased by proper use of low-pressure cuffs (88, 90).

Trauma during Insertion

Injuries ranging from simple abrasion to severe laceration and perforation have been reported with intubation (203). They may be caused by the laryngoscope, endotracheal tube, or a protruding stylet.

Intubation trauma is increased when it is performed roughly, hurriedly, or by inexperienced personnel. Poor visualization of the anatomy and blind intubation make misdirection of the tube more likely. Hyperextension of the neck may increase the possibility of trauma by stretching the pharyngeal tissues. Unusual anatomy, poor muscle relaxation and motion on the part of the patient may be contributing factors.

With nasotracheal intubation, tearing of the mucosa with bleeding is common. The nasal septum may be dislocated or perforated and the mucosa of the nasopharynx abraded or lacerated (203–205). Fragments of adenoid tissue or nasal polyps may be dislodged (206). Underlining of nasal tissues with creation of a submucosal pouch may occur (207).

Injuries to the larynx include hematomas, contusions, lacerations, puncture wounds, cord avulsions and arytenoid dislocations and fractures (208–211). Most of these lesions heal quickly, usually without consequence.

Perforation of the pharynx or hypopharynx is a serious complication of intubation (173, 212–

222). Cervical subcutaneous and/or mediastinal emphysema is frequently seen. Pneumothorax may be seen, but is less common than with rupture of the lower airways. An abscess or fistula of the neck may develop.

Tracheal laceration can occur during tracheal tube insertion (203, 223–228). It may be more likely in elderly and emphysematous patients with a thin, friable, posterior tracheal membrane. Subcutaneous emphysema, hemorrhage, pneumomediastinum and pneumothorax may develop. Unless recognized and treated quickly, death can result.

Esophageal perforation is a rare but potentially fatal complication of intubation (216, 229–232). Subcutaneous cervical emphysema appears early. Dysphagia and temperature elevation are consistently present. The prognosis is poor if diagnosis is delayed (232).

The best way to avoid trauma is never to apply more than gentle pressure during intubation. Muscle relaxants should be used to avoid patient movement. Stylets should be flexible and never extend beyond the tip of the tube.

A vasoconstrictor should be used before nasal intubation. Tubes used for nasal intubation should be smaller than considered optimal for oral intubation and should be well lubricated along their entire length.

Swallowed Endotracheal Tube

There are several case reports in the literature of a tracheal tube being lost in the esophagus (233–239). All cases occurred during newborn resuscitation. The tubes were removed from the esophagus and no permanent sequelae occurred.

This complication can be prevented by using a connector that fits firmly in the tube. The tube should be long enough that it protrudes from the mouth when correctly placed. Placing a suture around the tube (240) or a safety pin through the wall of the tube (235) may be helpful.

If this complication does occur, removal of the tube need not be immediate (238). Resuscitation should continue and the patient's condition stabilized first.

Inadvertent Esophageal Intubation

Esophageal intubation is a potentially disastrous complication that can occur even with an experienced anesthesiologist. In a study of catastrophic anesthesia accidents in the United

Kingdom between 1970 and 1977, it was found to be the most common fault in technique (241).

Recognition that this has occurred and prompt correction are necessary to prevent dire consequences (242). Therefore it is mandatory that immediately after intubation the position of the tube be checked to determine if it is in the tracheobronchial tree. There are a number of commonly used tests available to determine this (243).

1. Sighting of the tube passing between the vocal cords. If actually seen, this is reassuring, but frequently the glottis cannot be visualized. The tube may be displaced when the laryngoscope is withdrawn or with various movements of the head and neck (244).

2. The characteristic feel of the reservoir bag associated with normal lung inflation and deflation. Decreased compliance and expiratory time may be seen with esophageal intubation (245). Unfortunately, this test is also unreliable (243, 244).

3. Hearing of normal breath sounds on auscultation of the chest while compressing the bag. Auscultation should be performed in the apices and bases bilaterally, not the anterior chest. The quality of the sounds is important. A gurgling sound of fluid in the tube ("death rattle") (246) should alert the anesthesiologist to possible esophageal placement. This test is not totally reliable, since similar sounds can be generated by gas moving through the esophagus (243, 244).

4. Visual and/or manual confirmation of bilateral chest expansion on inflation. Movement of the chest can occur with the tube in the esophagus (241), especially in patients whose respiration is primarily abdominal (243, 244, 246).

5. Lack of gas escaping around the tube. This test also has failed (243).

6. Absence of borborygmi on epigastric auscultation. Such sounds may be confused with breath sounds often heard in the epigastric area, especially of thin individuals (242).

7. Movement of the reservoir bag in time with the patient's respiratory effort after the muscle relaxant has worn off. This can be difficult to detect since the amount of bag movement will depend on the strength and coordination of the patient's ventilatory effort and the degree of distension of the bag. Tidal volumes can be generated with the tube in the esophagus (243). Lack of movement may be misinterpreted as chest wall spasm (244). Frequently patients are given such large doses of muscle relaxants that they cannot resume spontaneous ventilation for some time.

8. Appearance of moisture from expired gases in transparent tracheal tubes (245). Moisture can, however, appear with esophageal intubation.

9. Absence of changes in blood pressure or heart rate. Unfortunately neither blood pressure nor heart rate is a reliable indication of hypoxia or hypercarbia (247, 248). The electrocardiogram also cannot be relied upon.

10. Persistence of good patient color. Color changes will be delayed with esophageal intubation if preoxygenation has been performed, so any signs of hypoxia developing within 15–20 min following intubation must be regarded as due to accidental intubation of the esophagus until disproved.

11. Escape of gas from the lungs through the open end of the endotracheal tube when the sternum is abruptly depressed. This test can be misleading for a variety of reasons (243).

12. Confirmation of placement by chest x-ray. But this can be misleading (249). Routine chest x-ray after each intubation is not practical.

13. Lack of distention of the stomach. This test can fail, even in a thin patient (243, 246).

14. Palpation of the cuff in the suprasternal notch (76, 77, 187). Reliability of this test in detecting esophageal placement has not been confirmed.

15. Confirmation of placement by fiberoptic bronchoscopy or laryngoscopy (79). This requires special instruments and training, takes time, and cannot be used with small tubes.

16. Presence of carbon dioxide in the exhaled gases (250). This is unquestionably the best method available. Tube placement can be reliably checked on the first breath. It can be used either with the patient breathing spontaneously or with controlled ventilation. Unfortunately, it is not available in all operating rooms.

There is a widespread impression that accidental placement of a tracheal tube in the esophagus can be readily detected. In the vast majority of patients distinguishing between esophageal and tracheal intubation is not difficult. In a small number of patients, however, some signs can so closely resemble tracheal placement that they can deceive even a careful, experienced anesthesiologist. In most of the reported incidents involving esophageal intubation, one or more of the above-described tests have been performed and were misleading (242–244, 246, 249).

If there is the slightest doubt as to where the tube has been placed, and the patient's condition permits, a check of tube position by direct laryngoscopy should be made. Since misplacement is often associated with difficult laryngoscopy in the first place, this is not often helpful. If the patient's condition is deteriorating, or direct laryngoscopy is not helpful, the tube should be removed. The dictum "When in doubt, take it out," is a good rule to follow. Alternately, the patient can be ventilated using a mask placed over the open tube and mouth. Cyanosis relieved by this maneuver is evidence of tube misplacement (244).

Endobronchial Intubation

Insertion of an endotracheal tube into a mainstem bronchus is a relatively common and sometimes fatal complication (250–258).

It can occur either at the time of initial insertion or subsequently. If not firmly anchored the tube may descend into a bronchus as a result of the weight of the attachments or from frequent suctioning (259). The tube will move toward the carina with neck flexion (81, 260, 261) and going from an erect to a recumbent position (253). Trendelenburg position, placement of upper abdominal packs, lithotomy position, and compression of the abdomen will move the carina upward (255). The margin of safety in children is less because of the shorter trachea.

If an endotracheal tube is inserted so far that the tip impinges on the carina, persistent coughing and bucking will result. More commonly the tube enters the right mainstem bronchus. This will result in varying degrees of obstruction of the left main bronchus and decreased or absent ventilation of the left lung. Perfusion of the unventilated lung may also be interrupted (262). A tube inserted into the right main bronchus may also occlude the bronchus to the right upper lobe (263). Subsequent overventilation of the right lower lobe may be associated with alveolar rupture, interstitial emphysema and tension pneumothorax (258, 264).

The signs will depend on the length of time the tube is left in place. Improper placement may be manifested by incomplete (usually expiratory) obstruction and excessive or persistent bucking. Dullness of breath sounds, tachypnea, hypotension, and cyanosis can occur (257, 259),

but massive atelectasis can exist without changes in vital signs or cyanosis (253, 254). Because of this variation in clinical features, a high index of suspicion should be maintained in every intubated patient.

Endobronchial intubation is best prevented by placing the tip of the tube in the middle third of the trachea with the neck in a neutral position (81, 260). A cuffed tube should be inserted until the cuff is 3–4 centimeters past the vocal cords in adults. This will allow for movement of the tip with head positioning and of the carina with respiration. The tube should then be securely anchored in place to avoid subsequent slippage. Fixation to the lower lip may be safer than fixation to the upper lip (261).

In pediatrics, measuring the tube before intubation and cutting it to the proper length according to a nomogram or special formula may decrease the incidence of this complication (70, 265), but these are based on averages and cannot be considered totally reliable (187).

After intubation, an attempt should be made to detect inadvertent endobronchial intubation. This should be repeated at intervals during long intubations, whenever changes in the patient's position are made, and whenever there is any indication of hypoxia. When a patient fails to "settle down" and continues to "cough on the tube," the anesthesiologist should suspect that the tube may be irritating the carina.

There are several methods used to detect endobronchial intubation. Visualization of symmetrical chest expansion is easily performed, but is not reliable.

The most commonly used method is auscultation of the lower and upper peripheral lung fields bilaterally. Unfortunately this may be inaccurate unless the tube is wedged firmly in a main bronchus (187, 254–256, 258), and a false sense of security may be generated if there is no difference between the two sides. When a tube is in a bronchus, some ventilation of the side opposite the tube tip may occur by air escaping around the tube so that breath sounds may be heard (256). Auscultation is of no value if the tube is at the carina.

Another method of detecting endobronchial intubation is to check the position of the tip of the tube radiographically. This is expensive, time-consuming, often not immediately available, and may be impractical because of interference with sterile technique.

The position of the tip may be checked by use

of the fiberoptic bronchoscope or laryngoscope (78, 79, 266) but this requires special equipment and training.

Rapid inflation and deflation of the cuff with palpation in the suprasternal notch is helpful (76, 77). With uncuffed tubes, the tip of the tube is palpated (187). This method is noninvasive, simple, rapid, and requires no special equipment. But the inflation and deflation can cause damage to the trachea. For uncuffed tubes a stylet and second person are required and the method requires some practice.

Other methods include use of a foil band on the tube with an electronic detector (267) and auscultation in the suprasternal notch after fluid has been injected into the cuff (268).

Exhaled carbon dioxide analyzers cannot be relied upon to diagnose endobronchial intubations. A transcutaneous oxygen monitor may be helpful, since sudden and immediate falls in arterial oxygen occur with endobronchial intubation.

When an endotracheal tube is believed to be in a bronchus, the cuff should be deflated, the tube withdrawn, the cuff reinflated, and the position rechecked. If reintubation would be difficult because of the patient's position or because the initial intubation was difficult, consideration should be given to advancing a fiberoptic bronchoscope or laryngoscope into the tube and withdrawing the tube under direct vision (266). Even if extubation should occur, the endotracheal tube can be quickly reinserted over the fiberoptic instrument.

Bronchial Obstruction

Bronchial obstruction secondary to endobronchial intubation has been discussed above. Bronchial obstruction can also occur as a result of an anomalous tracheal bronchus (269). Such bronchi are nearly always found on the right side, usually supplying the right upper lobe. In the reported case, cuff position above the sternal notch had been confirmed after intubation. It was postulated that the tube migrated downward with manipulation of the head.

Foreign Body Aspiration

While one of the functions of an endotracheal tube is to provide protection against the entry of material into the lungs, intubation itself may be the source of a foreign body in the tracheobronchial tree. This can cause blockage or check valve obstruction to an area of the lungs. In some reported cases, serious, life-threatening airway obstruction has occurred (270, 271).

A tracheal tube inserted nasally may dislodge a fragment of adenoid or nasal tissue during its passage. Similarly bulky tumors of the oral cavity, pharynx, or larynx may become fragmented and aspirated during intubation.

It is possible for a tracheal tube to become separated from its connector and be aspirated into the trachea (271, 272). This can be avoided by making certain that the connector fits firmly into the tube. The tube should be long enough that the tape or other device used to fix the tube can be attached to the tube, not the connector. Use of a Cole tube may also prevent such distal migration (271).

In two reports, a defective endotracheal tube had the punched-out area forming the Murphy eye still in situ (273, 274). In one case this was discerned on inspection prior to intubation; in the other case, the piece was aspirated. Cases have been reported where a portion of a ruptured cuff fell into a bronchus (275–279).

Other foreign bodies have included a cottonoid used to protect the cuff from a laser beam (280), the distal portion of a flexometallic tube (281), pieces of aluminum used to protect the tube from ignition by a laser beam (270), parts of defective connectors (282, 283), and the sheared off covering of a stylet (284).

Careful inspection of connectors, tubes, and stylets before use will help to avoid this problem. These should also be checked after use. Damaged cuffs should be examined carefully to see if any portions are missing. Foreign body aspiration should always be suspected whenever obstructive signs or symptoms appear after extubation.

If foreign body aspiration is suspected, an immediate search of the patient's air passages should be made. This should include bronchoscopy if examination above the level of the larynx proves fruitless.

Bacteremia

Bacteremia may occur after intubation. Some reports suggest that the risk may be greater with nasotracheal than orotracheal intubation (285, 286), but another study showed little difference (287).

Endotracheal Tube Damage

Damage to the cuff system or the tube itself is uncommon. It may occur before, during, or after intubation. It may be more frequent with prolonged or difficult intubations (258) and with high-volume cuffs, which are more bulky and fragile and therefore more liable to be torn than low volume cuffs (288).

There are many causes. The cuff, inflating tube, or the tube itself may be torn by sharp jagged teeth, a turbinate, the laryngoscope blade, or forceps during insertion. A tube may be damaged by the sharp edge of a stylet as it is withdrawn (289).

Local anesthetic sprays may cause holes in the cuff (290). The cuff can rupture or become separated from the tube while in place (291). Puncture of a cuff has occurred during internal jugular and subclavian intravenous cannulation (292, 293).

There are many times when the surgical site is adjacent to the endotracheal tube and damage can result. This is especially likely during orthognathic surgery (288, 294–299), but can also occur in operations such as tonsillectomy (300). Instruments designed to protect tubes from damage during oral surgery procedures have been developed (288, 295). A laser beam can perforate the cuff and cause a leak (280). This can be avoided by protecting the cuff with wet cottonoids.

A defective cuff or tube can usually be detected before use. The cuff should be discarded if it does not inflate uniformly since such a cuff may fail to create a seal (301). The cuff should be left inflated for several minutes to detect a slow leak.

Fortunately, most damaged tubes are only a nuisance. A leaking tube may make maintenance of adequate ventilation difficult, fail to protect against aspiration, and make surgery involving the oral cavity extremely difficult.

When a leak occurs, the position of the cuff should be checked, since it may not be completely below the cords. This is usually easily corrected by deflating the cuff and advancing the tube. If this is not the problem the anesthesiologist has several alternatives, depending on the situation: (*a*) do nothing (if the leak is small); (*b*) keep adding air to the cuff to compensate for the leak. An intravenous tubing connected to an air-filled plastic container under pressure may be useful for this purpose; (*c*) reintubate. If this is elected, consideration should be given to use of a stylet which is passed through the lumen of the tube well beyond the tip (302, 303). The damaged tube is then removed and the new endotracheal tube inserted over the stylet. A fiberoptic laryngoscope or bronchoscope may be useful when changing a tube (304, 305); (*d*) put a mask over the patient's face and the tube and ventilate. (*e*) remove the tube and ventilate with a mask; (*f*) use pharyngeal packing to control the leak; (*g*) establish an acceptable airway in another fashion (tracheostomy or cricothyroid membrane puncture); (*h*) increase the fresh gas flow to compensate for the leak.

Endotracheal Tube Ignition

Since its introduction in the early 1970s, the use of the carbon dioxide laser for laryngeal surgery has been increasing. A major complication of this procedure is ignition of the endotracheal tube. Damage to the trachea may be severe (306, 307).

The laser beam can directly penetrate and ignite a tracheal tube (306–310). Indirect ignition can also occur. The interior surface of a tube can be ignited by burning pieces of tissue inhaled into the tube (311).

The laser beam is an intense heat source capable of igniting almost all rubber and plastic materials (312). The ease with which this occurs depends on the material itself, the gas environment surrounding the material and the focus of the beam. There is controversy in the literature over which type of tube, red rubber or plastic, is more resistant to ignition (312). Both have been implicated in case reports of fires.

Three methods are currently available to minimize the risk (313): no tube in the airway, protection of the tube by wrapping the outside surface with a variety of materials, and use of a noncombustible tube (312).

A tube in the airway can be avoided by using jet (Venturi) ventilation, anesthesia by insufflation, or by ventilation through a tracheostomy.

The tube can be protected by wrapping it with aluminum foil or tape to at least 1 cm below the vocal cords so that the laser beam will be reflected and its energy dissipated. Moist muslin can also be used to protect the tube (314). Wrapping methods have several disadvantages (313). The thickness of the tube wall is increased. The wrapping material may come off and possibly obstruct the airway (270). Ignition of the unwrapped cuff (280, 310), or the tube by sparks in close proximity to the tip of the tube may still occur (311). Wrapping with aluminum foil can predispose to tube occlusion and may be traumatic (314). Concern has been expressed over the possibility of further tissue damage by deflection of the laser beam from the reflective surface of the covered tube.

Metal tubes have been developed as a solution to the problem (315, 316). Tubes specially coated with metal oxide particles mixed with an elastomer are available, (Fig. 13.10). These can withstand several impacts with a laser beam.

The tube should be loosely fixed to the patient so that rapid extubation is possible (309). If ignition occurs, the tube should be immediately removed. Investigation of the extent of the damage to the larynx and tracheobronchial tree should be made.

Tracheal Tube Obstruction

One of the reasons for insertion of an endotracheal tube is to provide a patent airway. Unfortunately, the tube itself may become the cause of obstruction. In one study, approximately 20% of endotracheal tubes in children were partially obstructed. General anesthesia was associated with an increased incidence (317).

The obstruction can be partial or complete. Partial obstruction may clinically resemble bronchospasm. It is likely that many cases of wheezing and difficulty in ventilation during anesthesia are due to tracheal tube obstruction. Tube obstruction may be more of a problem with spontaneous ventilation, since positive airway pressure may overcome some increased resistance, while negative pressure may tend to make the obstruction worse. It is also possible to have a ball valve obstruction in which case inspiration is unimpeded, but resistance to expiration is increased (48, 318, 319). Barotrauma may follow.

Endotracheal tube obstruction can occur during insertion or some time later during an anesthetic. A delayed appearance may be due to softening of the tube at body temperature or diffusion of nitrous oxide into the cuff or other air space.

CAUSES

Kinking

Kinking is one of the more common causes of endotracheal tube obstruction. It may occur in

the pharynx (320) or outside the patient's mouth or nose because of the weight of the breathing system or surgical drapes pulling on the tube. It is more common with smaller tubes. Tubes vary in their resistance to kinking (25). Some tube materials soften when warmed to body temperature. Kinking sometimes occurs when the position of the patient's head is changed (321). When tubes are wrapped for laser microlaryngeal surgery, they may become occluded as a result of compression by the foil as the tube accommodates to the curvature of the posterior pharynx (314).

Spiral embedded tubes have been used to overcome this problem, but if the connector is not inserted inside the spirals, kinking can occur at the patient end (322) (Fig. 13.7).

Biting

Unless protection in the form of an airway or bite block is provided, the patient may bite the tube, causing obstruction (35, 36). Care should be taken to prevent the tube from slipping between the molar teeth where occlusion may occur in spite of an airway or bite block.

Foreign Body

Another cause of an obstructed endotracheal tube is a foreign body. This may be dried mucus, blood clots, pus, debris, or granulation tissue (323–332). It is possible for a tube to pass submucosally during nasal intubation.

Other foreign bodies reported have included foam rubber from a mask (333), an inflating valve (334), the end of a cleaning tube (329), a cleaning brush (335), an adaptor from an intravenous set (336), an intravenous needle (337), a stop from a stylet (338), a cork (339), a glass ampule (340), pieces of plastic (341, 342), tumor tissue from lung resection (343), dried lubricants (344, 345), and a dead cockroach (346).

Transparent tubes allow immediate identification of any material or objects blocking the lumen.

Defective Tubes

Spiral embedded tubes have a high incidence of defects. In one case insertion of a connector caused the inside of the tube to pucker up and occlude the lumen (44). During manufacture latex spiral tubes are dipped repeatedly until the desired wall thickness is attained. During this process, air bubbles may be formed within the wall between the layers. It is essential that these tubes not be gas-sterilized or steam-autoclaved with vacuum because these processes may cause blebs to form (347). During anesthesia, nitrous oxide may diffuse into an air bubble and cause swelling (45, 46). If inward herniation into the tube lumen occurs, obstruction may result (47). A tear can develop along the inner wall and form a flap valve (348). Air from the cuff can enter the space between layers (48, 49, 349).

Aberrant inflation of the cuff can push the bevel against the wall of the trachea (Fig. 13.13) (318, 322, 350–352). In infants when the tube orifice faces in one direction and the infant's head is turned to the other direction, the orifice may abut the tracheal wall (353). This occurs more readily with higher tube positions. The direction of the bevel may make it vulnerable to obstruction by an inappropriately placed throat pack (354) or assumption of certain head positions (355, 356).

It is possible for an overinflated cuff to balloon over the tip of the tube (319, 357, 358) (Fig. 13.13). Too short a distance from the distal end of the cuff to the bevel can predispose a cuff to herniate over the bevel if the cuff is overinflated or when anesthetic gases increase the volume of a properly inflated cuff (110).

Inflation of the cuff may cause it to compress the lumen of the tube (Fig. 13.14) (43, 359–366). This is more likely to occur if the cuff is over-inflated and may be more common with use of smaller tubes since a smaller tube frequently requires a high cuff pressure to seal the airway. Nitrous oxide diffusion into the cuff may cause

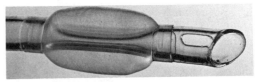

Figure 13.14. Reduction of tube lumen by cuff. Inflation of the cuff caused narrowing of the tube lumen which persisted after the cuff was deflated.

further narrowing of the lumen. Sterilizing methods utilizing heat may damage the tube and predispose to obstruction. Air trapped in the inflating tube and cuff may expand upon heating and cause the area under the cuff to weaken (Fig. 13.14) (361).

A case has been reported in which an aneurysmal dilatation of the inflating tube herniated into the lumen of the tube and obstructed flow (368). Defective connectors have been the source of obstruction (283, 369, 370).

PREVENTION

Prevention of tracheal tube obstruction requires constant vigilance on the part of the anesthesiologist. A non-kinking tube may be advisable if an operation involves turning the head or other maneuvers which may induce kinking. Biting of the tube may be prevented by using an oral airway or a bite block, maintaining an adequate level of anesthesia, and fitting the endotracheal tube to the center of the mouth. Use of a fenestrated (Murphy) tube may avoid some cases of obstruction.

The endotracheal tube should be examined carefully before use and the patency of the lumen checked. Large foreign bodies inside the lumen can be detected by inserting a stylet. The cuff should be examined to make certain that it is securely attached and inflates symmetrically. The lumen should not be reduced nor should the cuff balloon over the end of the tube when the cuff is inflated and compressed.

After insertion, the cuff should be inflated slowly as described in the section on use. Cuff pressure should be readjusted frequently, especially if nitrous oxide is used. When an x-ray is taken, the position of the orifice and the configuration of the cuff should be examined.

Traction on the tube should be avoided. Once inserted the tube should not be withdrawn while the cuff is inflated because this may cause the cuff to balloon over the end of the tube. Atten-

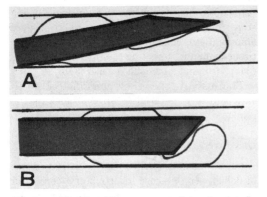

Figure 13.13. Two causes of tracheal tube obstruction. *A*, the bevel of the tube is pushed against the wall of the trachea by an eccentrically inflated cuff. *B*, the cuff has ballooned over the end of the tube.

tion should be paid to tidal volumes and airway pressures to detect early obstruction. When secretions are heard, they should be removed with a suction catheter. Humidifying the inspired gases will prevent drying of secretions.

Sterilizing methods utilizing heat may damage tubes (361). Other methods of disinfection should be used.

TREATMENT

When an obstructed endotracheal tube is encountered, immediate steps need to be taken to reestablish tube patency or the tube removed. Digital pressure on the site of a kink may relieve the obstruction (186). Simple alteration of the patient's head position may also help. If these simple maneuvers are unsuccessful, the cuff should be deflated. If the obstruction is still not relieved, the tube should be removed. If the obstruction is mild and/or it would be difficult to change the tube, the situation may be improved by eliminating nitrous oxide from the inspired mixture. Stenting of the tube with a smaller tube may be feasible (186).

A number of the reported cases of tracheal tube obstruction have ended disastrously (371–373, 351). Two mistakes are commonly made. First, the anesthesiologist does not consider that the tube is the source of obstruction and attributes it to bronchospasm or some other condition. The second mistake is wasting precious time trying to pass a suction catheter down a completely or almost completely blocked tube. If a tube is completely blocked by a defect in the tube, a suction catheter will not relieve the obstruction. If the tube is blocked by a foreign body, chances are also good that a suction catheter will not relieve the obstruction.

Pulmonary Aspiration

Although it is generally assumed that an endotracheal tube will protect the lungs from the entry of foreign material, this is not always the case. Since the morbidity and mortality rates following documented aspiration are high, aspiration of even small amounts of material should be prevented whenever possible (92). Aspiration may occur while the cuff is in place, upon extubation, or following extubation.

The chances of significant aspiration with the tube in place are increased by the following factors.

1. Use of low-pressure cuffs (92, 133). Many low-pressure, high-volume cuffs wrinkle despite proper inflation (136). Fluid can pass through channels formed along the folds of the cuff. The number and size of the folds are determined by the intracuff pressure, cuff wall thickness and the cuff-to-trachea diameter ratio (374).

Infolding can be decreased by increasing the pressure in the cuff (137), using a thin walled cuff (92), and using a tube whose cuff diameter approximates the internal diameter of the trachea when inflated to residual volume (137, 374).

2. Improper inflation. Inflating a low pressure cuff to the point of no leak when positive pressure is applied to the airway may not protect against aspiration (133, 375).

3. Spontaneous ventilation. With thin walled cuffs, a negative airway pressure will be transmitted to the cuff during inspiration with spontaneous ventilation (135, 374). In addition, the trachea tends to dilate during spontaneous inspiration. Therefore higher cuff pressures may be required to prevent aspiration in spontaneously breathing patients (137).

4. Accumulation of fluid above the cuff. Frequent suctioning to maintain a clear oropharynx will decrease the the pressure exerted by fluid above the cuff.

It has been suggested that the cuff should be placed just below the vocal cords, reasoning that the shorter the distance between the top of the cuff and the vocal cords, the smaller the volume of fluid that cannot be removed by suctioning. If the cuff is just below the cords, however, movement of the head may cause the tube to move upward, causing the cuff to exert pressure on the cords. Further, it has been suggested that a cuff placed just below the cords may compress nerve endings against the thyroid cartilage, resulting in vocal cord paralysis (376). Finally, inadvertent spontaneous extubation may be more likely if the cuff is placed in this position.

5. Head-up position. If the pharynx fills with fluid with the patient sitting up, the hydrostatic pressure exerted from above on the cuff will be higher than if the patient is supine.

6. Use of uncuffed tubes (377). Use of continuous positive airway pressure may offer some protection in this situation (378).

7. Oral feedings or tube feedings (378, 379).

Pulmonary aspiration can be minimized by proper extubation procedures. Fluid accumulated above the cuff can find its way into the lungs when the cuff is deflated prior to extubation (380). This can be avoided by (a) placing the cuff just below the vocal cords (136) (this has the disadvantages mentioned above); (b) using a head-down tilt before deflation (380); (c) aspirating through the tube during extubation. This maneuver has been criticized because severe hypoxia can result (381, 382); (d) deflation of the cuff during the application of positive airway pressure (381, 382). This will blow any materials collected above the cuff up into the pharynx where they can be removed by suctioning.

Laryngeal incompetence may follow extubation (383, 384). Unfortunately, the problem appears to have been incompletely studied, especially following short term intubations.

Tracheal Dilatation

Tracheal dilatation is a recognized complication of cuffed tubes. It occurs in 2–5% of patients receiving long-term ventilatory support and may occur after brief use of a soft cuff (385). It appears to be less severe with a sponge cuff than an air-filled cuff (146). Spontaneous ventilation appears to be associated with less tracheal dilatation than positive pressure ventilation.

Dilatation results from sustained pressures from the cuff, which causes deformation and stretching of tissues. Other factors include high airway inflation pressures, infection, loss of elastic tissues associated with obstructive airway disease, and steroid therapy (386, 387, 388).

This complication presents two problems: the preservation of an airtight seal for adequate ventilation and protection of the lungs; and the danger of respiratory obstruction by a tube slipping into the dilated part of the trachea (389). In extreme cases, a tracheal diverticulum may be formed and rupture into the esophagus (388). It seems to be of little clinical significance after the termination of respirator treatment (388).

Prophylaxis consists of use of low-pressure cuffs for prolonged intubation and strict observance of proper cuff inflating techniques.

Meteorism

Massive gastric dilatation, or meteorism, has been reported in several cases in which a nasotracheal tube was used for prolonged intubation (170). This problem has not been seen associated with oral intubation and rarely with a tracheostomy.

Inadvertent Extubation

Accidental dislocation of an endotracheal tube from the trachea into the pharynx is an infrequent but life-threatening complication.

It can occur when the tube is not fixed properly. Secretions or disinfecting solutions can loosen the tape.

Another cause is positioning the cuff between or just below the cords. Distension of the cuff due to overinflation or diffusion of nitrous oxide may cause it to herniate upward. This may result in failure to achieve a seal. In this case the anesthesiologist's most likely response is to inject more air into the cuff. If the cuff is at or just above the vocal cords, the addition of more air will serve to push the tube farther out of the trachea.

Tubes with high-volume cuffs can dislocate spontaneously (139). During positive pressure ventilation a force is exerted from below upward on the cuff. If the tube is not stiff enough to resist this force, it may be dislocated from the trachea. This usually occurs in orally intubated patients and not in those intubated nasally (140).

Use of anti-disconnect devices may increase the danger of spontaneous extubation. Before these devices are used, the dangers of disconnection must be weighed against those of extubation. It can be argued that it is preferable for the connection between the tube and the breathing system to give way under strain than to permit the tube to be pulled out or cause unnecessary trauma to the patient secondary to movement of the tube.

Neck extension and lateral rotation of the head may each contribute to inadvertent extubation by causing the tip of the tube to move upward (81, 261, 390).

To avoid accidental extubation, the tube should be positioned with the tip in the middle third of the trachea with the neck in a neutral position (81). Once properly positioned, the tube should be well secured at the nose or mouth to avoid subsequent slippage. Fixation to the lower lip may be safer than fixation at the upper lip (261). Leverage on the tube should be avoided.

A cuff that requires frequent inflation should alert the anesthesiologist that it may be situated between instead of completely below the level of the cords.

The anesthesiologist should guard against accidental extubation, especially during procedures that involve repositioning of the head or neck.

Difficult Extubation

Extubation is usually a benign, uneventful procedure. Occasionally, however, the tube is difficult or impossible to remove. Trauma to the larynx may result if the tube is forcefully removed.

One cause of this problem is placement of too large a tube (391). The cuff may be held by tense vocal cords.

Another reason for difficult extubation is that the tube is anchored to the respiratory tract. This has been reported with maxillofacial surgery (392, 393) and pulmonary resection (394).

Cases of difficult extubation have been reported where the inflating tube became twisted around a nasogastric tube or a turbinate (395, 396). A fold or flange in the cuff may impede extubation (397–400).

With sponge cuffs, deflation of the cuff will be difficult if the inflating tube is cut or becomes detached (401). With a spiral embedded tube, air from the cuff may pass into the wall between layers. When the cuff is deflated air will be trapped in the wall of the tube (50).

The most common cause of difficulty in extubation is failure of the cuff to deflate. This is frequently due to obstruction of the inflating tube. If the obstruction is distal to the pilot balloon, the balloon will offer no clue that the cuff has not deflated. One case has been reported where heat from a drill melted the inflating tube, occluding both distal and proximal parts (294). Clamping or biting by the patient may cause the inflating tube to adhere to itself. With some spiral embedded tubes, insertion of the connector into the spirals may pinch off the inflating tube.

If there is resistance to extubation, the possibility of a suture through the tube should be considered if there has been surgery of the upper airways. The inflating tube should be cut as close to the tube as possible. If the cuff still remains inflated, the tube should be pulled until the cuff is close to the surface of the vocal cords. A needle can then be introduced through the cricothyroid membrane, puncturing the cuff. If tube is too large, removal may be accomplished by relaxing and abducting the vocal cords and/or rotation of the tube (391, 402).

Sore Throat and Laryngitis

Minor symptoms including sore throat, pain and/or difficulty in swallowing, hoarseness, and aphonia are common after intubation. These usually abate within 24–48 hr without any special treatment. Persistent symptoms deserve further study, including laryngoscopy.

The reported incidence of post-intubation sore throat varies from 6–70% of intubations (403–411). It has also been reported in 10–15% of nonintubated patients (104, 409). It is more common in females and after operations involving the head and neck or with the patient in the prone position. Use of muscle relaxants for intubation lowers the incidence slightly. Some studies have shown a higher incidence with "difficult" intubations but others have shown no correlation. Duration of surgery has been found to have no effect. Straining on the endotracheal tube may increase the number of complaints.

Attempts to reduce the frequency by using lubricants have not been successful (104, 412) and depending on the lubricant may increase the incidence and severity (104). Use of local anesthetic sprays has no effect.

Several investigators have looked at the relationship between endotracheal cuff design and the incidence of sore throat (33, 100, 103, 104, 413). Most studies have shown that high-pressure, low-volume cuffs were associated with a lower incidence of sore throat than low-volume, high-pressure cuffs of similar design, although one study showed no statistical difference. The incidence is high with sponge cuff and Lindholm tubes (33). If a "narrow" low-pressure cuff having a low tracheal contact area is used, the incidence of sore throat is quite low (103).

Airway Edema

Airway edema (post-intubation croup, laryngeal edema, post-intubation inflammation, acute edematous stenosis, stridor, subglottic edema) may occur along the path of the tube. Those areas commonly involved are the epiglottis, aryepiglottic folds, ventricular folds, vocal cords, and the retroarytenoid and subglottic spaces. Uvular edema has been reported (414, 415). The most serious area for post-intubation edema is the subglottic space. Here the fragile epithelium, loose submucosal tissue and complete cartilaginous ring that prevents external expansion make it particularly subject to obstruction.

Acute edema is more common in infants than in older children or adults, with a peak incidence between one and three years of age. It is most commonly seen after surgery involving the head and neck or that performed with the patient in a prone position (158, 416).

SYMPTOMS

Acute edema may manifest itself anytime during the first 48 hr after extubation. Usually, the first signs are evident 1–2 hr postoperatively, with a peak at 8 hr (416).

In its mildest form, it is evidenced by hoarseness or croupy cough persisting for several hours. In more severe cases, respiratory obstruction will occur. The clinical picture is one of dyspnea, inspiratory stridor, tachypnea, tachycardia, and suprasternal retractions. Decompensation may be rapid and may lead to cardiac arrest unless treated.

ETIOLOGIES

There are multiple possible etiologies of airway edema. They can be divided into three categories: inflammatory, mechanical, and allergic.

Inflammation

Inflammatory conditions include pre-existing inflammation of the larynx, bacterial contamination, and chemical irritation. It is generally acknowledged that the presence of infection in the tracheobronchial tree before intubation predisposes to an increased inflammatory response. A history of infection or post-intubation croup significantly increases the incidence of post-intubation croup (417). Bacterial contamination may be caused by lubricants, sprays, or the endotracheal tube itself. Chemical irritation may occur from lubricants, sprays, the endotracheal tube itself, or from substances formed during cleaning and sterilization of the tube.

Mechanical Trauma

Trauma during intubation may result from inadequate depth of anesthesia or muscle relaxation, unnecessary roughness or trying to insert too large a tube (417, 418). Too tight a fit or a high intracuff pressure may cause ischemia of the mucosa, with resultant edema when the tube is removed. Excessive motion secondary to rotation of the head, bucking, and swallowing will contribute to the piston effect.

Allergy

An allergic reaction to the tube itself or materials used in lubrication or sterilization has been postulated as a mechanism.

PREVENTION

Whenever possible, endotracheal intubation should be avoided in patients having upper respiratory infections. Endotracheal tubes which have the markings "IT" or "Z-79" on them should be used. Tubes, sprays, and lubricants used on the tubes should be sterile. Intubation should be gentle and atraumatic. An adequate anesthetic depth and/or good muscle relaxation should be maintained to prevent movement of the tube. Movements of the head should be kept to a minimum. Cuffs should not be overinflated.

TREATMENT

Treatment of acute laryngeal edema consists first of reassurance and careful observation. Humidified oxygen should be given. Intravenous steroids will prevent further edema and hasten resolution of the existing edema (419). Aerosol therapy or intermittent positive pressure breathing treatments combining high humidity with a vasoconstrictor may prove to be of value (420, 421).

Occasionally when these conservative measures fail, reintubation may be required. Tracheostomy may be necessary if airway obstruction occurs after repeat intubation (169).

Vocal Cord Dysfunction

Vocal cord paralysis and paresis have been reported after endotracheal intubation in spite of the intubation being atraumatic and the site of the surgery being unrelated to the neck area (209, 376, 422–430). It may be unilateral or bilateral. It has been reported with both high-pressure and low-pressure cuffs.

The mechanism of vocal cord dysfunction is unclear. The most common explanation is compression of the recurrent laryngeal nerve by the cuff (424). The nerve runs submucosally on the medial aspects of the thyroid lamina. Here it is susceptible to a cuff inflated just below the cords. Other proposals include an asymmetric and/or overinflated cuff, acute or prolonged hyperextension of the neck, stretch or trauma to soft tissue during laryngoscopy, anomalies of recurrent laryngeal nerve distribution, toxic substances from sterilization and mechanical trauma during intubation.

If the dysfunction is unilateral, respiratory obstruction does not usually occur and voice change and aspiration may be the only manifestations. The aspiration could be catastrophic, however. Bilateral paralysis will result in respiratory distress and tracheostomy is often required.

Most cases of vocal cord dysfunction resolve spontaneously, usually within a week. Posterior commissure fibrosis may occur (422).

Laryngeal Dilatation

Two cases of dilatation of the larynx caused by a Cole tube pressing against the glottis have been reported (31). Both involved patients intubated for 8 days. This complication has not been reported after short-term use of the Cole tube.

Paranasal Complications

Cases of maxillary sinusitis and otitis during and following nasotracheal intubation have been reported (431–436). Symptoms include temperature elevations, purulent drainage, and pain on the intubated side.

Nasal Damage

Nostril damage including stenosis of the nares, septal erosion, necrosis of the alae nasi, and ulceration of the inferior turbinate have been reported (188, 437–444). These appear to be caused by ischemia secondary to pressure on the nose, and may be prevented by attention to fixation and support of the tube.

Dental and Oropharyngeal Complications

Gingival and dental complications are commonly the result of trauma during intubation. Oral intubation in the infant has been found to cause damage to the unerupted teeth (445). Palatal deformities associated with prolonged orotracheal intubation in infants have been reported (446, 447).

Ulcerations

Ulcerations (erosions) of the larynx and trachea can occur secondary to intubation trauma or while the tube is in place. They are probably very common, even when a tube has been in place for only a short time. The incidence and severity increase with the duration of intubation (448–450). They are less frequent and severe when tubes with soft cuffs are used.

Ulcers are commonly found on the posterior parts of the larynx and the anterior and lateral aspects of the trachea at the sites of the cuff and the tube tip (171, 202, 449, 451). They vary from superficial lesions involving only the mucosa to deep ones in which the underlying cartilage is exposed (449, 452). The end result will depend on the location, severity as well as other factors, such as infection, that affect the healing process. Most superficial ulcers heal completely. More severe ones may result in formation of granulation or fibrous tissue. Healing of tracheal ulcers may result in the normal ciliated epithelium being replaced with a stratified squamous epithelium (449). Such a zone may be a barrier to removal of particulate matter from the tracheobronchial tree. An ulcer may erode into a vessel and cause severe bleeding (453) or may erode through the wall of the trachea.

Most ulcerations are believed to be caused by either pressure ischemia or mechanical trauma (449). Mechanical trauma may occur during intubation or from movement (either spontaneous or transmitted from the ventilator) while the tube is in place.

The shape of the tube and head position are important in the etiology of ulcer formation. The curve of the usual shaped tube tends to bring the tip forward toward the larynx as it passes through the hypopharynx. Since the airway turns abruptly posterior at the level of the vocal cords, the tip will tend to strike the anterior wall of the lower larynx or upper trachea. The resilience of the tube will cause pressure at the posterior commissure of the larynx. Lowering and extending the head will increase the curve at the vocal cords and the pressure on the larynx and trachea.

Symptoms of ulceration include pain and hoarseness. Vocal exertion usually aggravates these symptoms.

Prevention of ulcer formation is accomplished by limiting the duration of intubation as much as possible. Use of low pressure cuffs for long term intubation will reduce (but not eliminate) the incidence and severity of ulcerations at the cuff level. Raising and flexing the head will lessen the curve of the tube at the larynx. Use of smaller and less stiff tubes and tubes with a short blunt tip distal to the cuff may prevent ulcerations on the anterior tracheal wall caused by the tube tip (454). Spiral embedded tubes may cause less pressure on the airway than other tubes. Use of a flexible tube from the Y-piece to the tube will allow free movement of the patient's head and neck and reduce movement between the trachea and the tube (455).

Any postoperative hoarseness lasting for more than a week should be investigated by laryngoscopy to look for the presence of ulceration. Conservative treatment with vocal rest will usually be effective in allowing the ulcers to heal.

Granuloma of the Vocal Cord (Post-Intubation Granuloma, Contact Ulcer Granuloma, Intubation Granuloma, Postanesthesia Granuloma)

Reports on the incidence of granulomas of the vocal cords vary from 1 in 800 to 1 in 20,000 intubations (456, 457). Most cases are in adults and they are far more frequent in women than in men. The greatest incidence is associated with head and neck surgery.

The most common location for vocal cord granulomas is on the posterior portions of the cords on or near the vocal processes of the arytenoids. The lesions usually are unilateral but are occasionally bilateral.

The initial lesion is most commonly believed to be an ulcer. Nonspecific granulation tissue forms in an attempt to cover the exposed tissues. Constant trauma from the opposite vocal process causes the granulation tissue to proliferate. It becomes epithelialized and develops into a sessile lesion. Healing takes place by fibrosis which narrows the base until the granuloma becomes pedunculated. This process may continue until the granuloma is shed and expelled.

The exact etiology is not known. A few granulomas apparently result from direct injury from the laryngoscope or tube during intubation. Most lesions, however, probably result from injury while the tube is in place. Head position and the natural curve on most endotracheal tubes forces the tube into the posterior commissures against the vocal processes. Irritation by the tube due to excessive size, toxic substances in its composition, and hardness or roughness have been implicated. Movement of the tube or larynx (with spasm, coughing, vomiting, straining, respiration, swallowing, or surgery) may cause friction between the tube and glottis. Infection has been implicated (457–459).

Symptoms commonly include persistent hoarseness, intermittent loss of voice, and pain or discomfort in the throat. Less common symptoms include a feeling of fullness or tension in the throat, chronic cough, hemoptysis, and pain extending to the ear. Some cases are symptomless (460). Occasionally respiratory obstruction with dyspnea and cyanosis may develop. Symptoms may start after intubation or may not develop for as long as several months later.

A number of prophylactic measures have been suggested. They include use of a proper sized tube, use of tubes that conform to the airway after insertion, raising and flexing the head during anesthesia, gentle atraumatic intubation and avoiding friction between the tube and larynx by establishment of a proper depth of anesthesia or with the use of muscle relaxants. It has been recommended that a short period of vocal rest succeed every intubation (461).

Persistent hoarseness after intubation warrants laryngeal examination to exclude the presence of an ulcer. If the examination reveals ulceration over the vocal processes, the development of a granuloma may be prevented by insisting on strict voice rest to allow healing to take place.

The granuloma may heal spontaneously and removal should be postponed until it is apparent this is not going to take place, unless the granuloma interferes with respiration. Operative removal is most likely to be successful when the lesion has reached the pedunculated stage. Attempts at removal during the sessile stage should be avoided unless there is respiratory embarassment, as recurrence is likely.

Laryngotracheal Membrane (Subglottic Membrane, Membranous or Pseudomembranous Laryngotracheitis, Pseudomembrane) Formation

Formation of a subglottic membrane is a relatively uncommon but serious and sometimes fatal postoperative complication (462, 463). Most cases follow an intubation lasting a few hours. In some cases the intubation was traumatic, but in others, no problems were encountered.

Clinically, the picture is one of respiratory obstruction resembling laryngeal edema with cough, hoarseness, stridor, dyspnea, and suprasternal retractions. However, the symptoms typically occur later than those associated with edema, usually 24–72 hr after extubation (462–464).

The membrane is believed to start with an injury to the laryngeal or tracheal mucosal, resulting in an ulceration. When the compressive forces on the tissue are reduced by removal of the tube or release of cuff pressure, exudates and inflammatory cells gain access to the damaged tissues and form a pseudomembrane that may become separated from the ulcerated mucosa (89). Several cases probably associated with use of glutaraldehyde have been reported (465).

The membrane typically forms on the anterior

aspect of the trachea. It may come in contact with the inferior surface of the vocal cords.

The membrane itself can form an obstruction to respiration. It may also produce reflex adduction of the vocal cords. A portion may become detached, causing sudden, sometimes fatal, respiratory obstruction (464). A similar situation has been reported in which mucosal slough caused acute respiratory obstruction (466, 467). If this is not immediately and appropriately treated, it may lead to sudden death (468).

The diagnosis is made by laryngoscopy, followed by bronchoscopy. Unless visualization of the larynx is performed, the condition may be erroneously diagnosed as edema and an unnecessary tracheostomy performed.

Treatment is immediate removal by suction. Removal may not be easy because areas of epithelium still attached to the underlying tissue may be present. If the entire membrane is not removed, it may recur in 24 hr (462).

Glottic Stenosis

Glottic stenosis of varying severity following intubation and caused by formation of fibrous tissue has been reported (77, 177, 467, 469–480). The most common locations are the interarytenoid area, the posterior commissure and the vocal processes (472).

Depending on the locations of the lesions, simple narrowing of the posterior commissure and minor restrictions of vocal cord mobility may result, synechiae and webs may develop, or a circumferential scar may form (203). Fibrous tissue formation may cause ankylosis of the cricoarytenoid joints and narrow the subglottic space, resulting in severe stenosis.

The clinical picture will depend on the location of the lesion and how much it obstructs the airway. The most common symptoms are hoarseness and dyspnea. Inspiratory stridor may occur. Respiratory obstruction may be life-threatening. Symptoms may occur anytime from a few hours to months or even years following intubation. Many cases are misdiagnosed as vocal cord paralysis (472). Surgical or laser treatment may be helpful (177, 472, 475, 481, 482).

Subglottic (Cricoid) Stenosis

Subglottic stenosis is a stricture of the airway at the site of the cricoid ring. It most commonly occurs after prolonged endotracheal intubation in infants and children (400, 482–484), but is also seen in adults (470).

Subglottic stenosis is believed to be the end result of a process beginning with inflammation and ulceration of the mucosa. The subglottic tissues in children are unusually intolerant of contact with foreign material (482). In addition, the cricoid ring is the smallest diameter of the main airway in children and because it is a complete ring, it cannot expand outward.

Inflammation caused by the presence of an endotracheal tube may cause ischemic pressure necrosis and increased trauma with resulting ulceration. This may be followed by perichondritis of the cricoid cartilage. Granulation tissue often develops and wounds heal by secondary intention with production of collagen. Because new collagen has a tendency to contract, stenosis ensues.

Symptoms may appear at the time of extubation or at a variable period afterwards. Most often they present days or weeks after extubation. They include cough, hoarseness, stridor (especially inspiratory), and recurrent or prolonged episodes of croup (483).

The important etiological factors appear to be pressure, movement, and infection (484). Pressure can result from too large a tube in relation to the lumen of the larynx and is increased with edema of the larynx. Constant movement between the tube and mucosa may produce ulceration. Airway disease may predispose to damage because the endotracheal tube acts as a foreign body and will irritate an already inflamed and edematous laryngeal mucosa. The duration and frequency of intubation are probably highly significant (444, 480). Chemical irritation and other factors appear to be of lesser importance.

Prevention includes gentle intubation, keeping the number of tube changes to a minimum, and keeping the duration of intubation as short as possible (482). The tube should be loose-fitting (485). Movement of the tube should be kept to a minimum.

Treatment of subglottic stenosis is usually by dilatation, especially in infants and young children. Tracheostomy may be indicated to temporize while the stenosis is treated with dilations or to allow for tracheal growth to ameliorate the stenosis (482). If the stenosis remains severe, resection may be required.

Subglottic Granulation Tissue

Just as ulceration on the vocal cords may be followed by formation of granulomas, ulcers in the subglottic region may give rise to granulation tissue and granulomas (18, 444, 467, 474, 478,

479, 481, 486, 487). Their principal importance is that they may cause respiratory obstruction. The onset of symptoms may be immediately after extubation or may be delayed for up to several weeks.

Diagnosis is made by laryngoscopy and/or bronchoscopy. Steroids should be administered. Usually the granulation tissue will regress and may disappear, but occasionally removal is required. Recurrence is quite common so that repeat bronchoscopies may be necessary.

Subglottic Cysts

Cases of upper airway obstruction resulting from cysts of the subglottic area following prolonged intubation have been reported (488, 489). The obstruction can be relieved by fracturing the cysts with a bronchoscope.

Tracheal Stenosis

Tracheal stenosis is one of the most serious complications of intubation. It is more common in adults than children. Most cases are associated with prolonged intubation. It is more common when high-pressure cuffs are used than when low-pressure cuffs are properly used.

The stenosis most commonly occurs at the site of the cuff but may also be seen at the site of the tube tip (93, 158, 455, 482, 490–495).

Stenosis represents the final stage of pathological events initiated by ulceration of the mucous membrane. The ulceration is followed by necrosis that extends into the underlying cartilage. Subsequent development of scar tissue converts the area into a circumferential fibrous stenosis.

The onset of symptoms may be immediately after extubation or weeks or even years after the tube is removed. Early symptoms include a dry cough and inability to raise sputum. The inability to raise sputum may result in an acute obstructive episode or an attack of pneumonia. The symptoms may progress to dyspnea and signs of respiratory obstruction (490).

Cuff pressure, movement of the tube, infection, chemical irritation and host factors such as systemic hypotension and steroid administration have been implicated in the etiology of tracheal stenosis. The duration of intubation is important.

Conservative measures, including dilatation, may be useful in the cases of mild stenosis or stenosis in the early formative stages. In severe mature fibrous stenosis these measures are unlikely to be successful and surgical correction will be necessary.

STYLETS

A stylet (introducer, guide, director, guiding catheter) is a device which fits inside an endotracheal tube. It facilitates insertion of the tube by making the tube more rigid and/or allowing its shape to be changed. It can also be used to check the patency of a tube before intubation and as an aid to change tubes (303).

A stylet should always be available when intubation is being performed. Many anesthesiologists routinely use a stylet while others reserve its use for difficult intubations. Certain endotracheal tubes (such as the spiral embedded tubes and those made of Silastic) usually require use of a stylet for insertion.

A stylet is often helpful during intubations where the larynx is difficult to visualize, when the operator recognizes the anatomical landmarks but cannot direct the tip of the endotracheal tube into the laryngeal inlet or when substantial movement of the head and/or neck is undesirable.

A variety of objects, including copper wires, coat hangers, crochet hooks, knitting needles, etc. have been used for stylets. Stylets are available from several manufacturers. Some of these have special non-friction coverings (496–498). A stylet should have enough malleability that its shape can be changed easily, yet enough rigidity that the endotracheal tube's shape will be maintained during insertion. It should be resistant to chipping and breaking.

The distal end of the stylet should be smooth so that trauma to soft tissues will be minimized if the tip should accidentally protrude from the bevel and the stylet will not damage the tube.

There should be a means to limit the stylet's advancement into the endotracheal tube. Bending the stylet acutely at the proximal end will also prevent advancement. The proximal end should be flared or have an attachment that will fit firmly into the endotracheal tube connector to prevent rotation of the tube on the stylet.

Unless the stylet has a nonstick coating, a thin film of lubricant should be spread over its length before insertion. Unless this is done, it may be difficult to remove the stylet after the tube is in place. The stylet should be inserted into the tube until the distal end is within ¼ inch of the tube tip and fixed so that the tip cannot advance. The tube and stylet should then be bent to the desired shape. For routine intubations a straight or slightly curved configuration is used. When an anterior larynx is encountered, a J shape or hockey stick configuration is usually desirable.

The larynx should be exposed in the usual manner and the endotracheal tube inserted. As soon as the distal part of the tube is inserted, the stylet is withdrawn.

Problems can occur with stylets. The increased rigidity of the tube may result in more trauma, especially during blind intubations. The tip may protrude from the end or through a Murphy eye, lacerating tissues. Part of the stylet may be sheared off during removal from the tube (284). Finally, the stylet may damage the endotracheal tube (289).

Flexible stylets with a mechanism to move the distal tip anteriorly, posteriorly, or laterally are available (499).

Lighted stylets are available to guide the endotracheal tube into the larynx by transillumination. With the room light dimmed, the position of the tip can be determined by the appearance of light shining through the tissues (500, 501). This works best with a transparent plastic tube (502).

An optical stylet has been described (503). It consists of a telescope with a built-in illuminator. Illumination is transmitted from an external light source via a flexible fiberoptic cable. It allows an unobstructed view through the endotracheal tube during the entire intubation procedure. It can be used alone or with a standard laryngoscope to keep the tongue out of the way. It may permit visualization of the larynx in difficult intubations where the glottic opening cannot be visualized with a standard laryngoscope.

FORCEPS

Forceps can be used to direct an endotracheal tube into the larynx or a nasogastric tube or other device into the esophagus. It can also be used to insert pharyngeal packing and to retrieve foreign objects. Forceps should be readily available whenever an intubation is performed.

The most popular type is the Magill forceps. These are designed so that when the grasping ends are in the axis of the tracheal tube, the handle is at a right angle. Thus the operator can have the larynx exposed by a laryngoscope held in the left hand, the tube in full view and hold the forceps in the right hand, out of the line of sight.

Cuff damage frequently occurs when forceps are used with high-volume cuffs. It is suggested that these tubes be picked up at the tip, not the cuff.

References

1. Wall MA: Infant endotracheal tube resistance: effects of changing length, diameter and gas density. *Crit Care Med* 8:38–40, 1980.
2. Boretos JW, Battis CG, Goodman L: Decreased resistance to breathing through a polyurethane pediatric endotracheal tube. *Anesth Analg* 51:292–296, 1972.
3. Baier H, Begin R, Sackner MA: Effect of airway diameter, suction catheters and the bronchofiberscope on airflow in endotracheal and tracheostomy tubes. *Heart Lung* 5:235–238, 1976.
4. Duckworth SI: The Oxford non-kinking endotracheal tube. *Anaesthesia* 17:208–214, 1962.
5. Brown ES: Resistance factors in pediatric endotracheal tubes and connectors. *Anesth Analg* 50:355–360, 1971.
6. Colgan FJ, Liang JQ, Barrow RE: Noninvasive assessment by capacitance respirometry of respiration before and after extubation. *Anesth Analg* 54:807–813, 1975.
7. Demers RR, Sullivan MJ, Paliotta J: Airflow resistances of endotracheal tubes. *JAMA* 237:1362, 1977.
8. Demers RR, Sullivan MJ, Paliotta J: The clinical importance of endotracheal tube resistance. *Resp Care* 22:919–921, 1977.
9. Haynes MS, Cornelius DB, Johnson RL Jr: The contribution of endotracheal tube resistance to total pulmonary resistance and the work of breathing. *Am Rev Resp Dis* 119:127, 1979.
10. Gal TJ, Suratt PM: Resistance to breathing in healthy subjects following endotracheal intubation under topical anesthesia. *Anesth Analg* 59:270–274, 1980.
11. Cave P, Fletcher G: Resistance of nasotracheal tubes used in infants. *Anesthesiology* 29:588–590, 1968.
12. Carroll RG, Kamen JM, Grenvick A, Safan P, Robison E, Stoner DL, Sheridan DS, McGinnis GE: Recommended performance specifications for cuffed endotracheal and tracheostomy tubes: a joint statement of investigators, inventors, and manufacturers. *Crit Care Med* 11:155–156, 1973.
13. Shupak RC, Deas TC: The ideal tracheal tube. Proceedings of a Workshop on Tracheal Tubes, Valley Forge, Pa., April 30–May 1, 1981, pp 103–106.
14. Guess WL: Tissue testing of polymers. *Int Anesthesiol Clin* 8:787–804, 1970.
15. Wu W, Arteaga M, Mlodozeniec AR, Popper PJ: Surface ultrastructure and pressure dynamics of tracheal tube cuffs. *Biomed Mat Res* 14:11–21, 1980.
16. Guess WL: Rubber for tracheal tubes. *Int Anesthesiol Clin* 8:815–821, 1970.
17. Guess WL, Stetson JB: Tissue toxicity from rub-

ber endotracheal tubes. *Int Anesthesiol Clin* 8:823–828, 1970.

18. Stetson JB, Guess WL: Causes of damage to tissues by polymers and elastomers used in the fabrication of tracheal devices. *Anesthesiology* 33:635–652, 1970.

19. Williams DP: The reactions of tissues to materials. *Biomed Eng* 6:152–156, 1971.

20. Guess WL: Plastics for tracheal tubes. *Int Anesthesiol Clin* 8:805–814, 1970.

21. Ingraham FD, Alexander E, Matson DD: Polyethylene, a new synthetic plastic for use in surgery. *JAMA* 135:82–87, 1947.

22. Rendell-Baker L: Members alerted to irritation resulting from some plastic endotracheal tubes. ASA Newsletter, Vol 32, No. 3, March 1968.

23. Eustace RR, Boucher RF, Horne M, Richards EG: A clinical appraisal of polyvinyl endotracheal tubes. *Anesthesiology* 24:366–372, 1969.

24. *American National Standard for Anesthetic Equipment—Tracheal Tubes.* ANSI Z79.14-1983, American National Standards Institute, 1430 Broadway, New York, N.Y. 10018.

25. Bernhard WN, Yost L, Turndorf H, Danziger F: Cuffed tracheal tubes—physical and behavioral characteristics. *Anesth Analg* 61:36–41, 1982.

26. Murphy FJ: Two improved intratracheal catheters. *Anesth Analg.* 20:102–105, 1941.

27. Cole F: An endotracheal tube for babies. *Anesthesiology* 6:627–628, 1945.

28. Cole F: A new endotracheal tube for infants. *Anesthesiology* 6:87–88, 1945.

29. Glauser EM, Cook CK, Bougas TP: Pressure-flow characteristics and dead spaces of endotracheal tubes used in infants. *Anesthesiology* 22:339–341, 1961.

30. Hatch DJ: Tracheal tubes and connectors used in neonates—dimensions and resistance to breathing. *Br J Anaesth* 50:959–964, 1978.

31. Brandstater B: Dilatation of the larynx with Cole tubes. *Anesthesiology* 31:378–379, 1969.

32. Lindholm CE: Experience with a new orotracheal tube. *Acta Otolaryngol* 75:389–390, 1973.

33. Loeser EA, Machin R, Colley J, Orr D, Bennett GM, Stanley TH: Postoperative sore throat—importance of endotracheal tube conformity versus cuff design. *Anesthesiology* 49:430–432, 1978.

34. Ring WH, Adair JC, Elwyn RA: A new pediatric endotracheal tube. *Anesth Analg* 54:273–274, 1975.

35. McTaggart RA, Shustack A, Noseworthy T, Johnston R: Another cause of obstruction in an armored endotracheal tube. *Anesthesiology* 59:164, 1983.

36. Adamson DH: A problem of prolonged oral intubation: case report. *Can Anaesth Soc J* 18: 213–214, 1971.

37. Walton WJ: An invaginated tube. *Br J Anaesth* 39:520, 1967.

38. Hedden M, Smith RBF, Torpey DJ: A complication of metal spiral-imbedded latex endotracheal tubes. *Anesth Analg* 51:859–862, 1972.

39. Dunn GL: Letters to the Editor. *Can Anaesth Soc J* 22:379–380, 1975.

40. Malone BT: A complication of Rusch armored endotracheal tubes. *Anesth Analg* 54:756, 1975.

41. Ng TY, Krimili BI: Hazards in use of anode endotracheal tube: a case report and review. *Anesth Analg* 54:710–714, 1975.

42. Birkhan HJ, Heifetz M: "Uninflatable" inflatable cuffs. *Anesthesiology* 26:578, 1965.

43. Jacobson J: A hazard of armored endotracheal anesthesia. *Anesth Analg* 48:37–41, 1969.

44. Robbie DS, Pearce DJ: Some dangers of armoured tubes. *Anaesthesa* 14:379–385, 1959.

45. Ohn K, Wu W: Another complication of armored endotracheal tubes. *Anesth Analg* 59:215–216, 1980.

46. Munson ES, Stevens DS, Redfern RE: Endotracheal tube obstruction by nitrous oxide. *Anesthesiology* 52:275–276, 1980.

47. Burns THS: Danger from flexometallic endotracheal tubes. *Br Med J* 1:439–440, 1956.

48. Kohli MS, Manku RS: Reinforced endotracheal tube-diversion of air from cuff balloon producing obstruction. *Anesthesiology* 27:513–514, 1966.

49. Catane R, Davidson JT: A hazard of cuffed flexometallic endotracheal tubes. *Br J Anaesth* 41:1086, 1969.

50. Davies RM: Faulty construction of a reinforced latex endotracheal tube. *Br J Anaesth* 35:128–129, 1963.

51. Rendell-Baker L: Reinforced tracheal tube hazard alert. *Anesth Analg* 59:519–520, 1980.

52. *Tracheal Tubes.* CSA Z168.1, Canadian Standards Association, 178 Rexdale Blvd., Rexdale, Ontario, Canada, 1970.

53. Cohen DD: Note on endotracheal tubes. *Anesthesiology* 33:463, 1970.

54. Cope RW, Anderson SM, Hawksley M, Glover WJ, Jackson DG: A "new" infant anaesthetic set. *Anaesthesia* 19:297, 1964.

55. Stenqvist O, Sonander H, Nilsson K: Small endotracheal tubes. Ventilator and intratracheal pressures during controlled ventilation. *Br J Anaesth* 51:375–381, 1979.

56. Mackenzie CF, Shin B, Whitley N, Schellinger D: The relationship of human trachea size to body habitus. *Anesthesiology* 51:S378, 1979.

57. Mackenzie CF, Shin B, Whitley N, Helrich M: Human tracheal circumference as an indicator of correct cuff size. *Anesthesiology* 53:S414, 1980.

58. Lindholm C: Prolonged intubation. Part I. Importance of cuff design and tube shape. Prevention of glottic and tracheal stenosis. In Proceedings of a Workshop on Tracheal Tubes, Valley Forge, Pa., April 30–May 1, 1981, pp 3–12.

59. Mostafa SM: Variation in subglottic size in children. *Proc R Soc Med* 69:793–795, 1976.

60. Fisk GC: Variation in sizes of endotracheal tubes for infants and young children. *Anaesth Intensive Care* 1:418–422, 1973.

61. Gregory GA: Respiratory care of newborn infants. *Pediatr Clin N Am* 19:311–324, 1971.

62. Downes JJ: Pediatric tracheal tube considerations. Part I. In Proceedings of a Workshop on Tracheal Tubes, Valley Forge, Pa; April 30–May 1, 1981, pp 62–81.

63. Steward DJ: Endotracheal tubes for infants and children. In Proceedings of a Workshop on Tracheal Tubes. Valley Forge, Pa; April 30–May 1, 1981, pp 82–90.

64. Penlington GN: Endotracheal tube sizes for children. *Anaesthesia* 24:494–495, 1975.
65. Corfield HMC: Orotracheal tubes and the metric system. *Br J Anaesth* 35:34, 1963.
66. Lane GA, Pashley RT, Fishman RA: Tracheal and cricoid diameters in the premature infant. *Anesthesiology* 53:S326, 1980.
67. Baby finger width shows endotracheal tube size. *JAMA* 228:960, 1974.
68. Gregory GA: Respiratory care of the child. *Crit Care Med* 8:582–587, 1980.
69. Zulliger JJ, Garvin JP, Schuller DE, Birck HG, Beach TP, Frank JE: Assessment of intubation in croup and epiglottitis. *Ann Otol Rhinol Laryngol* 91:403–406, 1982.
70. Tochen ML: Orotracheal intubation in the newborn infant: a method for determining depth of tube insertion. *J Pediatr* 95:1050–1051, 1979.
71. Saha AK: The estimation of the correct length of oral endotracheal tubes in adults. *Anaesthesia* 32:919–920, 1977.
72. Schellinger RR: The length of the airway to the bifurcation of the trachea. *Anesthesiology* 25:169–172, 1964.
73. Jackson-Rees G, Owen-Thomas JB: A technique of pulmonary ventilation with a nasotracheal tube. *Br J Anaesth* 38:901–906, 1966.
74. Mattila MAK, Heikel PE, Suutarinen, Lindfors EL: Estimation of a suitable nasotracheal tube length for infants and children. *Acta Anaesth Scand* 15:239–246, 1971.
75. Coldiron JS: Estimation of nasotracheal tube length in neonates. *Pediatrics* 41:823–828, 1968.
76. Chander S, Feldman E: Correct placement of endotracheal tubes. *NY State J Med* 79:1843–1844, 1979.
77. Smith BL: Confirmation of the position of an endotracheal tube. *Anaesthesia* 30:410, 1975.
78. Vigneswaran R, Whitfield JM: The use of a new ultra-thin fiberoptic bronchoscope to determine endotracheal tube position in the sick newborn infant. *Chest* 80:174–177, 1981.
79. Whitehouse AC, Klock LE: Evaluation of endotracheal tube position with the fiberoptic intubation laryngoscope. *Chest* 68:848, 1975.
80. Todres ID, deBros F, Kramer SS: Endotracheal tube displacement in the newborn. Papers, American Society of Anesthesiologists Meeting, 1975, pp 27–28.
81. Conrady PA, Goodman LR, Lainge F, Singer MM: Alteration of endotracheal tube position. *Crit Care Med* 4:8–12, 1976.
82. Frost PM: The design of disposable endotracheal tubes. *Anaesthesia* 32:387–388, 1977.
83. McGinnis GE, Shively JG, Patterson RL, Magovern GJ: An engineering analysis of intratracheal tube cuffs. *Anesth Analg* 50:557–564, 1971.
84. Magovern GJ, Shively JG, Fecht D, Thevoz F: The clinical and experimental evaluation of a controlled-pressure intratracheal cuff. *J Thorac Cardiovasc Surg* 64:747–756, 1972.
85. Kosanin R, Maroff M: Continuous monitoring of endotracheal intracuff pressures in patients receiving general anesthesia utilizing nitrous oxide. *Anesthesiol Rev* 8:29–32, 1981.
86. Brandt L: Pressures on tracheal tube cuffs. *Anaesthesia* 37:597–598, 1981.
87. Carroll RG: Evaluation of tracheal tube cuff designs. *Crit Care Med* 1:45–46, 1973.
88. Lewis FR, Schlobohm RM, Thomas AN: Prevention of complications from prolonged tracheal intubation. *Am J Surg* 135:452–457, 1978.
89. Leigh JM, Maynard JP: Pressure on the tracheal mucosa from cuffed tubes. *Br Med J* 1:1173–1174, 1979.
90. Nordin U: The trachea and cuff-induced tracheal injury: *Acta Otolaryngol Suppl* 345:1–74, 1977.
91. Dobrin P, Canfield T: Cuffed endotracheal tubes: mucosal pressures and tracheal wall blood flow. *Am J Surg* 133:562–568, 1977.
92. Bernhard WN, Cottrell JE, Sivakumaran C, Patel K, Yost L, Turndorf H: Adjustment of intracuff pressure to prevent aspiration. *Anesthesiology* 50:363–366, 1979.
93. Cooper JD, Grillo HC: Analysis of problems related to cuffs on intratracheal tubes. *Chest* 62:21S–27S, 1972.
94. Schneider JC, Main D, O'Connor TD, Garrard CC: Comparison of endotracheal tube cuff pressures using a minimal leak technique. *Crit Care Med* 10:235, 1982.
95. Wu W, Lim I, Simpson FA, Turndorf H: Pressure dynamics of endotracheal and tracheostomy cuffs. *Crit Care Med* 1:197–202, 1973.
96. Dunn CR, Dunn DL, Moser KM: Determinants of tracheal injury by cuffed tracheostomy tubes. *Chest* 65:128–135, 1974.
97. Carroll R, Hedden M, Safar P: Intratracheal cuffs: performance characteristics. *Anesthesiology* 31:275–281, 1969.
98. Ward CF, Gamel DM, Benumof JL: Endotracheal tube cuff herniation: a cause of delayed airway obstruction. *Anesth Analg* 57:114–116, 1978.
99. Jensen PJ, Hommelgaard P, Sondergaard P, Eriksen S: Sore throat after operation; influence of tracheal intubation, intracuff pressure and type of cuff. *Br J Anaesth* 54:453–457, 1982.
100. Loeser EA, Orr DL, Bennett GM, Stanley TH: Endotracheal tube cuff design and postoperative sore throat. *Anesthesiology* 45:684–687, 1976.
101. Loeser EA, Bennett G, Orr D, Stanley TH: Reduction of postoperative sore throat with new endotracheal tube cuffs. Papers, American Society of Anesthesiologists Annual Meeting, 1978, pp 213–214.
102. Loeser EA, Machin R, Colley J, Bennett G, Stanley TH: Post-operative sore throat: importance of endotracheal tube conformity versus cuff design. Papers, American Society of Anesthesiologists Annual Meeting, 1977, pp 655–656.
103. Loeser EA, Bennett GM, Orr DL, Stanley TH: Reduction of postoperative sore throat with new endotracheal tube cuffs. *Anesthesiology* 52:257–259, 1980.
104. Loeser EA, Stanley TH, Jordan W, Machin R: Postoperative sore throat: influence of tracheal tube lubrication versus cuff design. *Can Anaesth Soc J* 27:156–158, 1980.
105. Stanley TH, Loeser EA: Minimizing sore throat. *Anesthesiology* 51:488–489, 1979.
106. Black AMS, Seegobin RD: Pressures on endotra-

cheal tube cuffs. *Anaesthesia* 36:498–511, 1981.

107. Loeser EA, Hodges M, Gliedman J, Stanley TH, Johansen RK, Yonetani D: Tracheal pathology following short-term intubation with low- and high-pressure endotracheal tube cuffs. *Anesth Analg* 57:577–579, 1978.

108. Mamawadu BR, Miller R: Endotracheal cuff inflation. An improved technique. *Anesthesiol Rev* 4:46–47, 1977.

109. Chandler S: Air volume in endotracheal tube cuffs. *Anesthesiology* 53:437, 1980.

110. Bernhard WN, Yost LC, Turndorf H, Cottrell JE, Paegle RD: Physical characteristics of and rates of nitrous oxide diffusion into tracheal tube cuffs. *Anesthesiology* 48:413–417, 1978.

111. Brandt L: Nitrous oxide in oxygen and tracheal tube cuff volumes. *Br J Anaesth* 54:1238–1239, 1982.

112. Ikeda D, Schweiss JF: Tracheal tube cuff volume changes during extracorporeal circulation. *Can Anaesth Soc J* 27:453–457, 1980.

113. Mehta S: Effects of nitrous oxide and oxygen on tracheal tube cuff gas volumes. *Br J Anaesth* 53:1227–1231, 1981.

114. Revenas R, Lindholm CE: Pressure and volume changes in tracheal tube cuffs during anaesthesia. *Acta Anaesth Scand* 20:321–326, 1976.

115. Stanley TH: Effects of anesthetic gases on endotracheal tube cuff gas volumes. *Anesth Analg* 53:480–482, 1974.

116. Stanley TH, Kawamura R, Graves C: Effects of nitrous oxide on volume and pressure of endotracheal tube cuffs. *Anesthesiology* 41:256–262, 1974.

117. Stanley TH: Nitrous oxide and pressures and volumes of high and low-pressure endotracheal-tube cuffs in intubated patients. *Anesthesiology* 42:637–640, 1975.

118. Stanley TH, Liu W: Tracheostomy and endotracheal tube cuff volume and pressure changes during thoracic operations. *Ann Thorac Surg* 20:144–151, 1975.

119. Konchigeri HN, Lee YE: Preventive measure against nitrous oxide induced volume and pressure changes of endotracheal tube cuffs. Papers, American Society of Anesthesiologists Annual Meeting, 1977, pp 661–662.

120. Archibald C: Reduced tracheal damage from prestretched cuffs. *Resp Ther* 2:29–31, 1972.

121. Arola MK, Anttinen J: Post-mortem findings of tracheal injury after cuffed intubation and tracheostomy. *Acta Anaesth Scand* 23:57–68, 1979.

122. Grillo HC, Cooper JD, Geffin B, Pontoppidan H: A low-pressure cuff for tracheostomy tubes to minimize tracheal injury. A comparative clinical trial. *J Thorac Cardiovasc Surg* 62:898–907, 1971.

123. Mathias DB, Wedley JR: The effects of cuffed endotracheal tubes on the tracheal wall. *Br J Anaesth* 46:849–852, 1974.

124. Geffin B, Pontoppidan H: Reduction of tracheal damage by the prestretching of inflatable cuffs. *Anesthesiology* 31:462–463, 1969.

125. Ching NP, Ayres SM, Paegle RP, Linden JM, Nealon TF: The contribution of cuff volume and pressure in tracheostomy tube damage. *J Thorac Cardiovasc Surg* 62:402–410, 1971.

126. Cross DE: Recent developments in tracheal cuffs. *Resuscitation* 2:77–81, 1973.

127. Nealon TF, Ching N: Pressures of tracheostomy cuffs in ventilated patients. *NY State J Med* 71:1923–1928, 1971.

128. MacKenzie CF, Klose S, Browne DRG: A study of inflatable cuffs on endotracheal tubes. *Br J Anaesth* 48:105–110, 1976.

129. Tonnesen AS, Vereen L, Arens JF: Endotracheal tube cuff residual volume and lateral wall pressure in a model trachea. *Anesthesiology* 55:680–683, 1981.

130. Crawley BE, Cross DE: Tracheal cuffs. A review and dynamic pressure study. *Anaesthesia* 30:4–11, 1975.

131. MacKenzie CF, Shin B, McAslan TC, Blanchard CL, Cowley RA: Severe stridor after prolonged endotracheal intubation using high-volume cuffs. *Anesthesiology* 50:235–239, 1979.

132. Macrae W, Wallace P: Aspiration around high-volume, low-pressure endotracheal cuff. *Br Med J* 283:1220, 1981.

133. Cottrell JE, Bernhard WN, Sivukumaran C, Patel K, Turndorf H: Endotracheal aspiration associated with cuffed-tracheal tubes. Papers, American Society of Anesthesiologists Meeting, 1977, pp 179–180.

134. Egnatinsky J: Overinflating low-pressure-cuffs to prevent aspiration. *Anesthesiology* 42:114, 1975.

135. Routh G, Hanning CD, Ledingham IM: Pressure on the tracheal mucosa from cuffed tubes. *Br Med J* 1:1425, 1979.

136. Mehta S: Aspiration around high-volume low-pressure endotracheal cuff. *Br Med J* 284:115–116, 1982.

137. Pavlin EG, VanNimwegan D, Hornbein TF: Failure of a high-compliance low-pressure cuff to prevent aspiration. *Anesthesiology* 42:216–219, 1975.

138. Pippin LK, Short DH, Bowes JB: Long-term tracheal intubation practice in the United Kingdom. *Anaesthesia* 38:791–795, 1983.

139. Ripoli I, Lindhold C, Carroll R, Grenvik A: Spontaneous dislocation of endotracheal tubes: a problem with too soft tube material. *Crit Care Med* 6:101–102, 1978.

140. Ripoli I, Lindhold CE, Carroll R, Grenvik A: Spontaneous dislocation of endotracheal tubes. *Anesthesiology* 49:50–52, 1978.

141. Job CA, Betcher AM, Pearson WT, Fernandez MA: Intraoperative obstruction of endobronchial tubes. *Anesthesiology* 51:550–553, 1979.

142. Nakao MA, Killam D, Wilson R: Pneumothorax secondary to inadvertent nasotracheal placement of a nasoenteric tube past a cuffed endotracheal tube. *Crit Care Med* 11:210–211, 1983.

143. Sweatman AJ, Tomasello PA, Loughhead MO, Orr M, Datta T: Misplacement of nasogastric tubes and oesophageal monitoring devices. *Br J Anaesth* 50:389–392, 1978.

144. Stark P: Inadvertent nasogastric tube insertion into the tracheobronchial tree. A hazard of new high-residual volume cuffs. *Radiology* 142:239–240, 1982.

145. Sweatman AJ, Tomasello MG, Loughhead M,

Orr M, Datta T: Misplacement of nasogastric tubes and oesophageal monitoring devices. *Br J Anaesth* 50:389–392, 1978.

146. King K, Mandava B, Kamen JM: Tracheal tube cuffs and tracheal dilatation. *Chest* 67:458–462, 1975.

147. Leverment JN, Pearson PG, Rae S: Tracheal size following tracheostomy with cuffed tracheostomy tubes: an experimental study. *Thorax* 30:271–277, 1975.

148. Carroll RG, Grenvick A: Proper use of large diameter, large residual volume cuffs. *Crit Care Med* 1:153–154, 1973.

149. Ching NPH, Ayres SM, Spina RC, Nealon TF: Endotracheal damage during continuous ventilatory support. *Ann Surg* 179:123–127, 1974.

150. Bernhard WN, Yost L, Joynes D, Cavallo R, Steffee T: Just seal intracuff pressures during mechanical ventilation. *Anesthesiology* 57:A145, 1982.

151. Cox PM, Schatz ME: Pressure measurements in endotracheal cuffs: a common error. *Chest* 65:84–87, 1974.

152. Lawler PG, Rayner RR: The limitations of the Shiley pressure relief adaptor. *Anaesthesia* 37:865, 1982.

158. Kim J: The tracheal tube cuff pressure stabilizer and its clinical evaluation. *Anesth Analg* 59:291–296, 1980.

154. Stanley TH, Foote JL, Lu WS: A simple pressure-relief valve to prevent increases in endotracheal tube cuff pressure and volume in intubated patients. *Anesthesiology* 43:478–481, 1975.

155. Jacobson L, Greenbaum R: A study of intracuff pressure measurements, trends and behavior in patients during prolonged periods of tracheal intubation. *Br J Anaesth* 53:97–101, 1981.

156. Stoner DL, Cooke JP: Intratracheal cuffs and aeromedical evacuation. *Anesthesiology* 41:302–306, 1974.

157. Kamen JM, Wilkinsos CJ: A new low-pressure cuff for endotracheal tubes. *Anesthesiology* 34:482–485, 1971.

158. Trout C: Artificial airways: tubes and trachs. *Resp Care* 12:513–520, 1976.

159. Boyer FE, Crouch NB, Beekham RW: Comparison of endotracheal tube intracuff pressures. *Resp Ther* 7:57–58, 1977.

160. Lederman DS, Klein EF, Drury WD, Donnelly WH, Appleford JJ, Chapman RL, Downs J: A comparison of foam and air-filled endotracheal-tube cuffs. *Anesth Analg* 53:521–526, 1974.

161. Shapiro BA, Olson SF, Fleming RS, Harrison RA: Case study: myasthenia gravis. *Resp Care* 19:460–465, 1974.

162. Patterson RL: Correspondence. *Surv Anesthesiol* 22:500–501, 1978.

163. Tavakoli M, Corssen G: An unusual case of difficult extubation. *Anesthesiology* 45:552–553, 1976.

164. Kamen JM, Wilkinson C: Removal of an inflated endotracheal tube cuff. *Anesthesiology* 46:308–309, 1977.

165. *Tracheal Tube Connectors and Adapters.* ANSI Z79.2-1976, American National Standards Institute, 1430 Broadway, New York, N.Y. 10018.

166. Galloon S: The resistance of endotracheal connectors. *Br J Anaesth* 29:160–165, 1957.

167. Smith WDA: The effects of external resistance to respiration. Part II. Resistance to respiration due to anaesthetic apparatus. *Br J Anaesth* 33:610–627, 1961.

168. Questions and Answers. *Anesth Analg* 53:573–574, 1974.

169. Stauffer JL, Silvestri RC: Complication of endotracheal intubation, tracheostomy, and artificial airways. *Resp Care* 27:417–434, 1982.

170. Cooper JD, Malt RA: Meteorism produced by nasotracheal intubation and ventilatory assistance. *N Engl J Med* 287:652–653, 1972.

171. Dubick MN, Wright BD: Comparison of layrngeal pathology following long-term oral and nasal endotracheal intubations. *Anesth Analg* 57:663–668, 1978.

172. Pecora DV, Seinige U: Prolonged endotracheal intubation. *Chest* 82:130, 1982.

173. Seltzer AP: Complications of nasotracheal intubation. *J Natl Med Assoc* 61:415–416, 1969.

174. Scott M, Brechner VL: Retrobulbar hemorrhage from nasotracheal intubation. *Anesthesiology* 20:717, 1959.

175. Bennett EJ, Grundy EM, Patel KP: Visual signs in blind nasal intubation. A new technique. *Anesthesiol Rev* 5:18–20, 1978.

176. Tahir AH: A simple manoeuvre to aid the passage of nasotracheal tube into the oropharynx. *Br J Anaesth* 42:631–632, 1970.

177. Warner WA: Layngeal band: possible relation to prolonged nasotracheal intubation. *Anesthesiology* 28:466–467, 1967.

178. Dryden GE: Use of a suction catheter to assist blind nasal intubation. *Anesthesiology* 45:260, 1976.

179. Liew RPC: A technique of naso-tracheal intubation with the soft Portex tube. *Anaesthesia* 28:567–568, 197.

180. Tobias R: Increased success with retrograde guide for endotracheal intubation. *Anesth Analg* 62:366–367, 1983.

181. Bourke D, Levesque PR: Modification of retrograde guide for endotracheal intubation. *Anesth Analg* 53:1013–1014, 1974.

182. Dunn EJ, Lee CM, Graham WP, Roberts DH: Translaryngeal guide for tracheal intubation. *Anesthesiol Rev* 2:30–31, 1975.

183. Freilich JD, Sassano JL: Orotracheal intubation using modified Seldinger technique in an adult patient with tracheal stenosis. *Anesthesiol Rev* 9:25–26, 1982.

184. Harmer M, Vaughan R: Guided blind oral intubation. *Anaesthesia* 35:921, 1980.

185. Powell WF, Ozdil T: A translaryngeal guide for tracheal intubation. *Anesth Analg* 46:231–234, 1967.

186. Roberts KW: New use for Swan-Ganz introducer wire. *Anesth Analg* 60:67, 1981.

187. Bednarek FJ, Kuhns LR: Endotracheal tube placement in infants determined by suprasternal palpation: a new technique. *Pediatrics* 56:224–229, 1975.

188. Gowdar K, Bull MJ, Schreiner RL, Lemons JA, Gresham EL: Nasal deformities in neonates.

Their occurrence in those treated with nasal continuous positive airway pressure and nasal endotracheal tubes. *Am J Dis Child* 134:954–957, 1980.

189. Arrott JJ, Talley AW: Endotracheal tube holder. *Anesth Analg* 53:70–71, 1974.

190. Ayoub AH, Libby A, Stabilization of oral endotracheal tubes and airways in long-term intubation. *Resp Care* 22:744–745, 1977.

191. Bloch EC: Prolonged paediatric nasotracheal tube fixation. *Br J Anaesth* 45:995, 1973.

192. Cussell G, Levy L, Thompson RE: A method of securing orotracheal tubes in neonatal respiratory care. *Pediatrics* 53:266–267, 1974.

193. Dangel PH, Curarasamy N: Safe system for prolonged nasotracheal intubation. *Lancet* 1:916–918, 1973.

194. Epstein RA: A method of fixation of nasotracheal tubes in infants. *Anesthesiology* 33:458–459, 1970.

195. Edwards JM: A method of fixation of endotracheal tubes. *Br J Anaesth* 44:990–991, 1972.

196. Garcia-Tornel S, Martin JM, Carits J, Toberna L, Garcia ME: Method of fixating tubes in infants and children. *Resp Care* 22:58, 1978.

197. Konchigeri HN, Homi J: A simple technique of endotracheal-tube fixation. *Anesthesiology* 40:498, 1974.

198. Molho M, Lieberman P: Safe fixation of oro- and nasotracheal tubes for prolonged intubation in neonates, infants and children. *Crit Care Med* 3:81–82, 1975.

199. Richards SD: A method for securing pediatric endotracheal tubes. *Anesth Analg* 60:224–225, 1981.

200. Tahir AH, Adriani J: A method for anchoring oral endotracheal tubes during pediatric anesthesia. *Anesth Analg* 50:314–315, 1971.

201. Young TM: Securing the endotracheal tube. *Anaesthesia* 31:1094–1095, 1976.

202. Donnelly WH: Histopathology of endotracheal intubation. *Arch Pathol* 88:511–520, 1969.

203. Keane WM, Denneny JC, Rowe LD, Atkins JP: Complications of intubation. *Ann Otol Rhinol Laryngol* 91:584–587, 1982.

204. Gonty AA, Racey GL: Nasal endotracheal intubation for outpatient anesthesia. *J Oral Surg* 98:191–195, 1980.

205. Tintinalli JE, Claffey J: Complications of nasotracheal intubation. *Ann Emerg Med* 10:142–144, 1981.

206. Binning R: A hazard of blind nasal intubation. *Anaesthesia* 29:366–367, 1974.

207. Barnard J: An unusual accident during intubation *Anaesthesia* 3:126, 1948.

208. Jaffe BF: Postoperative hoarseness. *Am J Surg* 123:432–437, 1972.

209. Komorn RM, Smith CP, Erwin JA: Acute laryngeal injury with short-term endotracheal anesthesia. *Laryngoscope* 83:683–690, 1973.

210. Kambic V, Radsel Z: Intubation lesions of the larynx. *Br J Anaesth* 50:587–590, 1978.

211. Prasertwanitch Y, Schwarz JJH, Vandam LD: Arytenoid cartilage dislocation following prolonged endotracheal intubation. *Anesthesiology* 41:516–517, 1974.

212. Talbert JL, Rodgers BM, Felman AH, Moazam F: Traumatic perforation of the hypopharynx in infants. *J Thorac Cardiovasc Surg* 74:152–156, 1977.

213. Touloukian RJ, Beardsley GP, Ablow RC, Effmann EL: Traumatic perforation of the pharynx in the newborn. *Pediatrics* 59:1019–1022, 1977.

214. Smith RH, Pool LL, Volpitto PP: Subcutaneous emphysema as a complication of endotracheal intubation. *Anesthesiology* 20:714–716, 1959.

215. Stauffer JL, Petty TL: Accidental intubation of the pyriform sinus. A complication of "roadside" resuscitation. *JAMA* 237:2324–2325, 1977.

216. Wolff AP, Kuhn FA, Ogura JH: Pharyngeal-esophageal perforations associated with rapid oral endotracheal intubation. *Ann Otol* 81:258–261, 1972.

217. Richard RR, Burford JG, George RB: Subcutaneous crepitance occurring during mechanical ventilation. *Resp Care* 27:181–182, 1982.

218. Intubation hazards. *Br J Anaesth* 14:147–149, 1952.

219. Manhein A, Perez RE Jr., Nevin JE III: A rare complication from a not-so-rare occurrence (endotracheal intubation). *South Med J* 64:814–819, PASIM, 1971.

220. Myers EM: Hypopharyngeal perforation: a complication of endotracheal intubation. *Laryngoscope* 92:583–585, 1982.

221. Hawkins DB, Seltzer DC, Barnett TE, Stoneman GB: Endotracheal tube perforation of the hypopharynx. *West J Med* 120:282–286, 1974.

222. Adelman MH: Perforation of the pyriform sinus, a sequela of endotracheal intubation. *J Mt Sinai Hosp* 19:665–667, 1953.

223. Guernelli N, Bragaglia RB, Briccoli A, Mastrorilli M, Vecchi R: Tracheobronchial ruptures due to cuffed Carlens tubes. *Ann Thorac Cardiovasc Surg* 28:66–68, 1979.

224. Kumar SM, Pandit SK, Cohen PJ: Tracheal laceration associated with endotracheal anesthesia. *Anesthesiology* 47:298–299, 1977.

225. Orta DA, Cousar JE, Yergin BM, Olsen GN: Tracheal laceration with massive subcutaneous emphysema: a rare complication of endotracheal intubation. *Thorax* 34:665–669, 1979.

226. Serlin SP, Daily WJR: Tracheal perforation in the neonate: a complication of endotracheal intubation. *J Pediatr* 86:596–597, 1975.

227. Schild JP, Wuilloud A, Kollberg H, Bossi E: Tracheal perforation as a complication of nasotracheal intubation in a neonate. *J Pediatr* 88:631–632, 1976.

228. Thompson DS, Read RC: Rupture of the trachea following endotracheal intubation. *JAMA* 204:995–997, 1968.

229. Pembleton WE, Brooks JW: Esophageal perforation of unusual etiology. *Anesthesiology* 45:680–681, 1976.

230. Kanarek KS, David RF: Traumatic perforation of the esophagus in a newborn. *J Fla Med Assoc* 66:288–289, 1979.

231. Eklof O, Lohr G, Okmian L: Submucosal perforation of the esophagus in the neonate. *Acta Radiol* 8:187–192, 1969.

232. Dubost C, Kaswin D, Duranteau A, Jehanno C,

Kaswin R: Esophageal perforation during attempted endotracheal intubation. *J Thorac Cardiovasc Surg* 78:44–51, 1979. ·

233. Dickson JAS, Fraser GC: "Swallowed" endotracheal tube: a new neonatal emergency. *Br Med J* 1:811–812, 1967.

234. Abrahams N, Goldacre M, Reynolds EOR: Removal of swallowed neonatal endotracheal tube. *Lancet* 2:135–136, 1970.

235. Flynn GJ, Lowe AK: Endotracheal tube swallowed by a neonate. *Med J Aust* 1:62–63, 1973.

236. Kennedy S: Swallowed neonatal endotracheal tube. *Lancet* 2:264, 1970.

237. Mucklow ES: "Swallowed" endotracheal tube. *Br Med J* 2:618, 1967.

238. Prinn MG: "Swallowed" endotracheal tube. *Br Med J* 3:176, 1967.

239. Storch A, Calderwood GC: Endotracheal tube swallowed by neonate. *J Pediatr* 77:123, 1970.

240. Storch A: Swallowed neonatal endotracheal tube. *Lancet* 2:421, 1970.

241. Utting JE, Gray TC, Shelley FC: Human misadventure in anaesthesia. *Can Anaesth Soc J* 26:472–478, 1979.

242. Peterson AW, Jacker LM: Death following inadvertent esophageal intubation. A case report. *Anesth Analg* 32:398–401, 1973.

243. Pollard BJ, Junius F: Accidental intubation of the oesophagus. *Anaesth Intensive Care* 8:183–186, 1980.

244. Howells TH, Riethmuller RJ: Signs of endotracheal intubation. *Anaesthesia* 35:984–986, 1980.

245. Dhamee MS: Signs of endotracheal intubation. *Anaesthesia* 36:328–329, 1981.

246. Cundy J: Accidental intubation of oesophagus. *Anaesth Intensive Care* 9:76, 1981.

247. Knill RL, Gelb AW: Peripheral chemoreceptors during anesthesia: are the watchdogs sleeping? *Anesthesiology* 57:151–152, 1982.

248. Manninen P, Knill RL: Cardiovascular signs of acute hypoxaemia and hypercarbia during enflurane and halothane anaesthesia in man. *Can Anaesth Soc J* 26:282–287, 1979.

249. Batra AK, Cohn MA: Uneventful prolonged misdiagnosis of esophageal intubation. *Crit Care Med* 11:760–764, 1980.

250. Ionescu T. Signs of endotracheal intubation. *Anaesthesia* 36:422–423, 1981.

251. Taryle DA, Chandler JE, Good JT, Potts DE, Sahn SA: Emergency room intubations—complications and survival. *Chest* 75:541–543, 1979.

252. Dronen S, Chadwick O, Nowak R: Endotracheal tip position in the arrested patient. *Ann Emerg Med* 108:116–117, 1982.

253. Alberti J, Hanafee W, Wilson G, Bethune R: Unsuspected pulmonary collapse during neuroradiologic procedures. *Radiology* 89:316–320, 1967.

254. Hamilton WK, Stevens WC: Malpositioning of endotracheal catheters. *JAMA* 198:1113, 1966.

255. Heinonen J, Takki S, Tammisto T: Effect of the Trendelenburg tilt and other procedures on the position of endotracheal tubes. *Lancet* 1:850–853, 1969.

256. Kuhns LR Poznanski AK: Endotracheal tube position in the infant. *J Pediatr* 78:991–996, 1971.

257. Twigg HL, Buckley CE: Complications of endotracheal intubation. *Am J Roentgenol* 109:452–454, 1970.

258. Zwillich CW, Pierson DJ, Creash CE, Sutton FD, Schatz E, Petty TL: Complications of assisted ventilation. *Am J Med* 57:161–170, 1974.

259. Tisi GM, Twigg HL, Moser KM: Collapse of left lung induced by artificial airway. *Lancet* 1:791–793, 1968.

260. Todres ID, deBros F, Kramer SS: Endotracheal tube displacement in the newborn infant. *J Pediatr* 89:126–127, 1976.

261. Bosman YK, Foster PA: Endotracheal intubation and head posture in infants. *S Afr Med J* 52:71–73, 1977.

262. Cowan RJ, Short DB, Maynard CD: Nonperfusion of one lung secondary to improperly positioned endotracheal tube. *JAMA* 227:1165–1166, 1974.

263. Seto K, Goto H, Hacker DC, Arakawa K: Right upper lobe atelectasis after inadvertent right main bronchial intubation. *Anesth Analg* 62:851–854, 1983.

264. Loew A, Thiebeault DW: A new and safe method to control the depth of endotracheal intubation in neonates. *Pediatrics* 54:506–508, 1974.

265. Mattila MAK, Suutarinen T, Sulamaa M: Prolonged endotracheal intubation or tracheostomy in infants and children. *J Pediatr Surg* 4:674–682, 1969.

266. Moyers J, Gregory GA: Use of fiberoptic bronchoscopy to reposition an endotracheal tube intraoperatively. *Anesthesiology* 43:685, 1975.

267. Cullen DJ, Newbower RS, Gemer M: A new method for positioning endotracheal tubes. *Anesthesiology* 48:596–599, 1975.

268. Kopman EA: A simple method for verifying endotracheal tube placement. *Anesth Analg* 56:123–124, 1977.

269. Vredevoe LA, Brechner T, Moy P: Obstruction of anomalous tracheal bronchus with endotracheal intubation. *Anesthesiology* 55:581–583, 1981.

270. Kaeder CS, Hirshman CA: Acute airway obstruction: a complication of aluminum tape wrapping of tracheal tubes in laser surgery. *Can Anaesth Soc J* 26:138–139, 1979.

271. Tahir AH: Endotracheal tube lost in the trachea. *JAMA* 222:1061–1062, 1972.

272. Gaisford JC, Hanna DC, Monheim LM: Endotracheal anesthesia complications associated with head and neck surgery. *Plast Reconstr Surg* 24:463–471, 1959

273. Chiu T, Meyers EF: Defective disposable endotracheal tube. *Anesth Analg* 55:437, 1976.

274. Milstein J, Rabinovitz J, Goetzman B: A foreign body hazard in the neonate. *Anesth Analg* 56:726–727, 1977.

275. Doyle LA, Conway CF: A hazard of cuffed endotracheal tubes. *Anaesthesia* 22:140–141, 1967.

276. Davies A, Rowlands DE: Endotracheal tubes. *Anaesthesia* 26:79, 1971.

277. Kleine JW, Moesker A: Endotracheal tubes. *Anaesthesia* 27:104–105, 1972.

278. Loughrey JD: Danger of cuffed endotracheal tube

during tracheostomy. *Br J Anaesth* 39:692, 1967.

279. Smotrilla MM, Nagel EL, Moya E: Failure of inflatable cuff resulting in foreign body in the trachea. *Anesthesiology* 27:512–513, 1966.

280. Vourcih G, Tannieres ML, Freche G: Anaesthesia for microsurgery of the larynx using a carbon dioxide laser. *Anaesthesia* 34:53–57, 1979.

281. Yeung ML, Lett Z: An uncommon hazard of armoured endotracheal tubes. *Anaesthesia* 29:186–187, 1974.

282. Desmeules H: Defective tracheal tube connector. *Can Anaesth Soc J* 29:404, 1982.

283. Lahay WD: Defective tracheal tube connector. *Can Anaesth Soc J* 29:80–81, 1982.

284. Restall CJ: Plastic-covered wire stylet. *Anesth Analg* 55:755, 1976.

285. Berry FA, Blankenbaker WL, Ball CG: A comparison of bacteremia occurring with nasotracheal and orotracheal intubation. *Anesth Analg* 52:873–876, 1979.

286. Rowse CW: Bacteraemia induced by endotracheal intubation. *Br Dent J* 151:363, 1981.

287. Gerber MA, Gastanaduy AS, Buckley JJ, Kaplan EL: Risk of bacteremia after endotracheal intubation for general anesthesia. *South Med J* 73:1478–1480, 1980.

288. Pagar DM, Kupperman AW, Stern M: Cutting of nasoendotracheal tube: an unusual complication of maxillary osteotomies. *J Oral Surg* 36:314–315, 1978.

289. Munson ES, Lee R, Kushing LG: A new complication associated with the use of wire-reinforced endotracheal tubes. *Anesth Analg* 58:152, 1979.

290. Jayasuriya KD, Watson WF: P.V.C. cuffs and lignocaine-base aerosol. *Br J Anaesth* 53:1368, 1981.

291. Debnath SK, Waters DJ: Leaking cuffed endotracheal tubes: two case reports. *Br J Anaesth* 40:807, 1968.

292. Blitt CD, Wright WA: An unusual complication of percutaneous internal jugular vein cannulation, puncture of an endotracheal tube cuff. *Anesthesiology* 40:306–307, 1974.

293. Brown HI, Burnard RJ, Jensen M, Wightman AE: Puncture of endotracheal-tube cuffs during percutaneous subclavian-vein catheterization. *Anesthesiology* 43:112–113, 1975.

294. Fagraeus L, Angelillo JC, Dolan EA: A serious anesthetic hazard during orthognathic surgery. *Anesth Analg* 59:150–152, 1980.

295. Hought R, Zallen RD, Nathan R: Use of a metallic nasal tube protector during maxillary osteotomy. *J Oral Surg* 36:977, 1978.

296. Patel C, Cotten C, Turndorf H: Partial severance of an oronasotracheal tube during a le Fort I procedure. *Anesthesiology* 58:357, 1980.

297. Mosby EL, Messer EJ, Nealis MF: Intraoperative damage to nasotracheal tubes during maxillary surgery—report of cases. *J Oral Surg* 36:963–964, 1978.

298. Orr DL: Airway compromise during oral and maxillofacial surgery: case report and review of potential causes. *Anesth Prog* 25:161–168, 1978.

299. Tseuda K, Carey WJ, Gonty AA, Bosomworth PB: Hazards to anesthetic equipment during maxillary osteotomy: report of cases. *J Oral Surg* 35:47, 1977.

300. Bamforth BJ: Complications during endotracheal anesthesia. *Anesth Analg* 42:727–733, 1963.

301. Tahir AH, Adriani J: Failure to effect satisfactory seal after hyperinflation of endotracheal cuff. *Anesth Analg* 50:540–543, 1971.

302. Desai SP Fencl V: A safe technique for changing endotracheal tubes. *Anesthesiology* 53:267, 1980.

303. Finucane BT, Kipshik HL: A flexible stilette for replacing damaged tracheal tubes. *Can Anaesth Soc J* 25:153–154, 1978.

304. Rosenbaum SH, Rosenbaum LM, Cole RP, Askanazi J, Hyman AI: Use of the flexible fiberoptic bronchoscope to change endotracheal tubes in critically ill patients. *Anesthesiology* 54:169–170, 1981.

305. Watson CB: Use of fiberoptic bronchoscope to change endotracheal tube endorsed. *Anesthesiology* 55:476–477, 1981.

306. Cozine K, Rosenbaum LM, Askanazi J, Rosenbaum SH: Laser-induced endotracheal tube fire. *Anesthesiology* 55:583–585, 1981.

307. Oxygen fire during laser surgery: $5 million suit filed. *Biomed Safety Stand* 11:87, 1981.

308. Snow JC, Norton ML, Saluja TS: Fire hazard during CO_2 laser microsurgery on the larynx and trachea. *Anesth Analg* 55:146–147, 1976.

309. Vourcih G, Tannieres M, Freche G: Ignition of a tracheal tube during laryngeal laser surgery. *Anaesthesia* 34:685, 1979.

310. Burgess GE, LeJeune FE: Endotracheal tube ignition during laser surgery of the larynx. *Arch Otolaryngol* 105:561–562, 1979.

311. Hirshman CA, Smith J: Indirect ignition of the endotracheal tube during carbon dioxide laser surgery. *Arch Otolaryngol* 106:639–641, 1980.

312. Hermens JM, Bennett MJ, Hirshman CA: Anesthesia for laser surgery. *Anesth Analg* 62:218–229, 1983.

313. Wainwright AC, Moody RA, Carruth JAS: Anaesthetic safety with the carbon dioxide laser. *Anaesthesia* 36:411–415, 1981.

314. Patel V, Stehling LC, Zauder HL: A modified endotracheal tube for laser microsurgery. *Anesthesiology* 51:571, 1979.

315. Hirshman CA, Leon D, Porch D, Everts E, Smith JD: Improved metal endotracheal tube for laser surgery of the airway. *Anesth Analg* 59:789–791, 1980.

316. Norton ML, Vos P: New endotracheal tube for laser surgery of the larynx. *Ann Otol Rhinol Laryngol* 87:554–557, 1978.

317. Redding GJ, Fan L, Cotton EK, Brooks JG: Partial obstruction of endotracheal tubes in children. *Crit Care Med* 7:227–231, 1979.

318. Duffy BL: Delayed onset of respiratory obstruction during endotracheal anesthesia. *S Afr Med J* 50:1551–1552, 1976.

319. Johnson JT, Maloney RW, Cummings CW: Tracheostomy tube: cuff obstruction. *JAMA* 238:211, 1977.

320. Rao CC, Krishna G, Trueblood S: Stenting of the endotracheal tube to manage airway obstruction in the prone position. *Anesth Analg* 59:700–701, 1980.

321. Anonymous: Tracheal tube kinking. *Health Devices* 7:292–293, 1978.

322. Cohen DD, Dillon JB: Hazards of armored en-

dotracheal tubes. *Anesth Analg* 51:856–858, 1972.

323. Gold ML, Atwood JM: Respiratory obstruction. *Anesthesiology* 26:577–578, 1965.

324. Gilston A: Obstruction of endotracheal tube. *Anthesia* 24:256, 1969.

325. Carter GL, Holcomb MC: An unusual cause of endotracheal tube obstruction. *Anesthesiol Rev* 5:51–53, 1978.

326. Hitchen JE, Wiener AP: Unexpected obstruction of a nasotracheal tube: report of case. *J Oral Surg* 31:722–724, 1973.

327. Haselhuhn DH: Obstruction of nasotracheal tube by impacted nasal secretion. *Anesthesiology* 20:589, 1962.

328. Henzig D, Rosenblatt R: Thrombotic occlusion of a nasotracheal tube. *Anesthesiology* 51:484–485, 1979.

329. Peers B: Foreign bodies in endotracheal tubes. *Anaesth Intensive Care* 3:267, 1975.

330. Robinson BC, Jarrett WJ: Postoperative complication after blind nasotracheal intubation for reduction of a fractured mandible: report of case. *J Oral Surg* 29:340–343, 1971.

331. Tofany VI: Occlusion of endotracheal catheter. *Anesthesiology* 22:124–125, 1961.

332. Torres LE, Reynolds RC: A complication of use of a microlaryngeal surgery endotracheal tube. *Anesthesiology* 53:355, 1980.

333. Powell DR: Obstruction to endotracheal tubes. *Br J Anaesth* 46:252, 1974.

334. Stark DCC: Endotracheal tube obstruction. *Anesthesiology* 45:467–468, 1976.

335. Jenkins AV: Unexpected hazard of anaesthesia. *Lancet* 1:761–762, 1959.

336. Haselhuhn DH: Occlusion of endotracheal tube with foreign body. *Anesthesiology* 19:561–562, 1958.

337. Wittman FW: Airway obstruction due to a foreign body. *Anaesthesia* 37:865–866, 1982.

338. Dutton CS: A bizarre cause of obstruction in an Oxford non-kink endotracheal tube. *Anaesthesia* 17:395–396, 1962.

339. Stewart KA: Foreign body in endotracheal tube. *Br Med J* 2:1226, 1958.

340. Rainer EH: Foreign body in endotracheal tube. *Br Med J* 2:1357, 1958.

341. Goudsouzian NG, Ryan JF, Moench B: An unusual cause of endotracheal tube obstruction in a child. *Anesthesiol Rev* 7:23–24, 1980.

342. Shaw EA: Airway obstruction. *Anaesthesia* 26:368–369, 1971.

343. Barat G, Ascorve A, Avello F: Unusual airway obstruction during pneumonectomy. *Anaesthesia* 31:1290–1291, 1976.

344. McLellan I: Blockage of tracheal connectors with K-Y jelly. *Anaesthesia* 30:413–416, 1975.

345. Blitt CD: Case report: complete obstruction of an armored endotracheal tube. *Anesth Analg* 58:624–625, 1974.

346. Singh CV: Bizarre airway obstruction. *Anaesthesia* 32:812–813, 1977.

347. Rendell-Baker L: A hazard alert—reinforced endotracheal tubes. *Anesthesiology* 53:268–269, 1980.

348. Lall NG: Airway obstruction with latex armoured endotracheal tube. *Indian J Anaesth* 17:297, 1969.

349. Bachand R, Fortin G: Airway obstruction with cuffed flexometallic tracheal tubes. *Can Anaesth Soc J* 23:330–333, 1976.

350. Seuffert GW, Urbach KF: An additional hazard of endotracheal intubation. *Can Anaesth Soc J* 15:300–301, 1968.

351. Pryer DL, Pryer RLR, Williams AF: Fatal respiratory obstruction due to faulty endotracheal tube. *Lancet* 2:742–743, 1960.

352. Mirakhur RK: Airway obstruction with cuffed armoured tracheal tubes. *Can Anaesth Soc J* 21:251–258, 1974.

353. Brasch RC, Heldt GP, Hecht ST: Endotracheal tube orifice abutting the tracheal wall: a cause of infant airway obstruction. *Radiology* 141:387–391, 1981.

354. Gooneratne RS: Throat packing for oral surgery. *Anaesth Intensive Care* 11:79–80, 1983.

355. Saxena GC, Vittal K: Unusual cause of obstruction to endotracheal tube. *Indian J Anaesth* 17:295–296, 1969.

356. Thompson RC: Obstructed endotracheal tube demonstrated by roentgenogram. *JAMA* 162:194–196, 1956.

357. Hartnett JS: Aberrant inflation of disposable endotracheal tube with complete airway obstruction. *J Am Assoc Nurse Anesth* 38:57–58, 1970.

358. Stoneham FJR: Danger from cuffed endotracheal tubes. *Br Med J* 2:565, 1952.

359. Roland P, Stovner J: Brain damage following collapse of a "polyvinyl" tube: elasticity and permeability of the cuff. *Acta Anaesth Scand* 19:303–309, 1975.

360. Ketover AK, Feingold A: Collapse of a disposable endotracheal tube by its high-pressure cuff. *Anesthesiology* 48:108–110, 1975.

361. Muir J, Davidson-Lamb R: Apparatus failure—cause for concern. *Br J Anaesth* 52:705–706, 1980.

362. Patel K, Teviotdale B, Dalal FY: Internal herniation of a Murphy endotracheal tube. *Anesthesiol Rev* 5:60–61, 1978.

363. Chan MCY: Collapse of endotracheal tubes. *Anaesth Intensive Care* 9:289–290, 1981.

364. Dietz GW, Pierce AK, Christensen EE: Endotracheal tube compression demonstrated by roentgenogram. *JAMA* 206:2512–2518, 1968.

365. Bishop MJ: Endotracheal tube lumen compromise from cuff overinflation. *Chest* 80:100–101, 1981.

366. Perel A, Katzenelson R, Klein E, Cotev S: Collapse of endotracheal tubes due to overinflation of high-compliance cuffs. *Anesth Analg* 56:731–733, 1977.

367. Hoffman S, Freedman M: Delayed lumen obstruction in endotracheal tubes. *Br J Anaesth* 48:1025–1028, 1976.

368. Abramowitz MD, McNabb TG: A new complication of flexometallic endotracheal tubes. *Br J Anaesth* 48:928, 1976.

369. Chamberlin DA, Tatham PF: Defective adaptor delays resuscitation. *Lancet* 1:188, 1970.

370. Zebrowski ME: Buckled adaptor. *Anesthesiology* 51:276–277, 1979.

371. Harmel MH: Intubation of the trachea does not absolutely insure a patent airway. *NY State J Med* 56:2125–2126, 1956.

372. Forrester AC: Mishaps in anesthesia. *Anaesthesia* 14:388–399, 1959.

373. Choked by faulty Magill tube. *Br Med J* 2:1383, 1953.

374. Mehta S: Performance of low-pressure cuffs. An experimental evaluation. *Ann R Coll Surg Engl* 64:54–56, 1982.

375. Mostert JW: Cuffs do not seal the trachea airtight. *Anesthesiology* 46:309–310, 1977.

376. Hahn FW, Martin JT, Lillie JC: Vocal cord paralysis with endotracheal intubation. *Arch Otolaryngol* 92:226–229, 1970.

377. Browning DH, Graves SA: Incidence of aspiration with endotracheal tubes in children. *J Pediatr* 102:582–584, 1983.

378. Goodwin SR, Graves SA, Haberkern CM: Aspiration in premature infants with endotracheal tubes. *Anesthesiology* 59:A435, 1980.

379. Pinkus NB: The dangers of oral feeding in the presence of cuffed tracheostomy tubes. *Med J Aust* 1:1238–1240, 1973.

380. Mehta S: The risk of aspiration in presence of cuffed endotracheal tubes. *Br J Anaesth* 44:601–605, 1972.

381. Cooke JW: The risk of aspiration in presence of cuffed endotracheal tubes. *Br J Anaesth* 44:1335, 1972.

382. Cheney D: The risk of aspiration in presence of cuffed endotracheal tubes. *Br J Anaesth* 44:1335, 1972.

383. Burgess GE, Cooper JR Jr, Marino RJ, Peuler MJ, Warriner RA: Laryngeal competence after tracheal extubation. *Anesthesiology* 51:73–77, 1979.

384. Siedlecki J, Borowicz JA, Adamski M: Impairment of efficiency of laryngeal defensive reflexes after regaining full consciousness following endotracheal anaesthesia. *Anaesth Res Intensive Ther* 2:247–252, 1974.

385. Honig EG, Francis PB: Persistent tracheal dilatation: Onset after brief mechanical ventilation with a "soft-cuff" endotracheal tube. *South Med J* 72:487–489, 1979.

386. Fryer ME, Marshall RD: Tracheal dilatation. *Anaesthesia* 31:470–478, 1976.

387. Jacobsen E, Jensen J: Tracheal dilatation. A complication of tracheostomy. *Acta Anaesth Scand* 12:95–102, 1968.

388. Bain JA: Late complications of tracheostomy and prolonged endotracheal intubation. *Int Anesthesiol Clin* 10:225–244, 1972.

389. Lloyd JW, McClelland RMA: Tracheal dilation. An unusual complication of tracheostomy. *Lancet* 1:83–84, 1964.

390. Conrady PA, Goodman LR, Lainge F, Singer MM: Nasotracheal tube mobility with flexion and hyperextension of the neck. *Crit Care Med* 1:117, 1973.

391. Tashayod M, Oskoui B: A case of difficult extubation. *Anesthesiology* 39:337, 1973.

392. Lee C, Schwartz S, Mok MS: Difficult extubation due to transfixation of a nasotracheal tube by a Kirschner wire. *Anesthesiology* 46:427, 1977.

393. Hilley MD, Henderson RB, Giesecke AH: Difficult extubation of the trachea. *Anesthesiology* 59:149–150, 1983.

394. Dryden GE: Circulatory colapse after pneumo-

nectomy (an unusual complication from the use of a Carlens catheter): case report. *Anesth Analg* 56:451–452, 1977.

395. Fagraeus L: Difficult extubation following nasotracheal intubation. *Anesthesiology* 49:43–44, 1978.

396. Sklar GS, Alfonso AE, King BD: An unusual problem in nasotracheal extubation. *Anesth Analg* 55:302–303, 1976.

397. Lall NG: Difficult extubation. A fold in the endotracheal cuff. *Anaesthesia* 35:500–501, 1980.

398. Mishra P, Scott DL: Difficulty at extubation of the trachea. *Anaesthesia* 38:811, 1983.

399. Ng TY, Datta TD: Difficult extubation of an endotracheal tube cuff. *Anesth Analg* 55:876–877, 1976.

400. Pavlin EG, Nelson E, Pulliam J: Difficulty in removal of tracheostomy tubes. *Anesthesiology* 44:69–70, 1976.

401. Tavakoli M, Corssen G: An unusual case of difficult extubation. *Anesthesiology* 45:552–553, 1976.

402. Gould AB, Seldon TH: An unusual complication with a cuffed endotracheal tube. *Anesth Analg* 47:239–240, 1968.

403. Wolfson B: Minor laryngeal sequelae of endotracheal intubation. *Br J Anaesth* 30:326–332, 1958.

404. Wylie WD: Hazards of intubation. *Anaesthesia* 9:143–148, 1950.

405. Sobel AM, Sheiner B, Boyer R: Possible prevention of complications following endotracheal anesthesia. *Anesth Analg* 43:504–509, 1964.

406. Jones GOM, Hale DE, Wasmuth CE, Homi J, Smith ER, Viljoen J: A survey of acute complications associated with endotracheal intubation. *Cleve Clin Q* 35:23–31, 1968.

407. Hamelberg W, Welch CM, Siddall J, Jacoby J: Complications of endotracheal intubation. *JAMA* 168:1959–1962, 1958.

408. Gard MA, Cruickshank LFG: Factors influencing the incidence of sore throat following endotracheal intubation. *Can Med Assoc J* 84:662–665, 1961.

409. Conway CM, Miller JS, Sugden FLH: Sore throat after anesthesia. *Br J Anaesth* 32:219–223, 1960.

410. Campbell D: Trauma to larynx and trachea following intubation and tracheostomy. *J Laryngol Otol* 82:981–986, 1968.

411. Baron SH, Kohlmoos HW: Laryngeal sequelae of endotracheal anesthesia. *Ann Otol Rhinol Laryngol* 60:767–792, 1951.

412. Riding JE: Minor complications of general anaesthesia. *Br J Anaesth* 47:91–101, 1975.

413. Stenqvist O, Nilsson K: Postoperative sore throat related to tracheal tube cuff design. *Can Anaesth Soc J* 29:384–386, 1982.

414. Ravindran R, Priddy S: Uvular edema, a rare complication of endotracheal intubation. *Anesthesiology* 48:374, 1978.

415. Seigne TD, Felske A, DelGiudice PA: Uvular edema. *Anesthesiology* 49:375–376, 1978.

416. Waterman PM, Smith RB: Tracheal intubation and pediatric outpatient anesthesia. *Eye Ear Nose Throat Monthly* 52:173–177, 1973.

417. Lee KW, Templeton JJ, Dougal RM: Tracheal tube size and post-intubation croup in children. *Anesthesiology* 53:S325, 1980.

418. Koka BV, Jeon IS, Andre JM, MacKay I, Smith RM: Postintubation croup in children. *Anesth Analg* 56:501–505, 1977.
419. Biller HF, Harvey JE, Bone RC, Ogura JH: Laryngeal edema. An experimental study. *Ann Otol Rhinol Laryngol* 79:1084–1087, 1970.
420. Jordan WS, Graves CL, Elwyn RA: New therapy for postintubation laryngeal edema and tracheitis in children. *JAMA* 212:585–588, 1970.
421. Taussig LM, Castro O, Beaudry PH, Fox WW, Bureau M: Treatment of laryngotracheobronchitis (croup): use of intermittent positive-pressure breathing and racemic epinephrine. *Am J Dis Child* 129:790–793, 1975.
422. Prolonged intubation may cause vocal cord paresis. *JAMA* 242:15, 1979.
423. Cox RH, Welborn SC: Vocal cord paralysis after endotracheal anesthesia. *South Med J* 74:1258–1259, 1981.
424. Ellis PDM, Pallister WK: Recurrent laryngeal nerve palsy and endotracheal intubation. *J Laryngol Otol* 89:823–826, 1975.
425. Gibbin KP, Egginton MJ: Bilateral vocal cord paralysis following endotracheal intubation. *Br J Anaesth* 53:1091–1092, 1981.
426. Holley HS, Gildea JE: Vocal cord paralysis after tracheal intubation. *JAMA* 215:281–284, 1971.
427. Kennedy RL: Questions and answers. *Anesth Analg* 56:321–322, 1977.
428. Mass L: Another post-endotracheal vocal cord paralysis of uncertain etiology. *Anesthesiol Rev* 2:28–30, 1975.
429. Minuck M: Unilateral vocal cord paralysis following endotracheal intubation. *Anesthesiology* 45:448–449, 1976.
430. Salem MR, Wong AY, Barangan, Canalis RF, Shaker MH, Lotter AM: Postoperative vocal cord paralysis in paediatric patients. *Br J Anaesth* 48:696–699, 1971.
431. Arens JF, LeJeune FE, Webre DR: Maxillary sinusitis: a complication of nasotracheal intubation. *Anesthesiology* 40:415–416, 1974.
432. Caplan ES, Hoyt NJ: Sinusitis: a complication of nasal intubation in critically ill patients. *Crit Care Med* 9:261, 1981.
433. Pope TL, Stelling CB, Leitner YB: Maxillary sinusitis after nasotracheal intubation. *South Med J* 74:610–612, 1981.
434. Knodel AR, Beekman JF: Unexplained fevers in patients with nasotracheal intubation. *JAMA* 248:868–870, 1982.
435. Stauffer JL, Olson DE, Petty TL: Complications and consequences of endotracheal intubation and tracheotomy: a prospective study of 150 critically ill adult patients. *Am J Med* 70:65–76, 1981.
436. Berman SA, Balkany TJ, Simmons MA: Otitis media in the neonatal intensive care unit. *Pediatrics* 62:190–201, 1978.
437. Sherry KM: Ulceration of the inferior turbinate: a complication of prolonged nasotracheal intubation. *Anesthesiology* 59:148–149, 1983.
438. Zwillich C, Pierson DJ: Nasal necrosis: A complication of nasotracheal intubation. *Chest* 64:376–377, 1973.
439. Barkin ME, Trieger N: An unusual complication of nasal-tracheal anesthesia. *Anesth Prog* 23:57–

58, 1976.
440. Baxter RJ, Johnson JD, Geotzman BW, Hackel A: Cosmetic nasal deformities complicating prolonged-nasotracheal intubation in critically ill newborn infants. *Pediatrics* 55:884–886, 1975.
441. Jung AL, Thomas GK: Stricture of the nasal vestibule: a complication of nasotracheal intubation in newborn infants. *J Pediatr* 85:412–414, 1974.
442. Owen-Thomas JB: A follow-up of children treated by prolonged nasal intubation. *Can Anaesth Soc J* 14:543–550, 1967.
443. Pettet G, Merenstein GB: Nasal erosion with nasotracheal intubation. *J Pediatr* 87:149–150, 1975.
444. Hatcher CR, Calvert JR, Logan WD, Symbas PN, Abbott OA: Prolonged endotracheal intubation. *Surg Gynecol Obstet* 127:759–762, 1968.
445. Boice JB, Krous HF, Foley JM: Gingival and dental complications of orotracheal intubation. *JAMA* 236:957–958, 1976.
446. Duke PM, Coulson JD, Santos JI, Johnson JD: Cleft palate associated with prolonged orotracheal intubation in infancy. *J Pediatr* 89:990–991, 1976.
447. Saunders BS, Easa D, Slaughter RJ: Acquired palatal groove in neonates. A report of two cases. *J Pediatr* 89:988–989, 1976.
448. Hegendorfer U, Peter K, Ruckert U: Damage to the respiratory tract after prolonged intubation and tracheostomy in adults with special consideration to morphology. *Surv Anesthesiol* 16:219–220, 1972.
449. Paegle RD, Ayres SM, Davis S: Rapid tracheal injury by cuffed airways and healing with loss of ciliated epithelium. *Arch Surg* 106:31–34, 1973.
450. Rasche RFH, Kuhns LR: Histopathologic changes in airway mucosa of infants after endotracheal intubation. *Pediatrics* 50:632–637, 1972.
451. Burns HP, Dayal VS, Scott A, van Nostrand AWP, Bryce DP: Laryngotracheal trauma: observations on its pathogenesis and its prevention following prolonged orotracheal intubation in the adult. *Laryngoscope* 89:1316–1325, 1979.
452. Cooper JD, Grillo HC: Experimental production and prevention of injury due to cuffed tracheal tubes. *Surg Gynecol Obstet* 129:1235–1241, 1969.
453. Paegle RD: Fatal hemorrhage from airway tube tip. *JAMA* 246:40, 1981.
454. Benumof JL, Berryhill RE, Maruschak GF, Ozaki GT, Meathe EA: Tracheal wall pressure caused by endotracheal tube tip. *Anesthesiology* 51:S193, 1979.
455. Andrews MJ, Pearson FG: Incidence and pathogenesis of tracheal injury following cuffed tube tracheostomy with assisted ventilation. *Ann Surg* 178:249–263, 1971.
456. Howland WS, Lewis JS: Postintubation granulomas of the larynx. *Cancer* 9:1244–1247, 1956.
457. Snow JC, Harano M, Balogh K: Postintubation granuloma of the larynx. *Anesth Analg* 45:425–429, 1966.
458. Howland WS, Lewis JS: Mechanisms in the development of postintubation granulomas of the larynx. *Ann Otol Rhinol Laryngol* 65:1006–1011, 1956.
459. Epstein SS, Winston P: Intubation granuloma.

J Laryngol Otol 71:37–48, 1957.

460. Carruthers HC, Graves HB: The complications of endotracheal anaesthesia. *Can Anaesth Soc J* 3:244–252, 1956.

461. Bergstrom J: Post-intubation granuloma of the larynx. *Acta Otolaryngol* 57:113–118, 1964.

462. Etsten B, Mahler D: Subglottic membrane. A complication of endotracheal intubation. *N Engl J Med* 245:957–960, 1951.

463. Muir AP, Straton J: Membranous laryngo-tracheitis following endotracheal intubation. *Anaesthesia* 9:105–113, 1954.

464. Lewis RN, Swerdlow M: Hazards of endotracheal anaesthesia. *Br J Anaesth* 36:504–515, 1964.

465. Belani KG, Priedkalns J: An epidemic of pseudomembranous laryngotracheitis. *Anesthesiology* 47:530–531, 1977.

466. Ozdil T, von der Lage FC, Kattine AA, Duncan OJ: Postintubation acute respiratory distress due to annular slough of laryngotracheal mucosa. *Anesth Analg* 56:356–358, 1977.

467. Tonkin JP, Harrison GA: The effect on the larynx of prolonged endotracheal intubation. *Med J Aust* 2:581–587, 1966.

468. Lu AT, Tamura Y, Koobs DH: The pathology of laryngotracheal complications. *Arch Otolaryngol* 74:105–114, 1961.

469. Lindholm CE: Prolonged endotracheal intubation. *Acta Anaesth Scand (Suppl)* 33:1–131, 1969.

470. Hawkins B: Glottic and subglottic stenosis from endotracheal intubation. *Laryngoscope* 87:339–346, 1977.

471. Allen TH, Steven IM: Prolonged endotracheal intubation in infants and children. *Br J Anaesth* 37:566–573, 1965.

472. Cohen SR: Pseudolaryngeal paralysis: a postintubation complication. *Ann Otol* 90:483–488, 1981.

473. Fearon B, MacDonald RE, Smith C: Airway problems in children following prolonged endotracheal intubation. *Ann Otol Rhinol Laryngol* 75:975–986, 1966.

474. Harrison GA, Tonkin JP: Some serious laryngeal complications of prolonged endotracheal intubation. *Med J Aust* 1:605–606, 1967.

475. Hutcheon JR, Crosse WHB: Successful repair of intubation tracheal web. *J Otolaryngol Soc Aust* 22:90–91, 1967.

476. Klaustermeyer WB, Winn WR, Olsen CR: Use of cuffed endotracheal tubes for severe exacerbations of chronic airway obstruction. *Am Rev Resp Dis* 105:268–275, 1972.

477. Markham WG, Blackwood MJA, Conn AW: Prolonged nasotracheal intubation in infants and children. *Can Anaesth Soc J* 14:11–21, 1967.

478. Young N, Steward S: Laryngeal lesions following endotracheal anaesthesia: a report of twelve adult cases. *Br J Anaesth* 25:32–42, 1953.

479. Strome M, Ferguson CF: Multiple postintubation complications. *Ann Otol* 83:432–438, 1974.

480. Strong RM, Passy V: Endotracheal intubation. *Arch Otolaryngol* 103:329–335, 1977.

481. King EG: Aftermath of intubation. *Emerg Med* 154:201–209, 1983.

482. Harley HRS: Laryngotracheal obstruction complicating tracheostomy or endotracheal intubation with assisted respiration. A critical review. *Thorax* 26:493–533, 1971.

483. Holinger PH, Kutnick SL, Schild JA, Holinger LD: Subglottic stenosis in infants and children. *Ann Otol* 85:591–599, 1976.

484. Abbott TR: Complications of prolonged nasotracheal intubation in children. *Br J Anaesth* 40:347–353, 1968.

485. Battersby EF, Hatch DJ, Tomey RM: The effects of prolonged naso-endotracheal intubation in children. *Anaesthesia* 32:154–157, 1977.

486. Smith RO, Hemenway WG, English GM, Black FO, Swan H: Post-intubation subglottic granulation tissue: review of the problem and evaluation of radiotherapy. *Laryngoscope* 79:1227–1251, 1969.

487. Fine J, Finestone SC: An unusual complication of endotracheal intubation: report of a case. *Anesth Analg* 52:204–206, 1973.

488. Couriel JM, Phelan PD: Subglottic cysts: a complication of neonatal endotracheal intubation? *Pediatrics* 68:103–105, 1981.

489. Wigger HJ, Tang P: Fatal laryngeal obstruction by iatrogenic subglottic cyst. *J Pediatr* 72:815–820, 1968.

490. Geffin B, Grillo HC, Cooper JD, Pontoppidan H: Stenosis following tracheostomy for respiratory care. *JAMA* 216:1984–1988, 1971.

491. Miller DR, Sethi G: Tracheal stenosis following prolonged cuffed intubation: cause and prevention. *Ann Surg* 171:283–293, 1970.

492. Aberdeen E, Downes JJ: Artificial airways in children. *Surg Clin N Am* 54:1155–1170, 1974.

493. Som PM, Khilnani MT, Keller RJ: Tracheal stenosis secondary to cuffed tubes. *Mt Sinai J Med (NY)* 40:652–665, 1973.

494. Arola MK, Inberg MV, Puhakka G: Tracheal stenosis after tracheostomy and after orotracheal cuffed intubation. *Acta Chir Scand* 147:183–192, 1981.

495. Bradbeer TL, James ML, Sear JW, Searle JF, Stacey R: Tracheal stenosis associated with a low pressure cuffed endotracheal tube. *Anaesthesia* 31:504–507, 1976.

496. Linder GS: A new polyolefin-coated endotracheal tube stylet. *Anesth Analg* 53:341–342, 1974.

497. Linder GS: More on wire stylets. *Anesth Analg* 56:325, 1977.

498. Marshall J: Self-lubricated stylet for endotracheal tubes. *Anesthesiology* 29:385, 1968.

499. Rao TLK, Mathrubhutham M, Mani M, Salem MR: Experience with a new intubation guide in cases of difficult intubation. Papers, American Society of Anesthesiologists Meeting, 1977, pp 115–116.

500. Ducrow M: Throwing light on blind intubation. *Anaesthesia* 33:827–829, 1978.

501. Rayburn RL: "Light wand" intubation. *Anaesthesia* 34:677–678, 1979.

502. Ducrow M: Throwing light on blind intubation. *Anaesthesia* 35:81, 1980.

503. Katz RL, Berci G: The optical stylet—a new intubation technique for adults and children with specific reference to teaching. *Anesthesiology* 51:251–254, 1979.

CHAPTER 14

Equipment Checking and Maintenance

DAILY CHECKS BEFORE BEGINNING ANESTHESIA (1–4)

Introduction

Before anesthesia can be administered safely, all necessary equipment must be present, functional, calibrated, and leakproof. Just as an airline pilot goes through a system of checks of his aircraft before a flight, the anesthesiologist also needs to do a thorough and systematic check of his equipment before use, even if he was the last person to use it and is under pressure to start the next anesthetic.

Most injuries involving equipment can be avoided by a thorough examination before each use. Failure to perform a proper check has been found to be associated with a high percentage of critical incidents (5, 6) and will increase the possibility of injury or death. The anesthesiologist who has not checked his equipment will likely find his defense difficult after a patient has been harmed by its use.

The ANSI machine standard (7) requires the manufacturer to permanently and prominently affix to the machine a *simple* list of operation checks to be carried out prior to use of the machine. User manuals provided by manufacturers for newer machines have fairly complete and detailed directions. These manuals should be read carefully and the suggested procedures followed.

The following checking procedures are provided because older anesthesia machines may not have manuals with them and because most older manuals did not give complete checking procedures. Because of the great variety of machines and breathing systems available, it will not be possible to apply all of these procedures to some equipment. Changes or additions may be necessary, but the checks performed should always be as comprehensive as those described

here. It may be advantageous to put a copy of these procedures (amended as necessary for individual machines) in the drawer of the anesthesia machine or cart.

Anesthesia Machine

COMPONENT CHECKING

On-Off Switch

Many of the newer machines have an on-off switch which must be activated before gases can flow. In addition, alarms are usually activated when the switch is turned on. Checking cannot proceed unless this switch is in the ON position.

Gas Supplies

Before the gas supplies are inspected, all flow control valves should be closed by turning them clockwise. Excessive torque should be avoided. Opening a cylinder or connecting a pipeline hose when a flow control valve is open may cause the indicator to shoot up to the top of the tube and perhaps be damaged, stuck at the top, or not noticed (8–10).

Pipeline Pressures. If the hospital pipelines are to be the primary supply, the hoses should be securely connected to the machine. If the machine is fitted with pressure gauges for the piped gases, these should be observed to verify that the pressures are in the range of 50 psig.

As discussed in Chapter 3, a pipeline pressure gauge will register only pipeline pressure if it is positioned upstream of the check valve at the pipeline inlet, as required by the ANSI machine standard. If it is located downstream of the check valve, as it is on some machines, the pressure registered will reflect the pressure in the machine (11). With the pipeline hoses disconnected, turn on the cylinders for nitrous oxide and oxygen. If there are readings on the pipeline pressure gauges they are downstream of the check valve and will not reflect pipeline pressures while the cylinders are turned on. With the pipelines connected and the cylinders turned off, a reading significantly less than 50 psig indicates a problem with the pipeline supply.

Cylinder Pressures. Cylinder gauges should be checked to make certain that they read 0. Yokes should be scanned to make certain any not containing a cylinder are fitted with a yoke plug. All cylinders should be checked to determine that their tags indicate "full" or "in use."

Piped Gases in Use. If pipeline gas is in use and there are two backup cylinders on the machine, one should be designated as full, and the other as reserve. This will ensure that the cylinders will be rotated in use. Cylinder pressures are checked by turning each cylinder valve slowly counterclockwise while observing the related pressure gauge. If a hissing sound occurs when the cylinder valve is opened, the cylinder should be tightened in the yoke. The cylinders should contain sufficient gas so that in the event of a problem with the pipeline supply life support and/or anesthesia can be maintained until the pipeline problem can be corrected or more cylinders obtained. Empty or near-empty cylinders should be labeled as empty and replaced with full ones.

After the pressures are checked, the cylinder valves should be closed. If this is not done, leaks may cause loss of the entire supply. During use there will be pressure fluctuations in the machine and the pipeline hoses. This is especially true of oxygen when a ventilator is in use. As the ventilator cycles, there will be a transient lowering of the pressure in the machine. If the pressure falls below that present at the regulator while the cylinder valve is open, gas will be drawn from the cylinder until the pressure increases. Eventually the cylinder will empty and there may be no emergency supply available in the event of pipeline failure.

Piped Gases Not in Use. When piped gases are not available, the oxygen and nitrous oxide tanks become the source of supply. In this case a machine with double yokes for oxygen and nitrous oxide should be used and the pressures of all the tanks need to be checked. There should be a full oxygen and a full nitrous oxide cylinder and the valves on these should be closed after the pressures have been checked. The other

cylinders should be checked to make certain they have adequate pressures and the valves on these should be fully opened.

Other cylinders containing gases such as cyclopropane and carbon dioxide should also be checked. Their cylinder valves should be opened only if they are to be used. This will avoid problems if the gas is inadvertently turned on at the flow control valve and prevent leaks from depleting the cylinders and/or creating an explosion hazard.

Alarms

If the machine is equipped with an oxygen pressure failure alarm, this should be turned on and checked for proper function according to the manufacturer's instructions.

Flowmeters

Flowmeters should be examined with no gas flow to make certain that the indicator is at the 0 position. Each flow control valve should be opened and closed slowly while observing the indicator as it rises and falls within the tube. It should move smoothly and respond to small adjustments of the flow control valve. If the indicator is a rotameter or ball it should rotate freely (12). A sticking indicator or one that moves up and down in an irregular manner may be displaying erroneous flowrates and the machine should be taken out of service until the problem is corrected.

Vaporizers

Liquid levels should be checked and more agent added if needed. Control dials should be checked to determine that they move easily through the full range. Special care should be taken to confirm that vaporizer filler caps are tight.

TESTING THE MACHINE FOR LEAKS (7, 13–15)

This test must be performed separately from the test for leaks in the breathing system (13). Testing for leaks by pressurizing the breathing system frequently will not detect leaks in the machine. Most machines are equipped with unidirectional check valves, either near the common outlet or in a vaporizer, to prevent pressures in the breathing system from affecting the accuracy of the flowmeters or vaporizers. Testing the breathing system for leaks by pressurization will reveal only leaks downstream of these check valves. Important leaks, such as those associated with flowmeters, may go undetected.

When testing a machine for leaks, vaporizers on the machine should be turned to the ON position one at a time. Unless this is done, a leak in a vaporizer will be missed. The test should be repeated with each of the other vaporizers in the ON position.

Machine with a Low-Range Flowmeter

A pressure gauge (the gauge from a standard sphygmomanometer will do) is attached to the common gas outlet or the fresh gas hose (Fig. 14.1). The flow control valve of a flowmeter on the machine is slowly opened until the pressure on the gauge reaches 30 cm H_2O (22 mm Hg). If the machine has a measured-flow vaporizer, the flowmeter associated with that vaporizer should be used. If there is no measured-flow vaporizer, the oxygen flowmeter can be used. The flow is then lowered until a static equilibrium between the gas flow and the leak has been established at a pressure of 30 cm H_2O. The flow rate on the flowmeter is then equal to the leak rate in the machine. It should be less than 50 cc/min.

Machine without a Low-Range Flowmeter

If the machine does not have a flowmeter that reads as low as 50 cc/min, the following test may be used. A pressure gauge is attached to the machine outlet. The oxygen flowmeter is slowly turned on until a pressure of 30 cm H_2O is registered on the gauge. The flow is then turned off and the time it takes for the pressure to drop to 20 cm H_2O is observed. The time should be at least 10 sec. A shorter time implies an unacceptably high leak rate.

Special Test Devices

Some manufacturers supply a special device to aid pressure testing of components downstream of the flowmeters. One such device is a bulb that is squeezed until it is collapsed and then attached to the machine outlet. The bulb is then allowed to fill. The time it takes to fill is an index of the leak in the machine. It has been reported that the negative pressure used for testing could actually close some leaks and give a false negative result (16).

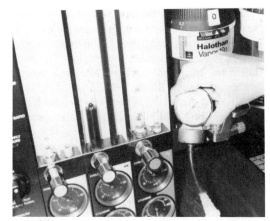

Figure 14.1. Leak testing of the anesthesia machine. A pressure gauge from a blood pressure cuff is attached to the delivery hose from the machine. Sufficient flow is established on a flowmeter to maintain a pressure of 22 mm Hg on the pressure gauge. The flow required to maintain that pressure should be less than 50 cc/min.

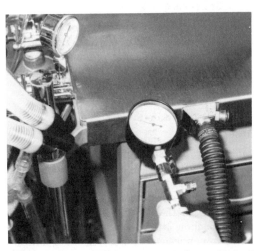

Figure 14.2. Back pressure inducer for leak testing. The back pressure inducer consists of a T-shaped device with a relief valve and a pressure gauge. It is attached to the machine outlet. Details for performing the leak test are given in the text.

The back pressure inducer (Fig. 14.2) is another special device for low-pressure leak testing. It has a pressure gauge and a relief valve. It is also installed on the common gas outlet. A flow of 5 liters/min is set on the anesthesia machine flowmeters. When the pressure reaches 3 psi, gas will be vented through the relief valve.

The oxygen flow is then turned off. If the pressure stabilizes above 1.5 psi, the machine can be considered to be leak tight. If the pressure continues to drop, but takes longer than 30 sec to fall from 1.5 psi to 1.25 psi, the leak rate is within acceptable limits.

After the machine has been checked for leaks, it is important that all vaporizers and vaporizer circuit control valves be turned to the OFF position. If the vaporizer or the vaporizer circuit control valve is left in the ON position, an increase in pressure in the machine (from the breathing system or from use of the oxygen flush valve) will be transmitted to the vaporizing chamber and a subsequent surge of vapor into the fresh gas line may occur (17).

ADDITIONAL TESTS

Some manufacturers recommend tests in addition to those above, which should be considered the minimum necessary.

Test for Leakage at Yoke

Some manufacturers recommend that after cylinder pressures have been checked and the valves closed, the cylinder pressure gauges be observed for 2–5 min. A drop in pressure of more than 50 psig indicates significant leakage.

Oxygen Failure Safety Valve

Many recommend that the oxygen failure safety valve be tested at the beginning of the day and/or each case. This test can be performed using either the pipelines or cylinders as the gas source and some recommend that it be performed with both sources. A cylinder of each gas on the machine is turned on, leaving the pipeline hoses disconnected. Flows of 2 liters/min are established on the flowmeters for each gas. The oxygen cylinder is then turned off. As the pressure of the oxygen falls the oxygen flowmeter indicator will fall. At a certain oxygen pressure, the indicators for each of the anesthetic gases should suddenly fall to 0. Reinstating the oxygen pressure should cause the indicators to return to their previous positions. To perform the test using pipeline gases, all cylinder valves should be closed and the flow control valves opened until the cylinder pressure gauges register 0 pressure. The pipeline hoses are then connected and flows established on both anesthetic gas and oxygen flowmeters. The oxygen hose is disconnected. The indicators of the anesthetic gases should fall to 0 with the oxygen indicator.

Breathing Systems

OXYGEN ANALYZER

No anesthetic should be started without a functioning oxygen analyzer in the circuit. Analyzers with polarographic sensors need to be calibrated in accordance with the manufacturer's instructions. The alarms should be checked and the probe placed in the breathing system.

CIRCLE SYSTEM

Pressure Gauge

The pressure gauge should be checked to make certain that it reads 0.

Absorber

The color of the absorbent should be noted and the absorbent changed if indicated (see Chapter 8). If a bypass is present, it should be determined that it is not in the ON position.

Unidirectional Valves and System Patency

The unidirectional valves should be examined to make certain they contain discs. Obstructions in the system can be detected by having someone (the patient or user) breathe through the system (Fig. 14.3A). Alternately, a bellows or other device (such as the hose from a ventilator) which can alternate volume displacement can be attached to the Y-piece (Fig. 14.3B). The discs in the unidirectional valves should rise and fall with respirations, the bag should inflate and deflate, and the pressure gauge should show positive and negative fluctuations. Negative pressure at the patient port will reveal obstructions in the inspiratory limb and positive pressure will indicate obstructions in the exhalation limb (18).

Failure to perform this test may result in missing a misconnection of the circle system with the scavenging system (19) or an obstruction in the system (18).

System Integrity

The hoses and bag should be checked to make certain they are firmly attached to the absorber. The selector valve, if present, should be placed in the bag position.

To check for leaks, the relief valve is closed and the patient port of the Y-piece occluded. The reservoir bag is filled using the oxygen flush

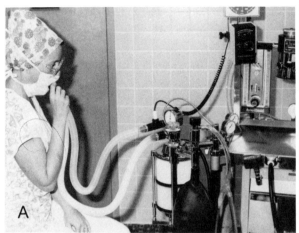
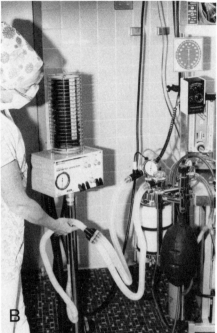

Figure 14.3. Checking for function of the unidirectional valves and system patency. *A*, system patency can be established by breathing through the patient port. The discs in the unidirectional valves should rise and fall with respirations and the bag should inflate and deflate. *B*, system patency can be established by observing the inflation and deflation of the bag and the action of the discs in the unidirectional valves while the patient port is attached to a cycling ventilator.

until a pressure of 30–40 cm H_2O water is indicated on the pressure gauge (Fig. 14.4). With no additional gas flow the pressure should not drop more than 5 cm H_2O in 30 sec. This corresponds to a leak of less than 50 cc/min. (The typical compliance for this circuit is 5 ml/cm H_2O (16), so a drop of 5 cm H_2O indicates leakage of 25 ml of gas. A drop of 25 ml in 30 sec corresponds to a leak of 50 cc/min.)

As an alternative test for leaks, the breathing system can be pressurized using the oxygen flush until the pressure gauge registers 30 cm H_2O, and the oxygen flow control valve turned on until that flowmeter registers 100 cc/min. If the pressure on the absorber gauge continues to increase, the leakage is within the acceptable range.

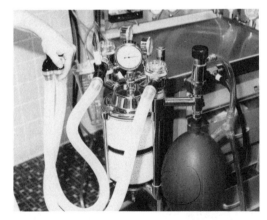

Figure 14.4. Test for system integrity. The relief valve is closed and the patient port occluded. The reservoir bag is filled with oxygen until a pressure of 30–40 cm H_2O is shown on the pressure gauge. With no additional gas flow the pressure should not drop more than 5 cm H_2O over a 30-sec period.

Relief Values

High-Pressure Relief Valve. After the system has been checked for leaks, the pressure should be released by slowly opening the relief valve. There should be a gradual loss of pressure from the system. This establishes proper function of the relief valve and patency of the trans-

fer tubing. The pressure should not be released at the Y-piece as this may cause a cloud of absorbent dust to fly into the breathing tubes (20, 21).

Low-Pressure Relief Valve. The low-pressure relief valve is checked by first closing the high-pressure relief valve and occluding the patient port of the Y-piece. The reservoir bag is partially filled using the oxygen flush. A 4-liter/min flow is set on the oxygen flowmeter. After 1 min, the bag should be filled, but not distended, and the pressure in the breathing system should not increase. The bag is then given a quick squeeze. The relief valve should close and the pressure in the system increase. Releasing the bag should cause the valve to open and the pressure to fall.

Spare Components

Extra components of the breathing system should be immediately available. These include an additional disposable system or individual components of reusable systems (Y-piece, tubings, and bag).

MAPLESON SYSTEMS

Pressure Gauge

The pressure gauge, if present, should be checked to make certain that it reads 0.

Leak Testing

System integrity is tested by occluding the patient port, closing the relief valve and activating the oxygen flush on the anesthesia machine to distend the bag. The bag should maintain the distension and not deflate. The relief valve, (with transfer tubing attached) should then be opened. The bag should deflate.

Special Test of the Bain System

Potential dangers with the Bain system include the inner tube having a hole, becoming detached at its proximal end, or not extending to the patient end of the outer tubing (Fig. 10.9). If this happens, the dead space is greatly increased. These problems can be detected by the following test (22, 23):

1. A 50-ml/min flow is set on one of the flowmeters.

2. The plunger from a small syringe is inserted into the distal (patient) end of the outer tube, occluding the inner tube (Fig. 14.5A). The flowmeter indicator should fall.

Alternate Test (24).

1. The reservoir bag is filled.

2. The patient port remains open to atmosphere (Fig. 14.5B).

3. The oxygen flush valve on the machine is activated while observing the reservoir bag. The high flow of gas through the inner tube will produce a Venturi effect which lowers the pressure in the larger outer tube. If there are no problems with the inner tube, the bag should deflate slightly. If the bag does not deflate or inflates slightly, check to see if the inner tube is properly attached at the machine or patient end. (*Note:* The authors prefer the first test because if the inner tube does not extend to the patient end of the outer tube or if the inner tube has been omitted, the second test may give no indication that anything is amiss (25). If the second test is used a visual check should be made to be certain that the inner tube extends to the distal end.)

Spare Components

As with any breathing system it is important that spare components be readily available.

SYSTEMS EMPLOYING NON-REBREATHING VALVES

Leak Testing

The relief valve, if present, should be closed and the patient port occluded. The bag is then inflated until it is distended, using the oxygen flush. The bag should maintain the pressure and not deflate. Pressure should then be applied to the bag so that the active component of the non-rebreathing valve moves to the inspiratory position. There should be no leak to atmosphere and the pressure should be maintained.

Relief Valve

Upon opening the relief valve, the bag should deflate. If a low-pressure relief valve is used in the system, it should be checked in the manner previously described.

System Patency

Obstructions and competency should be checked for either by breathing through the system or attaching a volume displacement device to the patient port. Negative pressure at the patient port should cause the bag to deflate. Resistance to exhalation should be minimal.

Spare Components

A complete extra breathing system should be immediately available.

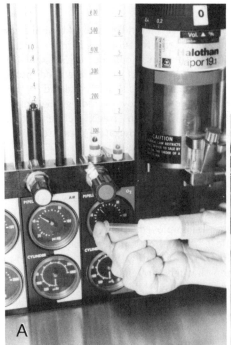
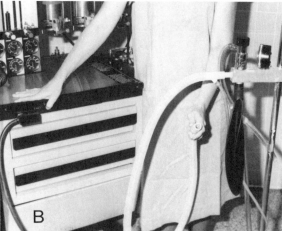

Figure 14.5. Tests of the Bain system. *A*, the plunger from a small syringe is inserted into the patient end of the system over the end of the inner fresh gas delivery tubing. The flowmeter indicator, previously set at 50 cc/min, should drop. *B*, with the patient port open to atmosphere, activation of the oxygen flush should cause the reservoir bag to collapse.

Ventilators

The manufacturer's instructions should be read and the procedures for checking followed. If there are no checking procedures given, the following tests should check most ventilator functions.

1. If the ventilator has a pressure gauge, verify that it reads 0.

2. Connect the ventilator to the power outlet of the anesthesia machine or the station outlet of the pipeline system, making certain that the scavenging transfer tubing is attached to the ventilator.

3. Form a customary breathing system, but place the bag on the patient port (Fig. 14.6). Close the relief valve.

4. Set a flow of 10 liters/min on the anesthesia machine flowmeters.

5. Connect the ventilator hose to the bag mount, or turn the selector valve (if present) to the ventilator position.

6. Turn on the ventilator and any independent pressure monitors. The bag should inflate and deflate and the pressure gauge should show deflections.

7. Check that the tidal volume and respiratory rate can be altered easily.

8. Disconnect the bag at the patient port and verify that the pressure alarm(s) sound.

9. Turn off the ventilator and flowmeters.

10. Test for leak in ventilator bellows.

Ascending Bellows

With this type of ventilator, the bellows descends during inspiration and rises during exhalation.

Machine with a Low-Range Flowmeter

Occlude the patient port in the breathing system. Open the oxygen flow control valve until the bellows reaches its full upright position, then decrease the flow until a pressure of 30 cm H_2O is just maintained on the system pressure gauge. The flow on the oxygen flowmeter after an equilibrium has been attained should be less than 100 cc/min.

Machine without a Low-Range Flowmeter

If a low flow cannot be set on the flowmeters,

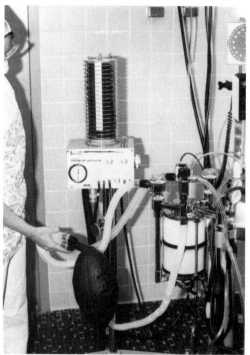

Figure 14.6. Ventilator function checks. The breathing system is slightly modified by placing the bag on the patient port. The ventilator hose is connected to the bag mount and the relief valve is closed. A flow is set on the flowmeters and the ventilator is turned on. The bag should inflate and deflate.

the ventilator bellows should be inflated using the oxygen flush. The ventilator hose is occluded (Fig. 14.7A). The bellows should remain inflated.

DESCENDING BELLOWS

With these ventilators the bellows moves downward and expands during exhalation and rises during inspiration.

The bellows is contracted upwards by inhaling gas from the ventilator hose and the end of the hose is occluded (Fig. 14.7B). The bellows should remain contracted.

Scavenging System

COLLECTION ASSEMBLIES AND TRANSFER TUBINGS

The transfer tubings should be checked to be certain that they are not obstructed and can be detached easily.

Interface

The interface should be checked to make certain that the transfer tubing is firmly attached. If there is a bag, it should be verified that this inflates and deflates as gas is exhausted into it. All scavenging systems should be tested for positive pressure relief by occluding the tubing downstream of the interface. Active systems should be checked for negative pressure relief.

DISPOSAL TUBING AND SYSTEM

It should be ascertained that the disposal system is connected to the interface and that the disposal tubing is not obstructed. If an active system is employed, the active components should be turned on and the adequacy of flow verified. With a high gas flow (8 liters/min) of oxygen through the relief valve, the sensor for an oxygen analyzer placed at the positive pressure relief of the interface should not indicate over 21%.

Endotracheal Tubes

A tracheal tube of size appropriate for the age and sex of the patient should be ready for use. One larger and one smaller tube should be readily available.

Patency of the lumen should be checked. With clear tubes, simple observation will suffice. With other tubes it is necessary to look in both ends or, better, insert a stylet.

When a cuffed tube is to be used, the cuff should be held inflated for at least a minute to verify that there are no leaks. It should inflate evenly and not stick to the wall of the tube or decrease the size of the lumen.

Laryngoscopes

Laryngoscope malfunction is a frequent problem (6). At least two laryngoscopes should be present, each fitted with the type of blade the user anticipates will be best for the patient (Fig. 14.8). The lights should be checked for adequate intensity. Blades of other sizes and shapes should be immediately available and checked for proper functions.

Accessory Intubation Equipment (Fig. 14.8)

A stylet should be immediately available (Fig. 14.8). If a "rapid sequence" intubation is planned, the stylet should be fitted to the tube,

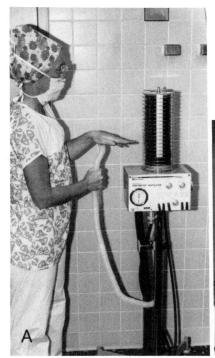

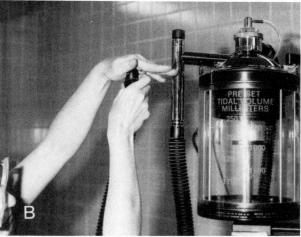

Figure 14.7. Tests of the ventilator bellows. *A*, ascending bellows. The bellows are inflated and the hose from the ventilator is occluded. If a leak is present, the bellows will drop. *B*, descending bellows. The bellows is drawn into the fully contracted position. In the absence of a leak the bellows will remain contracted with the hose occluded.

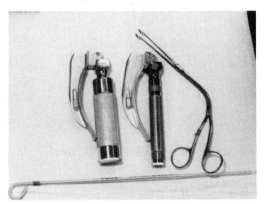

Figure 14.8. Intubation equipment. The minimum necessary intubation equipment includes two complete laryngoscopes an intubation forceps and a stylet.

if not actually in it. An intubating forceps should be immediately available.

Masks and Airways

An assortment of masks and airways in a variety of sizes should be readily available. It may be necessary to try several masks on the patient's face before finding a suitable one.

Suction Equipment

An inflexible suction catheter should be present. The adequacy of suction can be checked by placing the end of the suction tubing on the underside of the user's finger (Fig. 14.9). The tubing should stay without support.

Other Equipment

Standard equipment such as cardiac monitors, sphygmomanometers, etc. and special equipment required for particular cases such as extension pipeline hoses, hypothermia blanket, etc. should be present and checked prior to use.

Resuscitation Bag

Ideally, there should be an emergency self-inflating bag in every operating room. At the very least, there should be at least one in a location where it can be quickly obtained. If a problem occurs with the machine or breathing

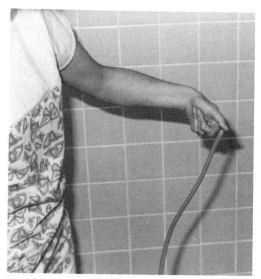

Figure 14.9. Suction check. The strength of the vacuum is tested by determining that the weight of the suction tubing can be supported at waist height by the seal between the tubing and the underside of a finger. If the vacuum is unsatisfactory, the tubing will not remain in contact with the finger.

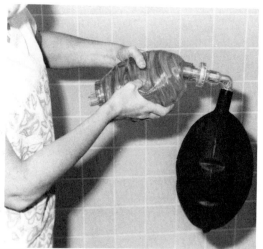

Figure 14.10. Tests of resuscitation bag. The resuscitation bag should be either in the room or in a readily accessible location. It is checked by placing the reservoir bag from the breathing system over the mask connection. Squeezing the resuscitation bag should cause the reservoir bag to inflate. The reservoir bag should then deflate easily when it is squeezed.

system which cannot be diagnosed or corrected quickly, this will allow the user to generate a positive pressure and ventilate the patient with room air while the problem is corrected or a new machine brought in.

It is important that the resuscitation bag be checked for proper function during both inflation and deflation (26). A reservoir bag is placed over the patient port (Fig. 14.10). Squeezing the resuscitation bag should cause the reservoir bag to inflate. After the resuscitation bag is released, patency of the exhalation path should be confirmed by squeezing the reservoir bag. It should deflate easily.

Emergency Airway and Ventilation System

There should be available a means to quickly establish an airway and emergency ventilation should a situation arise where it is not possible to intubate a patient or ventilate using a mask. One such system is shown in Figure 14.11. Several other systems have been described (27–32).

PROCEDURES AT THE END OF THE CASE

At the conclusion of a case, flowmeters, vaporizers, the oxygen analyzer, the on-off switch, alarms, monitors, suction, and other equipment should be turned off. The bypass valve on the

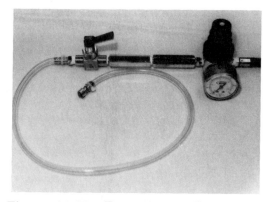

Figure 14.11. Emergency ventilation system. This system is designed to deliver oxygen at high flow through a small tubing. The regulator at the right is attached to a 50 psig oxygen source such as the pipeline system or the ventilator power outlet on the anesthesia machine. The pressure delivered can be adjusted by turning the knob over the pressure gauge. The flow is controlled by the toggle switch downstream of the regulator. The tubing is attached to a large bore needle or other device placed percutaneously into the trachea.

absorber should be left in the off position. The absorbent should be checked for signs of exhaustion and changed if indicated (see Chapter 8). Dirty equipment should be removed to the cleaning area.

PROCEDURE AT END OF DAY

Following the last case the pipeline hoses should be disconnected at the wall or ceiling (not at the back of the machine) and coiled over the machine. If the hoses are disconnected at the back of the machine, they will continue to be pressurized and gas may be lost into the room through leaks. Cylinder valves should be closed. Each flow control valve should be opened until the cylinder and pipeline pressure gauges read 0, then closed (33, 34). Closing the flow control valve will not conserve any gas, but if they are left open, restoration of the gas supply may forcibly raise the indicator to the top of the flowmeter, causing damage.

Vaporizers should be filled at the conclusion of the day after the operating room personnel have left the room. This will decrease their exposure to trace amounts of anesthetic agents.

Liquid should be drained from the base of the absorber. Care must be exercised as the liquid is caustic and should not come in contact with skin.

CHECKING NEW EQUIPMENT

Each new anesthesia machine, ventilator, or other complex piece of equipment should come with at least one user's manual. It will contain assembly and installation instructions, a list of accessories, spare parts numbers, maintenance requirements, and daily checking procedures. This should be read carefully by each member of the department. It should be kept in the central equipment files and reviewed periodically. It is advantageous to keep a copy of at least the daily checking procedures with the equipment.

The assembly and installation instructions should be carefully followed. The following series of tests designed to test the gas supplies should be performed on all new machines and at any time repairs or adjustments are made to the machine that involve disassembly and reassembly and/or the use of hand tools. In many states, this procedure is a legal requirement (35).

1. All hoses are detached and all cylinder valves are closed.

2. The oxygen pipeline hose is connected and the reading on the pipeline gauge checked to confirm that it reads between 45 and 55 psig.

3. The oxygen flush is actuated and flow from the common outlet is confirmed.

4. The ventilator power outlet is actuated and flow is confirmed.

5. The oxygen flow control valve is opened and flow on the oxygen flowmeter is verified. Flow control valves for other gases are opened to make certain no flow occurs.

6. The flow control valves on built-in vaporizer(s) are opened and flow on the flowmeter(s) verified.

7. The nitrous oxide pipeline hose is connected and it is verified that the reading on the pressure gauge is between 45 and 55 psig.

8. The oxygen hose is disconnected.

9. Steps 3, 4, 5, and 6 are repeated. There should be no gas flow from any flowmeters, the flush valve, or the power outlet.

10. The oxygen pipeline hose is reconnected and a suitably calibrated oxygen analyzer connected to the common outlet. The oxygen flow control knob is turned counterclockwise to the OFF position.

11. The oxygen flush valve is actuated. One hundred percent oxygen should be indicated on the oxygen analyzer.

12. The oxygen flow control valve is opened so that a flow of 5 liters/min is indicated on the flowmeter. One hundred percent oxygen should be indicated on the oxygen analyzer. The nitrous oxide flow control valve is opened so that 5 liters/min are indicated on the flowmeter. Fifty percent oxygen should be indicated on the oxygen analyzer.

13. All flow control valves are closed.

14. The pipeline hoses are disconnected and steps 2 through 13 repeated, except that the oxygen and nitrous oxide cylinders are used instead of the pipeline hoses. The results should be the same except for the pipeline pressure gauge readings.

After the special tests for new equipment are performed, the checking procedure described in the beginning of this chapter needs to be performed. In addition there may be special testing procedures recommended by the manufacturer.

PREVENTIVE MAINTENANCE

A supplement to the daily checks, but by no means a substitute for them, is the use of preventive maintenance contracts for major equipment such as ventilators and anesthesia machines. With this type of program, a trained service representative will come to the hospital and service the equipment at 3- to 4-month intervals. This includes inspection, testing, cleaning, lubrication, and adjustment of various components. Worn or damaged parts are fixed or replaced. Frequently such servicing can result in detection of deterioration before an overt malfunction occurs.

It is strongly recommended that anesthesia departments avail themselves of such manufacturer-authorized service agreements to ensure that equipment is maintained in an operational condition with the lowest possible breakdown rate unless qualified in-house biomedical personnel are available. Lack of a preventive maintenance program may lead to an unacceptably high rate of breakdowns, premature replacement of major equipment, and unnecessary accidents and hazards (36).

REPAIRS OR CHANGES BY USERS OF A MACHINE

In the past, when most anesthesia equipment was relatively simple, a few skilled and knowledgeable physician-mechanics successfully did their own repairs and preventive maintenance. With increased complexity of equipment, this is no longer feasible in the majority of cases. Some of the greatest hazards associated with anesthesia equipment have been due to repairs or modifications by an amateur. The literature contains many instances where parts were jumbled and upon reassembly have turned an anesthesia machine into a potentially lethal instrument (37). Unauthorized repairs or modifications not specifically approved by a manufacturer ordinarily void any warranties and place the consequences for malfunction on the user.

RECORD KEEPING

Record keeping for anesthesia equipment is frequently neglected. Many people assume that the manufacturer's service representative who does periodic preventive maintenance will take care of this task. Common experience does not support this. Record keeping is important for several reasons.

1. It provides proof that an effort has been made to keep the equipment in proper working order. This could have medicolegal significance.

2. It provides a means of communication with the service representative. Representatives frequently come in the late afternoon or evening when the anesthesia schedule is finished and personnel have departed. If there is no written record of problems that have occurred with the equipment, the service representative may not perform the indicated repair(s).

3. It provides a complete, up-to-date record for each piece of equipment. If one piece of equipment malfunctions more frequently than others, consideration should be given to replacing it.

4. It provides a written record that maintenance by a service representative was performed and shows what was done. Service representatives usually present only a bill for service and parts but usually no record of what was actually done to a specific machine is provided.

5. It provides a check on the service rendered by the representative. After equipment is serviced, it should perform well. If a machine develops a problem soon after servicing or if there is an increased frequency of repairs that can be traced to a change in service representatives, one may wish to question that representative's effectiveness.

6. With pieces of equipment such as vaporizers that need to be sent to the manufacturer periodically for servicing, or oxygen analyzers that need to have certain components replaced at intervals, it serves to remind the user when the equipment needs to be serviced or a component replaced. After a vaporizer is serviced, it may be held in reserve before being put into use. This would extend the time before servicing would be due. This can be noted on the form by recording the time when a vaporizer is received from the manufacturer and when it is actually put into service on a machine.

A sample check record is shown in Figure 14.12. It consists of identification data for the particular piece of equipment, date of purchase, instructions for servicing, and the name, address, and telephone number of the service representative. One of these forms should be used for each anesthesia machine, oxygen analyzer, direct-reading vaporizer, ventilator, monitor, or other important piece of equipment. If a problem with the equipment arises, the date and problem are entered in the first two columns. When some action is taken, it is recorded in the third column. If routine maintenance is performed, this should be noted, along with any problems found or parts replaced. Each entry should be signed by the person making it.

Figure 14.12.   Sample Record.
Department of Anesthesia Equipment Form

Equipment_____

Model No._____   Serial No._____   Hospital No._____

Date of Purchase_____

Manufacturer's Instructions for Servicing_____

Manufacturer's Service Representative:

Address:

Phone No.:

Date	Problems and/or Checks	Servicing

References

1. DeVore DT: How to check for proper installation of anesthetic equipment. *J Oral Surg* 35:955, 1977.
2. Murray B, Herr GP, Cullen BF, Hardy CA, Liv P, Miller EV, Murphy FL, Sivarajan M, Stevens WC, Willinkin R, Winter P: Anesthesia set-up and machine checkout skill examination. Abstracts of Scientific Papers, American Society of Anesthesiologists Annual Meeting, New Orleans, La., 1977, pp 699–700.
3. Ward CS: *Anaesthetic Equipment. Physical Principles and Maintenance.* Baltimore, Williams & Wilkins, 1975, pp 84–86.
4. Cundy J, Baldock GJ: Safety check procedures to eliminate faults in anaesthetic machines. *Anaesthesia* 37:161–169, 1982.
5. Craig J, Wilson ME: A survey of anaesthetic misadventures. *Anaesthesia* 36:933–936, 1981.
6. Cooper JB, Newbower RS, Lóng CD, McPeek B: Preventable anesthesia mishaps: A study of human factors. *Anesthesiology* 49:399–406, 1978.
7. *Minimum Performance and Safety Requirements for Components and Systems of Continuous-Flow Anesthesia Machines for Human Use.* Z79.8, 1979, American National Standards Institute, 1430 Broadway, New York, N.Y. 10018.
8. Lomanto C, Leeming M: A safety signal for detection of excessive anesthetic gas flows. *Anesthesiology* 33:663–664, 1970.
9. Dinnick OP: Accidental severe hypercapnia during anaesthesia. *Br J Anaesth* 40:36, 45, 1968.
10. Prys-Roberts C, Smith WDA, Nunn JF: Accidental severe hypercapnia during anaesthesia. *Br J Anaesth* 39:257–267, 1967.
11. Wilson AM: The pressure gauges on the Boyle International Anaesthetic machine. *Anaesthesia* 37:218–219, 1982.
12. Clutton-Brock C: Static electricity and rotameters. *Br J Anaesth* 44:86–90, 1972.
13. Comm G, Rendell-Baker L: Back pressure check valves a hazard. *Anesthesiology* 56:327–328, 1982.
14. Page J: Testing for leaks. *Anaesthesia* 32:673, 1977.
15. Wilson ME, Burleton AS: Leak tests. *Br J Anaesth* 54:572, 1982.

16. Anonymous: Anesthesia units. *Health Devices* 9:31–51, 1980.

17. Greenhow DE, Barth RL: Oxygen flushing delivers anesthetic vapor—a hazard with a new machine. *Anesthesiology* 38:409–410, 1973.

18. Grundy EM, Bennett EJ, Brennan T: Obstructed anesthetic circuits. *Anesthesiol Rev* 3:35–36, 1976.

19. Flowerdew RMM: A hazard of scavenger port design. *Can Anaesth Soc J* 28:481–483, 1981.

20. Debban DG, Bedford RF: Overdistention of the rebreathing bag, a hazardous test for circle-system integrity. *Anesthesiology* 42:365–366, 1975.

21. Ribak B: Reducing the soda-lime hazard. *Anesthesiology* 43:277, 1975.

22. Seed RF: A test for co-axial circuits. *Anaesthesia* 32:676–677, 1977.

23. Foex P, Crampton-Smith A: A test for co-axial circuits. *Anaesthesia* 32:294, 1977.

24. Pethick SL: Correspondence. *Can Anaesth Soc J* 22:115, 1975.

25. Petersen WC: Bain circuit. *Can Anaesth Soc J* 25:532, 1978.

26. Dolan PF, Shapiro S, Steinbach RB: Valve misassembly—manually operated resuscitation bag. *Anesth Analg* 60:66–67, 1981.

27. Scuderi PE, McLeskey CH, Comer PB: Emergency percutaneous transtracheal ventilation during anesthesia using readily available equipment. *Anesth Analg* 61:867–870, 1982.

28. Smith RB, Schaer WB, Pfaeffle H: Percutaneous transtracheal ventilation for anaesthesia and resuscitation: a review and report of complications. *Can Anaesth Soc J* 22:607–612, 1975.

29. Miller WL: Management of a difficult airway in obstetrics. *Anesthesiology* 53:523–524, 1980.

30. Dunlap LB: A modified, simple device for the emergency administration of percutaneous transtracheal ventilation. *JACEP* 7:42–46, 1978.

31. DeLisser EA, Muravchick S: Emergency transtracheal ventilation. *Anesthesiology* 55:606–607, 1981.

32. Smith RB, Babinsky M, Kalin M, Pfaeffle H: Percutaneous transtracheal ventilation. *JACEP* 5:765–770, 1976.

33. Bracken A: Deposits in cyclopropane flowmeter tubes. *Br J Anaesth* 48:52, 1976.

34. Russell FR: Deposits in the cyclopropane flowmeter. *Br J Anaesth* 33:323, 1961.

35. Compressed Gas Association: *Handbook of Compressed Gases*. New York, Van Nostrand Reinhold, 1981, pp 469–470.

36. Tamse JG: Preventive maintenance of medical and dental equipment. AAMI 13th Annual Meeting, March 28–April 1, 1978, Washington DC, p 261.

37. Nagel EL: Equipment hazards in anesthesia. In Saidman LJ, Moya F (eds): *Complications of Anesthesia*. Springfield, Ill., Charles C Thomas, 1970, pp 266–281.

CHAPTER 15

Cleaning and Sterilization

The possibility that infection could result from contaminated anesthesia equipment was ignored for a long time. In recent years, concern about the role played by equipment in the transmission of infections to patients undergoing anesthesia has increased, but the subject remains highly controversial.

THE STERILIZATION DILEMMA (1–4)

Those concerned with cleaning anesthesia equipment find themselves faced with a dilemma as to how much should be attempted. Most, if not all, would agree that sterilization of equipment is essential after use in a patient with a demonstrated or suspected infection of the respiratory tract or who is known to harbor a particularly virulent organism such as *Pseudomonas aeruginosa*. Likewise, most anesthesiologists would agree that patients whose resistance to infection is impaired should be anesthetized only with sterile equipment. However, the vast majority of patients do not fall into these categories and a less rigorous approach is usually adopted.

Those who argue that more vigorous approaches are not needed and feel that sterilization is being advocated to an unreasonable degree advance the following arguments.

1. Documented cross infection by contaminated anesthesia equipment is rare. Although it is recognized that equipment does become contaminated, periodic decontamination will reduce the number of organisms present so that the number actually transmitted to the patient is small. The macrophages of the normal healthy patient can then combat these organisms. Some recent studies have cast doubt on the likelihood of the anesthesia machine or breathing system causing postoperative respiratory infections (5, 6).

2. Sterilization is difficult, costly and may carry with it certain dangers to the patient and hospital personnel. Although certain items are easily sterilized, others, particularly bulky ones, do not lend themselves easily to present techniques. Sterilization entails a heavier capital outlay for equipment, increased work for personnel and requires increased storage space. Considerable indoctrination of aides is necessary. Many forms of sterilization can damage equipment. Liquid and gas chemical sterilization may leave residues in the equipment that can subsequently cause harm to the patient.

3. The very nature of maneuvers required in anesthesia makes sterility impractical (7).

4. Increased frequency of cleaning of equipment will increase the risks of mistakes in assembling and accidental disconnections.

Proponents for more vigorous attempts at sterilization argue as follows:

1. Cases of cross-contamination caused by anesthesia equipment have been reported (8, 9).

2. The risk of cross-contamination may be greater than is commonly believed because it is frequently difficult to pinpoint the exact cause of a postoperative infection.

3. The humid environments that frequently exist in anesthesia equipment provide a potentially favorable habitat for gram-negative organisms, which are assuming a greater role in nosocomial infections.

4. Patients undergoing anesthesia and surgery are more likely to develop respiratory infections than a normal population. Many have underlying diseases that reduce their resistance. Even relatively nonpathogenic organisms can cause secondary, or even primary, infection in an already debilitated individual (10). Anesthesia interferes with ciliary and mucus activity and surgery can impair the patient's ability to cough and deep breathe.

5. Although there is general agreement that sterilization of equipment is essential after use in a patient with a respiratory infection or a particularly virulent organism, it is frequently impossible to identify these patients at the time

they undergo anesthesia. Furthermore, the loss of distinction between pathogens and nonpathogens means that any organism is a potential cause of infection. Therefore, all patients are at risk and all equipment is suspect.

6. Even if the incidence of postoperative respiratory infections coming from anesthesia apparatus is low, the cost of a single such infection in terms of mortality, morbidity, and economics cannot be disregarded.

It is hoped that future development will provide some answers to the dilemma described above. In the meantime, serious thought should be given to upgrading the care at every facility. The different approaches will be discussed more fully in a later section.

DEFINITIONS

Bacteria: minute unicellular plant-like organisms which usually multiply by binary division. This term is usually applied to the vegetative (growing) forms (11).

Spore: the normal resting stage in the life cycle of certain bacteria. Spores are more difficult to kill than vegetative bacteria.

Viruses: infectious agents smaller in size than bacteria. Some are barely visible with the light microscope but most are beyond this range (11).

Sterilization: destruction of all forms of microorganisms, including bacteria, fungi, spores, and viruses. There is no such thing as "almost sterile" or "practically sterile." An object is either sterile or not sterile.

Disinfection: the destruction of many, but not all, microorganisms on inanimate surfaces. Formerly this was used to designate destruction of only pathogenic organisms but the terms "pathogen" and "nonpathogen" are no longer relevant (12, 13). Any microorganism can be pathogenic under certain circumstances.

Antiseptic: any substance that has a bactericidal or bacteriostatic effect and that can be safely applied to the skin.

Bacteriocide (Germicide): an agent which kills bacteria (14, 15).

Bacteriostat: an agent which will prevent bacterial growth but does not necessarily kill the bacteria (14).

Microbiocide: an agent that kills all organisms.

Fungicide: an agent which kills fungi.

Sporicide: an agent which kills spores.

Viricide: an agent that kills viruses.

Nosocomial: Pertaining to a hospital.

Bioburden (Microbial Load): The number of organisms with which an object is contaminated.

Biological Indicator: a calibration of microorganisms of high resistance to the mode of sterilization being monitored. Subsequent growth or failure of the microorganisms to grow under suitable conditions indicates the adequacy of sterilization.

Chemical Indicator: a device, usually with a sensitive chemical or dye, employed to monitor one or more process parameters of a sterilization cycle. Chemical indicators are not sterility indicators. They only indicate that the material has been subjected to one or more parameters of the sterilization cycle (16).

Mechanical Control (Physical) Monitors: sterilizer components that gauge and record time, temperature, humidity or pressure during a sterilization cycle.

Decontamination: Getting rid of a harmful substance. This is a general term encompassing cleaning, disinfection, and sterilization.

CLEANING OF EQUIPMENT

Cleaning of equipment means essentially the removal of foreign matter without any special effort to kill microorganisms. This subject is often neglected in comparison to disinfection and sterilization, but it is of equal importance. Unless an article is mechanically clean, there may not be sufficient surface contact between it and the decontaminating agent and sterilization will not be accomplished. Organic material (e.g., blood and protein) inactivates many disinfectants. Even if the material is rendered sterile, a patient may react to a protein or other substance in the residue. Cleaning will usually reduce the bacterial output but will not disinfect or sterilize.

Cleaning of anesthesia equipment should be performed in the anesthesia workroom, not at the surgical scrub sink (17). Personnel handling contaminated items should wear gloves. Items that do not lend themselves to cleaning by immersion often may be cleaned by a cloth soaked in detergent and water. Most items, however, are cleaned by immersion. This involves several steps:

Prerinsing

Items should be rinsed with cold water as soon as possible after use to prevent drying of organic material.

Preparing the Equipment

This involves disassembly, removal of tape, etc. In general, if an item can be disassembled, this should be done. Stylets should be removed and impermeable caps and plugs removed. Tubes should be free of obstructions.

Soaking

This will allow the water to penetrate, soften, and loosen soil. The equipment should be immersed in a solution of water and detergent. The detergent should be chosen for its surface-wetting action rather than disinfection activity. It should be low sudsing and noncorrosive to rubber and plastics. Ample soaking time should be permitted for the detergent solution to penetrate and loosen organic matter. Adhesive or oil on the equipment may require special solvent for removal.

Removal of Soil

During cleaning, particular attention should be paid to corners and grooves in which debris may be hidden. Most equipment cleaning is still done manually and requires the use of a stiff brush. An ordinary scrub brush used in surgery is adequate for cleaning most equipment. Test-tube brushes can be used for the lumens of tubes and airways.

In recent years, machines for washing equipment have come into widespread use (15, 17–19). One of these, the Cidematic, also disinfects the equipment.

Most operating room suites have at least one ultrasonic cleaner, in which high-frequency electrical energy is converted into mechanical energy in the form of sound waves. The waves, passing through a solvent, produce submicroscopic bubbles. These bubbles collapse on themselves, generating tiny shock waves that knock debris off surfaces. Ultrasonic cleaning is sometimes superior to scrubbing by hand, because it can remove soil from areas impossible to reach with a brush. It probably deserves more widespread use for cleaning anesthesia equipment.

Rinsing

This will remove the soil and keep it from resettling on the equipment. It will also remove residual detergent. Some items should be rinsed with distilled or demineralized water to remove minerals from tap water (16). After rinsing, each item should be inspected to ensure freedom from foreign matter.

Drying

Unless some form of heat sterilization is to be used, the cleaned item should be thoroughly dried. Even if an item is to undergo no further disinfection, drying is important because a humid environment may encourage the growth of gram-negative organisms. If a liquid chemical agent is used to disinfect or sterilize, any water on the equipment will dilute it and make it less effective. If water droplets are left on equipment that is to be gas sterilized, ethylene oxide will dissolve in the water and form ethylene glycol which is both difficult to remove and toxic.

Most items may be towel dried or air dried. Air-drying cabinets and hot air ovens are available. If an item is to undergo ethylene oxide sterilization, only unheated air should be used to prevent dehydration.

METHODS OF DISINFECTION AND STERILIZATION
Moist Heat

Heat causes coagulation and denaturation of cellular proteins, resulting in irreversible protoplasmic changes within the cell. Dry heat has little applicability for anesthesia equipment, but moist heat has been widely used.

PASTEURIZATION (BELOW 100°C)

Pasteurization as a means of disinfection is the rediscovery of an old method for treating milk. The equipment is immersed in water at an elevated temperature for a given time period. The time and temperature recommended vary (21–23). Specially designed dishwasher units with removable baskets are available.

This method is a disinfecting process but cannot be depended on for sterilization (21, 24). The treated equipment is wet and must still be dried and packaged.

The biggest advantage of this method is that the lower temperature is less damaging to equipment than higher temperatures employed in boiling and autoclaving.

BOILING (AT 100°C)

Boiling at 100°C is lethal to all vegetative forms of bacteria, most spores, and practially all viruses if the time is at least 30 min. A boiling time of 3–5 min at sea level kills most vegetative bacteria (14, 25). At higher altitudes where boiling occurs below 100°, a longer time is needed. It is recommended that the 30-min boiling time be extended 5 min for each 1000 ft of altitude (26).

The water should be made either acid or alkaline for best destruction of spores (26). All instruments should be covered by at least 1 inch of water. Use of soft water will prevent scale formation.

Boiling suffers from the same disadvantages as pasteurization, namely that the equipment is wet and cannot be prepackaged.

AUTOCLAVING (STEAM STERILIZATION) (ABOVE 100°C)

Moist heat in the form of saturated steam under pressure is a widely used, dependable method for the destruction of all forms of microbial life.

At normal atmospheric pressure at sea level, water boils at 100°C. When water is boiled within a closed vessel at increased pressure, however, the temperature at which it boils and that of the steam it forms will exceed 100°C, the extent of the increase depending primarily upon the pressure within the chamber. This is the basic principle of the autoclave. Pressure per se has little or no sterilizing effect. It is the moist heat at a suitable temperature, as regulated by the pressure in the chamber, that brings about sterilization.

The higher the temperature, the more rapidly sterilization can be accomplished. The minimum time for sterilization by steam at 121°C and 15 psig is 15 min (27). If the temperature is 126°C, the time is reduced to 10 min. It is 3 min at 134°C and only a few seconds at 150°C (28).

The presence of air in the chamber will impair sterilization. Air is a poor conductor of heat and retards the penetration of steam (29). The modern hospital autoclave provides for evacuation of much of the air before steam enters the chamber (25, 27, 30–32).

In addition to residual air, incomplete steam penetration can occur because of overloading and/or incorrect positioning of the packages in the sterilizing chamber (27).

Use of sterility indicators (monitors) is important when an autoclave is used. Physical and chemical monitors can be checked immediately after an item has been autoclaved, but none yet devised monitors completely all the parameters necessary for sterilization. Use of biological

monitors is more reliable, but takes several days. Most hospitals use physical and chemical monitoring with each load and supplement this with periodic use of biological indicators to detect problems in technique or failure of the autoclave to function properly.

Autoclaving kills all bacteria, spores and viruses. It offers high penetration capability and allows the interior of a wrapped package to be sterilized. Advantages include speed, penetration of fabrics, economy, ease of control, absence of toxic products or residues and reliability. The material can be prepackaged and kept sterile until used. A great advantage is that the autoclave is available in every modern operating theater. Since steam is the most effective and least expensive means of sterilizing items, it should be used whenever possible.

The principal disadvantage of autoclaving is that many pieces of equipment made from heat-sensitive materials (including rubber and plastic) are damaged if subjected to steam. Autoclaving can cause blunting of cutting edges, corrosion of metal surfaces, shortening of the life of electronic circuits, and degradation of drugs in ampules.

Gamma Radiation

Gamma radiation (gamma rays) is an electromagnetic wave produced during the disintegration of certain radioactive elements. Cobalt 60 is the most plentiful and useful source. If the dosage applied to a product is large enough, all bacterial spores and viruses will be killed.

There are many advantages to gamma radiation. The product can be prepackaged in a wide variety of impermeable containers before treatment. The package will not interfere with the sterilization process. The treated items then remain sterile indefinitely until the packaging seal is broken. As there is virtually no temperature rise during treatment, thermolabile materials can be sterilized and thermolabile packaging used.

Equipment may be used immediately after gamma radiation treatment with no risk from retained radioactivity.

Gamma radiation is not practical for everyday use in hospitals. It requires expensive equipment and is used only by large manufacturers to sterilize disposable equipment (33). The importance of gamma radiation is that it does cause changes in some plastics, especially polyvinyl chloride

(PVC). When PVC is sterilized by gamma radiation, chloride ions are liberated. This does not cause problems when the PVC comes into contact with tissues. However, if such an item is subsequently exposed to ethylene oxide gas for resterilization, the gas forms ethylene chlorohydrin. This substance is extremely toxic to tissues and cannot be easily eluted. Therefore, irradiated PVC items should not be resterilized with ethylene oxide (34).

Liquid Chemical Agents

Liquid chemical agents (cold sterilization) are especially useful for heat-sensitive equipment. Destruction of microorganisms is accomplished through a variety of mechanisms, including coagulation or denaturation of proteins, cell rupture or lysis, and enzyme degradation or binding.

Advantages of liquid chemical disinfection include economy, speed, and simplicity. However, it cannot be used for all types of equipment. Many devices cannot be soaked because their design prevents solution contact or because the aqueous solution would damage electrical circuitry and/or corrode metal components. Prepackaging is not possible and the equipment will usually be wet. Thus, there is an opportunity for recontamination during subsequent rinsing, drying, or wrapping. With most agents sterility cannot be guaranteed. Finally, some solutions are irritating to tissues and have unpleasant odors.

FACTORS INFLUENCING CHEMICAL STERILIZATION

Concentration of the Chemical Agent

The rate of kill of a bacterial population varies directly with the concentration of the disinfectant (35). Generally disinfectants of high concentration will be bactericidal and those of lower concentration bacteriostatic. Water left on equipment will dilute the liquid agent and render it less effective. For this reason, equipment to be sterilized must be dried after it is cleaned.

While it is usually true that the stronger the solution the more effective will be its disinfectant action, a strong solution may be more irritating to tissues and/or injurious to the item being disinfected. In such cases, weaker solutions must be used.

Temperature

While these agents are designed to be used at room temperature, increasing the temperature usually increases their effectiveness.

Cleanliness of Material

Cleanliness of the surface to be disinfected is essential for reliable germicidal action. Soiled equipment will require longer exposure and/or a stronger concentration or adequate disinfection may not be achieved.

Infecting Organisms

Liquid agents vary widely in their effectiveness against various types of contaminating microorganisms. Some organisms are more readily killed than others. Most bacteria with the exception of the acid-fast bacilli, are rapidly killed by most chemical disinfectants (35) while spores are generally not killed unless the contact time is quite long. Some microorganisms are particularly resistant to certain chemicals and contaminating organisms have been isolated from solutions of some disinfectants.

Time

The time required for the different chemical agents to function effectively as disinfectants varies from seconds to hours and will depend on the factors just mentioned. The degree of disinfection will be greater with increased time. Some microorganisms are killed faster than others. Generally it takes longer to kill spores than bacteria. It is essential that the minimum time of exposure to a specific chemical solution be known if disinfection is to be assured.

Nature of the Surface to be Disinfected

Uneven or porous surfaces resist chemical disinfection. Deeply situated resident flora are not affected by disinfectants applied to the surface (35). Air entrapment prevents contact between the liquid and bubble-covered regions.

AGENTS

Chemical disinfectants vary in their degree of effectiveness. Some are specific and destroy certain types of microorganisms but allow others to grow. Table 15.1 lists some of the commonly used liquid agents and some of their characteristics.

Soaps

Soaps are alkali salts of fatty acids. Their principal action is to lower surface tension and remove dirt. Most soaps are not bactericidal. Other agents are sometimes added to soap to impact bacteriostatic or bacteriocidal activity.

Detergents

Detergents are salts of synthetic aliphatic compounds. They act as surface-wetting agents and disperse oil and grease into aqueous solution.

Detergents are primarily cleansing agents but most have some bactericidal effect. They are more active against gram-positive than gram-negative bacteria. They are not effective against tubercle bacilli and many viruses. Bactericidal action is greatly reduced by contact with organic protein. Germicidal agents are sometimes combined with detergents and marketed as detergent-disinfectants, detergent sanitizers, or detergent germicides.

Quaternary Ammonium Compounds (Quats)

Quaternary ammonium compounds, or quats, are cationic detergents and possess the useful property of lowering the surface tension of the solution. They are relatively inexpensive and odorless. They are stable and non-irritating when used in recommended concentrations and do not damage instruments (36, 37). The best known are benzalkonium chloride (Zephiran, Roccal) and cetyltrimethyl ammonium bromide (Centrimide). When mixed with chlorhexidine, Centrimide is known as Savlon. Some quats are mixed with alcohol to form a tincture.

Quaternary ammonium compounds are inactivated by soaps and detergents (38, 39). If soaps or detergent have been used, they must be thoroughly rinsed off before exposing the equipment to a quarternary ammonium compound. Quats are selectively absorbed by organic materials including fabrics, absorbent cotton, and gauze so that a solution becomes less concentrated if one of these is placed in it (39, 40). Cork stoppers and certain dissolved minerals such as calcium, magnesium, and iron in the water to which these substances are added also decreases their effectiveness (36, 40, 41).

Quarternary ammonium compounds are effective against gram-positive bacteria. Most gram-negative organisms are less susceptible. These compounds are not effective against spore-forming bacteria. If a spore is coated with a quaternary ammonium compound it will not develop into vegetative cells as long as the coating of the

Table 15.1.
Liquid Chemical Agents

Disinfectant	Effective Against						Inactivated	Remarks
	Gram-Positive Bacteria	Gram-Negative Bacteria	Tubercle Bacillus	Spores	Viruses	Fungi		
Soaps	0	0	0	0	0	0		
Detergents	±	∓	0	0	0	0	Organic matter	
Quaternary ammonium compounds	+	±	0	0	±	±	Organic matter, soaps, detergents	Do not use gauze or cork stoppers
Chlorhexidine	+	+	∓	0	±	±	Plastics, organic matter	Do not use as an aqueous solution
Phenolic compounds	+	+	0	0	±	±		Best for furniture
Hexachlorophene	+	∓	0	0	±	±	Organic matter	Possible link to genetic defects
Alcohols	+	+	+	0	±	±		
Glutaraldehyde	+	+	+	±	+	+		

+, good; ±, fair; ∓, poor; 0, little or no activity.

germicide remains, but if the coating is removed, the cell can germinate (38, 39).

Many investigators have found various pseudomonas species residing in quaternary ammonium compound solutions (36, 41–47). The risks of contamination or inactivity may be lessened if a tincture (where alcohol is added) rather than an aqueous solution is used (36). If an aqueous solution must be used, it should be dispensed in unit-dose containers and sterilized after packaging. It must not be packaged with or come into contact with organic material such as cork or cotton.

Other reported problems include an allergic reaction of the tracheal mucosa after use of a quaternary ammonium compound to clean a tracheostomy tube (48) and contact dermatitis (49).

Chlorhexidine (Hibitane)

Chlorhexidine is effective against gram-positive and negative bacteria but not against spores (50). It can be mixed with alcohol as a tincture or with centramide (a quaternary ammonium compound) as Savlon. It has been incorporated into soap (51).

An aqueous solution might support such gram-negative organisms as Pseudomonas (52, 53). It is inactivated by many materials, including some plastics and organic matter (54).

Phenolic Compounds

Phenol (carbolic acid) is one of the oldest germicides. The hundreds of compounds derived from it constitute the phenolic compounds. They are good bactericides and are active against fungi. They are sometimes viricidal but are not sporicidal except at or above 100°C. They are active in the presence of organic matter and soap (55). They are sometimes combined with detergents to form detergent germicides. Phenolic compounds are very stable so that they remain after mild heating and prolonged drying. Subsequent application of moisture to a surface previously treated with a phenolic compound can redissolve the chemical so that it again becomes bactericidal.

Unfortunately, most phenolic compounds have a bad odor and are irritating to skin (38, 55). They are absorbed by rubber and may subsequently damage skin or mucous membranes they contact.

They are used mainly on floors and furniture (38), but may be useful on anesthesia equipment such as machines, carts, and cylinders which do not contact the patient. They have been used for reservoir bags but are absorbed by rubber and may irritate the anesthesiologist's hand. Facial burns may result from their use on masks (56). Depigmentation has been reported (57).

Hexachlorophene

Hexachlorophene is only a fair disinfectant. It is less active against gram-negative than gram-positive bacteria (55, 58, 59). Hexachlorophene has no effect against the tubercle bacillus or spores. It is inactivated by organic matter. Hexachlorophene is sometimes added to soap to impart bacteriostatic action. Phisohex is such a combination.

Hexachlorophene's action is slow. Its use results not only in an immediate reduction of the numbers of bacteria present on skin, but the bacteriostatic activity of the residual hexachlorophene significantly inhibits the growth of bacteria (60).

Hand cream containing hexachlorophene has been found to be contaminated with gram-negative bacilli (52, 59, 61–63).

Hexachlorophene is readily absorbed into the blood stream from normal skin and especially from abraded and burned skin. Frequent hand washing by nurses has been found to be associated with an increased incidence of birth defects in their offspring (64). The future of hexachlorophene is in doubt because of these findings and work indicating central nervous system changes (46). The Food and Drug Administration has taken action to limit its use.

Alcohol (Ethyl or Isopropyl)

Ethyl and isopropyl alcohol are effective, relatively inexpensive disinfectants (55). They are often combined with other agents to enhance the action of the other agent. This is known as a tincture. Ethyl alcohol is bactericidal in 50–90% concentrations (70% is best) and isopropyl alcohol in approximately 50% concentration.

Both kill most bacteria during an exposure of 1–5 min (65). They kill the tubercle bacillus rapidly and are among the best agents for this (55). They do not kill spores. Their action against viruses is variable. Ethyl alcohol is superior to isopropyl alcohol against viruses.

They have a cleansing action. Alcohols are inactivated by protein, but not by soap.

Both ethyl and isopropyl alcohol are quite volatile. Items to be disinfected should be soaked in alcohol. It is not necessary to rinse because alcohol evaporates rapidly. Care must be taken not to use alcohol in the presence of open flame or electrical sparks which could ignite the vapor.

Alcohol can damage certain types of materials (66). Prolonged and repeated exposure of rubber and certain plastic items causes swelling and hardening.

Glutaraldehyde (Pentanedial)

Glutaraldehyde is perhaps the most useful of the liquid chemical agents available today for disinfecting anesthesia equipment. It is available in alkaline, acid, and neutral formulations.

Alkaline Glutaraldehyde. Alkaline or buffered glutaraldehyde was the first of the chemical disinfectants using glutaraldehyde. It is marketed as a mildly acidic solution with a separate container of buffer which is mixed with the acid solution just prior to use. The resulting solution has a pH of 7.5 to 8.5. It may contain a rust inhibitor to protect metals (67). At least four alkaline glutaraldehyde solutions are available: one that must be discarded after 14 days, one that is effective for 28 days, a special solution for use in automatic machines, and one with a phenolic buffer added.

In 2% solution and at room temperature it is sporicidal in 3–10 hr, virucidal in 10 min and deals effectively with most bacteria (except tubercle bacilli) almost instantly (55, 68–77). It is effective in the presence of organic material and does not coagulate proteins (76, 77).

It is noncorrosive to metal with short exposure times and is not harmful to rubber or plastics. It can be used on rigid and flexible endoscopes. Alkaline glutaraldehyde should not be heated.

Disinfection can be carried out in a special automatic unit called Cidematic which is in effect a machine with several cycles that performs both cleansing with a detergent and cold disinfection with glutaraldehyde (15, 18, 78). The glutaraldehyde is held in a side tank and is automatically pumped into the tub. Upon completion of the disinfection cycle, the solution is returned to the side tank for reuse during later cycles.

Alkaline glutaraldehyde has an irritating odor and may irritate skin with repeated exposures. Rubber gloves should always be worn when handling this agent. Thorough rinsing of all exposed materials is mandatory because residual glutaraldehyde is irritating to tissues.

Pseudomembranous laryngitis has been linked to disinfection of endotracheal tubes with alkaline glutaraldehyde (79). Allergic contact dermatitis has also been reported (80). Sticking of relief valves may occur (81).

Acid Glutaraldehyde. Acid glutaraldehyde is used as a 2% solution and a pH of 2.7–3.7. It is scented with lemon oil. It comes ready for use and requires no premixing.

At room temperature it will kill most bacteria (except tubercle bacilli), viruses, and fungi in 10 min. Tubercle bacilli are killed in 20 min. It is not sporicidal at this temperature.

Its microbiocidal activity is increased at higher temperatures, up to 100°C. At 60°C (140°F) it is bacteriocidal, virucidal, and fungicidal in 5 min, tuberculocidal in 20 min, and sporicidal in 60 min.

Acid glutaraldehyde has wetting and penetrating properties. It does not coagulate blood. While it will not harm rubber, plastic, steel, or lensed instruments, it is not recommended for plated metal instruments. It does not stain or irritate the hands or irritate the eyes or nostrils. Gloves are not necessary when using it.

It can be used in open containers, automatic washing/disinfecting machines or ultrasonic cleaners. If processing is carried out at elevated temperatures, a closed container should be employed to reduce evaporation. It can be reused for up to 30 days (82).

Neutral Glutaraldehyde. Neutral glutaraldehyde solution has a pH from 7.0 to 7.5. It is used in a 2% solution but is effective down to a .2% solution. It requires liquid activation and has a useful life of 28 days.

Neutral glutaraldehyde is bactericidal, fungicidal, tuberculocidal, and effective against some viruses in 10 min. It is sporicidal in 10 hr.

A surfactant may be added to lower surface tension and give slight detergency, allowing surfaces to wet evenly. Special corrosion inhibitors to make it safe for steel and delicate lensed instruments may be added. It can be used on rigid and flexible endoscopes. Gloves should be worn when using it.

Chemical Gas Sterilization

Ethylene oxide (EtO) is a synthetic gas which is widely used to sterilize anesthesia equipment. It is especially useful for heat- and moisture-sensitive materials such as rubber and plastic. As a gas, EtO penetrates into crevices and through permeable bags. Items can be packaged before sterilization, and stored sterile for extended periods of time.

Ethylene oxide kills bacteria, spores, fungi, and at least the larger viruses. The mechanism of destruction is believed to be a chemical attack on the genetic nucleic acids.

Ethylene oxide is available commercially in high-pressure tanks and unit-dose ampules and cartridges. It is flammable and explosive in 3% or greater concentrations by volume in air. Manufacturers have dealt with the fire and explosion hazard in two ways (67). Some dilute the EtO with carbon dioxide or a fluorocarbon. Mixtures containing up to 12% EtO in these inert diluents are nonflammable, but retain their sterilizing capacity. Ready-made mixtures are available commercially as compressed gases in cylinders. Other manufacturers use 100% of EtO, but design equipment specially for gas containment and to minimize the risk of explosion.

PREPARATION FOR ETHYLENE OXIDE STERILIZATION

It is important to verify that the product is suitable for sterilization by ethylene oxide. The manufacturer's instructions for each device should be consulted. For example, some devices may need to be sterilized at a lower temperature. Disposable devices not recommended for reuse should not be resterilized.

Before packaging and loading, items must be disassembled, cleaned, and dried. Disassembly is important because all barriers to the gas's free movement must be removed to allow ethylene oxide to penetrate throughout the whole product. Caps, plugs, valves, and/or stylets must be removed. Hollow-bore products such as needles and tubes must be open at both ends and inspected to ensure an unobstructed lumen. Syringes should have the plunger outside of the barrel.

Items for gas sterilization must be free of visible water droplets. They may be allowed to dry in ambient air, towel dried, or dried by the forced passage of unheated air. The use of heated forced air drying cabinets or hot ovens should be avoided, since the ethylene oxide sterilization process depends on the presence of adequate (but not excessive) moisture. Extended exposure of products to this method of drying may result in organisms becoming hyperdesiccated and

more resistant to ethylene oxide (83). The small amount of humidity will not produce significant amounts of ethylene glycol (84).

The sterilizer manufacturer's instructions for loading should be carefully followed. Items should be loaded in a loose fashion to allow penetration of water vapor and gas throughout the load to be sterilized. Items should be loaded in such a fashion that packages will not contact the operator's hands when baskets or carts are transferred from the sterilizer to the aerator. The operator should strive to sterilize full loads of items having common aeration times (85).

STERILIZATION

Factors Affecting Ethylene Oxide Sterilization

Several parameters must be considered if ethylene oxide sterilization is to be safe and effective.

Concentration of the Gas. The concentration of ethylene oxide is usually measured in milligrams of gas per liter of space. For effective sterilization, 450 mg/liter or greater is needed.

Temperature. The sterilizing efficiency of ethylene oxide is greatly influenced by temperature. Exposure time can be decreased by increasing the temperature. Operating temperatures in automatic sterilizers are usually preset during manufacturing. Some sterilizer models provide a selection of two specific preset temperatures (16), generally 120–145°F (49–63°C) for a warm cycle and 85–100°F (29.4–37.8°C) for a cold cycle (16). A few sterilizers conduct sterilization at room temperature. This is equally efficacious if other factors (exposure time and concentration) are adjusted.

Humidity. The moisture content of the atmosphere immediately surrounding microorganisms and the moisture content of the microorganisms themselves are extremely important to the lethal action of ethylene oxide. Some water in the form of humidity is necessary to soften the walls of spores and to act as a catalyst for the reaction between ethylene oxide and bacterial proteins.

In most automatic sterilizers, humidity is injected into the sterilizer under vacuum before admitting the ethylene oxide, or a wet gauze or sponge may be placed in the sterilizer. Other sterilizers depend on ambient humidity. They must compensate for lower moisture by using a longer exposure time.

Articles and wrappings should be protected

from excessive drying before sterilization by storage in an atmosphere of at least 40% relative humidity, but this does not eliminate the need for humidifying the sterilizer.

Protective Barriers. Blood and other proteinaceous materials and dried saline can act as barriers to ethylene oxide. Equipment must therefore be thoroughly cleansed and rinsed with water before sterilization (86).

Packaging. The type of wrapping used is very important. It must be permeable to ethylene oxide gas and water vapor. In sterilizers which have a vacuum cycle, the material must allow the air inside the packages to escape.

Polyethylene is the most commonly used wrapping. It is transparent so one can see what is inside the package.

Period of Exposure. The time needed for sterilization will depend on the factors mentioned above. In automatic sterilizers, the time generally ranges from 105–260 min (16). Up to 12 hr may be required.

Sterilizers

Manufacturers of ethylene oxide sterilizers have developed highly sophisticated units to ensure that the EtO process is consistently reliable and safe. Sterilizers for hospitals range from small portable to large, permanently installed units. Chamber sizes range from 0.25–200 cubic feet. Most hospital models are 2–40 cubic feet in capacity. Although they may be referred to as portable or mobile units, in practice they become fixed in order to provide dedicated (local) exhaust to the outside atmosphere and to connect to utilities (16).

After the sterilizer chamber is tightly sealed and the controls set, a typical sterilization in a gas sterilizer includes the following phases: (*a*) warming the chamber; (*b*) evacuating residual air from the chamber and packaged items it contains to a predetermined vacuum; (*c*) introduction of moisture and maintenance for a "dwell" period to ensure that the water vapor penetrates the wrappings and materials to be sterilized; (*d*) introduction of the ethylene oxide; (*e*) raising the chamber pressure (in some sterilizers); (*f*) raising the temperature if required; (*g*) exposure for the time required; (*h*) release of the pressure in the chamber; (*i*) removal of the ethylene oxide mixture under vacuum. This is called a purge cycle or phase (16); some sterilizers are provided with several successive purge phases; (*j*) re-establishment of atmospheric pressure by introduction of filtered air into the chamber.

Although the design, appearance, and available accessories of gas sterilizers may differ from one manufacturer to another, they generally fall into two design classes: those that are manually operated and those that are automatic (16). Automatic sterilizers are designed to internally control and monitor the physical operation of the units. Operation of both sterilization and built-in safety features is monitored and controlled automatically. Some models have abort systems that ensure that the units will not continue to function in the presence of some adverse condition and alert the operator to possible malfunction or operator error (16).

In most automatic sterilizers a source of EtO gas is provided (usually by attachment of a cylinder of an EtO mixture or insertion of a unit dose cartridge of 100% EtO) and then a sterilization cycle is selected and begun. At this point the sterilizer proceeds to cycle to completion, following the above phases, without further operator attention, unless one of its safety features indicates a malfunction or error.

Gas sterilizers are available that carry out sterilization at room temperature and ambient humidity. No negative pressure phase is utilized. A typical sterilizer of this type provides a single use glass ampule of ethylene oxide sealed inside a small gas-release bag. When the ampule is broken, the liquid vaporizes and diffuses out of the gas-release bag into a larger bag into which the materials to be sterilized have been placed. These two bags act as a diffusing chamber and allow the gas to remain long enough for sterilization to be accomplished. A stainless steel container acts as an open flame and spark shield.

INDICATORS

Because of the many variables that affect ethylene oxide sterilization, it it advisable to have evidence that sterilization is being achieved. Three types of indicators (monitors)—physical, chemical, and biological—are available. For maximum value, they should be used in combination.

Physical (mechanical control) monitors include all sterilizer components that gauge and record exposure time, temperature, humidity, and/or pressure during each cycle. They should be examined for proper functioning at the beginning, middle, and at the end of each cycle.

Chemical indicators change color when certain conditions necessary for sterilization have been met. Color change varies with the product. They are available as tapes, strips, cards, and sheets. They may be implanted or attached to packaging material or enclosed in packages. There are two types of chemical indicators currently available: those that monitor the combination of gas plus moisture and those that monitor heat plus moisture (16).

Chemical indicators are not at present sterility indicators and should not replace biological monitors. They only indicate that the package has been subjected to some parameters of the sterilization cycle. Chemical indicators may change color under conditions inadequate for sterilization.

It is recommended that a chemical indicator be used with each article that undergoes ethylene oxide sterilization to prevent sterilized packages from being mixed with non-sterilized items and to detect some failures of sterilization. The user of an ethylene oxide-sterilized item should always check the chemical indicator for color change before use.

To achieve a high degree of certainty that a sterilizer is functioning properly, and to detect problems in techniques, biological indicators should be placed in the most inaccessible location in the sterilized load and then cultured. They provide positive assurance that each package has been subjected to proper sterilizing conditions. It should be noted that if the articles to be sterilized have not been properly cleaned before packaging, a biological indicator will not be a valid tool for determining sterility

The recommended frequency of use for biological indicators varies. Some experts recommend their use in every load, but most institutions use them only periodically. They should always be used after installation of a sterilizer and after any repairs.

AERATION

Ethylene oxide not only comes in contact with all surfaces of articles being sterilized, but also penetrates some items, which then retain varying amounts. These items need special treatment called aeration (degassing, desorption) to remove enough residual ethylene oxide that a level safe for both personnel and patient use is achieved.

Aeration may be done passively in air (ambient aeration) or actively in a mechanical aerator.

Ambient Aeration

Ambient aeration is highly variable because of the lack of control of temperature and air flow. It results in a slower reduction of residual ethylene oxide than mechanical aeration. It is possible that some of the toxicity problems encountered in the early hospital use of ethylene oxide resulted from failure to recognize this fact.

Items that require 8–12 hr of mechanical aeration may require 7 days of ambient aeration (87, 88). Some items take 5–6 weeks. Thus the hospital must maintain a large and often costly inventory of items. Ambient aeration may also result in hazardous exposure of workers to ethylene oxide.

If ambient aeration is unavoidable (for heat-sensitive items that cannot withstand the elevated temperatures of conventional aerator cabinets and when a closed vented cabinet especially designed for that purpose is not available), measures to minimize traffic in the aeration area and to ensure that personnel who must enter the area are not exposed to ethylene oxide at hazardous concentrations should be taken (85).

Mechanical Aerators (16)

In mechanical aerators a stream of filtered air is directed over the sterilized items. This reduces the necessary aeration time.

Factors Affecting Aeration

Composition of the Article. The amount of residual EtO and the length of time needed for it to dissipate depend on the type of material being sterilized. Hard-surfaced items such as metal and glass do not absorb ethylene oxide and require little or no aeration. Plastics, rubbers and other "soft" materials such as muslin and paper may absorb significant quantities. Items that consist of a combination of absorbent and nonabsorbent materials (e.g., a metal item with rubber parts) must be treated as though they were made entirely of absorbent material. Metal and glass items that are wrapped in EtO-absorbent material must be aerated.

The most common material retaining large amounts of EtO is polyvinyl chloride. The type and amount of plasticizer in the polyvinyl chloride will strongly influence the amount absorbed. Rubber absorbs less, and polyethylene and nylon still less. Teflon absorbs very little ethylene oxide. When the composition of a device is in doubt, it should be treated as if it were polyvinyl chloride (85).

Configuration of the Object. Thicker objects require longer aeration time than thin ones.

Diluent. The fluorocarbon mixture requires a longer aeration time than the carbon dioxide mixture.

Wrappings. Attention should be paid to the packaging material, as this must allow the transfer of gas. Most wrappings freely allow the transfer of ethylene oxide and thus do not present any problem of gas retention.

Temperature of Aeration. Increasing the temperature greatly accelerates the removal of ethylene oxide from items. The usual aeration temperature is 50 or 60°C (16). If these temperatures would be damaging to a device, aeration can be carried out at room temperature in a closed ventilated cabinet especially designed for that purpose or ambient aeration can be used.

Air Flow. Aeration is affected by the number of air changes per hour and the air flow characteristics.

Sterilizer Used. Use of sterilizers which subject materials to hot gases under elevated pressure can result in higher levels of ethylene oxide in the items sterilized (90).

Intended Use of the Device. Whether the item is to be external to the body, within a body cavity, intravascularly, or implanted will affect the acceptable level of residual ethylene oxide.

Time of Aeration. Unfortunately, it is impossible to establish a single aeration period required for the removal of ethylene oxide from every article which can be gas sterilized as this depends on so many factors. There is also a lack of definite information on the levels of ethylene oxide which are nontoxic to human tissues. Many device manufacturers provide specific aeration recommendations for their devices.

The minimum recommended times for devices that are difficult to aerate are 8 hr at 60°C or 12 hr at 50°C in a mechanical aerator and 7 days at room temperature (85). When in doubt about aeration requirements for a particular device, these recommendations may be followed as a general rule. It should be noted, however, that some items may require even longer periods.

COMPLICATIONS OF ETHYLENE OXIDE STERILIZATION

Patient Complications

Complications of ethylene oxide sterilization include skin reactions and laryngotracheal inflammation (91–95). When blood is exposed to ethylene oxide-treated materials, destruction of the red cells can occur (96–98). Sensitization and anaphylaxis from exposure to products sterilized with ethylene oxide have been reported (99).

These problems are caused by excessive levels of ethylene oxide or its byproducts, ethylene glycol and ethylene chlorhydrin, which are left after sterilization. EtO will remain a gas at room temperature and can be removed by allowing sufficient aeration time. Ethylene glycol is formed by the reaction of ethylene oxide and water. Since even dry materials contain some moisture, some glycol formation is unavoidable. Traces of glycols are generally regarded as relatively harmless and permissible for human exposure (100). Removing all visible water droplets from equipment before sterilization should prevent formation of excessive glycol.

Concern has been expressed over the use of EtO for rubber-stoppered vials or glass ampules, as the ethylene oxide might gain access to the interior of local anesthetic containers where, upon contact with water, it would be transformed to ethylene glycol (101, 102).

Ethylene chlorhydrin is formed when ethylene oxide comes into contact with chloride ions such as may be present in previously gamma-irradiated PVC items. The American National Standards Institute has recommended that PVC items which have been gamma-irradiated never be re-sterilized with ethylene oxide (88). Doubt has been cast on this, however, by some workers who have found very low levels of byproducts in gamma-irradiated products treated with ethylene oxide (103–105).

Alterations in Equipment

Repeated ethylene oxide sterilization may affect some equipment adversely. Repeated exposure of some plastics to ethylene oxide and heat may leach out plasticizers and weaken the structural integrity (106). Rubber and some plastic endotracheal tubes may soften and kink more easily (67) or become sticky. Blisters between layers in the walls of latex endotracheal tubes containing embedded spiral wires can occur, resulting in narrowing of the lumen (67). It is recommended that these tubes not be sterilized by this method (107). Reuse of a disposable esophageal stethoscope has been associated with detachment of the balloon (106).

Personnel Complications

Possible Hazards of Exposure to Ethylene Oxide. A fundamental problem with the use of ethylene oxide is exposure of the operator to the toxic sterilant. Scientific evidence and clinical studies suggest that acute and chronic exposure to ethylene oxide increases risks to the health of exposed personnel.

EtO acts as a vesicant, causing burns and irritation if confined against the skin (108). Acute toxic effects from inhalation of EtO in man and animals include respiratory and eye irritation, nausea and vomiting, diarrhea, blunting of taste or smell, peculiar taste, headache, incoordination, increased fatigability, memory loss, dizziness, difficulty swallowing, cramps, convulsions, encephalopathy, and peripheral neuropathies (109). Known chronic effects include respiratory infections, anemia, and altered behavior (100). In addition, there are concerns that EtO may be mutagenic and possibly carcinogenic to humans and that it may produce adverse effects on the reproductive system, including teratogenicity (85, 110).

Since some exposure to ethylene oxide is unavoidable, there is a need to establish tolerable limits for concentrations and exposure times. At the time of writing of this book, the Occupational Safety and Health Administration had proposed lowering the permissible average daily exposure rate to ethylene oxide over 8 hr from 50 to 1 ppm (111). A ceiling limit on one-time exposure was not proposed, but it is likely that some limit will be set before the final regulations go into effect. It is essential that each health care facility keep current with applicable federal regulations and voluntary guidelines. Limits on maximum exposure may be reduced as a result of ongoing research on the effects of EtO.

The presence of gaseous EtO in very high concentrations is easily detected, since it is irritating to the eyes and mucous membranes, but caution should be exercised in depending upon nasal sensory detection. About 600 ppm is the odor threshold, so it is possible to be in a room with dangerously high ethylene oxide concentrations without being aware of it (112).

Recommendations to Reduce Exposure (16, 67, 85, 110, 113, 114). The following steps can be taken to minimize occupational exposure to ethylene oxide.

1. Unnecessary use of EtO should be avoided. It should be reserved for those products which must be sterilized and cannot withstand autoclaving.

2. Each sterilizer and aerator should have preventive maintenance at least quarterly to ensure that malfunctions, especially leaks, are minimal and that any malfunctions that do occur are detected and corrected. Records should be kept on all malfunctions and repairs.

3. Cylinders of ethylene oxide should be stored in a designated area that meets building codes and OSHA regulations, conforms to the temperature specifications of the gas supplier/manufacturer and is out of the way of traffic. Tanks should be stored and used in an upright position and should be securely fastened to a solid structure (16).

4. EtO tanks should be transported on equipment designed to keep them secure during transit.

5. Caution should be exercised not to expose the technician to ethylene oxide when changing tanks. Use of appropriate personnel safeguards such as protective attire (e.g., goggles, heavy-duty gloves) and self-contained breathing apparatus should be considered (85). There should be check or shutoff valves in the EtO lines close to the connection point to limit the release of EtO into the atmosphere during cylinder changes.

6. The hospital should form an "action team" responsible for the development and exercise of written procedures to handle EtO leaks and spills (16, 85).

7. Sterilizers and aerators should be located in well-ventilated areas with limited access, away from work stations, storage areas, and employee traffic. Entrances to areas where EtO is used should be posted with signs warning that high levels of EtO are possible. No supplies or unnecessary equipment should be stored in the vicinity of sterilization/aeration equipment and the personnel permitted in those areas should be as few as possible. Personnel not involved in sterilizing must be routed away.

8. Rooms in which sterilizers or aerators are located should have a minimum volume of 1000 cubic feet and a non-recirculating ventilation system with at least 10 air changes per hour (85). The room air should be vented to the outside atmosphere, away from any intake ducts or pedestrian traffic (115). Ventilation rates should be monitored and documented at least every 3 months to ensure adequate performance. The effectiveness of ventilation should also be

checked soon after any change that might result in significant increases in airborne exposure to ethylene oxide (110).

9. Location of sterilization equipment in proper relationship to room air intakes and exhausts will help assure adequate ventilation of the area housing the sterilizer (85).

10. Sterilizers, aerators, and floor waste drains should be vented to the outside, by means of dedicated vent lines made of ethylene oxide-impervious material. Sponge-type or water tray "absorbers" must not be used (85).

11. Use of local exhaust ventilation systems to capture ethylene oxide before it can escape into the general work environment will reduce exposure (85). The ethylene oxide can be collected in a hood of suitable design located as close to the source of EtO as possible and exhausted to the outside atmosphere via a fan and duct system. The following are the most common areas where high EtO concentrations may occur, and where local exhaust systems are recommended: (a) the area immediately adjacent to the sterilizer door; (b) the area near the sterilizer pressure relief valve (where applicable); (c) the area immediately above the drain line into the sanitary sewer (for sterilizers that discharge to a sanitary system); and (d) EtO cylinder connection points.

12. Consideration should be given to purchase and use of newer sterilizers with special safety features. Each new generation of sterilizers is equipped with new components that can make the process safer. Some of these safety features can be added to certain existing models (16).

13. Employees operating sterilizers or aerators should be properly instructed in the hazards of ethylene oxide and appropriate safety procedures. They should be familiar with the sterilizer and techniques whereby EtO exposure can be reduced. If feasible, workers may be isolated from direct contact with the work environment by the use of automated equipment operated by personnel observing from a closed control booth or room (110).

14. Occupational exposure to EtO can be avoided by using a loading cart and/or wire baskets (16). These can be moved into and from the sterilizer, then directly into and from the aerator. Items should be loaded in such a manner that they will not touch the operator's hands when the cart or basket is transferred from the sterilizer to the aerator.

15. The single greatest source of employee exposure occurs when the sterilizer door is opened upon completion of a cycle (116). Exposure control at this point is essential. A purge or air flush cycle preceding opening of the sterilizer door is desirable (117). A local exhaust at the door opening is advisable (116–119). Employees should avoid being close to a sterilizer that has just finished a cycle, except as necessary to operate the unit.

Materials should not be left in a closed sterilizer after the cycle, as this will allow high concentrations of EtO to build up in the sterilizer and be released into the room when the door is first opened.

The chamber door should be opened 3–6 inches immediately following a cycle. A door-opening device on some large sterilizers allows the operator to push a button, then walk away, while the sterilizer door slowly opens (100).

The operator should leave the immediate sterilizer area for a minimum of 15 min after opening the door (85, 120). This time allows residual ethylene oxide to dissipate out of the chamber and be removed by the general ventilation system. A local exhaust ventilation system will significantly reduce the amount of time required for ethylene oxide to be removed from the sterilizer area.

It should be noted that purge characteristics of some newer sterilizers will prevent the buildup of ethylene oxide inside the chamber (85). These sterilizers should be unloaded immediately upon opening the door, since it is at this time that the EtO concentration within the chamber is lowest. When in doubt, the manufacturer's instructions should be consulted.

16. Sterilized items should be transferred without delay to the aerator with as little handling as possible. Transfer carts should be used to remove sterilized items from large sterilizers and gloves and forceps for items in small sterilizers. This will minimize the inhalation of EtO by the operator and the possibility of skin contact with EtO. Carts should be pulled, rather than pushed, to the aerator and the items immediately placed in the aerator. Unaerated items should never be left outside the aerator where they might contaminate the environment or be used inadvertently.

17. All ethylene oxide-sterilized items should be aerated prior to handling. A mechanical aerator is best. If ambient aeration is unavoidable, the aeration area should be segregated from general work areas and have limited access. It

should have good general ventilation and be at a negative pressure with respect to adjoining areas. Storage of supplies in the area must be prohibited. Alternately, aeration can be performed in dedicated, well-ventilated areas, such as hoods.

18. Personnel and/or environmental monitoring similar to that discussed in Chapter 9 should be practiced to ensure that recommended levels in the air are not exceeded. Instruments similar to those used for trace gas monitoring are available. Samples should be taken during periods of heavy use. Leak monitoring using a simple leak detector should be performed regularly (113).

Comprehensive surveys should be conducted annually and following major ventilation system changes, new equipment installation or substantive employee complaints, especially if accompanied by documented medical signs or symptoms. Quarterly monitoring of room air concentrations is recommended unless results indicate excessive exposure levels, in which case more frequent sampling should be performed until the cause is identified.

ADVANTAGES AND DISADVANTAGES

Ethylene oxide sterilization has many advantages. It is effective against all organisms. It is very reliable since the gas penetrates into crevices and regions blocked to liquids. It can be used on a wide variety of items including those which would be damaged by heat or moisture. Indeed, it is the only reliable and practical means for sterilizing many devices in common use today. Damage to most equipment is minimal. Items can be prepackaged and the package sealed. This eliminates the danger of recontamination that can occur during rinsing and packaging following "cold sterilization," and allows the items to remain sterile during long-term storage.

Ethylene oxide has a number of disadvantages. Fires and explosions involving sterilizers have been reported (121, 122). Flammable mixtures require special handling. Even with the diluted ethylene oxide mixtures, care must be exercised, since there is a possibility that the gas mixture may become stratified and create a fire or explosion hazard (67).

It is more costly than most other types of disinfection. Total processing time is long, so a large inventory is required. Installation of the necessary equipment is expensive and if large items are to be sterilized the equipment will take

a great deal of space. Personnel need to be highly trained and supervised to ensure proper sterilization and prevent complications. Frequent biological monitoring is required.

Equipment to be sterilized needs to be dry, which can be difficult to achieve with items such as corrugated tubings. Some materials deteriorate after repeated sterilization, especially at elevated temperatures. It cannot be used to sterilize any medical devices that have petroleum-based lubricants in or on them, since ethylene oxide cannot permeate these lubricants (123).

A PROGRAM FOR ANESTHESIA EQUIPMENT

Organization

The responsibility for decontamination of anesthesia equipment should be vested in one individual who devises and administers a comprehensive program. This person should be a member of the infections committee of the hospital.

A decontamination program which meets the needs of a given hospital usually results from tailoring several techniques to that hospital's needs. Factors to be considered include cost, types of equipment employed, available facilities and the importance attributed to sterilization in that hospital. A hospital which has many patients with reduced immunity must be more careful than a surgical center which handles only healthy outpatients. Whatever decontamination plan is devised, it is important that alternate methods be available in the event the primary system fails. Whatever system is devised, certain factors are essential for a successful program.

ADEQUATE PHYSICAL ARRANGEMENT

Areas for cleaning, drying, packaging for sterilization, disinfection, and/or sterilizing and storage should be clearly designated. The area where the equipment is cleaned should be separate from the others. It should be near to the operating rooms and should be organized in a fashion that permits an efficient flow of equipment. Signs showing where dirty equipment should be placed should be prominently displayed.

ADEQUATE AMOUNT AND CORRECT TYPE OF EQUIPMENT

While equipment is being cleaned it cannot be used. This necessitates a larger inventory.

Depending on the individual circumstances, disposable equipment may be utilized to a greater or lesser degree. Some disposable items should always be available for use with known infected cases.

GOOD ASSISTANCE

It is imperative that cleaning and disinfection or sterilizing of anesthesia equipment be delegated to conscientious, well-trained individuals who understand the principles of containment of contamination and the disinfecting or sterilizing process (124).

Depending on the individual hospital's circumstances, cleaning and/or sterilization may be done by an aide, the operating room staff, the central service, nurse anesthetists, or an anesthesiologist. Frequently, responsibilities are divided among several of these.

Most nurses are well indoctrinated in the principles of aseptic technique. However, frequently technicians caring for equipment are without a clinical hospital background. Such people need considerable indoctrination before they can be relied upon in practice.

SURVEILLANCE

The fourth factor necessary for a successful decontamination program is surveillance to check the efficiency of decontaminating techniques. This should include routine bacteriological checks of the equipment and monitoring the sterilizing procedures using bacteriological indicators.

Housekeeping during Administration of Anesthesia

Good housekeeping during the administration of anesthesia will limit potential sources of contamination. It is important to establish a routine whereby an article not used on a patient is kept free of contamination and secondly to be able to identify and isolate all articles which may have been contaminated.

The anesthesiologist should always work from a clean surface. At the start of each anesthetic those articles which are to be used on that patient should be placed there.

All used articles should be placed in a special receptacle that is physically separated from the clean area. This serves to identify anything dirty and saves further handling of the articles. It may contain water with detergent to prevent

drying of secretions. At the end of the operation, this receptable can be taken to the dirty wash-up area. This will keep handling of dirty items by personnel to a minimum. Disposable items that are not to be used again should be discarded in suitable containers in the operating room.

Handwashing between contacts with patients should be done by all persons who are involved in patient care, using an effective antimicrobial agent to reduce the bacterial count on the hands and thus lessen the risk of cross-infection.

Use of Bacterial Filters

Use of filters in the breathing system has been advocated to reduce the incidence of postoperative respiratory infections. A variety of filters are available (see Chapter 5).

Use of filters is controversial. Certain hazards, especially obstruction, are associated with their use. Recent studies (125–127) indicate that routine use of filters does not prevent postoperative pulmonary infections. Their use might occasionally be indicated in patients requiring respiratory isolation at the time of surgery or to protect patients at increased risk of developing an infection.

Disposable Versus Reusable Equipment (23)

A major consideration for anesthesiologists is the issue of disposable versus non-disposable (reusable) equipment. Factors to be taken into account include costs, convenience, quality of the equipment and decontamination procedures, and ecological concerns.

When reusable equipment is employed, it is essential that decontamination procedures have good quality control. In addition to the initial cost of an item, expenses for recycling, including labor and materials, must be examined. It must be remembered that there is a given life span for reusable equipment.

The advantages of disposable equipment center around convenience and time savings. However, many disposable items are not as well made as reusable ones. Costs of the equipment and inventory must be taken into account. Storage space can be a problem. The ecological problems of getting rid of disposable items after use must not be ignored.

The choice of which items to reuse and which to discard will depend on local circumstances and preferences. It is sometimes advisable to keep some disposable items for use on patients with known infections or in certain sections of the hospital while using reusable items most of the time.

Known Infected Cases

When anesthetizing patients with known or suspected communicable respiratory diseases, consideration should be given to one or more of the following:

RESTRICTING SPREAD OF ORGANISMS

Unnecessary equipment should be removed from the operating room. Traffic within the room should be kept to a minimum. The anesthesiologist should wear gloves plus an outer gown and shoe covers. The patient should wear a mask until the last possible moment. At the end of the procedure, all gowns, gloves, shoe covers, and masks should be removed and left in the contaminated operating room.

USE OF DISPOSABLE EQUIPMENT

One of the best ways of dealing with this problem is to use disposable equipment whenever possible. Most equipment is made disposable and a small supply can be kept on hand for such cases. After use the equipment should be placed in impervious disposal bags in the operating room and discarded or incinerated.

EMPLOYMENT OF BACTERIAL FILTERS

These will protect complex, difficult-to-sterilize equipment such as ventilators and absorbers from bacterial contamination. Then only the parts between the filters and the patient need be disinfected or discarded.

With a Mapleson system a single filter placed near the patient will protect most parts of the breathing system. With the circle system two filters must be used. Although placing the filters near the patient will protect the breathing hoses, this may be cumbersome, so it may be better to use disposable hoses and place filters at the machine end of the hoses.

USE OF SUITABLE REUSABLE EQUIPMENT

Reusable equipment should be selected at least partly on the basis of ease of dismantling, cleaning, and disinfecting or sterilizing.

Immediately after use, small pieces of equipment, such as masks, endotracheal tubes, airways, etc., should be submerged in a fresh solution of a detergent-germicide right in the operating room. If a ventilator or circle absorber has become contaminated, it should be disassembled, with the parts that can be submerged added to the solution. After it has soaked for at least 30 min, the equipment should be thoroughly cleaned, rinsed, and taken to the usual processing area where it should undergo standard cleaning and disinfection or sterilization. Alternatively, contaminated items can be double bagged at the point of use and taken to the processing area for decontamination. Employees who handle items before decontamination should wear protective attire.

The anesthesia machine, cart, monitors, and other equipment which cannot be sterilized should be wiped with a soft cloth soaked in liquid detergent-germicide immediately after the case.

In the past it has been recommended that items used in treating a patient with a communicable disease be subjected to a double exposure time of ethylene oxide before being aerated and reprocessed. However, such a procedure presents hazards in that items may contain soil not affected by EtO. These may then contaminate the sterilizer, the environment during the transfer from sterilizer to aerator, and the aerator itself. Therefore the use of ethylene oxide for this type of decontamination procedure should be undertaken with caution (16).

Cleaning and Sterilization of Anesthesia Equipment

GENERAL CONSIDERATIONS

Before an approach to a particular item can be decided upon, the following questions must be answered: What is the risk of the item becoming contaminated? What is the risk that the equipment will transmit organisms to the next patient on whom it is used?

Risk of Contamination of Items

No component of anesthesia equipment inevitably escapes contamination. However, certain components are affected more often and more heavily than others. Items which are inserted into the patient's mouth, i.e., laryngoscope blades, airways, endotracheal tubes, suction catheters, etc., constantly become contaminated. Items which are not inserted into the patient but which are used near the patient are frequently contaminated. These include masks, adaptors and the portions of the breathing system nearest the patient. Components remote from the patient have the least contamination.

Risk of Transmittal of Infection to Another Patient

There are four possible mechanisms whereby infectious particles can be transmitted to a patient: (a) aerosolization from surfaces in the breathing system to sterile parts of the respiratory tract; (b) spillage of condensate down into the mask or endotracheal tube; (c) direct trauma to the mucosa and (d) airborne wound contamination.

Aerosolization. It has been shown that organisms may travel 3 feet through corrugated tubes during anesthesia (1). Therefore, any part of the breathing system may transmit organisms to the respiratory tract, although the dosage will usually be small.

Condensate. Exhaled gases are warm and saturated with moisture. As they pass through connectors and the breathing system, they are cooled and water condenses on the sides of the equipment. This water may then run down into the mask or endotracheal tube, carrying with it any organisms present on the equipment.

Trauma to the Mucosa. The mouth and lower pharynx are always full of bacteria and have a stratified protective epithelium designed to withstand wear and tear. Therefore, many people feel that instruments for use in the mouth need be only as clean as one's spoon and fork at the table. On the other hand, inasmuch as the mucosa may be traumatized during maneuvers performed during anesthesia, the risk of infection is present, although experience suggests the incidence is not great.

In contrast, the nasal mucosa and the trachea are easily traumatized so that the risk of infection is great. The incidence of bacteremia with nasal intubation is quite high.

Airborne Wound Contamination. Although not usually considered, this is certainly an important consideration, particularly in prolonged surgical procedures.

APPROACHES TO CLEANING AND DISINFECTION OR STERILIZATION

The exact approach to decontaminating any component will vary, depending on the answers to the preceding questions, the ease of disinfection or sterilization, and the feelings of personnel about the sterilization dilemma. Approaches generally fall within one of the following categories:

Cleaning and Sterilization after Use, with the Item Maintained Sterile until the Next Use

This approach, reserved in equipment, is now frequently used for items placed in the trachea. It has also been advocated for such items as face masks (1).

Cleaning and Sterilization or Disinfection after Use, with the Article Kept Clean until the Next Use

This approach is often used for equipment to be placed in the patient's mouth and face masks. Inasmuch as the patient will be exposed to organisms present in the operating room anyway, it is unnecessary to keep the equipment sterile.

Cleaning after Use with Periodic Sterilization or Disinfection

This approach is frequently adopted for pieces of equipment that are difficult to sterilize. Infectiousness depends both on the virulence of organisms and the total dosage. Periodic sterilization or disinfection can reduce the incidence of infections by reducing the prevalence of bacteria to a point below the level of total dosage necessary to produce infection (128).

Cleaning after Use, with No Attempt at Disinfection of Sterilization

This approach is usually adopted for pieces of equipment such as anesthesia machines which are impossible to sterilize or disinfect.

CONSIDERATION OF INDIVIDUAL ITEMS

It should be obvious from the above discussion and that of the sterilization dilemma that no hard and fast rules can be laid down for decontaminating anesthesia equipment. What will be attempted in this section is to consider each item from the standpoint of risks, with suggestions for use, cleaning and, where applicable, disinfection or sterilization.

Anesthesia Carts

General Considerations. Anesthesia carts are used in many operating rooms as a repository for equipment and drugs used in anesthesia. Some attention should be given to the placement of equipment in the drawers. For instance, a blood pressure cuff that is used on several patients with no attempt to decontaminate it between cases should not be placed in the same drawer as airways or masks that are not kept in sterile containers, but it may be placed in a drawer containing items such as suction catheters and syringes that are kept in disposable containers. Equipment such as airways and masks that are not kept in sterile containers should be placed in drawers that are less frequently opened, e.g., not in the same drawer as frequently used drugs. Containers used to hold syringes, needles, etc., should be made of metal or plastic rather than cardboard to facilitate cleaning.

If a known contaminated case occurs, the items of equipment or drugs considered likely to be needed during the case should be removed from the cart and placed on the anesthesia machine or an easily cleaned operating room stand. The cart should then be placed just outside the operating room door.

Cleaning. The top, front and sides of the anesthesia cart should be wiped off with a detergent germicide once daily and a clean covering should be placed on the top at the start of each day. Blood or secretions should be wiped off promptly.

At least once a week, and following use on a patient with a known communicable disease, the entire cart should be cleaned. All equipment should be removed and the drawers washed with detergent and water and then wiped or sprayed with a germicide. Containers for syringes, etc., should be washed.

Gas Cylinders

General Considerations. Gas cylinders are transported to the hospital in open trucks and are frequently stored outside. Therefore, they should be considered dirty when received in the operating room area. Some are furnished in plastic or paper wrappers. Before taking a cylinder into an operating room, the wrapper, if present, should be removed.

Cleaning. The cylinder should be washed with water and detergent and wiped with a cloth soaked in germicide or sprayed with a germicidal spray. After placing the cylinder on the anesthesia machine, it may be considered part of the machine and treated accordingly.

Anesthesia Machines

General Considerations. Anesthesia machines usually remain in the operating room and are not transported to other areas. They are often used to store drugs and equipment and may provide the "clean" and/or "dirty" areas for equipment. The same principles for storage of equipment and separation of clean and dirty areas apply to machines as to carts. The top of an anesthesia machine is a convenient area for keeping equipment. Many machines have a shelf several feet above the table. This can be used for placing a tray holding "clean" equipment or a receptable for the "dirty" equipment. Equipment placed there will be separate from the rest of the equipment but readily available.

Cleaning. The cleaning of anesthesia machines is often neglected because (a) operating rooms strive for a minimum of time between cases and (b) prolonged indoctrination of attendants against tampering with the machine often fosters a "hands off" attitude. Anesthesia machines should be considered operating room furniture and receive the routine cleaning that other pieces of furniture do. The horizontal surfaces should be cleaned between cases (129). The machine should be subjected daily to a thorough surface wiping with a damp cloth containing a detergent with particular attention to cleaning around the knobs, vaporizers, cylinders, etc. At least once a week equipment should be removed from the drawers and the drawers cleaned. The final application should be with a cloth containing a disinfectant solution or a germicidal spray may be used.

After anesthetizing a patient with a known infection, the machine should be sprayed with a bactericidal aerosol and then cleaned as during the weekly cleaning.

The Circle System

Because the circle system is composed of many parts, some of which are not easily sterilized, it would seem advantageous to anesthetize a patient with a known pulmonary infection with another system. Alternately, one might use a completely disposable circle system or use bacterial filters to protect the parts of the system which are difficult to sterilize.

Absorber, Unidirectional Valves and Relief Value. *General Considerations.* Studies strongly suggest that regardless of prior upper airway colonization and duration of anesthesia, patients rarely contaminate these parts with significant levels of bacteria (5). Nevertheless, they can harbor dangerous organisms (130, 131). Disposable absorbers are available.

Cleaning. The manufacturer's instructions should be consulted with respect to disassembling, cleaning, and disinfecting.

The absorbent should be removed from the absorber. Absorbent cannot be sterilized. It combines chemically with ethylene oxide to change the chemical composition, change the indicator color, and reduce the carbon dioxide uptake capacity. Steam sterilization may cause granules to fragment and cause caking, which increases air flow resistance. Cold sterilization is also impossible.

The canisters should be cleaned with water and detergent to remove dust and other debris. The screens should receive particular attention as they are susceptible to the gumming film produced by absorbents. The absorber frame should be cleaned at this time by wiping with a cloth soaked in a detergent germicide. Unidirectional valves are usually easily disassembled and cleaned by wiping the disc, the inside of the plastic dome and the valve seat with alcohol or a detergent (132, 133). Relief valves can be cleaned by wiping with a detergent.

Disinfection and/or Sterilization. Some canisters will withstand autoclaving (132, 134) but most will not. Some can be boiled (135). Some relief valves may be autoclaved.

Most canisters can be sterilized by immersion in a liquid such as glutaraldehyde, as can most relief valves. However, use of glutaraldehyde on relief valves has been reported to cause stickiness and increase the opening pressure (81). Autoclaving was less harmful.

The entire absorber, unidirectional valves and relief valve can be sterilized using ethylene oxide (12, 136). A cold cycle should be used to prevent damage to plastic parts. A minimum of 7 days ambient aeration or 8 hr in an aerator is necessary (12). Before use on a pateint, the system should be operated for at least 3 min to remove any entrapped ethylene oxide (11).

The Reservoir Bag. The risk of the reservoir bag in a circle system becoming contami-

nated is much higher if it is placed on the expiratory side of the absorber than when it is on the inspiratory side (14). Also, in this position the inside of the bag is more likely to become wet. However, if placed on the inspiratory side, the risk of its transmitting infectious particles to the patient is greater.

Disposable rubber and plastic bags are available. Some come with disposable tubing or as parts of a completely disposable system. The reader is cautioned concerning the pressure-volume characteristics of some plastic bags (see Chapter 5).

Inasmuch as the bag is usually connected near the absorber, it is usually possible to protect it from contamination by use of filters.

Cleaning. Cleaning of the inside of the bag is not easy. However, because of its position, solid material should not get inside the bag often. Rinsing the inside with running tap water is probably sufficient in most cases or some water and detergent may be placed inside and the bag agitated, then rinsed under a running tap. The outside of the bag may be washed with water and detergent. The bag may also be cleaned in a washing machine. After cleaning, the bag should be dried, unless moist heat sterilization is to be used. A stream of compressed air may be used to help dry the bag.

Disinfection or Sterilization. Ethylene oxide is probably the most satisfactory means of sterilizing the bag. Aeration times should be carefully observed and the bag filled and emptied a few times before use on a patient.

Bags can be sterilized by autoclaving, provided an adequate wick is placed inside to ensure steam contact with all surfaces (137). However, autoclaving will cause rubber bags to deteriorate and will usually melt plastic bags. Bags may be boiled (135) or pasteurized (138) but this also will result in gradual deterioration.

Chemical disinfection can be used. The bag must be filled with liquid to remove pockets of air (139). Of the various agents used, glutaraldehyde is probably the most satisfactory, provided adequate rinsing is performed. Bags can be disinfected in a Cidematic (15).

Corrugated Tubings. *General Considerations.* The corrugated tubing of the circle system presents a difficult problem in decontamination of equipment. Numerous studies have shown that this tubing is contaminated after use. The closer to the patient, the heavier the contamination. Some studies suggest that anesthetic gases can pick up and transfer microorganisms from contaminated tubing (140). Other studies indicate that microbial contamination inherent in, or added to, tubing remains stationary along the corrugations and is not affected by gas flow or patient expirations (5). Another study showed that use of sterile tubings did not prevent postoperative pulmonary infections (6). Water commonly condenses in the expiratory tubing. If the tubings are lifted up, the water may run down into the mask or endotracheal tube. Because of their bulk and construction, tubings are difficult to clean and disinfect or sterilize. They also present a storage problem if frequent changes are made. Disposable tubings are available (141).

Cleaning. Corrugated hoses should not be heavily contaminated with soil, but if a patient coughs while under anesthesia particles of solid matter may travel far into the tubing. Tubes should be rinsed out under a running tap soon after use to prevent drying. They may then be soaked in a large container containing water and detergent.

The long length and ridges preclude a brush being effective in cleaning. Ultrasonic cleaning has been used to remove debris from corrugated tubing in respiratory therapy (142), and might be worthwhile trying. A washing machine with agitation may be used to wash the tubings. Other proposals include pouring detergent and water into one end of the tube and agitating in a seesaw manner (143).

After washing the tubings should be thoroughly dried unless moist heat is to be used for sterilization. Special tube dryers are available.

Disinfection and/or Sterilization. Autoclaving (132, 144), pasteurization (134, 138), and boiling (133) have all been used for corrugated tubings. With all of these the Y-piece should be removed beforehand. Otherwise, a loose fit may result. All of these procedures will shorten the life of the tubing.

Ethylene oxide may be used to sterilize the tubings. The tubings must be dry. Unfortunately, their bulk makes them unsuitable except for large sterilizers and only a few tubings can be put into a sterilizer at a time.

Chemical disinfection can be carried out using the Cidematic or by immersion in a liquid agent. It is important that the tube be inserted vertically, making sure it is filled on the inside and there are no air pockets.

The Y-Piece. Y-pieces are contaminated in a high percentage of cases (14, 26, 135, 138, 144).

Because of their proximity to the patient, the danger of cross-infection is great. Fortunately, they are relatively easy to sterilize. Disposable Y-pieces are available, usually attached to disposable tubings.

Cleaning. After use, the Y-piece should be removed from the corrugated tubings and rinsed out under a tap of running water. They should then be placed in a solution of water and detergent to soak. They may be scrubbed inside manually or placed in a washing machine. If chemical or ethylene oxide sterilization is to be used, the Y-piece should be thoroughly dried.

Sterilization or Disinfection. Metal Y-pieces may be boiled, autoclaved, pasteurized, immersed in liquid agents or sterilized with ethylene oxide. They should not be connected to the corrugated tubing during autoclaving, boiling, or pasteurizing. Plastic Y-pieces can undergo cold disinfection or ethylene oxide sterilization.

Systems Employing Non-Rebreathing Valves

General Considerations. The non-rebreathing valve is frequently contaminated (138) and because of its proximity to the patient carries a high risk of transmitting infection.

The bag, corrugated tubing, and relief valve should not become contaminated unless the non-rebreathing valve is incompetent but, because of their position directly in the inspiratory pathway, at least periodic sterilization or disinfection should be performed.

Cleaning. The manufacturer's instructions should be consulted before cleaning the non-rebreathing valve. Most can be disassembled.

Disinfection and/or Sterilization. The manufacturer's instructions should be consulted. A few non-rebreathing valves can be autoclaved. Most can be sterilized with ethylene oxide. The other components of the system may be disinfected or sterilized as described under the section on the circle system.

The Mapleson Systems

General Considerations. Any components into which the patient exhales are subject to contamination. Likewise, any components from which the patient inhales gases or which are near to the patient will represent a danger to the patient. The closer the component to the patient the greater these dangers. One study of Bain circuits found a contamination rate of 8% following single patient use (145).

Cleaning. After use the systems should be disassembled and the components cleaned.

Disinfection and/or Sterilization. The components may be disinfected or sterilized by one of the methods discussed. Metal components can undergo autoclaving. Rubber and plastic parts can undergo cold or gas sterilization.

Anesthesia Ventilators

General Considerations. A ventilator is a mechanical substitute for a reservoir bag. The bellows and other parts exposed to respired gases can become contaminated. Condensate which can act as a nutrient for organisms often accumulates in the bellows (4). Ventilators can be protected from contamination by use of a filter in the hose leading to the breathing system. This will also protect the patient from a contaminated ventilator.

Cleaning, Disinfection, or Sterilization. Some ventilators have metal poles to which the hose is attached. These poles can be autoclaved. The manufacturer's instructions should be consulted for treatment of other parts.

Face Masks

General Considerations. Face masks are among the most frequently and heavily contaminated pieces of equipment, being subject to microorganisms both from the mouth and airway and from the patient's skin. Frequently, mucus or vomitus gets onto them. Because of their proximity to the patient, transmittal of infection to the patient is a definite possibility. For obviously contaminated cases, disposable masks are available.

Asepsis should be practiced in the use of the face mask. They should not be allowed to drop onto the floor or be exposed to obvious contamination. After use the mask should be kept near the patient's head or with the dirty equipment.

Cleaning. Immediately after use the mask connector should be removed and the mask rinsed in cool tap water. Then it should be soaked and scrubbed. An ordinary scrub brush used in surgery is good for cleaning most masks. Some masks, however, are more difficult to clean and may require special brushes. They may be cleaned automatically in a washing machine. Masks should always be thoroughly rinsed and carefully dried, especially if ethylene oxide is to be used for sterilization.

Disinfection and/or Sterilization. Masks can be disinfected or sterilized by any of the methods described earlier.

Ethylene oxide offers the advantage that the mask can be maintained sterile for long periods of time. However, aeration must be adequate or facial burns may result (91, 93). Most automatic ethylene oxide sterilizers employ a vacuum at least once during the sterilization cycle. This vacuum may cause the pneumatic cushion of the mask to balloon and the mask may lose its cushion and conductivity (2). This can be prevented by removing the plug that seals the pneumatic cushion or by using a sterilizer not employing a vacuum phase.

Autoclaving is sometimes used for face masks. Steam will shorten the life of masks made of conductive rubber. Conductive neoprene face masks are available which will withstand steam sterilization (137). Autoclaving also involves a vacuum phase that will damage the inflated cushion, so before autoclaving the plug should be removed. Boiling (133, 134, 146) and pasteurization (26, 146) have also been used for face masks. The mask connector should be removed when any of these forms of heat sterilization are used.

Liquid chemical agents are widely used for face masks. Thorough rinsing is necessary to remove residual detergent. Facial injury can be caused by a mask improperly sterilized with liquid agents (56, 147). Phenolic compounds should not be used because they are absorbed by the rubber. Alcohol is advantageous because it does not leave residual chemical.

Headstraps

Headstraps should be subjected to periodic cleaning with a detergent, then soaked in a disinfectant solution or sterilized with ethylene oxide.

Airways

General Considerations. Airways are always heavily contaminated after use. Inasmuch as they are inserted into a relatively dirty portion of the patient, they are usually not sterile at the time of use. Disposable airways are available for contaminated cases or routine use.

Before use, airways should be treated as clean objects and not allowed to drop on the floor. After removal, they should be treated as dirty equipment.

Cleaning. As soon as possible after use, airways should be rinsed under a running tap of cold water and then placed in a solution of water and detergent. They should be washed mechanically with a brush both inside and out or washed in a machine (15, 18, 19). Thorough rinsing is essential to remove residual detergent.

Disinfection and/or Sterilization. Pasteurization, liquid chemical disinfection, or ethylene oxide sterilization can be used for airways. Metal airways may be autoclaved or boiled. Rubber airways may also be autoclaved or boiled but this will usually shorten their life.

Laryngoscope Blades, Stylets, and Intubating Forceps

General Considerations. Laryngoscope blades and forceps should be stored under clean conditions. Many people believe stylets should be kept sterile, since they are placed inside an endotracheal tube. All will be contaminated after use (148) and should be treated as dirty.

For known contaminated cases disposable laryngoscope blades are available.

Cleaning. For fiberoptic laryngoscopes, the manufacturer's instructions for cleaning and disinfection or sterilization should be consulted and followed.

Roberts (148) reported that simply wiping the blade thoroughly with 70% isopropyl alcohol after use killed most bacteria. However, most authors favor more mechanical cleansing.

As soon as possible after use, the blade, stylet, or forceps should be rinsed under a running tap or immersed in a pan of water and detergent. It should be washed mechanically with particular attention given to cleaning around the light bulb.

Disinfection and/or Sterilization. Blades, stylets, and forceps may be boiled, autoclaved, gas sterilized or treated with liquid chemicals. Of the liquid chemical agents, alcohol and glutaraldehyde are the most frequently used.

Roberts (148) found that autoclaving did not affect the bulb or wiring although Jenkins (138) reported that the electrical insulation on some blades would withstand autoclaving only a few times.

If ethylene oxide is used for sterilization, no aeration time is required.

Endotracheal Tubes and Connectors

General Considerations. The endotracheal tube is placed into an area of the body that is normally sterile. Most workers feel that it should be sterile.

If sterile, it should be kept in its package until just before use and the patient end of the tube should not be touched. Sterile lubricant should be used. If possible, the tube should not touch any part of the mouth or pharynx during insertion.

After use the tube is always heavily contaminated and should be treated as a dirty piece of equipment.

Disposable endotracheal tubes are available at relatively low cost.

Cleaning. It is important that secretions be prevented from drying by rinsing in cold running water and soaking in a detergent and water solution. Before immersion, the inflating tube should be plugged to prevent water from entering the inflating tube and cuff. The connector should be removed and tape, etc., taken off. The tube should then be brushed inside and out. While washing the tube, one should be careful not to catch the cuff on any sharp object. The tube should be rinsed thoroughly, making sure to flush the lumen. Endotracheal tubes may be cleaned in a washing machine.

Unless the tube is to be autoclaved, pasteurized, or boiled, the connector should be reinserted after cleaning. Thorough drying is important before chemical disinfection or gas sterilization.

Disinfection and/or Sterilization. Use of ethylene oxide is a popular method for sterilizing endotracheal tubes. The tube and connector must be free of water droplets. The end of the inflating tube should be open.

Cases of laryngeal irritation have been associated with improperly aerated tubes and PVC tubes sterilized with ethylene oxide after previous gamma radiation. Attention to proper aeration times and discarding used PVC tubes that have been gamma-irradiated will avoid these problems.

With repeated ethylene oxide sterilization, rubber and some plastic endotracheal tubes become softened and kink more easily (67, 149). Spiral latex endotracheal tubes should not be gas-sterilized or steam-sterilized with a vacuum applied in the sterilizing cycle, as the latex layers can separate. During anesthesia, anesthetic gases, especially nitrous oxide, may penetrate into the layers, resulting in partial or total occlusion of the inner lumen of the tube (107). These problems can be avoided by using a sterilizer that operates at room temperature and does not employ a vacuum phase (128, 150).

Autoclaving has been used in the past for sterilizing endotracheal tubes. It offers an advantage in that the tube may be left in its package and kept sterile until ready for use. However, repeated autoclaving makes endotracheal tubes more likely to kink and causes a decrease in the elasticity of the rubber composing the cuffs. Spiral embedded tubes are especially susceptible to damage from steam autoclaving. Most of the newer endotracheal tubes made of plastic will not withstand the high temperatures involved in autoclaving.

When packaging endotracheal tubes for autoclaving, the connector should be removed. Otherwise, a loose fit will result. The inflating tube end should be left open. Otherwise, the heat will cause the air in the cuff to expand and may cause the tube to narrow under the cuff.

Boiling (131, 134) and pasteurization (134) have been used for endotracheal tubes.

Liquid chemical disinfection of endotracheal tubes has been used. The inflating tube should be closed during immersion to prevent the solution from entering the cuff. The tube will frequently float and needs to be held down with an object which does not distort it or prevent the solution from reaching all surfaces. This method has the disadvantage of possible recontamination during drying and storage. Thorough rinsing is necessary after all agents except alcohol. Otherwise, tracheitis may result (151, 152).

Adaptors

General Considerations. Adaptors used near the patient are contaminated in a high percentage of cases. Fortunately, they are usually not difficult to clean or sterilize.

Cleaning. After use, adaptors should be rinsed under a running tap, then placed in a solution of detergent and water and soaked. They may be washed manually or in a washing machine.

Disinfection and/or Sterilization. Rubber and plastic adaptors may be sterilized with ethylene oxide or in a liquid such as glutaraldehyde. Metal adaptors may be boiled, autoclaved, or pasteurized.

Resuscitation Bags

Resuscitation bags should be disassembled, cleaned, and, if possible, disinfected or sterilized after each use.

Blood Pressure Apparatus

General Considerations. Blood pressure apparatus can be a reservoir of bacteria (153). It should, therefore, receive attention.

Cleaning. The bulb and tubing should be disconnected, Velcro straps should be brushed to remove any string or plastic that have adhered to the surface. The rubber bladder should be removed and wiped with a disinfectant solution. The cuff should be soaked in detergent solution and then washed in warm, soapy water.

Stethoscopes can be washed with soap and water and wiped with alcohol. Ear plugs can be cleaned with an alcohol-saturated appliance.

Disinfection or Sterilization. Most cuffs can be soaked in disinfectant solution. After rinsing, the bladder can be reinserted, air pumped into it and the cuff hung to dry. Alternately, the cuff can be dried and subjected to ethylene oxide sterilization.

References

1. Thomas ET: The sterilization dilemma: Where will it end? Clinical aspects. *Anesth Analg* 47:657–662, 1968.
2. Russell JP: The sterilization dilemma: Where will it end? Laboratory aspects. *Anesth Analg* 47:653–656, 1968.
3. Hamilton WK, Feeley TW: A need for aseptic inhalation anesthesia equipment for each case is unproven. In Eckenhoff JE (ed): *Controversy in Anesthesiology*. Philadelphia: W. B. Saunders, 1979.
4. Dryden GE: Inhalation anesthesia equipment should be aseptic for each use. In Eckenhoff JE (ed): *Controversy in Anesthesiology*. Philadelphia, W. B. Saunders, 1979.
5. Du Moulin GC, Saubermann AJ: The anesthesia machine and circle system are not likely to be sources of bacterial contamination. *Anesthesiology* 47:353–358, 1977.
6. Feeley TW, Hamilton WK, Xavier B, Moyers J, Eger EI: Sterile anesthesia breathing circuits do not prevent postoperative pulmonary infection. *Anesthesiology* 54:369–372, 1982.
7. Anonymous: Cross-infection during anaesthesia. *Br J Anaesth* 36:465, 1964.
8. Coulthard CE: The microbiological control of sterile pharmaceutical products. *JSCI* 67:441–444, 1948.
9. Joseph JM: Disease transmission by inefficiently sanitized anesthetizing apparatus. *JAMA* 149:1196–1198, 1952.
10. Albrecht WH, Dryden GE: Five-year experience with the development of an individually clean anesthesia system. *Anesth Analg* 53:24–28, 1974.
11. Smith DT, Conant NF, Overman JR: *Microbiol-*

ogy. New York, Appleton-Century-Crofts, 1964.

12. Anonymous: The sterilization of anesthesia equipment by ethylene oxide. *Anesth Analg* 49:957–964, 1970.

13. Thomas ET: The problem in practice. *Int Anesthesiol Clin* 10,2:11–22, 1972.

14. Nickel JA: The anesthetist's role in the prevention of nosocomial infections. *Am Assoc Nurse Anesthetists J* 38:209–216, 1970.

15. Wilson RD, Traber DL, Allen CR, Priano LL, Bass J: An evaluation of the Cidematic decontamination system for anesthesia equipment. *Anesth Analg* 51:658–661, 1972.

16. *Ethylene Oxide Use in Hospitals. A Manual for Health Care Personnel.* American Society for Hospital Central Service Personnel of the American Hospital Association, 840 N. Lake Shore Drive, Chicago, Ill. 60611, 1982.

17. Surgical scrub sinks. *JAMA* 164:1629–1630, 1957.

18. Borick PM, Dondershine FH, Hollis RA: A new automated unit for cleaning and disinfecting anesthesia equipment and other medical instruments. *Dev Ind Microbiol* 12:266–272, 1971.

19. Bennett PJ, Cope DHP, Thompson REM: Decontamination of anaesthetic equipment. *Anaesthesia* 23:670–675, 1968.

20. Barrow MEH, Meynell MJ: A method of disinfecting anaesthetic equipment. *Br J Anaesth* 38:907–910, 1966.

21. Roberts FJ, Cockcroft WH, Johnson HE: A hot water disinfection method for inhalation therapy equipment. *Can Med Assoc J* 101:30–32, 1969.

22. Rendell-Baker L, Roberts RB, Watson BM: Problems in Sterilization of Medical Equipment (Exhibit). Department of Anesthesiology, Mount Sinai School of Medicine, New York, N. Y.

23. Ahlgren EW: Decontamination of respiratory therapy equipment. ASA Workshop on Techniques of Respiratory Therapy, Atlanta, Ga., Nov. 17–18, 1973.

24. Nelson EJ, Ryan KJ: A new use for pasteurization: disinfection of inhalation therapy equipment. *Resp Care* 16:97–103, 1971.

25. Edgar WM, Wyman JB: Sterilization of apparatus and equipment. In Evans FT, Gray TC (eds): *General Anaesthesia*, ed 2. New York, Appleton-Century-Crofts, 1965, pp 530–538.

26. Schnierson SS: Sterilization by heat. *Int Anesthesiol Clin* 10,2:67–83, 1972.

27. Medical Research Council: Sterilization by steam under increased pressure. *Lancet* 1:425–435, 1959.

28. Rendell-Baker L, Roberts RB: Gas versus steam sterilization: when to use which. *Med Surg Rev* (4th Quart) pp 10–14, 1969.

29. Hoyt A, Chaney AL, Cavell K: Studies on steam sterilization and the effects of air in the autoclave. *J Bacteriol* 36:639–652, 1938.

30. Fallon RJ: Factors concerned in the efficient steam sterilization of surgical dressings. *J Clin Pathol* 14:505–511, 1961.

31. Howie JW, Allison VD, Bowie JH, Bruges EA, Darmady EM , Fallon RJ, Knox R, Shone JAV, Sykes G, Wells CA, Wylie GAP, Kelsey JC: Sterilization by steam under increased pressure. *Lancet* 2:1243–1244, 1960.

32. Kretz AP: High vacuum sterilization. *AORN J* 2:35–40, 1964.

33. Olander JW: New facilities and equipment for radiation sterilization. *Bull Parenteral Drug Assoc* 17:14–21, 1963.

34. Artandi C: Sterilization by ionizing radiation. *Int Anesthesiol Clin* 10, 2:123–130, 1972.

35. Rice HM: Testing of air-filters for hospital sterilizers. *Lancet* 2:1275–1277, 1958.

36. Dixon RE, Kaslow RA, Mackel DC, Fulkerson CC, Mallison GF: Aqueous quaternary ammonium antiseptics and disinfectants. *JAMA* 236:2415–2417, 1976.

37. Ederer GM, Matsen JM: Colonization and infection with Pseudomonas cepacia. *J Infect Dis* 125:613–618, 1972.

38. U. S. Dept. HEW: Selection and Use of Disinfectants in Health Facilities, HEW Publication No. HSM 72-4008. Selected Papers from a Training Course held in Albany, N.Y., Sept. 27–28, 1967.

39. Hussey HH: Benzalkonium chloride: failures as an antiseptic. *JAMA* 236:2433, 1976.

40. Kundsin RB, Walter CW: Investigations on adsorption of benzalkonium chloride USP by skin, gloves, and sponges. *Arch Surg* 75:1036–1042, 1957.

41. Anonymous: Bacteria in antiseptic solutions. *Br Med J* 2:436, 1958.

42. Lee JC, Fialkow PJ: Benzalkonium chloride—source of hospital infection with gram-negative bacteria. *JAMA* 177:708–710, 1961.

43. Malizia WF, Gangarosa EJ, Goley AF: Benzalkonium chloride as a source of infection. *N Engl J Med* 263:800–802, 1960.

44. Plotkin SA, Austrian R: Bacteremia caused by Pseudomonas sp following the use of materials stored in solutions of a cationic surface-active agent. *Am J Med Sci* 238:621–627, 1958.

45. Frank MJ, Schaffner W: Contaminated aqueous benzalkonium chloride. An unnecessary hospital infection hazard. *JAMA* 236:2418–2419, 1976.

46. Anonymous: Disinfectants and gram-negative bacteria. *Lancet* 1:26–27, 1972.

47. Anonymous: Failure of detergents to disinfect. *Lancet* 2:306, 1958.

48. Padnos E, Horwitz I, Wunder G: Contact dermititis complicating tracheostomy. *Am J Dis Child* 109:90–91, 1965.

49. Wahlberg JE: Two cases of hypersensitivity to quaternary ammonium compounds. *Acta Derm Venereol (Stockh)* 42:230–234, 1964.

50. Kelsey JC, Mackinnon IH, Maurer IM: Sporicidal aspects of hospital disinfectants. *J Clin Pathol* 27:632–638, 1974.

51. Kundsin RB, Walter CW: Antiseptics and disinfectants. *Practitioner* 200:15–22, 1968.

52. Burdon DW, Whitby JL: Contamination of hospital disinfectants with Pseudomonas species. *Br Med J* 1:153–155, 1967.

53. Mitchell RG, Hayward AC: Postoperative urinary-tract infections caused by contaminated irrigating fluid. *Lancet* 1:793–795, 1966.

54. Lumley J: Decontamination of anaesthetic equipment and ventilators. *Br J Anaesth* 48:3–8, 1976.

55. Spaulding EH: Chemical disinfection and anti-

sepsis in the hospital. *J Hosp Res* 9:7–31, 1972.

56. Herwick RP, Treweek ON: Burns from anesthesia mask sterilized in compound solution of cresol. *JAMA* 100:407–408, 1933.

57. Kahn G: Depigmentation caused by phenolic detergent germicides. *Arch Dermatol* 102:177–187, 1970.

58. Holland BF, Anderson RW: Selecting hospital disinfectant agents. *Hosp Form Manag*, Sept., 1967.

59. Ayliffe GAJ, Barrowcliffe DF, Lowbury EJL: Contamination of disinfectants. *Br Med J* 1:505, 1969.

60. Burrows W, Moulder JW: *Textbook of Microbiology*, ed 19. Philadelphia, W. B. Saunders, 1968, pp 178–197.

61. Bassett DCJ, Stokes J, Thomas WRG: Contamination of disinfectant solutions. *Lancet* 2:218, 1970.

62. Bassett DCJ: The effect of pH on the multiplication of a pseudomonad in chlorhexidine and cetrimide. *J Clin Pathol* 24:708–711, 1971.

63. Bassett DCJ, Stokes KJ, Thomas WRG: Wound infection with Pseudomonas multivorans. A water-borne contaminant of disinfectant solutions. *Lancet* 1:1188–1191, 1970.

64. New study shows hexachlorophene is teratogenic in humans. *JAMA* 240:513–514, 1978.

65. Spalding EH: Principles and application of chemical disinfection. *AORN J* 1:36–46, 1963.

66. Spaulding EWH: Alcohol as a surgical disinfectant. *AORN J* 2:67–71, 1964.

67. Ethylene oxide sterilization. *Health Devices* 5:27–50, 1975.

68. Borick PM: Chemical sterilizers (chemosterilizers). *Adv Appl Microbiol* 10:291–312, 1968.

69. Borick PM, Dondershine FH, Chandler VL: Alkalinized glutaraldehyde, a new antimicrobial agent. *J Pharm Sci* 53:1273–1275, 1964.

70. Borick PM: Antimicrobial agents as liquid chemosterilizers. *Biotechnol Bioeng* 7:435–443, 1965.

71. Kelsey JC, Mackinnon IH, Maurer IM: Sporicidal activity of hospital disinfectants. *J Clin Pathol* 27:632–638, 1974.

72. Haselhuhn DH, Brason FW, Borick PM: "In use" study of buffered glutaraldehyde for cold sterilization of anesthesia equipment. *Anesth Analg* 46:468–474, 1967.

73. Pepper RE, Chandler VLI: Sporicidal activity of alkaline alcoholic saturated dialdehyde solutions. *J Appl Microbiol* 11:384–388, 1968.

74. Roberts RB: The anaesthetist, cross-infection and sterilization techniques—a review. *Anaesth Intensive Care* 1:400–406, 1973.

75. Richards M, Levitsky S: Outbreak of Serratia marcescens infections in a cardiothoracic surgical intensive care unit. *Ann Thorac Cardiovasc Surg* 19:503–513, 1975.

76. Snyder RW: Cheatle EL: Alkaline glutaraldehyde as effective disinfectant. *Am J Hosp Pharm* 22:321–327, 1965.

77. Stonehill AA, Krop S, Borick PM: Buffered glutaraldehyde, a new chemical sterilizing solution. *Am J Hosp Pharm* 20:458–465, 1963.

78. Iddenden FR: New decontamination procedure cuts costs--reduces staff time. *Can Hosp* 49:26–28, 1972.

79. Belani KG, Priedkalns J: An epidemic of pseudomembranous laryngotracheitis. *Anesthesiology* 47:530–531, 1977.

80. Fisher AA: Reactions to glutaraldehyde with particular reference to radiologists and x-ray technicians. *Cutis* 28:113, 114, 119, 1981.

81. Mostafa SM: Adverse effects of buffered glutaraldehyde on the Heidbrink expiratory valve. *Br J Anaesth* 52:223–227, 1980.

82. Boucher RMG: Cidex and Sonacide compared. *Resp Care* 22:790–799, 1977.

83. *Effective Sterilization in Hospitals by the Ethylene Oxide Process*. CSA Standard Z314.2-M1977, Canadian Standards Association, 78 Rexdale Blvd., Rexdale, Ontario, Canada, M9W 1R3.

84. Ethylene oxide sterilization. *Hospitals* 45:99–100, 1971.

85. *Good Hospital Practice: Ethylene Oxide Gas-Ventilation Recommendations and Safe Use*. AAMI EO-VRSU, 1981, Association for the Advancement of Medical Instrumentation, 1901 N. Ft. Myer Drive, Suite 602, Arlington, Va., 22209.

86. Ernst RR, Doyle JE: Sterilization with gaseous ethylene oxide: a review of chemical and physical factors. *Biotechnol Bioeng* 10:1–31, 1968.

87. Rendell-Baker L: Ethylene oxide. II. Aeration. *Int Anesthesiol Clin* 10,2:101–122, 1972.

88. American National Standards Institute Sectional Committee Z-79 and ASA Subcommittee on Standardization: Ethylene oxide sterilization of anesthesia apparatus. *Anesthesiology* 33:120, 1970.

89. Deleted in proof.

90. Andersen SR: Ethylene oxide residues in medical materials. *Bull Parenteral Drug Assoc* 27:49–57, 1973.

91. The physician and the law. *Anesth Analg* 49:889, 1970.

92. Lipton B, Gutierrez R, Blaugrund S, Litwak RS, Rendell-Baker L: Irradiated PVC plastic and gas sterilization in the production of tracheal stenosis following tracheostomy. *Anesth Analg* 50:578–586, 1971.

93. Hazards associated with ethylene oxide sterilization. *NY State J Med* 69:1319–1320, 1969.

94. Royce A, Moore WKS: Occupational dermatitis caused by ethylene oxide. *Br J Ind Med* 12:169–171, 1955.

95. Aeration of anesthesia equipment. *Hosp Top* 44:115, 1966.

96. O'Leary RK, Guess WL: The toxiogenic potential of medical plastics sterilized with ethylene oxide vapors. *J Biomed Mater Res* 2:297–311, 1968.

97. Clarke CP, Davidson WL, Johnston JB: Haemolysis of blood following exposure to an Australian manufactured plastic tubing sterilized by means of ethylene oxide gas. *Aust NZ J Surg* 36:53–56, 1966.

98. Hirose T, Goldstein R, Bailey CP: Hemolysis of blood due to exposure to different types of plastic tubing and the influence of ethylene oxide sterilization. *J Thorac Carciovasc Surg* 45:245–251, 1963.

99. Poothullil J, Shimizu A, Day RP, Dolovich J: Anaphylaxis from the product(s) of ethylene oxide gas. *Ann Intern Med* 82:58–60, 1975.

100. Glaser ZR: Special occupation hazard review with control recommendations for the use of ethylene oxide as a sterilant in medical facilities. U.S. Dept. HEW, DHEW (NIOSH), Publication No. 77-200, August, 1977.

101. Abram SE, Ho K, Doumas BT: Ethylene oxide sterilization of local anesthetics: a potential hazard? *Regional Anesthesia* 4:2–3, 1979.

102. Rendell-Baker L: Sterilization of ampoules by ethylene oxide. *Anesth Analg* 56:743–744, 1977.

103. Roberts RB: Gamma Rays + PVC + EO = OK. *Resp Care* 21:223–224, 1976.

104. Stetson JB, Whitbourne JE, Eastman C: Ethylene oxide degassing of rubber and plastic materials. *Anesthesiology* 44:174–180, 1976.

105. Bogdansky S, Lehn PJ: Effects of gamma-irradiation on 2-chloro-ethanol formation in ethylene oxide-sterilized polyvinyl chloride. *J Pharm Sci* 63:802–803, 1964.

106. Bryson TK, Saidman LJ, Nelson W: A potential hazard connected with the resterilization and reuse of disposable equipment. *Anesthesiology* 50:370, 1979.

107. Rendell-Baker L: A hazard alert—reinforced endotracheal tubes. *Anesthesiology* 53:268–269, 1980.

108. Anderson SR: Ethylene oxide toxicity. *J Lab Clin Med* 77:346–355, 1971.

109. Gross JA, Haas ML, Swift TR: Ethylene oxide neurotoxicity: report of four cases and review of the literature. *Neurology* 29:978–983, 1979.

110. NIOSH Current Intelligence Bulletin 35: Ethylene Oxide (EtO), U.S. Department of Health and Human Services, DHSS (NIOSH), Publication No. 81-130, May 22, 1981.

111. Tougher rule on exposure to ethylene oxide proposed. *Americal Medical News*. May 6, 1983.

112. Manheimer A: Ethylene oxide: the silent hazard. *Resp Ther* 8:19–22, 74, 1978.

113. *Ethylene Oxide Sterilization*. Guideline Report No. 8, AHA Technology Series, American Hospital Association, Division of Management and Technology, 840 N. Lake Shore Drive, Chicago, Ill. 60611, 1982.

114. Daley WJ, Morse WA, Ridgway MG: Ethylene oxide control in hospitals. American Society of Hospital Central Service Personnel and American Society for Hospital Engineering of the American Hospital Association, 1979.

115. Revised guidelines for EO sterilization. *AORN J* 24:1086–1088, 1976.

116. Samuels TM: Personnel exposures to ethylene oxide in a central service assembly and sterilization area. *Hosp Top* 56:27–33, 1978.

117. Barron WR, Gunther DA, Durnick TJ, Young JH: Sterilizer modifications to minimize environmental ethylene oxide. Presented at the 16th Annual Meeting, AAMI, Washington D.C., May 11, 1981.

118. Samuels TM: Local exhaust and cycle purges reduce ETO release. *Hopitals* 55:67–69, 1981.

119. Samuels TM: Reduce operator environmental levels. Utilization of a unique local. *Hosp Top* 57:48–53, 1979.

120. Gunther DA, Barron WR, Durnick TJ, Young JH: Sources of environmental ethylene oxide gas contamination in a simulated sterilization facility. Presented at the 16th Annual Meeting, AAMI, Washington D.C., May 11, 1981.

121. Hazard: Amdek Boekel sterilizer. *Health Devices* 5:50–51, 1975.

122. Hazard: 3M models 100 and 200 sterilizers. *Health Devices* 5:51, 1975.

123. Halleck FE: Hazards of EO sterilization in hospitals. *Hosp Top* Nov./Dec., 1975, pp 45–52.

124. Standards for cleaning and processing anesthesia equipment. *AORN J* 25:1268–1274, 1977.

125. Pace ML, Webster C, Epstein B, Matsumaya S, Coleman M, Britt MR, Garibaldi RA: Failure of anesthesia circuit bacterial gas filters to reduce postoperative infections. *Anesthesiology* 51:S362, 1979.

126. Garibaldi RA, Britt MR, Webster C, Pace NL: Failure of bacterial filters to reduce the incidence of pneumonia after inhalation anesthesia. *Anesthesiology* 54:364–368, 1981.

127. Ping FC, Oulton JL, Smith JA, Skidmore AG, Jenkins LC: Bacterial filters—are they necessary on anaesthetic machines. *Can Anaesth Soc J* 26:415–419, 1979.

128. Snow JC, Anderson ML: How anesthesiologists can lessen infection. *Mod Hosp* 103:128–133, 1965.

129. American Society of Anesthesiologists: Practice advisory for infection control by anesthesia personnel. ASA Newsletter, May, 1976.

130. Beck A, Zadeh JA: Infection of anaesthetic apparatus. *Lancet* 1:533–534, 1968.

131. Stafford BC, Clark RR, Dixson S: The disinfection of anaesthetic apparatus. *Br J Anaesth* 36:471–476, 1964.

132. Ziegler C, Jacoby J: Anesthetic equipment as a source of infection. *Anesth Analg* 35:451–459, 1956.

133. Winge-Heden K: Bacteriologic studies on anaesthetic apparatus. *Acta Chir Scand* 124:294–303, 1962.

134. Clark R: Sterilization of anaesthetic apparatus. In *Proceedings of the Third Asian and Australian Congress of Anesthesia*, 1970. Butterworth, London, 1971,

135. Pecora DV, Richter D: Air contamination during anesthesia. *Am Surg* 35:619–621, 1969.

136. Snow JC, Mangiaracine AB, Anderson ML: Sterilization of anesthesia equipment with ethylene oxide. *N Engl J Med* 266:443–445, 1962.

137. Gibbons CP: Care of anesthesia equipment. *Hosp Top* 44:109–115, 1964.

138. Jenkins JRE, Edgar WM: Sterilization of anesthetic equipment. *Anaesthesia* 19:177–190, 1964.

139. George RH: A critical look at chemical disinfection of anaesthetic apparatus. *Br J Anaesth* 47:719–722, 1975.

140. Nielsen H, Vasegaard M, Stokke DB: Bacterial contamination of anaesthetic gases. *Br J Anaesth* 50:811–814, 1978.

141. Thomas CGA: Sterilization by ethylene oxide. *Guys Hosp Rep* 109:57–74, 1960.

142. Baker R: Sonic energy cleaning in inhalation therapy. *Inhal Ther* 13:56, 1968.

143. Maltais EA, Webber IM: Disinfection of anes-

thesia equipment—why not? *AANA J* 38:217–218, 1970.

144. Hope T: Prepackaging and sterilization of anesthetic equipment. *Nurs Times* 60:251–252, 1964.

145. Enright AC, Moore RL, Parney FL: Contamination and resterilization of the Bain circuit. *Can Anaesth Soc J* 23:545–549, 1976.

146. MacCallum FO, Noble WC: Disinfection of anaesthetic face masks. *Anaesthesia* 15:307–309, 1960.

147. Facial injury from anesthesia mask. *NY State J Med* 62:1246–1247, 1962.

148. Roberts RB: Cleaning the laryngoscope blade. *Can Anaesth Soc J* 20:241–244, 1973.

149. Bosomworth PP, Hamelberg W: Effect of sterilization techniques on safety and durability of endotracheal tubes. *Anesth Analg* 44:576–584, 1965.

150. Warren V: Effective technic for care of anesthetic equipment. *Hosp Top* 44:147–148, 1966.

151. Bamforth BJ: Questions & answers. *Anesth Analg* 42:658, 1963.

152. Keenleyside HB: Reaction to improperly cleaned endotracheal catheter. *Anesthesiology* 18:505–506, 1957.

153. Beard MA, McIntyre A, Rountree PM: Sphygmonamometers as a reservoir of pathogenic bacteria. *Med J Aust* 2:758–760, 1969.

Index

Abortions, spontaneous, 248–249
  in spouses, 249
Absorbents, 213–217
  barium hydroxide lime, 215
  compatibility with anesthetic agents, 215
  changing, 216–217
  dust, aspiration, 308
  efficiency of utilization, 217
  failure, 296
  indicators, 215
    absence of, 296
  indices of performance, 217–218
  soda lime, 213–214
  storage, handling and use, 216
Absorber, 210–218
  bypass, 212–213
  bypassed, 296
  checking before use, 404
  cleaning and sterilization, 434
  construction, 210–213
  failure, 296
  indices of performance, 217–218
  leaks, 300
  obstruction of, 303
Absorption capacity, 217
Accident
  investigation, 315–316
  prevention, 316–317
Accumulators, 20
Acetone, in circle system, 241
Active duct system, 264
Adaptors, 142
  cleaning and sterilization, 438
Adiabatic compression, 13, 314–315
Adjustable pressure-limiting valve (see Relief valve
    assembly)
Adsorption devices, 262–263
Aeration, 425–426
  ambient, 425
  factors affecting, 425–426
  mechanical, 425
Aerosol generator (see Nebulizers)
Aftercooler, 21
Agent-specific filling device, 122–124, 267, 309–310
Air compressors, 19–21
Air dilution, effect on inspired concentrations, 139
Air leak into system, 296
Air space, 215
Airway(s), 331–336
  checking before use, 409
  cleaning and sterilization, 436–437
  emergency, 410
  nasopharngeal, 333–335

Bardex, 334
  binasal airway technique, 335
  complications, 335–336
  insertion, 334–335
  Rusch, 334
  Saklad, 334
  obstruction caused by airway, 335
  oropharyngeal, 331–333
  Berman, 333
  Connell, 333
  Guedel, 332–333
  insertion, 333
  Waters, 333
Airway edema, 383–384
Alarm(s)
  gas piping systems
    central supplies, 21
    pipeline distribution system, 23–24
    testing after installation, 31
  oxygen analyzers, 153–154
  oxygen pressure failure, 51–52
    checking before use, 402
  oxygen/nitrous oxide flow rate, 59
  pressure (see Pressure alarms)
Alberts laryngoscope blade, 342
Alcohol, 421–422
Allergic reactions
  to endotracheal tube, 384
  to ethylene oxide, 426
  to glutaraldehyde, 422
  to quaternary ammonium compounds, 421
Ambu E2 valve, 199–200
Ambu Hesse valve, 199–200
Ambu transparent mask, 328
Ambu valve, 198–199
American National Standards Institute, (see Stand-
    ards)
Analyzing, of pipeline system, 30–31
Anaphylaxis to ethylene oxide, 426
Anatomical mask, 326
Anesthesia carts, cleaning, 433
Anesthesia machines (see Machines)
Anesthetic agent(s)
  breakdown products, inhalation of, 241, 309
  concentration in circle system, 235–236
  condensation in breathing system, 311
  diffusion, 311
  effects of rebreathing, 138
  estimation of uptake, 240
  inadvertent administration, 310–311
  incorrect, in vaporizer, 127–129
  liquid, in delivery line, 129–130
  monitoring, 158–160, 239

Anesthetic agent(s)—*continued*
  overdosage, 309–313
    causes, 309–313
    detection, 313
    treatment, 313
  release from system, 140
  underdosage, 313–314
  uptake by system, 139
Anode tubes (*see* Spiral embedded tubes)
ANSI (*see* American National Standards Institute)
Anti-confusion test, 30
Anti-disconnect devices, 302, 382
Anti-pollution valve (see Gas-collecting assembly)
Antiseptic, 416
Armored tubes (*see* Spiral embedded tubes)
Artificial nose (*see* Heat and moisture exchangers)
Aspiration
  foreign body, 350, 377
  pulmonary, 381–382
Assembly, improper
  Bain system, 298
  circle system, 302–303, 306
  flowmeters, 64
  Magill system, 298
  scavenging system, 266, 306, 307
Atomizers (*see* Nebulizers)
Autoclaving, 418
Awareness (*see* Anesthetic agent, underdosage)

Back pressure
  and flowmeters, 64
  and vaporizers, 88–92
  inducer, 403–404
Backlash, 145
Bacteremia, 377
Bacteria, 416
Bacterial filters, 222–223
  compressed air system, 21
  in yoke, 40
  obstructed, 306
  piped gases, 34–35
  placement in circle system, 229–230
  use of, 430, 431
Bacteriocide, 416
Bacteriostat, 416
Bag (*see* Reservoir bag)
Bag-ventilator switch valves (*see* Selector valves)
Bain system, 187
  checking before use, 406
  hazards, 190, 298, 301–302
  humidity, 190
Balancing valve or device (*see* Interface)
Ball floats, 56
Balloon
  McGinnis, 364–365
  pilot, 364–365
Bardex airway, 334
Barium hydroxide lime, 215
Barotrauma, 33, 304–308
Bennett laryngoscope blade, 342–343
Benzalkonium chloride, 420
Berman airway, 333
Binasal airway technique, 335
Bioburden, 416
Biological indicators, 416, 425
Birth defects
  and hexachlorophene, 421

and trace gases, 249–250
Bite block, 335
Bizarri-Guiffrida laryngoscope blade, 341
Blood pressure apparatus, cleaning and sterilization, 438
Bloomquist pediatric circle system, 237
Blow-off valve (*see* Relief valve assembly)
Blower system, dedicated, 264
Bobbin, 55
Boiling, 417–418
Boiling point, 78
Boom, swinging, 27
Bourdon tube, 43
Branch lines, 22
Breathing bag (*see* Reservoir bag)
Breathing system(s)
  circle system, 210–242
  classification, 172–176
  dysfunction, and capnometry, 165
  Mapleson, 182–196
  with non-rebreathing valves, 197–209
Breathing tubes, 145–146
  circle system, 219–220
  cleaning and sterilization, 434–435
  kinking, 303, 306
  leaks, 301
  moistening, 169
  standard, 145
  supports, 146
Bridgeless mask, 328
Bronchial obstruction, 377
Bulk oxygen system, 17
Burn(s)
  facial, 216, 421
  from laryngoscope, 351
Bushings, 142
Bypass, absorber, 212–213
Bypassed absorber, 296

Caking, 213
Calibration, improper, of flowmeters, 64
Cancer, 251–252
Canister(s), 210–218
  contents, 215–216
  heat, 217
  indices of performance, 217–218
Capnography, 166–167
Capnometry, 161–166, 239, 298, 308
  and circulation, 162–163
  breathing system dysfunction, 165
  disconnections, 302
  esophageal intubation, 375
  effects of respiration, 163–165
  in diagnosis hypoventilation, 304
  instruments, 161–162
    aspiration devices, 161–162
    flow-through devices, 161
  interpretation, 162–165
  metabolic effects, 162
Caps, valve protection, 12
Carbolic acid, 421
Carbon dioxide
  absorption, 213–218
  addition to fresh gas flow, 296–297
  arterial versus end-tidal, 165–166
  concentration in circle system, 233–234
  effects of rebreathing, 138–139

piped, central supplies, 21
Carbon monoxide in circle system, 241
Carden bronchoscopy tube, 361
Cardiac disease, and trace gas levels, 253
Carts, anesthesia (*see* Anesthesia carts)
Cell culture testing, 354
Central vacuum systems, for gas disposal, 263–264
Centrimide, 420
Cetyltrimethyl ammonium bromide, 420
CGA (*see* Compressed Gas Association)
Channeling, 217, 296
Checking
  before use, 401–410
    absorber, 404
    accessory intubation equipment, 408–409
    airways, 409
    Bain system, 406
    circle system, 404–406
    cylinder pressures, 402
    emergency airway and ventilation system, 410
    endotracheal tubes, 370–371, 408
    face masks, 409
    flowmeters, 402
    gas piping system pressures, 401–402
    laryngoscopes, 408
    leaks in anesthesia machine, 402–404
    Mapleson systems, 406
    non-rebreathing valves, 406
    oxygen analyzer, 404
    oxygen failure safety valve, 404
    oxygen pressure failure alarm, 402
    pressure gauge, 404
    relief valves
      high-pressure, 405
      low-pressure, 406
    resuscitation bag, 409–410
    scavenging equipment, 408
    suction equipment, 409
    systems with non-rebreathing valves, 406
    unidirectional valves, 404
    vaporizers, 402
    ventilators, 407–408
  new equipment, 411
Chemical agents, liquid, 419–422
Chemical indicator(s), 416, 424–425
Chlorhexidine, 421
Cidematic, 422
Circle system
  absorber, 210–218
  advantages, 242
  arrangement of components, 224–231
  bacterial filters, 222–223, 229–230, 431
  breathing tubes, 219–220
  circulators, 221–222, 230
  cleaning and sterilization, 433–435
  dead space, 232
  disadvantages, 242
  fresh gas inlet, 218, 226–227
  heat and humidity, 232–233
  in-system vaporizer, 223, 230, 236
  inspired versus delivered concentrations, 233–236
    anesthetic agent, 235–236
    carbon dioxide, 233–234
    nitrogen, 233
    oxygen, 234–235
  pediatric, 237–238
  pressure gauge, 219

relief valve, 219, 228–229
reservoir bag, 220, 227
resistance, 231–232
selector valves, 223–224
sensor, oxygen monitor, 221, 230
sensor, pressure alarm, 231
spirometer, 225, 231
unidirectional valves, 218–219, 227–228
use with low flows, 238–241
Y-piece, 220–221
Circulation, and capnometry, 162–163
Circulators, 221–222
  and humidity, 232
  hazards, 312
  placement in circle system, 230
Clark electrode, 152
Classification
  breathing systems, 172–176
  non-rebreathing valves, 198
  vaporizers, 81–87
Clayton yellow, 215
Cleaning, 416–417
  and sterilization (*see* individual components)
  approaches to, 432
Closed system anesthesia, 238–241
Cold sterilization, 419
Cole tube, 357
Collecting (collection) valve (*see* Gas-collecting assembly)
Color coding of cylinders, 4–5
Columbia pediatric valve circle system, 238
Column, rigid, 27–28
Combustible substance, 315
Common gas outlet, 70
Complications (*see* Hazards)
Compressed gas, definition, 1
Compressed Gas Association, 1, 16–17
Compressed gas container(s)
  checking before use, 402
  cleaning, 433
  color coding, 4–5
  construction, 1
  contents and pressure, 1–2, 3
  filling limits, 3–4
  hazards
    attachment of wrong cylinder to oxygen yoke, 293
    empty oxygen cylinder, 290
    improper installation, 291
    inability to use, 290–291
    no handle, 290–291
    valve problems, 291
    wrong contents in oxygen cylinder, 293
  labeling, 5, 6
  large
    valve outlet connections for, 10, 11
    valve protection caps, 12
  marking, 5
  placement in yoke, 42
  plugged, 5
  pressure gauge, 43
  safe use of, 10–14
  sizes and capacities, 1
  spun, 5
  tags, 5
  testing, 2–3
  transfilling, 14
  valves, 5–10

Compressed gas container(s)—*continued*
  attachment to cylinder, 5
  bodies, 6
  conical depression, 9
  cracking, 13
  diaphragm, 6–7, 8
  direct-acting, 6
  handles, 7–8, 9
    hazard, 8
  handwheels, 7–8
  large, 6
  noninterchangeable safety systems, 9–10
    pin index safety system, 10
    valve outlet connections, 10, 11
  packed, 6, 7
  port, 6
  safety relief devices, 8–9
    frangible disc assembly, 8, 9
    fusible plug, 8–9
    safety relief valve, 9
  small, 6, 7
  stem, 6–7
  visual inspection, 3
  washer, 5
  weight, 1, 2–3
Concentration-calibrated vaporizer (*see* Vaporizers, variable bypass)
Concentrations of gases, 78–79
Condenser humidifier (*see* Heat and moisture exchangers)
Conical depression, 9
Connecting assemblies, low-pressure (*see* Hoses)
Connectors, 142–144
  definition, 142
  size and sequence, 143–144
  tracheal tube, 370
    defective, 380
Connell airway, 333
Contact dermatitis
  due to quaternary ammonium compound, 421
  from glutaraldehyde, 422
  from mask, 330
Contact ulcer granuloma, 386
Contaminants
  cylinder, inhalation of, 308
  piping system, inhalation of, 308
Contamination
  of piped gases
    bacterial, 34
    gaseous, 34
    particulate, 34
  risk of, 431–432
  risk of transmission, 432
Continuity test, 30
Copper Kettle vaporizer, 92–94
Corrugated tubings (*see* Breathing tubes)
Cricoid stenosis, 387
Crossover of gases, 33–34, 292–293
  testing for, 30
Croup, post-intubation, 383
Crystal oscillation method, 159–160
Cuffs, endotracheal, 365–370
  causing obstruction, 380
  high-pressure, 365–366
    characteristics, 365–366
    evaluation, 366
    use, 366

low-pressure, 366–369
  characteristics, 366–367
  evaluation, 367–368
  hazards, 381
  use, 368–369
  sponge, 369–370
Cut-out control (*see* Absorber, bypass)
Cylinders (*see* Compressed gas containers)
Cysts, subglottic, 388

Dead space, 138
  circle system, 232
  endotracheal tubes, 354
  face masks, 330
Decontamination, 416
Denitrogenation, 233
Dental damage, 336
Department of Transportion, 1, 3
Depigmentation, 421
Depletion of reserve supply, 35
Dermatitis, contact (*see* Contact dermatitis)
Detergents, 420
Dial-controlled vaporizer (*see* Vaporizers, variable bypass)
Diameter Index Safety System, 24–26
Diaphragm valve, 6–7
Digby Leigh valve, 203–204
Diluent gas, loss of, 312
Direct duct or vent, 262
Direct-acting valve, 6
Direct-reading vaporizer (*see* Vaporizers, variable bypass)
Directional valves (*see* Unidirectional valves)
Director, 388–389
Dirt, in flowmeters, 64
Disc valve, 198
Discharge channel, 8
Disconnect alarm (*see* Pressure alarms, low-pressure)
Disconnections, 143, 302, 313
Disinfection, 146
  approaches to, 432
Disposable versus reuseable equipment, 430–431
Disposable line, direct, 262
Disposal route (*see* Gas disposal assembly)
Dome valves (*see* Unidirectional valves)
Droplines (*see* Hoses)
Duct system
  active, 264
  low-velocity specialized, 264
  specialized, 262
Ducted expiratory valve (*see* Gas-collecting assembly)
Dump valve (*see* Relief valve assembly)

Edema
  airway, 383–384
  laryngeal, 383
  subglottic, 383
  uvular, 336, 383
Educated hand, 148
Efficiency
  carbon dioxide absorption, 218
  of absorbent utilization, 217
  of vaporization, 83–84
Electrical equipment, defective, 314
Electricity, static
  and fires and explosions, 314
  and flowmeters, 64

Electrosurgical unit, 314
Elimination system or route (*see* Gas disposal assembly)
Emergency airway, 410
Emergency auxiliary supply, piped gas systems, 33
Emergency plan, inadequate pressure in gas piping system, 32–33
Emergency ventilation system, 410
EMMA (*see* Engstrom multigas monitor for anesthesia)
Endobronchial intubation, 376–377
Endotracheal tubes, 353–388
  anode (*see* Spiral embedded tubes)
  armored (*see* Spiral embedded tubes)
  biting, 379
  Carden bronchoscopy tube, 361
  checking before use, 370–371, 408
  checking position, 373
  cleaning and sterilization, 437–438
  Cole, 357
  complications, 374–388
    airway edema, 383–384
    aspiration, 381–382
    bacteremia, 377
    bronchial obstruction, 377
    dental and oropharyngeal, 385
    difficult extubation, 382–383
    endobronchial intubation, 376–377
    esophageal intubation, 374–376
    foreign body aspiration, 377
    glottic stenosis, 387
    ignition, 378–379
    inadvertent extubation, 382
    kinking, 379
    laryngeal dilatation, 385
    laryngotracheal membrane, 386–387
    meteorism, 382
    nasal damage, 385
    obstruction, 299, 379–381
    paranasal, 385
    sore throat and laryngitis, 383
    subglottic cysts, 388
    subglottic granulation tissue, 387–388
    subglottic stenosis, 387
    swallowed tube, 374
    tracheal dilatation, 382
    tracheal stenosis, 388
    trauma during insertion, 374
    ulcerations, 385–386
    vocal cord dysfunction, 384–385
    vocal cord granuloma, 386
  connectors, 370
  cuff systems, 364–370
    cuffs (*see* Cuffs, endotracheal)
    inflating lumen, 365
    inflating tube, 364
    inflating valve, 364
    pilot balloon, 364–365
  damaged, 378
  dead space, 354
  defective, 379–380
  description, 356–357
  Endotrol tube, 361
  fixation, 373
  flexometallic (*see* Spiral embedded tubes)
  foreign body in, 379
  Hi-low jet tube, 361
  insertion, 371–373
  laser-shield, 361
  length, 363
  Lindholm, 357
  Magill, 357
  markings, 364
  Murphy, 357
  preparation, 371
  RAE preformed, 357–358
  reactions to, 354
  reinforced (*see* Spiral embedded tubes)
  removal, 373–374
  resistance, 353–354
  size, 361–363
  spiral embedded (*see* Spiral embedded tubes)
  substances used in, 354–356
  use, 267, 370–374
Endotrol tracheal tube, 361
Enfluramatic, 104–106
Enflurane
  cancer, 251
  dangers to unborn offspring, 249–250
  involuntary infertility, 249
  lack of mutagenic effects, 252
  spontaneous abortions, 248
  trace gas levels, 247
Enfluratec, 97–101
Enfluratec 4, 101–104
Engstrom multigas monitor for anesthesia, 159–160
Epidemiological studies, 248
Epistaxis, 335–336, 374
Equipment, new, checking, 411
Erosions, 385–386
Esophageal intubation, inadvertent, 374–376
Esophageal perforation, 374
Esophageal stethoscope, and ethylene oxide sterilization, 426
Ethanol, concentration in circle system, 241
Ethermatic, 104–106
Ethyl orange, 215
Ethyl violet, 215
Ethylene chlorhydrin, 426
Ethylene glycol, 426
  aspiration, 308
Ethylene oxide
  aspiration, 308
  measures to reduce exposure to, 427–429
  sterilization, 422–429
    advantages and disadvantages, 429
    aeration, 425–426
    complications, 426–427
      alterations in equipment, 426
      hazards of exposure to personnel, 427
      patient, 426
    factors affecting, 423–424
    preparation for, 423
    sterilizers, 424
Evacuator (*see* Gas-collecting assembly)
Evaporators, 19
Eversole laryngoscope blade, 343
Excess gas valve (*see* Relief valve assembly)
Exclusion device, 125, 132
Exhaust route (*see* Gas disposal assembly)
Exhaust tubing (*see* Transfer tubing)
Exhaust valve (*see* Gas-collecting assembly; Relief valve assembly)
Exhaustion time, canister, 218

Expiratory valve (*see* Relief valve assembly)
Expiratory valve (*see* Unidirectional valves)
Explosions (*see* Fires and explosions)
Extracorporeal pump oxygenators, scavenging, 257
Extubation
    difficult, 382–383
    inadvertent, 382

Face masks, 326–331
    Ambu transparent, 328
    anatomical, 326
    bridgeless, 328
    checking before use, 409
    cleaning and sterilization, 436
    complications, 330–331
    dead space, 330
    fit, 266–267, 328–329
    Fleximask, 328
    Flotex antistatic, 328
    holding, 329–330
    Rendell-Baker-Soucek, 328, 330
    SCRAM, 328
    selection, 329
    Stephen-Slater non-rebreathing mask, 328
    Trimar, 326–327
Face plate, 24
Facial burns (*see* Burns, facial)
Fail safe (*see* Oxygen failure safety valve)
Fanning equation, 136
Fiberoptic laryngoscope, 345–347
    use, 348–349
Fiberoptic light source, 314
Filling density, 4
Filling ratio (*see* Filling density)
Filters (*see* Bacterial filters)
Fine adjustment valve (*see* Flow control valve)
Fink laryngoscope blade, 340–341
Fink valve, 200–201
Fires
    and explosions, 314–315, 429
        action in response to, 315
        prevention, 315
    and piped gases, 35
Fishmouth valve, 198
Flagg laryngoscope blade, 342
Flaking, metallic, 308
Flap valve(s) (*see* Unidirectional valves), 198
Fleximask, 328
Flexometallic tubes (*see* Spiral embedded tubes)
Float (*see* Machines, flowmeter assembly)
Flotex antistatic mask, 328
Flow, laminar, 136
Flow, turbulent, 136–137
Flow control valve(s), 53–54
    hazards, 63–65, 293–295
    mechanically linked, 59
    touch coded control knob, 58
Flowmeter-controlled vaporizer systems (*see* Vaporizers, measured-flow)
Flowmeters (*see* Machines)
Fluomatic, 104–106
Fluotec 4 vaporizer, 101–104
Fluotec Mark II vaporizer, 87–90, 94–97
Fluotec Mark III vaporizer, 97–101
Flush valves, 6
Flutter valves (*see* Unidirectional valves)

Foaming in vaporizers, 129, 312
Fome cuff, 369–370
Food and Drug Administration, 1
Forceps, 389
    cleaning and sterilization, 437
Foreign body(ies)
    aspiration, 350, 377
    causing obstruction in breathing system, 306
    in endotracheal tube, 379
Foreign substances, aspiration, 308–309
Fortec, 97–101
Fortec 4, 101–104
Frangible disc assembly, 8
French scale, 361
Fresh gas flow
    failure, 301–302
    high, 305
    inadequate, causing rebreathing, 297–298
Fresh gas inlet
    circle system, 218
    placement in circle system, 226–227
Frumin valve, 201–202
Fuel cell, 152
Fungicide, 416
Fusible plug, 8–9

Galvanic cell, 152
Gamma radiation, 418–419
    and PVC items, 426
Gas chromatography, 274
Gas disposal assembly
    active systems
        active duct system, 264
        central vacuum systems, 263–264
    choice, 264–265
    passive systems, 261–263
        adsorption devices, 262–263
        room ventilation system, 261–262
        through-the-wall system, 262
        venting to the floor, 261
Gas piping systems
    central supplies, 17–21
        air, 19–21
        alarms and safety devices, 21
        carbon dioxide, 21
        crossover of gases, 33–34, 292
        nitrogen, 21
        nitrous oxide, 19
        oxygen, 17–19
        testing after installation, 31
    checking pressures before use, 401–402
    design, 16
    hazards, 32–35
        alarm dysfunction, 33
        crossover of gases, 33–34, 292–293
        depletion of the reserve supply, 35
        excessive pressure, 33
        fires, 35
        gaseous contamination, 34
        inadequate pressure, 32–33
        leaks, 35
        particulate contamination, 34
    maintenance, 31–32
    pipeline distribution system, 21–24
        alarms, 23–24
        crossover of gases, 34

piping, 21–22
safety devices, 22–23
station outlet(s), 24–28
  crossover of gases, 34
  face plate, 24
  nitrogen outlet, 28
  noninterchangeable connections, 24–27
  primary valve, 24
  retaining device, 24
  secondary valve assembly, 24
testing after installation, 29–31
  procedures, 30–31
  responsibility, 30
Gas-capturing assembly (*see* Gas-collecting assembly)
Gas-collecting assembly, 255–257
Gas-loaded regulator, 50
Gasifiers, 19
Gasket (*see* Washer)
Gauge, pressure (*see* Pressure gauge)
Georgia valve, 149–150
Germicide, 416
Glottic stenosis, 387
Glutaraldehyde, 422
Government, federal, and trace gases, 277–279
Granular space, 215
Granulation tissue, subglottic, 387–388
Granuloma, vocal cord, 386
Guedel airway, 332–333
Guedel laryngoscope blade, 342
Guide, 388
Guiding catheter, 388

H float, 56
Hagen-Poiseuille Law, 136
Halothane
  alteration by heated humidifier, 172, 309
  cancer due to, 251
  dangers to unborn offspring, 250
  decomposition, 309
  involuntary infertility, 249
  mutagenic effects, 252
  reaction with absorbent, 241
  spontaneous abortions, 248
  trace gas levels, 247
Handles, cylinder (*see* Compressed gas containers, valves)
Hanger yoke assembly, 38–42
  checking for leaks, 269, 404
  placement of cylinder in, 42
Hazards
  absorbent, 296, 308
  absorber, 213, 296, 303
  airways, 335–336
  Ambu E valve, 200
  anesthetic agent overdose, 309–313
  anesthetic agent underdosage, 313–314
  aspiration of foreign substances, 216, 308–309
  bacterial filters, 222, 306
  Bain system, 190, 298, 301–302
  blockage of
    both inspiration and expiration, 299
    expiratory limb, 306
    inspiratory pathway, 302–303
  cylinder handle, 8
  cylinders, 10–14, 290–291, 293
  disconnections, 302

endotracheal tubes (*see* Endotracheal tubes)
ethylene oxide sterilization, 426–427
excessive pressure, 304–308
face masks, 330–331
fires and explosions, 314–315, 429
flowmeters, 63–65, 293–295, 300, 310, 313–314
fresh gas flow failure, 301–302
gas piping systems, 32–35, 289–290, 292–293
high inflow, 305
humidifiers, 171–172
hypercarbia, 241, 296–298
hyperventilation, 304
hypoventilation, 298–304
hypoxia, 289–296
in-system vaporizers, 312
inadvertent administration, 310
inadvertently low tidal volume, 299–304
kinking of tubes, 303, 306
Lack system, 185
Laerdal valve, 202
laryngoscopes, 350–351
leaks, 295, 300–301, 313
low outflow, 305–306
machine, 291, 293, 295–296, 300, 313, 314
Mapleson A system, 185, 298, 306
Mapleson D system, 190
Mapleson E system, 192, 306
Mapleson F system, 192, 306
Mapleson systems, 297–298
misassembly of components, 298, 302–303, 306, 307
non-rebreathing valves, 207, 297, 307
Ohio No. 100 inhaler valve, 220–221
oxygen flush valves, 305
pressure regulators, 48
quick connect fittings, 289, 293
rebreathing, 297–298
relief valve assembly, 148, 300, 306, 422
Ruben valve, 205
scavenging equipment, 255, 265–266, 303, 306, 307
selector valves, 223–224, 306
suction applied to breathing system, 303
transfilling of cylinders, 14
unidirectional valves, 218–219, 297, 303, 306
valved Y-piece, 219, 228, 303, 306
vaporizers, 127–132, 309–314
  Copper Kettle, 94, 309
  Enfluratec, 101
  Fluotec Mark III, 101
  Foregger "matic," 106, 311
  Modulus Verni-Trol, 122
  Ohio DM 5000, 111
  Ohio No. 8, 110, 301, 311
  sidearm Verni-Trol, 120–121, 309, 312–313
  Tec 3, 101
  Vapor, 114
  Vapor 19.1, 117
  Verni-Trol, 118, 309, 312–313
ventilators, 296, 301, 303, 306, 313
yoke block, 43, 293
Head strap, 330
Head-restraining strap, 330
Headband, 330
Heat
  circle system, 232–233
  clinical considerations, 141–142
  effect of rebreathing, 138

Heat—*continued*
    in a canister, 217
    low-flow techniques, 240–241
    of vaporization, 79–80, 141
    specific, 80–81, 140
    supplied to vaporizer, 86
Heat and moisture exchangers, 169–170
Hematological problems, and trace gas levels, 252–253
Hexachlorophene, 421
Hi-low jet tube, 361
Hibitane, 421
High-pressure system, 38–48
    leakage, 269
Hose assemblies (*see* Hoses)
Hoses, 28–29
    crossover of gases, 34, 293
    disconnection at end of day, 411
    leaks, 270, 289
Housekeeping, during administration of anesthesia, 430
Howland lock, 345
Huffman prism, 344
Humidification methods, 169–172
Humidifiers, 170–172
    leaks, 298, 301
Humidity, 140–142
    absolute, 140
    Bain system, 190
    circle system, 232–233
    clinical considerations, 141–142
    effect of rebreathing, 138
    effects on oxygen analyzers, 154
    low-flow techniques, 240–241
    relative, 140
Hydrogen, concentration in circle system, 241
Hypercarbia, 241, 296–298
Hypopharyngeal perforation, 374
Hypoventilation, 298–304
Hypoxia, 289–296

Ignition, sources of, 314–315
Immune response, alterations in, 253
In-system vaporizers (*see* Vaporizers)
Inaccuracy, in flowmeters, 63–64
Indicator(s)
    absorbent, 215
        absence of, 217, 296
        color change, 216–217
    biological, 416, 425
    chemical, 416, 424–425
    flowmeters (*see* Machines, flowmeter assembly)
    for ethylene oxide sterilization, 424–425
    physical (*see* Physical indicators)
Infection(s)
    associated with nasal airway, 336
    known, 431
    risk of transmittal, 432
Infertility, involuntary, 249
Inflammation, post-intubation, 383
Inflating tube, 364
    aneurysm, 380
Inflating valve (*see also* Non-rebreathing valves), 364
Infrared analysis
    anesthetic agents, 160
    trace gases, 273
Inhaler retainer, 330
Inspiratory pathway blockage, 302–303

Inspiratory valve (*see* Unidirectional valves)
Inspired gas composition
    discrepancy from delivered concentration, 139–140
    effects of rebreathing, 138–139
Interface, 257–259
Interlock devices, 125, 132
Intermediate pressure system, 48–67
    leakage, 269–270
Intermediate site (*see* Interface)
Intratracheal tube (*see* Endotracheal tubes)
Introducers, 388–389
Intubating forceps (*see* Forceps)
Intubation
    blind, 372–373
    endobronchial, 376–377
    equipment, checking before use, 408–409
    granuloma, 386
    inadvertent esophageal, 374–376
    nasal, 371–373
    oral, 371
    translaryngeal, 373
Investigation of accidents, 315–316
Ionizing leak detector, 273–274
Isofluramatic, 104–106
Isoflurane
    cancer due to, 251
    lack of mutagenic effects, 252
Isolating valve, 23
IT, 356

Jack, 27
Jackson-Rees system (*see* Mapleson F system)
Joint Commission on Accreditation of Hospitals, 16, 279

Kamen-Wilkinson cuff, 369–370
Kettle type vaporizer (*see* Vaporizers, measured-flow)
Keyed filling device, 122–124, 311
Kieselguhr, 213
Kinking
    breathing tubes, 303, 306
    endotracheal tubes, 360, 379

Lack system, 182
    hazards, 185
Laerdal valve, 202
Laminar flow, 136
Laryngeal dilatation, 385
Laryngeal edema, 383
Laryngeal incompetence, 382
Laryngeal irritation, 437
Laryngitis, 383
Laryngoscopes, 338–351
    accessories, 344–345
    blades, 338–344
        Alberts, 342
        Bennett, 342–343
        Bizarri-Guiffrida, 341
        cleaning and sterilization, 436
        Eversole, 343
        Fink, 340–341
        Flagg, 342
        Guedel, 342
        Macintosh, 339
            left-handed, 340
        Michaels, 342

Miller, 341
Oxford infant, 343–344
oxyscope, 344
polio, 340
Robertshaw, 343
Schapira, 342
Seward, 343
Siker mirror, 344
Snow, 342
Wis-Foregger, 341
    Whitehead modification, 341–342
Wis-Hipple, 342
Wisconsin, 341
checking before use, 408
complications, 350–351
fiberoptic, 345–347
    use, 348–350
handle, 338
prism, 344
stylet, 347
use, 347–349
Laryngospasm, 336
Laryngotracheal membrane, 386–387
Laser, 314, 378–379
Laser-shield tracheal tube, 361
Laterals, 22
Leakmeter (*see* Ionizing leak detector)
Leaks, 300–301, 313
causing anesthetic agent underdosage, 313
causing hypoventilation, 300
checking for, 402–404, 404–405
control, 268–272
effects on inspired concentrations, 139
gas piping systems, 35
hoses, 270, 289
of air into system, 296
vaporizers, 130–131
Left-handed Macintosh blade, 340
Lewis-Leigh valve, 203–204
Light, operating room, 314
Lindholm endotracheal tube, 357
Lip damage, 336
Liquified compressed gas
definition 1
pressure in cylinder, 1–2
Liver diseases, trace gas levels and, 252
Locking device, 24
Low-flow techniques, 238–241, 268
Low-pressure guardian system (*see* Oxygen failure
    safety valve)
Low-pressure system, 67–70
leakage, 270–272

Machine(s), 38–74
back pressure safety devices, 70, 90
cabinetry, 70–71
checking before use, 401–404
choice of, 73–74
cleaning, 433
common gas outlet, 70
cylinder pressure gauge, 43
flowmeter assembly, 52–65
    absence of fine control, 65
    arrangement, 56–57
    back pressure and, 64
    blockage of tube outlet, 65
    care and cleaning, 65

changes in float position, 65
conventional blocks, 53–59
dirt in, 64
float damage, 65
flow control valve (*see* Flow control valve)
flowmeter tubes, 52–53, 54–55
hazards, 63–65, 293–295, 300, 310, 313–314
improper alignment, 64
improper assembly or calibration, 64
inaccuracy, 63–65
indicator at top of tube, 55–56, 65
loose flow control valve knob, 65
on-off switch, 56
oxygen-nitrous oxide proportioning devices, 59–63
physical principles, 52–53
reading of wrong flowmeter, 65
safety devices, 58–59
scale, 56
sequence, 57–58
static electricity, 64
stop, 56
temperature and pressure effects, 53
transposition of parts, 295
hanger yoke assembly, 38–42
hazards, 291–296, 300, 313–314
high-pressure system, 38–48
intermediate pressure system, 48–67
leaks, 295, 300, 313
low-pressure system, 67–70
Ohio DM 5000, 83, 131, 310
on-off switch, 56, 401
oxygen flush valve, 65–67, 305, 313
oxygen pressure failure devices, 49–52
pipeline inlet connections, 49
pipeline pressure gauge, 49
pressure regulator, 43–48
pressurizing valve, 70, 90
procedures at end of day, 411
repair or changes by users, 412
servicing, 71–73, 74
standard, 38, 40, 43, 49, 50, 51, 54, 56, 57, 58, 66, 67,
    68, 73, 74, 81, 82, 90, 102, 114, 122, 125, 129,
    130, 401
unidirectional valve, 70, 90
vaporizer circuit control valve, 67–69
ventilator power outlet, 49
Macintosh laryngoscope blade, 339
left-handed, 340
Magill attachment (*see* Mapleson A system)
Magill endotracheal tube, 357
Magill forceps, 389
Magill system (*see* Mapleson A system)
Maintenance, preventive, 411–412
Maintenance valve, 24
Manometer (*see* Pressure gauge)
Mapleson A system, 149, 182–185
hazards, 185, 298, 306
Mapleson B system, 185–186
Mapleson C system, 186
Mapleson D system, 186–190
hazards, 190
Mapleson E system, 190–192
hazards, 192
Mapleson F system, 192–193
hazards, 193, 306
scavenging, 256

Mapleson systems
  bacterial filter, 431
  checking before use, 406
  cleaning and sterilization, 435–436
  evaluation, 193–194
  hazards, 297–298
Mask(s) (*see* Face masks)
  harness, 330
  retainer, 330
  straps, 330
    cleaning, 436
Mass spectrometry, 167–169
Mass spectroscopy for trace gas levels, 274
McGinnis balloon system, 364–365
McGinnis cuff pressure regulator, 368
MDM (*see* Monitored dial mixer)
Measured-flow vaporizers (*see* Vaporizers, measured-flow)
Mechanical control monitors (*see* Physical indicators)
Medico-legal considerations, trace gas levels, 279–280
Membrane, laryngotracheal, 386–387
Membranous laryngotracheitis, 386–387
Metabolism, and capnometry, 162
Metal spiral tubes (*see* Spiral embedded tubes)
Metallic flaking, 308
Meteorism, 382
Methane, concentration in circle system, 241
Methoxyflurane
  dangers to unborn offspring, 250
  lack of mutagenic effects, 252
  spontaneous abortions, 248
  trace gas levels, 247
Michaels laryngoscope blade, 342
Microbial load, 416
Microbiocide, 416
Microfuel cell, 152
Miller laryngoscope blade, 341
Mimosa Z, 215
Misassembly of components (*see* Assembly, improper)
Mode selector valves (*see* Selector valves)
Modulus Verni-Trol, 121–122
Moistening breathing tubes, 169
Monitor(s)
  anesthesia circuit (*see* Pressure alarms)
  mechanical (*see* Physical indicators)
  oxygen (*see* Oxygen analyzers)
  physical (*see* Physical indicators)
  pressure (*see* Pressure alarms)
  respiratory (*see* Pressure alarms)
Monitored dial mixer, 59–61
Monitoring personnel, for trace gas levels, 276–277
Mortality studies, 248
Mounts, 142
Murphy endotracheal tube, 357
Mushroom valve, 198
Mutagenicity testing, 251

Narkotest, 159
Nasal airways (*see* Airways, nasopharyngeal)
Nasal damage, 385
National Fire Protection Association, 1, 16–17
National Formulary, 1
National Institute for Occupational Safety and Health, 278–279
Nebulizers, 172
Necrosis, of tongue, 336
Needle valve (*see* Flow control valve)

Neff circulator, 221, 222
Neurological symptoms, and trace gas levels, 253
NFPA (*see* National Fire Protection Association)
NIOSH (*see* National Institute for Occupational Safety and Health)
Nipple, yoke, 40
Nitrogen
  concentration in circle system, 233
  in oxygen storage tank, 292
  piped, central supplies, 21
  piping station outlet, 28
Nitrous oxide
  cancer due to, 251
  contamination with oxygen, 313
  dangers to unborn offspring, 250
  involuntary infertility, 249
  lack of mutagenic effects, 252
  monitoring of trace levels, 276
  piped, central supplies, 19
  regulators, freezing, 33
  spontaneous abortions, 248
  supply failure, 313
  supply pressure variations, 292
  trace gas levels, 247
  whistles, 51
Non-rebreathing valves, 197–206
  Ambu valve, 198–199
  Ambu E valve, 199–200
  Ambu E2 valve, 199–200
  Ambu Hesse valve, 199–200
  checking before use, 406
  classification, 198
  cleaning and sterilization, 435
  Digby Leigh valve, 203–204
  Fink valve, 200–201
  Frumin valve, 201–202
  hazards, 207, 297, 307
  Laerdal valve, 202
  leaks, 301
  Lewis-Leigh valve, 203–204
  Ruben valve, 204–205
  scavenging, 256
  Stephen-Slater valve, 205–206
  terminology, 197–198
Non-return valves (*see* Unidirectional valves)
Nonpositional valve, 198
Nonrotating float, 55–56
Norry valve, 307
Nosocomial, 416

Obstruction
  breathing tube, 303
  endotracheal tube, 379–381
  expiratory limb, 306
  inspiration and expiration, 299
  inspiratory pathway, 302–303
  relief valve, 306
  reservoir bag, 303
  scavenging system, 265, 307
Occupational Safety and Health Administration, 278–279
Ohio calibrated vaporizer, 106–109
Ohio DM 5000 electrically heated vaporizer, 110–111
Ohio DM 5000 machine, 300, 310
Ohio infant circle absorber system, 237–238
Ohio No. 8 bottle vaporizer, 109–110, 311
Ohio No. 100 inhaler valve, 220–221

Ohio 30/70 proportioner, 61–63
One-way valves (*see* Unidirectional valves)
Oral airways (*see* Airways, oropharyngeal)
Organotin compounds, 355
Oropharyngeal airways, 331–333
OSHA (*see* Occupational Safety and Health Administration)
Out-of-system vaporizers (*see* Vaporizers)
Outlet, common gas, 70
Outlet assembly (*see* Station outlets)
Outlet point (*see* Station outlets)
Outlet station (*see* Station outlets)
Overfilled vaporizer, 129, 309
Overflow valve (*see* Relief valve assembly)
Overspill valve (*see* Relief valve assembly)
Oxford infant laryngoscope blade, 343–344
Oxygen
   concentration in circle system, 234–235
   effects of rebreathing, 138
   empty cylinder, 290
   estimation of consumption, 240
   piped, central supplies, 17–19
   shunted from machine, 295–296
   storage tank filled with nitrogen, 292
   supply problems, 289–292
Oxygen alarms (*see* Oxygen pressure failure alarms)
Oxygen analyzer(s), 151–156
   checking before use, 404
   desirable features, 153–154
   leak in connector, 301
   placement in circle system, 221
   position in circle system, 230
   types, 151–153
   use, 154–156
   with low-flow techniques, 239
Oxygen bypass (*see* Oxygen flush valve)
Oxygen failure safety valve, 50–52, 291–292
   checking before use, 404
   checking for, 51
   limitations, 51–52
Oxygen flow
   mandatory minimum, 58
   minimum, in proportion to total flow, 59
Oxygen flush valve (*see* Machines)
Oxygen monitors (*see* Oxygen analyzers)
Oxygen pressure failure alarm(s), 51, 292
   checking before use, 402
Oxygen pressure failure devices, 49–52
Oxygen supply pressure failure protection device (*see* Oxygen failure safety valve)
Oxygen whistles, 51
Oxygen-nitrous oxide proportioning devices, 59–63
Oxyscope laryngoscope blade, 344

Packed valve, 6
Paranasal complications, 385
Partial pressure, 78–79
Passive humidifier (*see* Heat and moisture exchangers)
Pasteurization, 417
Peaking, 214
Pediatric circle systems, 237–238
PEEP pressure alarm, 158
Pentanediol, 422
Pentec Mark I vaporizer, 94–97
Pentec Mark II vaporizer, 97–101
Pentomatic, 104–106

Percentage type vaporizer (*see* Vaporizers, variable bypass)
Personnel monitoring, 276–277
Pharmacopoeia of the United States, 1
Pharyngeal perforation, 374
Phenolic compounds, 421
Phenolphthalein, 215
Physical disconnection devices, 125–126, 132
Physical indicators, 416, 424
Physical monitors (*see* Physical indicators)
Physics
   pressure regulators, 44–46
   resistance, 136–137
   vaporizers, 77–81
Pilot balloon, 364–365
Pin Index Safety System, 10, 40, 43
   problems, 293
Pin safety system (*see* Agent-specific filling device)
Pin valve (*see* Flow control valves)
Pipeline inlet connections, anesthesia machine, 49
Pipeline outlet (*see* Station outlets)
Pipeline pressure gauge, 49
Piping systems (*see* Gas piping systems)
Plenum vaporizer (*see* Vaporizers, variable bypass)
Plug, 27
Plumb-bob float, 55
Polarographic cell, 152–153
Polio laryngoscope blade, 340
Pollution
   environmental, 240
   operating room, 240
Polyethylene, use in endotracheal tubes, 355
Polymer extract testing, 354
Polysiloxane (*see* Silicone)
Polyvinyl chloride
   and gamma radiation, 418–419
   gamma radiated and ethylene oxide, 426
   use in endotracheal tubes, 355
Pop-off valve (*see* Relief valve assembly)
Pore space, 216
Positional valve, 198
Postanesthesia granuloma, 386
Post-intubation croup, 383
Post-intubation granuloma, 386
Pressure
   back (*see* Back pressure)
   barometric, effects on vaporizers, 87–88
   from face mask, 330–331
   high, 304–308
      alarm, 158
      causes, 305–307
      detection, 308
      prevention, 307–308
      treatment, 308
   negative, as a hazard of scavenging equipment, 266
   partial, 78–79
   positive, as a hazard of scavenging equipment, 265
   rated bursting, 8
   service, 2
   subambient, 158, 303
   sustained elevated, 158
   terminology, 268
   vapor, 77–78
Pressure alarm(s), 156–158
   high-pressure, 158, 308
   low-pressure, 156–158, 302
   PEEP, 158

Pressure alarm(s)—*continued*
  placement of sensor in circle system, 231
  subambient, 158
  sustained elevated, 158
Pressure gauge
  breathing system, checking before use, 404
  circle system, 219
  cylinder, 43
  pipeline, 49, 289–290
Pressure inversion, 46
Pressure monitors (*see* Pressure alarms)
Pressure opening, 8
Pressure regulator, 43–48
  direct-acting, 46
  gas-loaded, 50
  hazards, 48
  indications, 44
  indirect-acting, 46
  modern, 47–48
  physics, 44–46
Pressure release valve (*see* Relief valve assembly)
Pressure relief device(s)
  anesthesia machine, 70, 90
  gas piping system, testing after installation, 31
Pressure sensor system (*see* Oxygen failure safety valve)
Pressure-balancing valve or device (*see* Interface)
Pressure-equalizing valve, 150–151
Pressure-limiting devices, 307
Pressure-limiting valve, adjustable (*see* Relief valve assembly)
Pressure-proportioned reduction, 46
Pressurizing effect, 91, 92
Pressurizing valve, 70, 90
Prevention of accidents, 316–317
Preventive maintenance, 411–412
Probe, 27
Procedures
  at end of case, 410–411
  at end of day, 411
Pseudomembrane, 386–387
Pseudomembranous laryngitis, 422
Pseudomonas
  in chlorhexidine solution, 421
  in quaternary ammonium compounds, 421
Pumping effect, 88–90, 91–92
Purging of pipeline system, 30
PVC (*see* Polyvinyl chloride)

Quaternary ammonium compounds, 420–421
Quats (*see* Quaternary ammonium compounds)
Quick connects (*see* Quick couplers)
Quick couplers, 26–27
  hazards, 293

RAE preformed endotracheal tube, 357–358
Rated bursting pressure, 8
Ratiometers (*see* Oxygen-nitrous oxide proportioning devices)
Rebreathing, 137–139
  effects, 138–139
  hypercarbia secondary to, 297–298
  hypoxia secondary to, 296
Record keeping
  equipment, 412–413
  leakage, 269, 270, 272
  trace gas levels, 278

Rees system (*see* Mapleson F system)
Regeneration, 214
Regeneration humidifier (*see* Heat and moisture exchangers)
Regulator (*see* Pressure regulator)
Reinforced tubes (*see* Spiral embedded tubes)
Release valve (*see* Relief valve assembly)
Relief valve
  safety, 9
  scavenging, 255–256
Relief valve assembly, 146–151
  cleaning, 434
  in circle system, 219, 228–229
  hazards, 148, 300, 306, 422
  high-pressure, 146–149
    checking before use, 405
    placement in circle system, 228
  low-pressure, 307–308, 149–151
    checking before use, 406
    placement in circle system, 229
Renal disease, trace gas levels, 252
Rendell-Baker-Soucek mask, 328, 330
Reserve supply depletion, 35
Reservoir bag(s), 144–145
  adaptor, 144
  as buffer, 304–305
  circle system, 220
  cleaning and sterilization, 434
  extension, 220
  holder, 144
  improperly connected, 302
  leaks, 301
  moistening, 169
  mount, 220
    breakage, 301
  obstructed, 303
  placement in circle system, 227
  standard, 145
Reservoirs, compressed air, 20
Resistance
  circle system, 231–232
  connectors, 143
  effects, 137
  endotracheal tubes, 353
  physics, 136–137
Respiration, and capnometry, 163–165
Respiratory alarm (*see* Pressure alarms)
Respiratory meters (*see* Spirometers)
Respiratory monitor (*see* Pressure alarms)
Respirometers (*see* Spirometers)
Resuscitation bag, 304
  checking before use, 409–410
  cleaning and sterilization, 438
Retaining screw, 40
Revell circulator, 221
Risers, 22
Robertshaw laryngoscope blade, 343
Roccal, 420
Rotameters, 55
Rotor, 55
Rubber, use in endotracheal tubes, 354–355
Rubber-gas partition coefficients, 79
Ruben valve, 204–205
Rusch airway, 334

Safe-T-Lor (*see* Oxygen failure safety valve)
Safety block (*see* Interface)

Safety devices, gas piping systems
  central supplies, 21
  pipeline distribution system, 23–24
Safety relief valve (*see* Relief valve assembly), cylinder, 9
Saklad airway, 334
Sampling
  area, 277
  continuous, 275
  end-tidal, 275–276
  grab, 274–275
  instantaneous, 274–275
  integrated personnel, 275
  periodic, 274
  room, 277
  single shot, 274
  snatch, 274
  time-integrated, 275
  time-weighted average, 275
Savlon, 420, 421
Scale, flowmeter, 56
Scavenging, 254–266
  equipment
    checking before use, 408
    gas-collecting assembly, 255–257
    gas disposal assembly, 259–265
    gas disposal assembly tubing, 259
    hazards, 255, 265–266, 303, 306, 307
    interface, 257–259
    transfer tubing, 257
  exhale valve (*see* Gas-collecting assembly)
  trap or valve (*see* Gas-collecting assembly)
Schapira laryngoscope blade, 342
SCRAM mask, 328
Sealing washer (*see* Washer)
Selector valve(s)
  absorber-mounted, 149, 223–224
  vaporizer, 125, 132
  ventilator mounted, 224, 306
Service outlet (*see* Station outlets)
Service pressure, 2
Seward laryngoscope blade, 343
Shunt valve (*see* Machines, vaporizer circuit control valve)
Shutoff valves
  gas piping system, central supplies, 21
  testing, 31
Sidearm Verni-Trol vaporizer, 118–121, 309, 312–313
Siker mirror laryngoscope blade, 344
Silicone, use in endotracheal tubes, 355
Silicone rubber relaxation, 159
Skirted float, 55
Sleeves, 142
Snow laryngoscope blade, 342
Soaps, 420
Socket, 27
Soda lime, 213–214
Sore throat, 383
Specific heat, 80–81
Spill valve (*see* Relief valve assembly)
Spiral embedded tubes, 358–361
  and ethylene oxide sterilization, 426
  hazards, 358–361, 379–380, 383
Spirometers
  placement in circle system, 231
  to detect hypoventilation, 303–304
  to detect ventilation, 308

Sponge cuff, 369–370
  difficult extubation, 383
Spore, 416
Sporicide, 416
Standards
  breathing tubes, 145
  humidifier, 170
  machine (*see* Machines)
  oxygen analyzer, 153
  reservoir bag, 145
  scavenging equipment, 255
Static increment, 45
Station outlets, 24–28
  incorrect, 293
  testing, 31
Steam sterilization (*see* Autoclaving)
Steen valve, 150–151
Stenosis
  acute edematous, 383
  cricoid, 387
  glottic, 387
  subglottic, 387
  tracheal, 388
Stephen-Slater non-rebreathing mask, 328
Stephen-Slater valve, 205–206
Sterilization
  approaches to, 432
  definition, 416
  dilemma, 415–416
  gas (*see* Ethylene oxide, sterilization)
  steam (*see* Autoclaving)
Sterilizers, ethylene oxide, 424
Stop, at top of flowmeter, 56
Storage receivers, compressed air, 20
Strap
  head, 330
  head-restraining, 330
  mask, 330
Stridor, acute edematous, 383
Striker, 27
Stylet laryngoscope, 347
  use, 349–350
Stylets, 388–389
  cleaning and sterilization, 437
Subambient pressure alarms (*see* Pressure alarms)
Subglottic cysts, 388
Subglottic granulation tissue, 387–388
Subglottic membrane 386–387
Subglottic stenosis, 387
Suction equipment, checking before use, 409
Suction system, dedicated, 264
Swedish nose (*see* Heat and moisture exchangers)
Swinging gate yoke, 40
Switching valves (*see* Selector valves)
Switch valve (*see* Selector valves)
Swivel gate yoke, 40
Systems (*see* Breathing systems)

T-piece system (*see* Mapleson E system)
T-tube interface, 258
Tags, cylinder, 5
Teeth, damage to (*see* Dental damage)
Teflon, use in endotracheal tubes, 355
Teratogenicity (*see* Trace gases, possible effects)
Terminal outlet (*see* Station outlets)
Testing
  cell culture, 354

Testing—*continued*
    gas piping systems, after installation, 29–31
    leakage, 268–272, 404–405
    polymer extract, 354
    tissue, 354
    tissue implantation, 354
Thermal conductivity, 81
Thorpe tube, 52
Tidal volume, low, 299–304
Tipping of vaporizers, 129, 309–310
Tissue implantation testing, 354
Toggle handle yoke, 40
Tongue necrosis, 336
Touch coding, oxygen flow control knobs, 54, 58
Trace gases
    control, 254–272
        alterations of work practices, 266–268
        leakage, 268–272
        scavenging, 254–266
    definition, 247
    levels, 247
    methods of investigation, 247–248
    monitoring, 272–277
        agents, 276
        continuous, 275
        end-tidal, 275–276
        frequency, 277
        gas chromatography, 274
        infrared, 273
        instantaneous, 274–275
        ionizing leak detector, 273–274
        mass spectroscopy, 274
        sampling methods, 274–276
        sites, 276–277
            area sampling, 277
            personnel, 276–277
        time-weighted average, 275
        venous blood sampling, 276
    possible effects, 248–254
        alterations in immune response, 253
        cancer, 251–252
        cardiac disease, 253
        dangers to unborn offspring, 249–250
        hematological problems, 252–253
        impairment of skilled performance, 250–251
        involuntary infertility, 249
        liver diseases, 252
        miscellaneous, 253
        neurological symptoms, 253
        spontaneous abortions, 248–249
            in spouses, 249
        teratogenicity, 240–250
Tracheal dilatation, 382
Tracheal laceration, 374
Tracheal stenosis, 388
Tracheal tubes (*see* Endotracheal tubes)
Transfer tubing, 257, 307
Transfilling, of compressed gas containers, 14
Trauma
    from endotracheal tube insertion, 374
    laryngoscopy, 350
Trimar mask, 326–327
Tube-within-a-tube, 258
Tubes, flowmeter (*see* Machines, flowmeter assembly)
Turbulent flow, 136–137

Ulcerations
    from airways, 336

from endotracheal tubes, 385–386
Ultraviolet analysis, 160
Unidirectional valves
    anesthesia machine, 70, 90
    circle system, 218–219
        checking before use, 404
        cleaning, 434
        hazards, 218–219, 297, 303, 306
        placement, 227–228
U. S. Department of Transportation, 2
Uvular edema, 336, 383

Valve(s)
    adjustable pressure-limiting (*see* Relief valve assembly)
    Ambu, 198–199
    Ambu E, 199–200
    Ambu E2, 199–200
    Ambu Hesse, 199–200
    anti-pollution (*see* Gas-collecting assembly)
    automatic shutoff, 24
    bag-ventilator switch (*see* Selector valves)
    balancing (*see* Interface)
    blow-off (*see* Relief valve assembly)
    Digby Leigh, 203–204
    directional (*see* Unidirectional valves)
    disc, 198
    dome (*see* Unidirectional valves)
    ducted expiratory (*see* Gas-collecting assembly)
    dump (*see* Relief valve assembly)
    excess gas (*see* Relief valve assembly)
    exhaust (*see* Gas-collecting assembly; Relief valve assembly)
    expiratory (*see* Relief valve assembly; Unidirectional valves)
    fine adjustment (*see* Flow control valves)
    Fink, 200–201
    fishmouth, 198
    flap (*see also* Unidirectional valves), 198
    flow control (*see* Flow control valve)
    flutter (*see* Unidirectional valves)
    Frumin, 201–202
    gas-capturing (*see* Gas-collecting assembly)
    Georgia, 149–150
    inflating, 364
    inspiratory (*see* Unidirectional valves)
    isolating, 23
    Laerdal, 202
    Lewis-Leigh, 203–204
    maintenance, 24
    mode selector (*see* Selector valves)
    mushroom, 198
    needle (*see* Flow control valves)
    non-rebreathing (*see* Non-rebreathing valves)
    non-return (*see* Unidirectional valves)
    nonpositional, 198
    Norry, 307
    Ohio No. 100 inhaler, 220–221
    one-way (*see* Unidirectional valves)
    overflow (*see* Relief valve assembly)
    overspill (*see* Relief valve assembly)
    pin (*see* Flow control valves)
    pop-off (*see* Relief valve assembly)
    positional, 198
    pressure release (*see* Relief valve assembly)
    pressure-balancing (*see* Interface)
    pressure-equalizing, 150–151
    pressure-reducing (*see* Pressure regulator)

pressurizing, 70, 90
protection caps, 12
release (*see* Relief valve assembly)
relief (*see* Relief valve assembly)
Ruben, 204–205
safety relief (*see also* Relief valve assembly), 9
scavenging (*see* Gas-collecting assembly)
secondary, 24
secondary shutoff, 24
selector (*see* Selector valves)
self-sealing, 24
shutoff, 24
  testing, 31
spill (*see* Relief valve assembly)
Steen, 150–151
Stephen-Slater, 205–206
switch (*see* Selector valves)
switching (*see* Selector valves)
terminal stop, 24
terminal unit, 24
unidirectional (*see* Unidirectional valves)
Vapor, 111–114
Vapor 19.1, 114–117
Vapor pressure, 77–78
Vaporization
  efficiency of, 83–84
  heat of, 79–80, 141
Vaporizer capability, 86
Vaporizer chamber bypass arrangement (*see* Vaporizers, variable bypass)
Vaporizer circuit control valve, 67–69, 83
  hazards, 295–296, 314
Vaporizer concentration, 86
Vaporizer output, 86
Vaporizer selector switch (*see* Vaporizer circuit control valve)
Vaporizers
  agent-specific filling devices, 122–124, 267, 309–311
  arrangement, 125–126
  automatic plenum (*see* Vaporizers, variable bypass)
  bubble-through, 84
  checking before use, 402
  choice of, 132–133
  classification 81–87
  concentration-calibrated (*see* Vaporizers, variable bypass)
  Copper Kettle, 92–94, 309
  dial-controlled (*see* Vaporizers, variable bypass)
  direct-reading (*see* Vaporizers, variable bypass)
  effect of altered barometric pressure, 87–88
  effects of back pressure, 88–92
  Enfluramatic, 104–106
  Enfluratec, 97–101
  Enfluratec 4, 101–104
  Ethermatic, 104–106
  exclusion device, 125, 132
  flow-over, 84
  flowmeter-controlled (*see* Vaporizers, measured-flow)
  flowmetered (*see* Vaporizers, measured-flow)
  Fluomatic, 104–106
  Fluotec Mark II, 87, 90, 94–97
  Fluotec Mark III, 97–101
  Fluotec 4, 101–104
  Foregger "matic," 104–106, 311
  Fortec, 97–101
  Fortec 4, 101–104
  hazards, 127–132, 309–314

control knob turned wrong way, 130, 312
cross contamination, 125, 311
discharge of agent into fresh gas line, 129–130, 312–313
empty, 314
foaming, 129, 312
inaccuracy, 312
inadvertently turned on, 310–311
incorrect agent, 127–129, 311–312, 314
incorrect calculation, 310, 314
incorrect dial setting, 130, 314
incorrect flowmeter readings, 310
incorrect installation, 312
leaks, 130–131, 313
overfilling, 129, 309
reflux of liquid anesthetic into vaporizer flowmeter, 130
reversed flow, 130
tipping, 129, 309–310
turned off, 314
vapor leak into the fresh gas line, 131–132, 311
in-system, 85–86, 169, 236
  leaks, 300–301
  placement in circle system, 230
interlock devices, 125, 132
Isofluramatic, 104–106
kettle type (*see* Vaporizers, measured-flow)
keyed filling devices, 122–124, 311
leaks, 130–131, 300–301, 313
  into fresh gas, 131–132, 311
liquid oxygen, 19
measured-flow, 82–83, 87, 88, 90, 312
Modulus Verni-Trol, 121–122
multiple-agent, hazards, 312
Ohio calibrated, 106–109
Ohio DM 5000 electrically heated vaporizer, 110–111
Ohio No. 8 bottle, 109–110, 311
out-of-system, 84–85, 86
Pentec Mark I, 94–97
Pentec Mark II, 97–101
Pentomatic, 104–106
percentage type (*see* Vaporizers, variable bypass)
physical disconnection devices, 125–126, 132
physics, 77–81
pressurizing effect, 91, 92
pumping effect, 88–89, 311
regulation of output concentration, 81–83
selector valve, 125, 132
servicing, 132
sidearm Verni-Trol, 118–121, 309, 312–313
tec
  newer models, 97–101
  old models, 94–97
Tec 4, 101–104
Vapor, 111–114
Vapor 19.1, 114–117
variable bypass, 81–82, 87, 88–90
Verni-Trol, 117–118, 309, 312–313
when to fill, 411
with low flows, 239
Variable bypass vaporizers (*see* Vaporizers, variable pass)
Vent, direct, 262
Ventilation, wasted, 145, 299–300
Ventilation failure alarm (*see* Pressure alarms)
Ventilation system(s)
  emergency, 410

Ventilation system(s)—*continued*
  room, 272
    for disposal of trace gases, 261–262
    non-recirculating, 261
    recirculating, 261
Ventilator alarms (*see* Pressure alarms)
Ventilator monitor (*see* Pressure alarms)
Ventilator power outlet, 49
Ventilators
  checking before use, 407–408
  cleaning and sterilization, 436
  descending bellows, 303
  desirable characteristics, 239, 300, 308
  hazards, 296, 301, 303, 306, 313
  leaks, 301, 313
  scavenging, 256–257
  with low flows, 239
Verni-Trol vaporizer, 117–118
Vigilance aids, 151
Viricide, 416
Viruses, 416
Vocal cord dysfunction, 384–385
Vocal cord granuloma, 386
Void space, 215–216
Volumes percent, 79
Vomiting and aspiration, 331

Wall outlets, 27
Washer, 13, 40

Wasted ventilation, 145, 299–300
Waters airway, 333
Whistles
  nitrous oxide, 51
  oxygen, 51
Wis-Foregger laryngoscope blade, 341
  Whitehead modification, 341–342
Wis-Hipple laryngoscope blade, 342
Wisconsin laryngoscope blade, 341
Wood's metal, 8
Woven tube (*see* Spiral embedded tubes)

Y-connector (*see* Y-piece)
Y-piece, 220–221
  cleaning and sterilization, 435
  leaks, 301
  septum, 226
  valved, 219
    hazards, 219, 228, 303, 306
Yoke (*see* Hanger yoke assembly)
Yoke adapter (*see* Yoke block)
Yoke block, 42–43
  hazards, 43, 293
Yoke insert (*see* Yoke block)
Yoke plug, 13, 14, 41

Z-79, 356
Zephiran, 420